Disaster Management

Medical Preparedness, Response and Homeland Security

Dedication

This book is dedicated with adorations and salutations to

Lord Shiva

The Consort of Uma, Gauri or Parvati.
The Bestower of Eternal Bliss, Knowledge and Immortality.

O Destroyer of Tripuras,
My silent adorations unto Thee,
Thou art Rudra, the destroyer,
Thou art the bestower of Immortality,

O Lord Shiva! Silent adorations unto Thee!
Thou art the only refuge, the only object of adoration,
the one Governor of the Universe, the self-effulgent Being.
Thou art the creator, preserver and destroyer of the universe. Thou art the Highest,
the Immovable, the Absolute.

Om Namah Shivaya.

Disaster Management

Medical Preparedness, Response and Homeland Security

Editors

Rajesh Arora
Preeti Arora

www.cabi.org

CABI is a trading name of CAB International

CABI
Nosworthy Way
Wallingford
Oxfordshire OX10 8DE
UK

Tel: +44 (0)1491 832111
Fax: +44 (0)1491 833508
E-mail: info@cabi.org
Website: www.cabi.org

CABI
38 Chauncey Street
Suite 1002
Boston, MA 02111
USA

T: +1 800 552 3083 (toll free)
T: +1 (0)617 395 4051
E-mail: cabi-nao@cabi.org

A catalogue record for this book is available from the British Library, London, UK.

Library of Congress Cataloging-in-Publication Data

Disaster management : medical preparedness, response, and homeland security / editors, Rajesh Arora and Preeti Arora.
p. ; cm.
Includes bibliographical references and index.
ISBN 978-1-84593-929-8 (hbk : alk. paper)
I. Arora, Rajesh. II. Arora, Preeti. III. C.A.B. International.
[DNLM: 1. Disaster Planning. 2. Civil Defense--methods. 3. Disaster Medicine--methods. 4. Emergency Medical Services--methods. 5. Relief Work. WA 295]

RA645.9
363.34'8--dc23

2013014239

ISBN: 978 1 84593 929 8

Commissioning editor: Rachel Cutts

Printed and bound in the UK from copy supplied by the editors by CPI Group (UK) Ltd, Croydon, CR0 4YY

Contents

Section 4: Disasters and Mass Casualty Incidents: Incident Site Command and Control, Point-of-Care Testing

Section 5: Medical Management of Complex Disasters and MCI Victims in Hospitals

Section 6: Securing the Homeland: The Medical Way

Contributors

Jameel Ali, Professor of Surgery, University of Toronto, 55 Queen St East, Suite 402, Toronto, Ontario M5C 1R6, Canada

David Allen, Emergency Management Coordinator, South Canterbury District Health Board, Christchurch, New Zealand

Preeti Arora, Formerly at the Center for Disaster Management Studies, Guru Gobind Singh Indraprastha University, Delhi, India and currently affiliated with the Bharathiar School of Management and Entrepreneur Development, Bharathiar University, Coimbatore, Tamil Nadu–641046, India

Rajesh Arora, Office of the Distinguished Scientist and Chief Controller Research and Development (Life Sciences and International Cooperation), Room No. 339, DRDO Bhawan, Rajaji Marg, New Delhi–11001, India

Itamar Ashkenazi, Surgery B Department, Hillel Yaffe Medical Center, PO Box 169, Hadera, 38100, Israel

Jean B. Bail, Associate Professor, 9 Devon Drive, Newtown Square, Philadelphia, PA 19073, USA

Jiri Bajgar, Department of Toxicology, Faculty of Military Health Sciences, UO, Trebesska 1575, 500 01 Hradec Kralove, Czech Republic

Miklosh Bala, Senior Surgeon, Department of General Surgery and Trauma Unit, Hadassah-Hebrew University Medical Centre, Ein Karem, PO Box 12000, Jerusalem, Israel

Gilles Barrier, Service Départemental d'Incendie et de Secours (SDIS) 06, 140 av. Maréchal de Lattre de Tassigny, BP99, 06271 Villeneuve Loubet – Cedex, France

Benjamin W. Berg, SimTiki Simulation Center, John A. Burns School of Medicine, 651 Ilalo St, Honolulu, HI 96813, USA

J.R. Bhardwaj, Former Member, National Disaster Management Authority (NDMA) Bhawan, A-1, Safdarjung Enclave, New Delhi, India

Raman Chawla, Division of CBRN Defence, Institute of Nuclear Medicine and Allied Sciences, Defence Research and Development Organization, Brig. S.K. Mazumdar Road, Timarpur, Delhi–110054, India

Anish V. Cherian, Department of Psychiatric Social Work, National Institute of Mental Health and Neuro Sciences (Deemed University), Hosur Road/Marigowda Road, (Lakkasandra, Wilson Garden), Bangalore–560029, India

Robert P. Chilcott, Professor, School of Pharmacy, University of Hertfordshire, College Lane Campus, Hatfield, Hertfordshire AL10 9AB, UK

Ayush Chowdhary, Division of CBRN Defence, Institute of Nuclear Medicine and Allied Sciences, Defence Research and Development Organization, Brig. S.K. Mazumdar Road, Timarpur, Delhi–110054, India

Maria Nirmala Christine, Head, Content and Research, Strategic Human Resource Management, #325, 5th Main, 1st Block, Koramangala, Bangalore–560034, India

Chris Cocking, Senior Lecturer, Department of Psychology, London Metropolitan University, Calcutta House, Old Castle St, London E1 7NY, UK

Ronald S. Cohen, Clinical Professor of Pediatrics, Stanford University School of Medicine, Director – PICN, 725 Welch Road, MC 5611, Palo Alto, CA 94304, USA

Timothy P. Cohen, The Institute of Terrorism Research and Response, PO Box 56555, Philadelphia, PA 19111, USA

Corbin Curtis, Point-of-Care Testing Center for Teaching and Research (POCT•CTR) and UC Davis Point-of-Care Technologies Center (NIBIB, NIH), Pathology and Laboratory Medicine, 3455 Tupper Hall, School of Medicine, One Shields Avenue, University of California, Davis, CA 95616, USA

Tahir Ahmed Dar, Government Bone and Joint Hospital, Srinagar-190010, Kashmir, India

Shabir Ahmed Dhar, Consultant, Sher-i-Kashmir Institute of Medical Sciences (SKIMS), Bemina, Srinagar, Jammu and Kashmir–190011, India

Joseph O. Prewitt Diaz, CEO, Center for Psychosocial Support in Disasters, 4107 Sequoia Court Alexandria, VA 22312

Christophor Dishovsky, Professor, Military Medical Academy, 3 St G. Sofiiski Str., Sofia 1606, Bulgaria

Christopher R. Foerster, The University of Queensland, Brisbane QLD 4072, Australia

Anju Goel, Marin County Deputy Public Health Officer, 2178 Williams St, Palo Alto, CA 94306, USA

Rajeev Goel, Division of CBRN Defence, Institute of Nuclear Medicine and Allied Sciences, Defence Research and Development Organization, Brig. S.K. Mazumdar Road, Timarpur, Delhi–110054, India

Rupa Gunaseelan, Bharathiar School of Management & Entrepreneur Development, Bharathiar University, Coimbatore-641046, Tamil Nadu, India

James C. Hagen, Professor and Program Coordinator, Graham School of Management, Saint Xavier University, 3825 West 103rd Street, Chicago, IL 60655, USA

Scott P. Hagen, College of Social Work, Governor's State University, 1 University Parkway, University Park, IL 60484-0975, USA

Arshiya Hamid, District Hospital Ganderbal- 190001, Srinagar, Kashmir, India

Mahmood Hosseini, Associate Professor, Head of Lifeline Engineering Department, International Institute of Earthquake Engineering and Seismology (IIEES), PO Box 19395/3913, Tehran, Iran

Mark K. Huntington, Assistant Director, Sioux Falls Family Medicine Residency Training Program, Center for Family Medicine, Associate Professor, Department of Family Medicine, Sanford School of Medicine of the University of South Dakota, Center for Family Medicine, 1115 East Twentieth Street, Sioux Falls, SD 57105, USA

Michael Hust, Institut für Biochemie und Biotechnologie, Technische Universität, Braunschweig, Spielmannstr. 7, D-38106 Braunschweig, Germany

Yasamin O. Izadkhah, Assistant Professor, Risk Management Research Centre, International Institute of Earthquake Engineering and Seismology (IIEES), PO Box 19395/3913, Tehran, Iran

Denis Josse, Institut de Recherche Biomédicale des Armées, Antenne de La Tronche, Département de Toxicologie et Risques Chimiques, Unité Protection et Décontamination, 24 avenue des Maquis du Grésivaudan, 38700 La Tronche, France

Kamen Kanev, Professor, Military Medical Academy, 3 St G. Sofiiski Str., Sofia 1606, Bulgaria

Levent Kenar, Associate Professor, and Specialist in Clinical Biochemistry, Department of Medical CBRN Defence, Gulhane Military Medical Academy, 06018 Etlik, Ankara, Turkey

Gerald J. Kost, Point-of-Care Testing Center for Teaching and Research (POCT•CTR) and UC Davis Point-of-Care Technologies Center (NIBIB, NIH), Pathology and Laboratory Medicine, 3455 Tupper Hall, School of Medicine, One Shields Avenue, University of California, Davis, CA 95616, USA

Rostislav Stefanov Kostadinov, Joint Medical Coordinator, NATO Joint Force Command Headquarters Naples, Viale della Liberazione, 180124 Napoli, Italy

Naveen C. Kumar, Assistant Professor, Department of Psychiatry, National Institute of Mental Health and Neuro Sciences (Deemed University), Hosur Road/Marigowda Road (Lakkasandra, Wilson Garden), Bangalore–560029, India

Richard Louie, Point-of-Care Testing Center for Teaching and Research (POCT•CTR) and UC Davis Point-of-Care Technologies Center (NIBIB, NIH), Pathology and Laboratory Medicine, School of Medicine, One Shields Avenue, University of California, Davis, CA 95616, USA

Suresh Bada Math, Associate Professor, Department of Psychiatry, National Institute of Mental Health and Neuro Sciences (Deemed University), Hosur Road/Marigowda Road (Lakkasandra, Wilson Garden), Bangalore–560029, India

Nandini Mukherjee, Department of Computer Science and Engineering, Jadavpur University, Kolkata, 700032, West Bengal, India

Mesut Ortatatli, Assistant Professor and Specialist in Infectious Diseases and Clinical Microbiology, Department of Medical CBRN Defence, Gulhane Military Medical Academy, Ankara, Turkey

Steven J. Parrillo, Professor, 35 Harvard Rd, Plymouth Meeting, PA 19462-7177, USA

Douglas Paton, Professor, School of Psychology, University of Tasmania, Newnham Campus, Building O, Tasmania 7250, Australia

Thibaut Pelat, Unité de biotechnologies des anticorps et des toxines, Institut de Recherche Biomédicale des Armées (IRBA-CRSSA), 24 Avenue des Maquis du Grésivaudan, 38702 La Tronche, France

Kai-Lit Phua, School of Medicine and Health Sciences, Monash University (Sunway Campus), Jalan Lagoon Selatan, 46150 Bandar Sunway, Selangor, Malaysia

Nibedita Ray-Bennett, Lecturer in Risk Management, University of Leicester, Civil Safety and Security Unit, 14 Salisbury Road, Leicester LE1 7QR, UK; Formerly: Lecturer in Disaster and Emergencies, Department of Management and Security, Cranfield University, UK. Also Research Affiliate at the Disaster and Development Centre (DDC), Northumbria University, UK

Aaron Richman, Co Director, Targeted Actionable Monitoring Center, The Institute of Terrorism Research and Response, PO Box 45059, Jerusalem 91450, Israel

Monideepa Roy, Department of Computer Science and Engineering, Jadavpur University, Kolkata, 700032, West Bengal, India

Anders Rüter, Associate Professor and Senior Lecturer, Sophiahemmet University College, PO Box 5605, S-114 86 Stockholm, Sweden

Ann Sakaguchi, Specialist/Director, UHPA Faculty Representative (PAU 043), University of Hawaii at Manoa, Anthropology/Pacific Emergency Management, Preparedness and Response Information Network and Training Services (Pacific EMPRINTS), 1960 East-West Road, Biomed A108, Honolulu, HI 96822, USA

Rakesh Sharma, Division of CBRN Defence, Institute of Nuclear Medicine and Allied Sciences, Defence Research and Development Organization, Brig. S.K. Mazumdar Road, Timarpur, Delhi–110054, India

Pallavi Thakur, Division of CBRN Defence, Institute of Nuclear Medicine and Allied Sciences, Defence Research and Development Organization, Brig. S.K. Mazumdar Road, Timarpur, Delhi–110054, India

Philippe Thullier, Unité de biotechnologies des anticorps et des toxines, Institut de Recherche Biomédicale des Armées (IRBA-CRSSA), 24 Avenue des Maquis du Grésivaudan, 38702 La Tronche, France

Stoian Tonev, Professor, Military Medical Academy, 3 St G. Sofiiski Str., Sofia 1606, Bulgaria

Marcia Trainer, 940 Congress Street, Costa Mesa, CA 92627, USA

Fernando Turégano, Head, General Surgery and Emergency Surgery, University Hospital Gregorio Marañón, c/Dr Esquerdo, 46 28040 Madrid, Spain

Dale S. Vincent, Program Director, Internal Medicine Residency Program, MCHK-DM, Department of Medicine, 1 Jarrett White Road, Tripler Army Medical Center, Honolulu, HI 96859-5000, USA

Edward Joseph Waller, Professor, Faculty of Energy Systems and Nuclear Science, University of Ontario Institute of Technology, 2000 Simcoe Street North, Oshawa, Ontario L1H7K4, Canada

Yoram G. Weiss, Associate Professor and Chair, Department of Anaesthesia, Hadassah-Hebrew University Medical Centre, Ein Karem, PO Box 12000, Jerusalem, Israel

Yuval Weiss, Director, Central Management, Hadassah University Hospital, Ein Kerem, PO Box 12000, Jerusalem, Israel

Foreword

Disasters, either natural or man-made, often cause substantial damage to environment and infrastructure, and result in the loss of a large number of lives. It is possible to prevent the damage caused to human lives to a substantial extent through proper planning. The ultimate goal of disaster management is mitigation of the effects of disasters.

Some of the major disasters of this century, including the Indian Ocean tsunami in South-east Asia, Hurricane Katrina in the USA, the cyclone in Myanmar, the novel H1N1 pandemic of 2009, the 2011 Tōhoku Japan Earthquake, etc. have highlighted the importance of disaster management and reinforced the need for developing and employing newer strategies. The changing security landscape and terror incidents, especially 9/11, the London bombings and the Mumbai incident, have further accentuated the need for effective disaster management tools and methods. Man-made disasters like chemical, biological, radiological and nuclear (CBRN) disasters pose a veritable threat to homeland security and there is an urgent need to take appropriate steps to manage the mass casualties that might result from such untoward incidents. The task of saving human lives takes priority following disasters and mass casualty incidents (MCIs). With a view to developing better strategies for management of disasters and MCIs, stress has been put in recent years on medical preparedness and response.

Since it is imperative to save a maximum number of human lives, all endeavours are usually focused in this direction. With rapid advances in the medical sciences, it is possible to effectively treat victims of disasters and MCIs. However, sometimes the whole medical system can become overwhelmed due to the magnitude of disasters, and quite often medical infrastructure too can be obliterated as a result of the disaster.

This unique and comprehensive book with a focus on disaster management is a well-timed effort undertaken by the editors, who have carefully selected the international subject experts in the area and brought them to a common platform to share their thoughts on issues that confront mankind. I congratulate the editors for envisaging this book, which certainly is a welcome step in the direction of documenting the current state of the art and emerging trends in the field of disaster management.

I am sanguine that this book will go a long way in improving disaster response globally and will greatly benefit disaster planners, medical professionals, military personnel and emergency responders, international agencies, government and non-governmental organizations (NGOs) and other agencies engaged in disaster mitigation and management, disaster management professionals, planners, researchers, environmentalists, academicians and students.

Dr W. Selvamurthy
Chief Controller Research and Development and Distinguished Scientist
Defence Research and Development Organization (Government of India), New Delhi, India

Acknowledgements

Our sincere thanks from the core of our hearts to all those who help save lives during disasters, thereby bringing smiles to the faces of their near and dear ones and to the face of humanity!

We would like to thank one and all who have helped make this book possible.

We would consider our efforts worthwhile if this work helps improve the quality of lives of affected people and save some precious lives during times of disasters!

Editors

The Editors

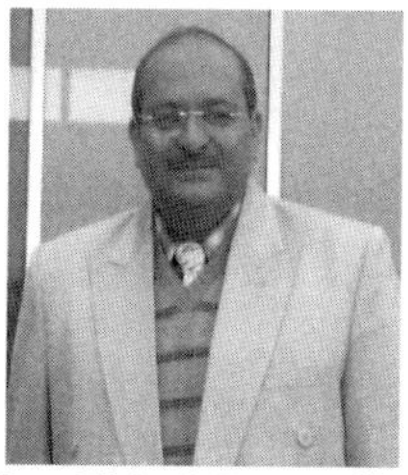

Dr Rajesh Arora is Staff Officer to the Chief Controller R&D and Distinguished Scientist in the Defence Research and Development Organization (DRDO), Government of India. He is actively associated with CBRN defence-related programmes and has steered numerous specialized training courses for the Armed Forces (Army, Navy and Air Force), Elite and Special Forces. He was an expert member associated with the development of National Disaster Management Guidelines by the National Disaster Management Authority – the apex body of the Indian Government. Dr Arora was a Visiting Scientist in the European Union during 2009–10 and is an alumnus of the George C. Marshall European Center for Security Studies, Germany. Dr Arora's name is included in the *Who's Who of the World, USA*, *Who's Who in Science and Engineering, USA* and *International Biography, UK*. He is a recipient of several prestigious fellowships and awards, including the DRDO Laboratory Scientist of the Year Award (2010). Dr Arora has more than 150 publications, 12 patents and 14 books to his credit. e-mail: rajesharoradr@gmail.com

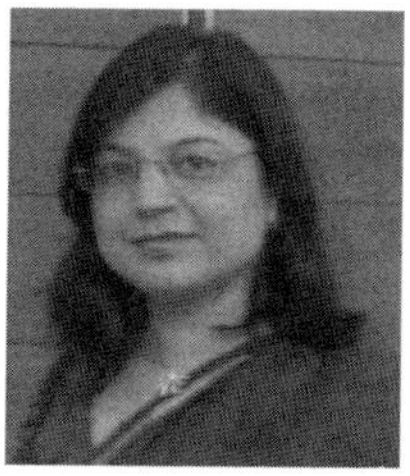

Ms Preeti Arora has an MBA in disaster management and has experience in several cross-cutting issues of disaster management. She has participated in the 'Training of Trainers' programme at the National Institute of Disaster Management (NIDM), New Delhi, and other programmes in diverse areas of disaster management. She has participated in/presented several papers at international/national conferences and has also published papers in international peer-reviewed journals. She has working experience in NGOs at grassroots level in disaster management, particularly involving the underprivileged children and women, and special needs people in the rural/urban sector. In the aftermath of the Japan 2011 disaster, she visited Japan and conducted a study evaluating the impact of the disaster on directly and affected community and India's Rescue and Relief Team, namely the National Disaster Response Force (NDRF), which was sent to Japan following the 2011 Tōhoku earthquake and tsunami. Ms Preeti Arora is an alumnus of the National Women's Education Center (NWEC), Japan and a select Visiting Researcher of the Japan Institute for Labour Policy and Training, Tokyo, Japan (2013). e-mail: preetisethiarora@gmail.com; website: preetisethiarora.tripod.com

Section 1

Disaster Management and Homeland Security:

A Prologue

Chapter 1

Prologue:

A Holistic View to Managing the Inevitable in High-tech and Resource-poor Settings

Rajesh Arora and Preeti Arora

Introduction

Extensive preparedness for management of both natural and man-made disasters is the need of the hour. While natural disasters are inevitable, man-made disasters are avoidable to some extent and their impact can be mitigated to a large extent with proper management. With appropriate and well-timed preparedness, it is possible to mitigate the effects of both natural and man-made disasters and change the face of disasters. The increase in the number of man-made disasters has made it imperative that they be circumvented or their impact reduced by employing newer methods and tools.

Though disasters have been ubiquitous throughout history, the last decade has seen several disasters inflicting extensive financial and infrastructural damage. Some of the disasters have struck developing nations and others developed nations and some both. But the impact of nature's fury on both types of nations has been substantial – what has been different is the way disasters have been managed. The costliest hurricanes that hit the US economy substantially include: Katrina (2005),which crossed southern Florida and struck Louisiana with great intensity, devastating New Orleans and resulting in damage that has been estimated to cost over US$108 billion, followed by Andrew (1992), which caused damage estimated to cost US$46 billion; Ike (2008) caused damage estimated at US$28 billion; Wilma (2005) resulted in damage estimated at US$29.5 billion; and Ivan (2004) inflicted damage estimated at US$19.8 billion. Just months before this book was envisaged, March 2011 witnessed a mega-disaster – the Tōhoku earthquake (and tsunami) – the costliest disaster of this century; while a few months prior in 2010 the Haiti earthquake inflicted extensive damage. While this book is nearing completion, the US has been struck by the 2013 Moore tornado, and man-made disasters like the West Fertilizer Company explosion and Boston marathon bombings have shook the world's oldest surviving federation. As the final days of this book approach, it is June 2013 and the North Indian states of Uttarakhand and Himachal Pradesh, some regions of Western Nepal and their adjoining areas have experienced heavy rainfall due to cloud bursts, which has triggered devastating floods and landslides. Kedarnath, Badrinath and several areas in Uttarkashi in Uttarakhand (nearly 40,000 sq. km) have been severely hit by the floods. The incident has been dubbed the 'Himalayan Tsunami'. Rescue and relief work is currently under way to evacuate nearly 100,000 people from the area. Twelve teams of National Disaster Response Force (NDRF) battalions have been deployed to various locations for response and relief operation in the states of Uttarakhand, Himachal Pradesh and Uttar Pradesh. The Indian Army has deployed about 5500 personnel, the Indo-Tibetan Border Police (ITBP) 2000 personnel and the Border Roads Organization 3000 personnel. Thirteen teams, comprising 300 personnel from the NDRF, have also been deployed. So far, the Indian Air Force has provided one C-130J aircraft, eight MI-17s, ten ALH, one AN-32 and one Avro to carry out rescue work. Almost 50 helicopters of the Indian defence forces have been deployed in Uttarakhand state for rescue missions, which are still ongoing. Disasters such as these pose a number of concerns that need to be addressed in earnest in times to come.

As per the World Health Organization (WHO) Collaborating Centre for Research on the Epidemiology of Disasters (CRED) Emergency Events Database (EM-DAT), during the first few months of 2012, over 143 natural disasters occurred, killing over 2500 people, affecting almost 61 million others and causing more than US$6.9 billion of economic damage. Over the same period, 86 countries have experienced at least one natural disaster, with the most affected countries being Afghanistan, the USA and the Philippines (CRED CRUNCH. No. 29 'Disaster Data: A Balanced Perspective', September 2012). As per early estimates, the economic damages inflicted by Hurricane Sandy – a tropical cyclone of the 2012 Atlantic hurricane season that severely affected several regions of the Caribbean, mid-Atlantic and north-eastern USA in October 2012 as this book was being written, with lesser effects in the south-eastern and Midwestern states and eastern Canada – could reach US$50 billion in the USA alone. That would make the storm the second costliest in American history, after Hurricane Katrina. It is estimated that 8.5 million homes and businesses lost power during Hurricane Sandy.

In view of the widespread damage caused by disasters in recent years, there has been a worldwide upsurge of interest in disaster management, and it is now well recognized that only a proactive approach can help in mitigation of the deleterious effects of disasters and mass casualty incidents. Both natural and man-made disasters need to be managed and overall preparedness is indispensable since disasters are inevitable. Rapid advances in the area have been the hallmark of this ever-growing field; advances which, if documented, could lead to saving of precious human lives in critical moments. Keeping this in mind, the present book was envisaged.

Covering a wide span of disaster fundamentals, this book presents the state-of-the-art in the area. The content of the book ranges from disaster/mass casualty management, homeland security concerns, incident command systems, planning and preparedness of hospitals for disasters, emergency medical services, improving patient outcomes, communication and IT tools for medical disaster response, psychosocial issues, coordination between pre-hospital and hospital care, triage planning, use of state-of-the-art training tools and research in disaster management and chemical, biological, radiological and nuclear (CBRN) disasters – response, rescue and relief.

This book is divided into ten sections. The first section of this book is an introductory section that provides a prelude to disasters and mass casualty incidents (MCIs), the problems associated with them and their management, and summarizes the key issues in disasters and homeland security with a focus on medical management of disasters and MCIs.

Covering a range of cross-cutting issues, the book should interest a wide audience, including those involved in disaster rescue, response and relief.

Mitigation, Training and Medical Preparedness

The second section of this book discusses the importance of mitigation and how training and medical emergency preparedness can solve problems associated with disasters; modern state-of-the-art training tools are discussed. This section also covers the importance of primary care physicians, who often have to handle disaster victims in close proximity with limited resources, yet they play an important role in saving human lives.

All disasters are said to be local. As primary care forms the foundation of effective healthcare, during disasters or MCIs usually such primary healthcare centres can do wonders by saving precious human lives. The second chapter of this book by Mark K. Huntington discusses the important role of primary healthcare. Some areas that have been discussed in detail in the chapter are highlighted in the following section. The provision of comprehensive, compassionate, patient-centred care; the first point of contact interfacing between the patient and the often complex health system, is a hallmark of the work of primary care physicians. This is even more the case in extreme circumstances. When a disaster strikes, it is the local primary care physicians who are the first to respond, and it is they who continue to provide care when the outside response and relief agencies leave. In resource-poor settings, the primary care physician plays a cardinal role in disaster management. Chapter 2 addresses the role of primary care physicians during each phase of a disaster, both as the local care provider and as a part of an outside response effort. Aspects of involvement of the primary care physician in all phases of the disaster cycle, including preparedness and prevention, response, recovery and mitigation have been reviewed. Key areas of knowledge for disaster medicine include triage, emergency medical and trauma care, chronic disease management, basic maternity care, paediatric care, geriatric care, psychological care and care for injuries from CNRN causes; these are all concisely covered in this chapter. In addition, this chapter focuses on community preparation activities, special practice considerations and opportunities for more extensive involvement. The foundational skills, knowledge and philosophy of the primary care physician are ideally suited for involvement in a variety of capacities in disaster medical response, both locally, and as part of a larger concerted effort in areas outside their home community. The important role played by the primary care physician has been highlighted.

Natural and man-made disasters are increasing worldwide, creating a need to train healthcare workers to respond to MCIs. Chapter 3 of this book by Dale S. Vincent and Benjamin W. Berg discusses the significant role of simulation-based medical education (SBME) as an effective methodology for this purpose, creating an experiential, interactive and realistic educational environment that engages learners and effectively transfers new knowledge and skills. These authors opine that the analysis, design, development, implementation and evaluation (ADDIE) instructional design model can provide a useful template for the development of MCI training courses using SBME. Novice and experienced learners may be trained individually or in groups, depending on the objectives of the course. Equipment and faculty resources are significant drivers in the design of simulation scenarios. This chapter also deliberates on curriculum considerations, which must include the type of disaster to be modelled, the types of injuries to be simulated and whether teaching life-saving interventions will be included in the programme. Scenarios have to be tested to ensure that they trigger appropriate learner responses, and faculty must be trained to evaluate learners and provide feedback during debriefing sessions. Evaluation methods need to be developed and put into place to determine whether individual as well as institutional goals are being achieved. Lastly, it is possible to gain new insights into the development of MCI training programmes by reviewing the experiences of educators in conducting programmes with similar goals. The use of SBME techniques has great potential to engage learners, transfer knowledge and skills, and measure educational outcomes in programmes that train healthcare workers to respond effectively to natural and man-made disasters. With rapid advances in virtual reality and artificial intelligence, SBME will change the way disasters are handled by medical professionals and paramedics and greatly improve survival of disaster and MCI victims.

For training purposes, manikins have been of great use and can be utilized quite effectively to simulate real environments. The authors suggest that experiential learning using manikin-based simulation may be an effective way to train healthcare providers for MCIs. Experts have identified the applicability of simulation-based education to disaster health education. Educators who are planning a MCI training programme using manikins can use instructional design principles to guide course development. A systematic approach to the design of MCI training using manikin-based simulation may help to ensure the successful transfer of knowledge and skills to both novice and experienced learners. The cost constraint, however, currently restricts its usage as an effective and efficient training tool in developing and underdeveloped nations. With decrease in cost, it should be possible to introduce manikins for training in resource-poor nations. The usage of manikins for the training related to management of CBRN emergencies is another area where attention is being focused in several countries. However, more attention is needed in this area to make it affordable and accessible for the resource-poor developing nations. This would enable more effective training of medical and paramedical professionals.

Crucial Role of Communication in Disaster Management and Homeland Security

Section 3 of the book focuses on new developments in medical disaster preparedness and communication during/immediately after the disaster utilizing web-based applications and the mobile grid. Ways to improve communication to expedite the movement of patients and resources between entities in the event of a regional disaster event that impairs the ability of one of more major medical centres to care for its patients are also discussed in the three chapters of this section.

When any community suffers a disaster, the shock and destruction to its system drive that community into chaos, threatening its individuals and its social institutions. The community's ability to recover is dependent on its resilience capability. Due to its hierarchical management systems, traditional disaster communications have wrestled with multiple issues of effective communication with the public, including trust. Marcia Trainer and Anju Goel in Chapter 4 of the book discuss the finer nuances of social networking in disaster management and homeland security. Recent technological innovations, advancements in Web 2.0 and peer-to-peer social networking have changed modes of communication all around the globe. Social networking's webbed horizontal structure has democratized information sharing, and its multiple applications are defined by social connections. These various generally inexpensive, user-friendly tools have fast become a normal conduit for both routine and extraordinary communications between people, groups and public and private institutions, changing the world in the process. However, disaster preparedness and response fields have not kept pace with the rapid development and use of social networking. With a few exceptions, social networking has not yet been assessed or routinely incorporated into many plans for disaster management. Consequently, little research has been done to systematically evaluate its utility in this context. Despite this, anecdotal information exists of successful public spontaneous social networking emergency response in multiple types of disasters. The authors of this chapter propose that social networking should be incorporated into disaster management plans to help address well researched and persistent problems in effective communication during disaster response. Its nature, breadth and widespread use lend to its potential as a powerful tool for disaster response communities worldwide. This chapter examines the considerable social research in public response to disasters that demonstrates its utility; problems in conventional disaster communication; social networking's definition and applications; its recent spontaneous successes in contemporary disasters; how to incorporate social networking into disaster plans; and disaster medicine applications built on Web 2.0 technology. This technology can be effectively used for better communication leading to efficient disaster response.

The communications and resource needs and allocations for high-risk and high-tech patients form the focus of the fifth chapter by Ronald S. Cohen. The chapter focuses on developing a resource-based triaged tool acceptable to all the hospitals in a region, and developing a region-wide approach to surge capacity. It is well recognized that disasters pose different threats and raise different issues for specialized medical professionals like neonatologists to those for physicians in surgery, emergency medicine or adult intensive care units. There are no likely scenarios that would result in a large number of preterm or term newborns, not already in hospital, becoming mass casualties. Thus far, no epidemic or pandemic has resulted in massive numbers of neonatal cases. There are, however, significant issues in disaster planning for those who work in newborn intensive care units. Specifically, neonatologists are likely to face one of three possible disaster scenarios: (i) the need to evacuate their own unit; (ii) the need to receive large numbers of neonates from neighbouring hospitals forced to evacuate; and (iii) the need to continue functioning in the face of marked depletion of staff. This chapter discusses possible ways to mitigate such scenarios. Preparing neonatal intensive care units (NICUs) for possible large-scale disasters, such as an earthquake or tsunami is essential. Clearly, this is an area of concern as far as neonatologists are concerned. Ways to improve collaboration and communication between NICUs to expedite the movement of patients and resources between units in the event of a regional disaster event that impairs the ability of one of more major medical centres to care for its patients are discussed. In addition, protocols to codify communications and focus on resource needs and allocations for high-risk and high-tech patients are evaluated.

Well organized responses to disasters like earthquakes, floods, terror incidents, etc. usually involve efficient coordination and collaboration among public safety/medical organizations, and sharing of emergency alerts and incident-related data between disparate systems. During the 2001 Gujarat earthquake and the 2004 Indian Ocean tsunami, as well as in the recent 2011 Great Eastern earthquake of Japan, the communication systems were severely disrupted for days together. During such emergencies, quite often extensive disruption of most infrastructure-based communication systems is witnessed. During such emergencies, rescue groups from different locations and medical departments gather together to implement their respective rescue operations. It is pertinent that these groups quickly establish networks among themselves, and exchange data, so as to complete their missions speedily and efficiently. Under such circumstances, mobile ad hoc networks (MANETs) are increasingly being perceived as the preferred types of networks because of their unique characteristics of independent network organization, dynamic topology, ease of deployment and no central nodes (see Chapter 6 of this book). A synergy of the resource-sharing potential of grid computing with the flexible, ubiquitous availability of MANETs can be used to create a mobile grid environment. A mobile grid would allow the networked mobile devices to accomplish a specific mission that maybe beyond an individual's computing or communication capacity due to their inherent constraints in terms of processing power, node life or low resources, etc. The sixth chapter of this book by Monideepa Roy and Nandini Mukherjee covers the application of mobile grid for medical emergency management/disasters and terror incidents. The authors present in this chapter a unique perspective of a mobile grid application for the setting up of an efficient disaster recovery system. These technologies, when used appropriately, can effect better communication leading to efficient disaster relief, response and recovery.

Social networking can significantly improve disaster response and help to obtain contact information, speeding reunions for people, as has been evident from the 2011 Japan mega-disasters, Hurricane Sandy, the EF5 tornado that devastated Moore, Oklahoma in 2013 and the recent MCIs like the 2013 Boston Marathon bombings and the June 2013 Uttarakhand landslides/floods (Himalayan Tsunami), and needs incorporation in future disaster plans. Social media can significantly empower individuals, providing them a platform to share their experiences and information irrespective of time and place. The application of IT tools can make information management during the disaster support planning and execution phases faster and more reliable, affordable and accessible.

Disasters and Mass Casualty Incidents: Incident Site Command and Control, Point-of-care Testing

Section 4 of the book focuses on the role of Incident Command and Control Systems in the management of disasters and MCIs, and highlights practical guidance in planning and implementing reliable, clinically useful and cost-effective point-of-care procedures and systems. The role of the Incident Command System (ICS) is discussed and similar systems from other nations are also reviewed. Applications of point-of-care (POC) testing in disaster settings, benefits, limitations and cost-effectiveness of point-of-care testing are also highlighted.

In a changed global scenario, POC testing is being pushed forward as a useful modality in the management of emergencies of diverse nature. POC testing is performed at or near the site of care and is an ideal approach to accelerate decision-making in emergencies, disasters and public health crises. The seventh chapter of this book, by Gerald J. Kost, Corbin Curtis, Richard Louie and Ann Sakaguchi, provides fundamental conceptual principles and value propositions that will enable new POC technologies to be assimilated into challenging sites when infrastructure is severely compromised. At the same time, it proposes developing professional competence and team experience cost-effectively in the context of existing small-world networks of healthcare delivery. There is a need for environmental limitations to be addressed, since use of current POC devices and test kits must adhere to manufacturer specifications, which to date are not robust enough for the hot, cold and humid conditions encountered during field operations. The author presents strategic alternatives for placement of POC testing in appropriate settings that readers will find useful as they adopt solutions to fulfil critical need. Overall, POC testing promises to transform crisis standards of care by bringing enhanced evidence-based diagnosis and treatment to the sites most in need and by accelerating process steps, such as screening and triage, that are critical to effective emergency and disaster responses. The chapter highlights practical guidance in planning and implementing reliable, clinically useful and cost-effective POC procedures and systems. Applications in disaster settings, benefits, limitations and cost-effectiveness of POC testing are discussed. Potential operational benefits of POC testing include: more rapid decision-making and triage, reduced operating times, reduced high-dependency, post-operative care time, reduced emergency room time, reduced number of outpatient clinic visits, reduced number of hospital beds required and ensuring optimal use of professional time. These are crucial and life-saving issues during disasters. It is anticipated that POC testing could have widespread implications particularly in CBRN disaster management, where it can help in early detection, thereby greatly improving treatment outcomes of the affected people (first responders, military personnel and even civilian populations).

The eighth chapter, by Steven Parrillo and Jean Bail, reviews salient features of the Incident Command System (ICS) as it is used in the USA, and outlines several systems from other nations. It points out similarities despite different naming conventions among national models. Effective and efficient management requires a system that allows leadership to establish and maintain command and control through guidance and structure.

Although many such systems are in use throughout the world, the most effective ones share the features of standardization and flexibility. As far as the ICS is concerned, there is a lot to learn from the USA. ICS was first used to deal with the common occurrence of western US wildfires; since then the ICS has become the national model in the USA by which virtually every significant event is managed. Hospitals use a version modified to meet the needs of healthcare facilities. The system allows for diverse agencies – emergency medical services, fire fighting and law enforcement – to interact, communicate and cooperate when the need arises. Shortly after the 9/11 terror attacks and motivated by those attacks, the Federal Government used the ICS as the basis for the National Incident Management System. Lessons learnt from the effective usage of ICS in the USA can be adopted by developing countries for effective management of disasters and terror incidents.

Continuing the theme from Chapter 8, in Chapter 9 Anders Rüter from Sweden further goes on to highlight command and control during the response to a disaster or an MCI as an area in disaster medicine where there is lack of sufficient evidence. He opines that although the processes involved are many and sometimes complex, they must be made very easy and comprehensive in order to be functional when a disaster strikes. There must be knowledge within the healthcare organization on how to build up a command and control system, often called a management system, what functions and roles must be included and how and when the system should be alerted. Standard operating procedures (SOPs) should be developed as well as quality indicators for evaluating an MCI response as well as the command and control system. Involved healthcare professionals must have proper training and must be familiar with the processes and skills involved in staff work. Action cards must be present during a response, and all processes must be based on simplicity and resemble as much as possible how the staff work during their daily work. Information is important, and staff must be trained to seek information, which then must be analysed. Information within the healthcare organization should be prepared in the form of templates for reports.

Coordination with other agencies is necessary and important issues should be solved in liaison. All involved healthcare personnel should have the possibility to receive training, and key position holders such as staff personnel must have the possibility of repeated training using various pedagogic tools. Research in this field is sparse and results from training as well as MCIs must be documented, analysed and, whenever possible, should be published so that it can be utilized during disasters/MCIs.

In Chapter 10 Douglas Paton from Australia and David Allen from New Zealand deliberate on disasters in medical care contexts and the role of planning for resilience in incident command personnel and systems in hospitals. When disaster strikes, healthcare settings have a significant and prolonged role to play in the recovery process. Geological hazards such as earthquakes and pandemics can create health demands that persist for weeks, months and possibly longer. When considering the role that healthcare staff play in disaster response the focus is typically on their medical and professional skills. However, to effectively use these skills, healthcare staff must be able to apply their professional skills in highly stressful circumstances over what may be long periods of time. It is thus important to develop the capability of hospitals and their staff to function effectively in challenging and threatening circumstances and at the same time maintain as high a level of personal and group well-being as possible. This chapter discusses factors that contribute to capacity building in hospitals and medical professionals, and further development and implementation of this capability. One important issue that arises in this context is the need for staff to function and to manage the consequences of disasters within empowering settings. This setting is defined by the actions of the incident coordination process and the existence of specially developed disaster management systems. This chapter specifically discusses how the integration of operational, coordinating and strategic functions can be accomplished. The issues to be considered when developing each of these levels of response management are discussed, as is the need for organizational learning and dedicated disaster management training.

Information management during the disaster medical support planning and execution phases is of great importance in modulating the outcome of disasters. Irrespective of their origin, whether natural or man-made, disaster events always require rapid mobilization of all community resources to meet the demand for proper assistance and delivery of resources and relief material to the devastated area. In the great majority of disasters, urgent provision of medical care is of utmost importance. Disaster medical support managers have to make their decisions in a constantly dynamic situation and under time constraints – time is the crucial factor in life-saving actions; often the golden hour and platinum minutes determine the difference between life and death. Therefore, providing accurate and up-to-date information is a prerequisite for efficient and adequate medical response.

When disaster strikes, medical information flow is required to be not only accurate, appropriate, but also timely. For this reason, establishing comprehensive and clear medical information management procedures is mandatory for fulfilling the disaster medical support ultimate objective – preserving the life, health and preventing residual disability of a maximum number of people harmed by the disaster event. Chapter 11 by Rostislav Kostadinov highlights the importance of information flow management, which could be defined as implementation of management techniques to collect medically meaningful data and convert them into medical information that is communicated to enable medical managers to make quicker and better decisions on disaster medical support planning and execution. A practical seven-step algorithm for disaster medical information flow management is presented by the author. Templates for exchange of information tools (questionnaires, reports, observations, etc.), already approved by practice, are provided in order to facilitate the algorithm implementation. Ideally, proper management of disaster occurs in an environment of preparedness and with prior planning. The unpredictable nature of disasters, however, almost always precludes such prior preparation. In these circumstances many pre-existing protocols with established pre-hospital and hospital liaison involving already trained physicians and paramedical personnel could be accessed and modified to accommodate the requirements of disaster management. Such pre-existing protocols and programmes not specifically designed for disaster management are described in this chapter as well as the manner in which they may be modified to facilitate disaster management. Even where there is a well-established disaster management system, these pre-existing programmes could prove important in supporting the principles of effective disaster management. Rapid advances and the use of modern IT tools will make information management during the disaster medical support planning and execution phases faster, reliable, affordable and accessible to the masses, especially for use in resource-poor scenarios.

Medical Management of Complex Disasters and MCI Victims in Hospitals

Quite often it has been observed that due to lack of coordination between pre-hospital and hospital interventions, precious lives are lost during emergencies. Issues concerning the synergy between two crucial points of treatment for emergency patient management have been discussed, taking examples from the developed and developing world. This section focuses on the medical management of disasters and MCI victims in hospitals. Hospitals are often considered to be the crux of a community's medical resilience in a disaster or MCI. A surge of patients, however, could overwhelm the resources and human resource so much that the hospitals themselves may need to reach outwards. This has often been observed in the aftermath of major terror strikes, particularly in Asia (India, Pakistan and Afghanistan). Looking at surge capacity at the hospital level can help identify what triggers would lead to the need for external resources, as well as what those resources would likely be. With this knowledge, the community can prepare to offer support and care for the patients when conditions challenge the normal healthcare delivery system. Contingency plans should be devised in such a manner that despite the constraints, they can operate effectively and efficiently. Proper integration of synergy of pre-hospital and protocols can go a long way in effective emergency patient management. Chapter 12 by Jameel Ali, a leading specialist in trauma programmes, explores methods by which existing synergistic pre-hospital and hospital protocols could be adapted to meet the needs of disaster management to complement other systems specifically designed for disaster management. In the area of trauma there are many internationally well-established programmes that involve aspects of training relevant to disaster management. These include the Advanced Trauma Life Support (ATLS®), the Pre-hospital Trauma Life Support programme, the Advanced Trauma Course for Nurses (ATCN), the Rural Trauma Team Development Course (RTTDC) and the Trauma Evaluation and Management (TEAM) courses. Several communities have in place systems geared towards timely pre-hospital management of stroke victims and those with suspected acute myocardial ischaemic syndromes. Existing protocols of this nature include components that could be modified to meet the needs of disaster management. There is an urgent need for adoption of such programmes in developing nations/underdeveloped countries. However, it might not be easy to accomplish this and this exercise would require support from international organizations like the United Nations (UN) and NGOs and the corporate sector under corporate social responsibility. Steps towards adopting existing protocols to meet the needs arising during disasters or disaster-like situations have been taken up in India under the aegis of the National Disaster Management Authority (NDMA) by establishing a Trauma Center at the premier All India Institute of Medical Sciences (AIIMS) in New Delhi, India.

It is a fact that no place is immune to man-made (transportation accidents and acts of terrorism) or natural (tornadoes and earthquakes) disasters, and this can culminate in a MCE scenario. Most disasters occur with little or no warning, hence the importance of preparedness. Miklosh Bala, Yuval Weiss and Yoram G. Weiss from Israel discuss process management of MCEs in Chapter 13, and bring to light a specific scenario that occurred nearly a decade ago wherein Jerusalem was the site of recurrent multiple MCEs; most of them related to the Israeli-Palestinian conflict. However, the most significant event was man-made; the collapse of the Versailles Wedding hall. Within a matter of 2 hours more than 250 injured were evacuated to the Jerusalem-area hospitals. Events such as these provide a rare chance to re-examine the effectiveness of MCE preparedness and MCE process control. The focus of this chapter is on the organizational steps needed to provide adequate hospital-wide preparedness and operational flexibility, emphasizing the importance of forward deployment of medical personnel to the trauma bay and emergency room, and the existence of a chain of command to limit chaos. Specific issues related to a multiple casualty process control, such as patient flow, information gathering, over- or under-triage are described. This chapter emphasizes the importance of a multidisciplinary team-approach in caring for these patients.

Securing the Homeland: The Medical Way

Homeland security is increasingly perceived as being critical to the overall security of any country. Homeland security of all nations is important in view of the changing world scenario and the emergence of ever new threats. Terror threats, including those from CBRN agents, pose immense challenges in a dynamically changing world order. Appropriate planning and interventions can mitigate the deleterious effects of CBRN agents, both in military and civil settings. Critical management issues include: training of healthcare providers; honing of medical response teams; emergency department preparedness; modern tools for analysis and detection; self- and collective protection through protective paraphernalia and decontamination strategies; provision of prophylactic and therapeutic stockpiles (antibiotics, antidotes, vaccines); and, most importantly, interlinking healthcare facilities with medical surveillance systems.

This section focuses on key issues involved in homeland security and prevention, medical response, and incorporates a few case studies, including those related to suicide terrorism. Medical planning for CBRN events requires careful and specialized planning. This section also discusses the key issues involved in medical planning, particularly for managing CBRN incidents in a military and civil setting. This section also focuses on the important role that military hospitals can play for CBRN events. Proper planning and medical interventions can go a long way in mitigating the deleterious effects of CBRN events. The key issues involved in decontamination of CBRN agents are also discussed. In the case of MCIs, decontamination would be indispensable. This section discusses some of the finer nuances of civilian and military decontamination, as well as touching on triage and treatment tools specifically for terrorist attacks and chemical, biological and radiological incident management. The role of triage cannot be understated as it is essential to sort patients based on their extent of injury as under such situations the medical facilities would already be overwhelmed. Quite often it has been observed that due to lack of synergy between pre-hospital and hospital interventions, precious lives are lost during MCIs. This section focuses on issues concerning the synergy between two crucial points of treatment for emergency patient management. This section also dwells upon crucial issues such as the history of suicide terrorism, causes, types, and their prevention, medical response and a few case studies.

It is apparent that homeland security against various kinds of terror strikes is the need of the hour. Terror incidents, including suicide bombings pose a serious concern. Richman *et al.* in chapter 14 opine that first responders, first receivers and emergency managers must be prepared to respond to suicide bombings. Staging safe and effective responses to these incidents requires knowledge of a number of unique considerations. This chapter uses examples from past suicide bombing cases to help convey these important considerations. The authors present a common framework that can help facilitate a coordinated and effective response from all agencies involved. Civilians and private security guards can play an important role in detecting the planning and execution of suicide attacks, and sometimes even in their interdiction in the imminent attack phase. The suspicions of civilians must be taken seriously and citizens should be encouraged to report these suspicions immediately. The first responding emergency services personnel must be able to effectively begin their agency's response to the attack, while maintaining strong situational awareness. Also, strong frontline commanders are needed on the scene to work together to lead a coordinated response. Interagency communication and using a scaled response is of increased importance at these incidents when first responders could be targeted by the secondary attacks or an initial threat that has not yet been declared safe. In the terror attacks on India and Pakistan this kind of strategy (secondary strikes) has been employed against first responders to dissuade them from carrying out their duties, often resulting in the loss of several lives. First responders can take the initial steps to promote the return to normalcy that is so important after terrorist attacks. First receivers must have adequate surge capacity plans to deal with the influx of trauma patients while guarding against the threat of the hospital being a target for attack. In the aftermath of attacks, efforts should be made to establish a collective knowledge within the emergency services community to share lessons learned in the response. Understanding these important considerations will allow for an effective and safe response to suicide bombings by all agencies. There indeed are number of lessons to be learnt from nations that have handled terror at close quarters.

Fernando Turégano and Itamar Ashkenazi in Chapter 15 highlight the issue of civilian hospital preparedness for MCIs following terrorist attacks, which is a growing concern throughout the world. The controversies surrounding the objective of the hospital response to an MCI in accordance to the caseload, and the metrics used to assess the efficacy of that response, as well as the triage process and some computer simulation models developed to aid in increasing the surge capacity of the receiving institution are discussed. Over-triage, the rate of non-critically injured being evacuated or hospitalized, and under-triage, the rate of critically injured who are mistriaged, can both be life-threatening in a large-scale MCI in a civilian setting. A certain degree of over-triage to the closest hospital is an unavoidable occurrence because of self-referrals of many casualties, and the frequent uneven distribution of casualties by the emergency medical services (EMS). Bottlenecks to the flow of casualties are the main concern during large-scale MCIs. The number of trauma teams and trauma resuscitation bays, radiology facilities, operating theatres and intensive care unit (ICU) beds constitute those potential bottlenecks. Published reports from large-scale MCIs in urban settings in the last two decades, together with the considerable experience gained from the high number of small-scale MCIs reported from Israel, have shed considerable light in this still rather new field of disaster medicine. Nevertheless, there is much that needs to be done to keep communities safe from this increasing global threat. This chapter discusses the finer nuances of hospital triage in mass casualties resulting from terror attacks. The lessons learnt from Israel can also be utilized in other parts of the globe. CBRN agents pose one of the biggest challenges in today's dynamically changing world order. In Chapter 16, Mesut Ortatatli and Levent Kenar discuss the role of military hospitals in handling chemical and biological disasters. In anticipation of the use of CBRN agents by adversaries, most military hospitals around the world were conventionally geared to handle such eventualities. They highlight the important role military hospitals can play during such disasters/incidents. The role of detectors and analytical measures, medical management and treatment of casualties, and antidote administration are discussed. They highlight that in cases involving the intentional release of chem-bio agents, the response should include a rapid and coordinated response amongst state, local and military foundations. This is a sine qua non for effective management of CBRN incidents. From the perspective of disaster planning and preparedness, some critical issues that need consideration include training of medical care providers, establishment of a chem-bio medical response team, emergency department preparedness, provision of a pharmaceutical stockpile consisting of antibiotics, antidotes, vaccines and self-protection by means of personal protective equipment (PPE), setting up medical care and a decontamination unit including a shower system, analytical and detection laboratories, linkage with other military healthcare facilities in addition to the surveillance system of long-term medical sequelae. The authors circumspectly present an account of the Turkish Military Medical Academy, which has established a medical CBRN response team in order to provide medical first aid and perform medical procedures in the event of a CBRN incident.

Major incidents may be caused by the accidental or deliberate release of chemical, biological or nuclear/radiological materials, of which chemicals arguably pose the greatest challenge. In Chapter 17, Robert P. Chilcott discusses the finer details of response to a CBRN threat. Recognizing the onset of a MCI is key to implementing an effective response. In the first instance, evacuation and cordoning of the affected area(s) should be undertaken, with appropriate triage and administration of emergency medical treatment as appropriate if sufficient personal protection is available to first responders. When the safety of casualties and responders has been established, disrobing of contaminated individuals should be undertaken as soon as practically possible, followed rapidly by decontamination. The author opines that following transfer to a safe area, personal details should be acquired in preparation for subsequent health surveillance to counter any potential chronic health effects. The civilian aspect of decontamination is as important as the military decontamination, rather more important since it would involve decontamination of a large section of population as compared with restricted personnel in the case of a military setting. Some such critical issues form the basis of this chapter.

Denis Josse and Gilles Barrier in Chapter 18 enumerate the emergency decontamination (ED) principles, procedures and systems, and discuss ED guidelines that could be provided to first responders as well as to victims in low-resource settings. In a scenario of military or civilian exposure to chemical, biological or radiological contaminants, the emergency (life-saving) procedures include the extraction of victims from the contaminated area, body surface decontamination and medical treatment, wherever necessary. Its objectives are to reduce both the intoxication of victims and the contamination transfer to care units and unexposed populations. ED consists of quick removal or neutralization of contaminants that are still present on the first layer of clothes and the exposed body surface (intact or wounded skin, hair and eyes). This is later on followed with complete disrobing and body surface washing, i.e. thorough decontamination. The authors present a pragmatic perspective for ED. In low-resource settings, i.e. in the absence of specifically dedicated equipments such as decontamination shelters, or fast transportation vehicles to hospitals, or large water supplies (pool, river, carwash site, etc.) in the vicinity, the victims themselves and emergency responders, possibly not equipped with decontamination kits or informed on the agent's identity, might have to find or design and use as quickly and effectively as possible any potential decontamination systems present on site to perform ED. Such scenarios are likely in developing countries, where even basic equipment is not available or even in emergency situations in developed nations, where ED equipment might not be available for various reasons, e.g. a really bad traffic jam or disruption of roads in a major city may preclude the emergency responders and dedicated equipment and transportation vehicles from reaching the incident site. In such cases, innovative decontamination methods would have to be resorted to. The chapter makes a strong case for loss-cost ED procedures and protocols for practical use during emergencies.

Radiological incident management assumes significance in today's scenario since there is a threat of usage of radiological agents by state-sponsored and non-state actors. In Chapter 19, Edward Joseph Waller, an expert in radiological incident management from Canada, discusses triage and treatment tools for radiological incident management. An accidental or intentional (malicious) release of radiological material may result in airborne contamination that can spread large distances from the source endangering human and animal life as well as the environment. This material may be inhaled directly or deposited on vegetation or water and ultimately be consumed as has been witnessed in the aftermath of the Chernobyl incident and the recent Fukushima incident. On the other hand, terrorist use of radiological materials for 'dirty bombs', radiological exposure devices or as radiological poisons can yield significant radiation doses to diverse populations jeopardizing lives. The author states that in both accidental and malicious releases, large numbers of persons may be affected, either through contamination or through the phenomenon of the 'worried well'. In all cases involving mass casualties, it is important to consider the emergency response in terms of planning, resource management, triage, treatment and patient follow-up. Three phases of medical management are important to the radiological disaster scenario: (i) pre-event (management plan, training and exercising the plans, treatment stockpiles and vulnerable populations); (ii) event (triage, treatment and decedents); and (iii) post-event (long-term care, dose reconstruction and epidemiology). Consideration of the unique challenges of radiological contamination to a classical disaster scenario from a medical management perspective is vital to ensuring first responders, nurses and physicians will be prepared to appropriately respond to all medical conditions presented without undue 'fear of radiation'. Waller goes on to highlight in this chapter that the challenge for the emergency management organization includes generating radiological disaster management plans, interfacing plans from disparate agencies that may be involved in the disaster response, training and exercising the plans (multi-agency preferred), addressing treatment pharmaceutical stockpiling for internal contamination management, addressing medical management for both localized and acute radiation injury, and considerations for dosimetry and health physics assets.

Defeating Emerging Health Threats: Managing by Prophylactic and Therapeutic Approaches

CBRN threats have become quite alarming in view of their ease of access and ability to create mass hysteria, if used. In addition, the emergence of newer health threats, particularly influenzas like bird 'flu and novel H1N1 in recent years has necessitated planning from a medical perspective. Systematic medical planning involving prophylactic and therapeutic approaches is needed. This section focuses on medical support to handle CBRN emergencies, prophylactic and therapeutic possibilities.

Biological agents can inflict damage to humans, animals and plants and pose a grave concern because new and rapid developments in biotechnology can transform them into potent bioweapons. Even small quantities of biological agents possess the ability to affect large areas and can cause far more casualties than the conventional chemical weapons. To counter such agents, there is an urgent need to devise preventive and protective strategies. The first line of defence against a terror attack with a bioweapon could be vaccination. Vaccines against biological threats can play a very important role in providing protection against natural emergence of diseases or the deliberate use of biological agents. There is an urgent need to have a strategic approach for developing suitable new generation vaccine candidates or developing technologies that can be readily used in case of emerging disease outbreaks and pandemics. Vaccines that are fairly stable for long periods and easy to administer would be necessary for the rapid large-scale immunization of populations following an attack of bioterrorism. In recent years, with a view to addressing this problem, recombinant DNA technology has been harnessed for the development of vaccines against a wide assortment of pathogenic microbes, including bacteria, fungi and viruses.

Recombinant antibodies are a highly successful therapeutic class of molecules and they are particularly well adapted for use against bioweapons as they act immediately, are often synergistic with other existing therapeutic molecules, have a long half-life and are well tolerated. Anthrax is a biological agent that can be used as one of the most potent bioweapons. However, its pathogenic properties depend on toxins that can be neutralized by antibodies. These toxins are formed by combining three different sub-units (PA, LF, EF). Chapter 20 elaborates on super-humanized antibodies and their role in biodefence. The chapter specifically discusses several recombinant anti-PA antibodies that have been developed utilizing an original approach starting from a hyper-immunized non-human primate (*Macaca fascicularis*). The humanization of this macaque Fab (35PA83) was then performed using human germline antibody sequences as a template, to reduce its potential immunogenicity. This approach resulted in a 'better than human' Fab and was called germline humanization or 'super-humanization'. An anti-PA antibody is also described along with an anti-LF antibody.

The emerging trends in this direction are many. It is felt that development of recombinant and multivalent vaccines could be optimized to enable a single oral dose to rapidly stimulate high levels of immunity to provide protection against various biological agents. Another strategy that could be utilized is immunomodulation by using potent adjuvants and immunomodulators, particularly of natural origin. Such immunomodulators can non-specifically stimulate the immune system and be of immense use in achieving improved survival in the aftermath of a bioterror attack. Transcriptome and proteome analysis of various human pathogens can lead to identification of critical genes that are important in infectivity and, therefore, could be possible targets for vaccine development. These are some of the several such approaches that can be utilized. Many other approaches are possible but they do not fall in the purview of this book and hence have deliberately not been discussed further.

Kamen Kanev and co-authors in Chapter 21 discuss the various facets of medical support in the case of chemical and biological incidents. It is a fact that chemical and biological incidents can occur during their development, production, transportation or use in different areas. The use of sarin by Aum Shinrikyo during the terrorist attack on Tokyo metro and the city of Matsumoto in Japan, as well as the use of anthrax and other agents in subsequent attacks has shown that these agents could be used by terrorists to kill people and disrupt society. Today, people around the globe believe that the danger of use of chemical and biological substances for terrorist goals is increasing. The continuous increase in the number of synthesized chemical substances (including highly toxic ones), as well as the development of genetic engineering and other high-tech technologies, has attracted a lot of attention at the hands of the scientists. Protection against biological and chemical substances is the need of the hour and attention needs to be paid to medical treatment of the victims of these substances. The authors feel that chemical and biological agents are becoming easier to carry around and are more difficult to track. The problem of medical treatment of chemicals and biological incidents also increases due to the fact that during terrorist acts or disasters, different types of toxic chemicals or biological agents could be released from plants, industrial and scientific facilities. In such an accident, the act of terrorism or disaster consequences turns into mass traumatism. The medical treatment of chemical and biological agent incidents has some common principles, but at the same time there exist a lot of differences connected with different types of agents. Some of these issues form the framework of this chapter.

In Chapter 22, Arora *et al.* delineate the various issues related to the medical management of CBRN emergencies as well as gearing medical paraphernalia for handling any such eventuality. The state-of-the-art in the area of managing CBRN emergencies is discussed along with the basic concepts, the history of nuclear and radiological emergencies, radiological terrorism, radiation syndromes, incident site management and the role of emergency response centres. The critical issues in the medical management of CBRN emergencies are discussed along with the currently available medical countermeasures for sociological/nuclear emergencies, besides the potential medical countermeasures under development or under approval by the Food and Drug Administration (FDA), including decorporation agents.

Disasters can occur anytime and anywhere, without any prior warning. The likelihood of release of toxic chemicals also cannot be excluded in any situation. Nerve agents belong to the category of the most dangerous chemical warfare agents and have been misused by terrorists in the past. Therefore, prophylaxis against the effect of nerve agents is both interesting and a complicated problem at the same time. In Chapter 23 Jiri Bajgar summarizes the basic principles of prophylaxis against intoxication with organophosphates (OP)/nerve agents, and highlights why keeping acetylcholinesterase (AChE, EC 3.1.1.7) the target enzyme for toxic action of OP/nerve agents (protection of cholinesterases) is a basic requirement for effective prophylaxis. This is achieved using reversible inhibitors (preferably carbamates), which are able to inhibit AChE reversibly. AChE inhibited by carbamates is resistant to OP/nerve agent inhibition. After spontaneous recovery of activity, normal AChE serves as a source of the active enzyme. Detoxification is realized by administration of the enzymes splitting the nerve agent or evaluating specific enzymes (cholinesterases). OP/nerve agent is bound to the exogenously administered enzyme and thus the nerve agent level in the organism is decreased ('scavenger' effect). The enzyme acts at the very beginning of the toxic action, without interaction with target tissues and without side-effects. The antidotes currently used for the treatment of OP/nerve agents poisoning have been tested as prophylactics. Standard antidotes have been evaluated in this respect, i.e. anticholinergics, reactivators, anticonvulsants etc. The problem with their use is the timing, duration and achievement of sufficient levels of these antidotes after their administration. At present, pyridostigmine seems to be a common prophylactic antidote, and PANPAL (tablets with pyridostigmine, trihexyphenidyle and benactyzine) and TRANSANT (a transdermal patch containing HI-6) are other prophylactics introduced to the armies of a number of countries. Future developments in the area are focused on scavengers and other drugs – either reversible cholinesterase inhibitors (e.g. huperzine A, physostigmine, acridine derivatives, etc.) or other compounds.

Handling Psychosocial Issues: A Difference in Perspective (Developed and Developing Nations)

The psychosocial aspects of disasters and MCIs have been the focus of attention in recent years since it has been observed and felt that such incidents result in psychological trauma amongst not only the immediate victims, but, both directly and indirectly, amongst the affected communities. While disasters and MCIs do affect both developed and developing nations, the question is whether the impact is felt much more by developing nations as compared with developed nations. Do people who are already in a deprived state perceive a disaster as an additional burden to cope with or are they more immune to such situations? In general, it has been felt that the ability of developed nations to cope with disaster aftermath is much better than developing nations. Reasons for this may be many and this is open to debate. The issue is whether psychosocial interventions should be employed accordingly. Resource-crunched developing nations simply cannot afford to employ resources for this, even if they wished to. Then who does? Such issues raise important questions in today's scenario. This section attempts to answer some of these contemporarily relevant questions, though many more still remain unanswered.

In Chapter 24, Chris Cocking presents an interesting account of collective resilience versus collective vulnerability after disasters from a social psychological perspective. Traditional accounts of the psychological impact of disasters propose a vulnerability model suggesting those affected by disasters are vulnerable to mass panic and psychological trauma in their aftermath. However, this notion of vulnerability is not supported by evidence from studies of behaviour during emergencies, and a wealth of research suggests instead that communities affected by disasters are more likely to show collective resilience than vulnerability. The social identity model of collective resilience argues that this is because disasters create a common identity through a sense of shared fate that encourages cooperative rather than selfish behaviour. This common identity can also be effective in shielding people from trauma after disasters. Therefore, it is recommended that plans for disaster preparation and mitigation should adopt a resilient rather than vulnerable approach to the public's response to mass emergencies and disasters. The debate continues!

In Chapter 25, Joseph O. Prewitt Diaz of Peru discusses how a community-based psychosocial support programme increases participation of disaster-affected people in their reconstruction as a result of an improvement in their psychosocial well-being. The chapter is divided into three parts. The first segment introduces a functional definition of psychosocial support, presents a theoretical overview and introduces the current international standards in support of the programme. The second part proposes a schematic for psychosocial support as a platform for community-based programmes, while the third segment integrates theory and practice by providing a case study from the psychosocial support programme implemented in Sri Lanka as a result of the 2004 South Asia earthquake and tsunami.

In Chapter 26, Suresh Bada Math and colleagues lay the background for preventive psychiatry. They address the current state of contemporary disaster mental health practice, which is based on the principles of 'preventive medicine'. This has necessitated a paradigm shift from relief-centred post-disaster management to a holistic, multidimensional integrated community approach of disaster prevention, preparedness and mitigation. The chapter aims to define, classify and elaborate on the various phases of disaster. This chapter also discusses the human responses, psychiatric morbidity and management of disasters from a mental health perspective. Mental health professionals will have to play multidimensional roles ranging from educating the public, training the trainers, coordinating with the administration and NGOs, advocating promotion of mental health and planning long-term rehabilitation.

Recent years have witnessed several major disasters. However, the earthquake of magnitude 9.0 on 11 March 2011 in Tōhoku, Japan and a number of aftershocks of 6, 7 and 8 on the Richter scale caused significant destruction and damage to human and animal lives, property, economy and the environment. It resulted in a tsunami with a maximum height of 40.4 metres in Japan. The 2011 Japan Tōhoku earthquake has been labelled as one of the major disasters of this century and resulted in the loss of 15,867 lives, and left 6109 injured and 2909 people missing. Over 300,000 people were displaced. The tsunami levelled 130,000 houses and severely damaged more than 260,000. Approximately 270 railway lines ceased operation immediately following the disaster, and 15 expressways, 69 national highways and 638 prefectural and municipal roads were closed for days. The World Bank estimated the economic cost of the disaster to be US$235 billion, making it the most expensive natural disaster in world history. Japan lies on 'the Pacific ring of fire' (intersection of three major tectonic plates) and thereby faces 90% of the earth's earthquakes. The earthquake and the subsequent massive tsunami resulted in a nuclear emergency situation at the Fukushima Daiichi (no.1) nuclear power plant that had to be reported to the International Atomic Energy Agency (IAEA). The emergency was caused due to failure of cooling of fuel rods because of damage of back-up diesel generators despite the existence of numerous tsunami protection strategies. This led to a cascade of reactions resulting in the IAEA declaring it an international nuclear and radiological event scale (INES) level 7 incident. The disaster led to increased radiation levels in the environment, food, milk and tap water far beyond the demarcated 30–40 km evacuation zone. The socioeconomic impact of the disaster has been tremendous as has been the psychosocial impact. As a part of rescue and relief operations, various countries extended their help to Japan to promote recovery efforts. India too sent an equipped and self-sustainable National Disaster Response Force (NDRF) team to Japan. This team contributed a lot by saving lives and extricating dead bodies and other economic assets.

The Japan 2011 multiple disasters have brought to the fore the role of leveraging human resource (HR) functions in alleviating the impact of the disaster. Preeti Arora along with co-authors in Chapter 27 presents a first-hand account of the societal impact of the 2011 Japan Tōhoku earthquake and ensuing multiple disasters on the community from an on- and off-ground perspective. The chapter presents a leveraging systems approach to HR management for efficient disaster management in the wake of the multiple disasters that severely affected Japan. The disaster led to a number of psychological problems amongst children, women and elderly people requiring specific attention. Some of the common problems faced by the population included: (i) fear that disaster will strike again; (ii) fear psychosis related to radiation contamination; (iii) psychological trauma (post-traumatic stress disorder – PTSD); (iv) loss of families, friends, relatives, property and belongings, which in turn led to stress and depression; (v) abuse and harassment; (vi) anxiety; (vii) lack of sleep; (viii) phobia; and (ix) feeling of helplessness, etc. There are a number of lessons to be learnt from the Japanese. Their close-knit community, cultural resilience and existence of family and strong social and professional values, besides support from the Japanese government, NGOs and also the international community helped in early recovery from the initial psychosocial problems that would have manifested otherwise to a great extent. Prior experience of the Indian Ocean tsunami of 2004 has shown this evidently. There is an urgent need to learn from the best practices followed by the Japanese so that the deleterious effects of disasters on humans and other life forms can be averted to the best possible extent. Psychological distress and post-traumatic stress responses have recently been confirmed by Japanese researchers in the Fukushima Nuclear Power Plant workers (2 to 3 months after the disaster – see Chapter 27). The prevalence of such disorders was higher than that reported in other studies, possibly due to the complexity of their experience. These findings highlight the intricacies involved in post-disaster scenarios and the need for psychosocial interventions to avert full blown psychological distress. The chapter proposes a simplistic model for integrating HR framework with a systems approach for efficient disaster management.

Bridging the Great Divide: The Challenge of Managing Disasters and MCIs in Resource-poor Settings

Managing disasters and MCIs in resource-poor settings is indeed a difficult enterprise. However, most developing nations struggle to manage disasters and MCIs despite all odds. There are several lessons to be learnt from such situations, particularly low-resource settings, though it is acknowledged that the necessity to bridge the great divide exists.

Nibedita Ray-Bennett in Chapter 28 discusses the issue of managing disasters through a health security approach. Health security in the context of disaster vulnerability is understood as not only access to health but also people's resilience to and agentive capabilities of coping and surviving recurrent shocks. Central to this, how health security can enhance different phases of disaster management is highlighted and also tasks are recommended for achieving health security, which is currently lacking in developing nations highly exposed to multiple disasters. The key issues of gender, sociology, development, health and disaster risk, which have serious policy implications are highlighted. She states that managing disasters from a health security perspective will have three important implications: (i) it will indicate an inroad to better specify the intersection of disaster and development activities; (ii) it will build the capacity of households and communities living with risk; and (iii) it will prioritize disaster management as a national security concern. Disaster management through a health security perspective should prioritize disaster management as a national security concern with the potential for improved innovation and securitization. Securitization of disaster management needs to be understood at the level at which it can have most impact, requiring the spread of know-how, to meet local conditions of disaster avoidance and development. Securitization is also a communicative process to promote a disaster-resilient culture by enhancing people's capability. The key to operationalizing disaster management through health security is underpinned by communication and communicating processes that take place between different institutions and local level day-to-day realities. To understand these communicative processes that are the lynchpins for successful disaster management and health security, Nibedita Ray-Bennett suggests that more sociological and anthropological research is needed that can engage with the ever-growing community of scholars, policy-makers, practitioners and civil societies that are engaged with the mainstreaming of Disaster Risk Reduction (DRR) to explore communicative processes, whilst being grounded in the local experiences of day-to-day adaptation and resilience in pursuit of reduced vulnerability and sustainable development.

Chapter 29, authored by Preeti Arora *et al.*, discusses the chain of events that led to the immense losses resulting from the 2011 Great Eastern Japan earthquake and the ensuing multiple disasters. The chapter lays emphasis on the lessons learnt from management of this mega disaster. The efforts made for mitigation and management of disasters in Japan prior to this disaster helped in saving many lives. An on- and off-ground assessment of the situation in Japan is also reported, along with the international efforts in the direction of relief, rescue and recovery. The chapter also briefly touches upon the role of the international rescue teams and the Indian NDRF in rescue and recovery operations in the aftermath of the disaster. The chapter also highlights the crucial role played by women and the gender sensitivity shown by the Japanese government. The lessons learnt will go a long way in mitigating the deleterious effects of future disasters. In addition to discussing the role of various agencies during the disaster, the chapter also sheds light on the importance of disaster resilience and discusses some finer nuances of managing disasters in resource-constrained settings based on the Japan experience.

In Chapter 30, Shabir Ahmed Dhar and colleagues view mass casualties from a hospital window and discuss some relevant issues for the developing world, where resources are constrained and mass casualties can affect hundreds to hundreds of thousands of people. They go on to highlight the range of possible mass disasters, which is worrisome to say the least, and can include scenarios such as nuclear detonation, radiological and biological (anthrax) attacks, pandemic influenza, plague and sulphur mustard attacks, etc. They state that the goal of disaster health preparedness and response is for resource-crunched communities to 'take simple steps to ensure that they have a sustainable supply of food, water and medicine, a reliable first aid kit and a plan to find relatives and friends if communication and transportation networks are disrupted'. Most underdeveloped or developing countries have insufficient critical care staff, medical equipment and ICU space to provide timely usual critical care to a surge of injured patients, with the main limitations being communications, sustainability of peak operations, education, cooperation and funding. In the developing countries, the problem particularly is the lack of an effective command centre, poor communication, lack of cooperation between the civil and the military establishments, delayed pre-hospital care, hospital overloading, inadequate staffing and mismanagement of public health resources. Local and regional mass casualty exercises should develop contingency plans to redistribute less injured patients away from the urban trauma epicentre to maintain availability. The hospitals should prepare triage and surge policies in advance. It is important that the developing countries develop an all hazards approach that can be used in a resource-constrained setting as well. The chapter also presents solutions to the problems, giving some examples.

Post-disaster Relief, Rehabilitation and Recovery

Disasters leave a long trail of destruction and suffering lasting several days to years. After disasters are over in terms of inflicting the damage, the genuine challenge begins. It is post-disaster that the preparedness of the community and responders is really tested. Then begin the efforts aimed towards relief, rehabilitation and recovery. The challenges posed are many and the real concern of governments and communities is to provide succour to the affected population. In terms of managing health issues, one area of great interest has been the use of alternative medical care facilities in times of disaster. This includes needs that arise due to damage of healthcare facilities, surge and other issues. This section deals with post-disaster relief and rehabilitation issues. Relevant post-disaster psychosocial health issues are also discussed in the last section of the book.

In Chapter 31, James C. Hagen and Scott P. Hagan highlight the several lessons to be learnt from the most recent catastrophes that have assaulted our world, including the 2011 Japanese earthquake and tsunami, the 2005 Hurricane Katrina, the 2004 Indian Ocean tsunami, flooding in Pakistan, earthquakes that occurred in India and China and a myriad of others. They go on to discuss that beyond the physical and economic devastation such events cause, there are extremely vulnerable populations that must be considered and 'invisible' factors that are of utmost importance in determining survival of 'community'. Recent global disasters highlight the extreme vulnerability of the human population, as well as its incredible capacity for recovery and reconstruction. Those most adversely affected are always the poor and vulnerable. An often-neglected area of study concerns the immediate post-disaster recovery period, and the importance of sociological factors that define 'community'. It is attention to these 'invisible' factors that helps define resilience and sustainability, and enhances the likelihood of community survival. An important location where reconstruction begins is the alternative care facility, where the 'invisible' factors may be acknowledged and addressed. In planning, responding to and recovering from disasters in this setting, special attention must be paid to psychological factors that compound the problems encountered and the levels of competency needed to address them. Cross-cultural lessons learned must be respected as we continue to experience catastrophes and share global best practices. This is extremely relevant as rescue operations these days are becoming more international in nature. Of particular importance are the impacts on, and the lessons that can be learned from, indigenous populations around the world. Hagen and Hagen opine that there is real value in organizing our alternative care facilities with an appreciation and acknowledgement of the value they have in stimulating and enhancing the recovery/reconstruction efforts and in regaining a sense of community. Post-disaster relief, rehabilitation and recovery continue to pose a major challenge in modern-day disasters.

In the aftermath of disasters and MCIs, a major problem encountered is that of the management and identification of the dead. The role of some of the important tools and techniques and critical operational issues in managing the dead are highlighted in Chapter 32 by Arora and co-authors. Though it might appear to be an easy task, it is one that requires great skill and deployment of trained HRs and proper management techniques to manage the dead since usually it is difficult to identify the dead post-disaster. Managing the dead and looking for missing persons is a humanitarian act that gives solace to the bereaved families from the state of uncertainty and continued distress, as nothing can be more stressful than living with an uncertain feeling about the welfare of near and dear ones. The various natural disasters like tsunamis, earthquakes, cyclones, hurricanes, and man-made disasters including fires, explosions, CBRN emergencies, etc. pose a significant burden of management of the dead during MCIs. CBRN emergencies, in particular, pose the additional challenge of managing the contaminated dead, who need to be handled using specialized procedures and protocols. While managing such events, there are numerous governing factors inclusive of religion, local and sociocultural issues in the recovery process that need to be kept in mind. It is pertinent to have systematic procedures in place that should be practised with great caution, fully respecting the deceased and providing appropriate care and empathy to their families. The major steps include body recovery, control of the recovered body by controllers of law and order, identification of the dead body by way of associated and non-associated articles, visual or circumstantial evidences, identification approaches including odontology, X-ray, medical history, genetics, DNA finger printing and matching with missing profiles, etc. These identification procedures require a legal post-mortem, followed by matching this with ante-mortem data. After identification, proper infrastructures should be in place to preserve the body and reconstruct its facial and other body features prior to repatriation or cremation (burial or exhuming or incineration). During such events, mass burial/cremation is also a conflicting issue due to the associated religious factors and sociocultural norms of society. The fear of spreading of epidemics is also a cause of major concern. The fear of contamination can be mitigated by providing protective clothing to those who are managing it, and all contaminated bodies need to be decontaminated prior to adoption of systematic procedures of management of dead bodies. In India, the Disaster Management Act, 2005 empowers the District Collector to take critical decisions on various vital issues related to management of the dead during mass casualty events. The District Collector has the right to bypass the existing systematic procedures or alternatively can adopt fast procedures of identification based on the disaster scenario. The basic premise of management of the dead includes the following: (i) the dead should not cause infection; (ii) victims should not be buried in common graves; and (iii) mass cremation should be avoided, it is better to develop temporary trenches to bury prior to complete identification. This chapter provides first-hand information on the critical challenges in this area and also an Indian perspective on the subject matter concerned.

Kai-Lit Phua in Chapter 33 highlights the socioeconomic dimension of disaster management. Social factors can affect the success of disaster management and emergency relief operations even if most of the benchmarks are already in place at satisfactory levels, e.g. if people with good intentions from outside the disaster area and from overseas attempt to assist by pouring into the area in large numbers but they are not properly managed by local authorities. This has been observed in many post-disaster situations in the South Asian region. In the aftermath of the Kosi floods of 2008 in India, such a problem was faced by local authorities. Similar problems were encountered during previous disasters in other countries, e.g. during the 1995 Hanshin-Awaji (Great Kobe) earthquake of Japan, there was a large influx of volunteers in the affected area and as a consequence the roads were blocked and hindrances were posed to the relief and rescue operations. There were also problems faced in crowd management. This is also the case with unsolicited donations of physical goods that may give rise to severe logistical challenges for disaster management and emergency relief personnel already in the field. Social factors that can mitigate or magnify the effects of disasters on individuals, families, communities and the larger society include the pre-disaster political situation; the economic resources available to the individuals and families living in the community and larger society; and pre-existing social tensions, social cleavages and resulting degree of social solidarity and cultural norms affecting cooperative behaviour. These social factors can at times make recovery from the disaster, and rebuilding of communities, more problematic. Some such issues form the basis of this chapter.

Community resilience against natural disasters is one of the most important concerns in all sustainable development programmes worldwide. One of the most effective ways to achieve disaster resilience is through education and training of various vulnerable groups of society such as children and women. In Chapter 34, Yasamin O. Izadkhah and Mahmood Hosseini address the vulnerability of these two groups of society. Next, they go on to discuss different aspects of disaster management phases including disaster preparedness, emergency response, recovery and restoration, and special problems of developing countries in facing disasters. Subsequently, the roles of children and women in developing a safety culture in the community as well as fostering disaster management activities are discussed. Finally, various issues with regard to educating these two groups, including materials, tools, time and methods are addressed in detail.

Final Comments and Preparing for the Future

The ten sections of this book containing 34 chapters cover the key facets of disaster management and homeland security from a medical perspective. The medical management of disasters is a steadily evolving area and the 9/11 terror attacks and Hurricane Katrina in the USA, and also the recent 2011 Japan earthquake and tsunami and 2012 Hurricane Sandy, the 2013 EF5 tornado that devastated Moore, Oklahoma and the recent MCIs like the Boston Marathon bombings have underscored the need for proactive disaster management strategies and development of state-of-the-art tools and techniques. Disasters most often spring surprises and pose challenges that test our ultimate preparedness levels, patience and community resilience.

Unfortunately, disasters – especially extreme-weather related disasters – are likely to increase in the future due to rapid global warming, as a result of the increase in human activities severely jeopardizing the climate of the planet and affecting millions of human lives. Several parts of the globe will witness severe changes in climate, leading to drought, large-scale massive flooding of coastal areas due to rising sea levels, heavy rainfall in discrete areas in a short time (cloud bursts), extreme heat events, etc. These events will become commonplace in unimaginable proportions in different parts of the globe if attention is not paid in earnest. Such disaster events will affect poor people the most, especially in thickly populated developing countries and resource-constrained settings. If poor people who are just able to eke out a living lose their livelihoods due to disaster events, it can only be imagined how they would be able to survive. In developing countries, people live in densely populated areas, unsafe housing and mostly in precarious living conditions with poor health and hygiene circumstances. The emergence of new pandemics will also pose problems in both high-tech as well as highly populated resource-poor settings.

Each disaster event is unique and endeavours to manage them inevitably lead to the development of novel expertise, and the experience thus gained proves useful in managing future disasters and MCIs and eventually achievement of a disaster-resilient society. The learning experience from each and every disaster goes a long way in developing better strategies for disaster management. It remains a fact that it is impossible to avoid, avert or control disasters totally, however, their impact can certainly be significantly reduced through preparedness in a dynamically changing world. Medical preparedness can help in effectively dealing with such disaster related issues. In addition, endeavours towards disaster management also lead to development of effective strategies for homeland security. This has been amply exemplified when humanity has faced the onslaught of terror on various fronts.

It is our firm belief that with preparedness and resilience in the community, the face of disasters and MCIs can be changed! This book is a humble step in that direction.

Section 2

Training, Mitigation and Medical Preparedness

Chapter 2

The Role of the Primary Care Physician in Disasters

Mark K. Huntington

Introduction

All disasters are local. When the unthinkable happens, it is the local primary care physicians who are at the forefront of the response. Local physicians are the first to respond, and they are the ones who will remain when all of the national and international disaster response resources leave. They are the ones who initiate the provision of aid to disaster victims, it is they that work diligently through the immediate aftermath to minimize the medical consequences of the calamity, and it is they that will deal with the recovery and long-term consequences after the event. Consequently, these physicians should be involved in the planning and preparation of disaster contingencies prior to such events. The involvement of primary care physicians in disaster medicine is inevitable; being equipped for this involvement is imperative.

Table 2.1. Types of disasters.

Natural	Accidental	Intentional
Meteorological (hurricane, blizzard, etc.)	Transportation (plane crash, etc.)	Explosive (bombing, shooting)
Geological (earthquake, flood, etc.)	Structural (building collapse, etc.)	Nuclear or radiological (fissile weapon, 'dirty bomb', etc.)
Other (pandemic, wildfire, etc.)	Industrial or agricultural (chemical spill, reactor meltdown, etc.)	Chemical or biological (nerve gas, bacterial release, etc.)

Disaster phases

Disasters come in many types (Table 2.1). Whatever their type, they may be divided into four phases (Fig. 2.1). The first is *preparation*, the inter-event time when planning, training and exercises, stockpiling of critical resources and vigilance occur. Although this phase lacks the adrenalin-driven activity of other phases, it is perhaps the most important phase. When activity in this phase is neglected, outcomes in subsequent phases are much bleaker. The second phase is *response*: the period during and immediately following the disastrous event itself. It is a period of triage, stabilization, emergency care and evacuation. It is followed by *recovery*, when the affected region rebuilds and attempts to return to normal. There is often significant overlap between the recovery phase of one disaster and the preparation phase for the next. The final phase is *mitigation*, when efforts to minimize the effects of the disaster are made. Primary care physicians play critical roles in each of these phases of disaster.

Patient-centred medical home

The primary care physician may be defined as a physician whose scope of practice is not limited by the patient's age, sex, affected organ system or the setting of care. They are generalists, or better, comprehensivists (Huntington, 1999). In recent years, increased attention has been given by various primary care specialties to the concept of the Patient-centred Medical Home (PCMH) of primary care (Kellerman and Kirk, 2007). Among the principles of the PCMH is a personal physician who is the first point of contact, provides continuous and comprehensive care, leads the team of healthcare professionals, has a whole-person orientation and integrates care across both the complex healthcare system and the resources in the community. In the context of disasters, the primary care physician can embody these principles throughout all the phases of the disaster: the first to respond to the needs of the local population, providing the needed care in collaboration with other local healthcare professionals who are also on-scene. The primary care physician understands the implications of the disaster for the individual, their family and the community, and facilitates the integration of the initial local response with that of the outside relief agencies and organizations that arrive to lend aid.

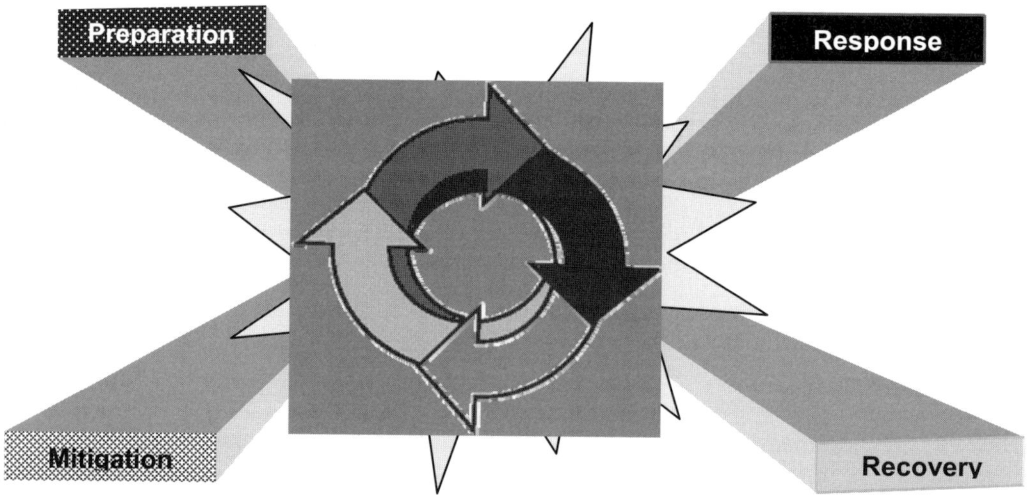

Fig. 2.1. The different phases of disasters.

Prevention

One of the foci of primary care physician's efforts is prevention, not merely treatment of disease. The primary care physician's approach to disaster medicine is no different. The adage 'an ounce of prevention is worth a pound of cure' applies throughout all areas of medicine; no less so to disaster medicine. There are several ways in which prevention may be applied in disaster medicine.

Baseline patient health

There is a positive correlation between pre-disaster morbidity and disaster mortality: healthy people are more likely to survive a disaster, and to survive intact (Greenough *et al.*, 2008; Hutton, 2009). As the primary care physician cares for their patients each day, seeking to optimize their health, they are also decreasing the vulnerability of their patients to disasters. Poverty and disenfranchisement are also associated with increased morbidity and mortality in disasters (Chen *et al.*, 2007); the socially conscious and active primary care physician further decreases patient risk in disasters through such involvements. In addition to achieving and maintaining a baseline of optimum health, patients may be further encouraged to decrease their vulnerability by personally planning for the contingencies of a disaster.

Patient disaster plans

One of the most important things a primary care physician can do is discuss disaster preparedness with their patients. A plethora of evidence exists that the simple act of physicians talking with their patients results in behavioural change for a host of health-related activities (Jepson *et al.*, 2010); disaster preparedness is no different.

Those families who have had a discussion with their doctor about disaster preparedness are much more likely to have a personal or family disaster plan in place than those who have not (Olympia *et al.*, 2010). Anticipatory guidance and disease prevention are essential components of the primary care physician's practice; most conditions are more easily prevented than remedied. So, too, are disasters. Encouraging patients to take steps to avoid becoming the victim of a disaster has the potential to reduce the number of casualties and thus the post-event burden on the medical system. Of course, not all hazards can be predicted – let alone avoided – but a well-considered plan can improve one's odds of survival.

Patients should develop a disaster plan. This begins with identifying the risks: what type(s) of disasters are possible or probable in their locale. Identify how they might become aware of the disaster; for example, what form of public warning system is present locally. Are there any members of the household who have special vulnerability, such as the elderly, young children, persons with disabilities or domestic pets (in some cultures)? Once these are all identified, a personalized disaster plan can be developed. This is outlined in Table 2.2.

More detailed information on this topic is available from a variety of sources, including www.disastercenter.com/guide/family.htm. Disaster kits, outlined in Table 2.3, are an essential component of the personal disaster plan, and should be prepared and maintained in advance of any event.

Table 2.2. Components of a family disaster plan.

Develop and discuss with the entire household • *Select meeting places:* one nearby in case the house needs to be evacuated, one further away in case the neighbourhood needs to be evacuated. • *Communication plan:* in case members become separated, include an out-of-town contact in case of more widespread chaos or disaster. Keep a list of emergency telephone numbers. • *Evacuation destinations:* in the event an evacuation is ordered, have somewhere to go planned in advance. • *Escape routes:* map several, depending on the nature of the disaster. Include not only routes out of the area, but also routes out of the home. • *Shelter-in-place locations:* identify safe places within the home, which will be different for differing types of disasters. • *Gas and water:* make sure everyone knows how to turn them off. • *Insurance:* if you have it, clarify what is covered. • *Emergency supply kits:* see Table 2.3. • *Vital documents:* keep copies of critical documents somewhere away from home.
Practise and maintain the plan, replace food and water stores regularly.

Clinic disaster plans

In addition to preparing one's patients for the event of a disaster, the primary care physician must prepare their practice for such an occasion. Without a plan for continuity, the physician's ability to aid their patients rapidly dissipates. In studies of primary care physicians' attitudes towards disaster response, the majority identify caring for their regular patients as their principal obligation (Shaw *et al.*, 2006). This is entirely appropriate, for in the event of a disaster there will be a variable period of time between the event and the arrival of outside responders and resources during which the local physician may be the sole source of care for the local population. This lag time may be accentuated in more rural locations, which typically receive attention substantially later than areas of higher population density in situations where a disaster affects a widespread geographical area.

A number of challenges face the physician hoping to maintain their practice in the face of a disaster (Collins *et al.*, 2006), and plans must be made to address them. Among the critical issues confronting non-hospital healthcare facilities are the development of a written plan, determining communication strategies, coping with affected staff and procuring essential supplies (Wineman *et al.*, 2007; Ablah *et al.*, 2008; Lauer *et al.*, 2008).

A written disaster plan is extremely valuable. The development of such a plan requires significant thought and effort. This investment, prior to a catastrophic event, is most worthwhile. Produced when there is adequate time to contemplate a myriad of circumstances, responses and consequences of each, it offers guidelines for appropriate priorities and actions in a time when the 'fog of disaster' can preclude clear thinking. It should be prepared with knowledge of the disaster plans of the local community and the state/provincial governments (Lauer *et al.*, 2008). Knowing what may be reasonably expected from these entities outside of the non-hospital healthcare facility – and what they may expect from the local physicians – can greatly aid in developing a plan that can coordinate with response efforts on the broader scale. A written disaster plan should include considerations of each of the other critical issues mentioned in the preceding paragraph.

Table 2.3. Components of disaster kits. (Used with permission from www.disastercenter.com/guide/kit.html).

Basic emergency kit

- A portable, battery-powered radio or television and extra batteries.
- Torch and extra batteries.
- First aid kit and first aid manual.
- Supply of prescription medications.
- Credit card and cash.
- Personal identification.
- An extra set of car keys.
- Matches in a waterproof container.
- Signal flare.
- Map of the area and phone numbers of places you could go.
- Special needs, for example, nappies or formula, prescription medicines and copies of prescriptions, hearing aid batteries, spare wheelchair battery, spare eyeglasses or other physical needs.

Evacuation supplies kit

- Three gallons (14.6 l) of water per person.
- Three-day supply of non-perishable food.
- Kitchen accessories: manual tin opener; mess kits or paper cups, plates and plastic/disposable utensils; utility knife; a can of cooking fuel if food must be cooked; household liquid bleach to treat drinking water; sugar, salt, pepper; aluminium foil; plastic resealable bags.
- One complete change of clothing and footwear for each family member, sturdy shoes or work boots, raingear, hat and gloves, thermal underwear, sunglasses;
- Blankets or sleeping bag for each family member.
- Tools and other accessories: paper, pencil; needles and thread; pliers, shut-off wrench, shovels and other useful tools; tape; medicine dropper; whistle; plastic sheeting; small canister, A-B-C-type fire extinguisher; emergency preparedness manual; tube tent; compass.
- Sanitation and hygiene items: toilet paper, towelettes; soap, hand sanitizer, liquid detergent; feminine supplies; personal items such as shampoo, deodorant, toothpaste, toothbrushes, comb and brush, lip balm; plastic garbage bags (heavy-duty) and ties (for personal sanitation uses); medium-sized plastic bucket with tight lid; disinfectant; household chlorine bleach; small shovel for digging an expedient latrine.
- Entertainment, such as games and books.

Remember to consider the needs of very young and older family members, such as infants and elderly or disabled persons.

- For babies: formula, nappies, bottles, powdered milk, medications.
- For adults: prescription drugs, denture needs, contact lenses and supplies, extra eyeglasses and hearing aid batteries.

The plan should include isolation measures in the event of a pandemic or other biological event. A simple example of the most basic of measures is separate waiting – and possibly care – areas for patients with symptoms of infection and those with non-infectious illnesses. These measures may be implemented with benefit during non-disaster periods, as well, such as during seasonal illnesses such as influenza. Such implementation benefits routine patients, and also offers the opportunity to train staff for infectious disasters.

A plan for decontamination of victims following chemical – and in some areas, radiation – exposures should be considered as well. A well-designed layout, separating 'hot' from 'cold' patients, is essential to avoid endangering both patients and responders. Although somewhat controversial, there is a trend towards including an urgent treatment area within the 'hot' zone for patients not yet stable enough to pass through the decontamination process (Baker, 2004). An example of a well-designed decontamination area is shown in Fig. 2.2.

In the absence of specialized decontamination fluids, a chlorine solution may be employed. Two concentrations are required: a 5% solution to decontaminate gloves, litters, scissors and other non-skin contact areas, and a 0.5% solution for skin, splints and wound irrigation. Regular household bleach is a 5% solution; diluting 100 ml in 900 ml of water will yield the 0.5% solution. Use of a washcloth provides additional benefit over irrigation alone (Amlot *et al.*, 2010). Detailed descriptions of decontamination procedures are available from a variety of sources, among the best are those produced by the military (US Army, 2000).

A related issue is personal protective equipment (PPE). Studies have found that healthcare providers are much more reluctant to care for disaster victims when adequate PPE is not available (Alexander *et al.*, 2006). Gloves, masks, gowns and sanitizing chemicals are important and should be stockpiled in adequate quantities to continue medical care during a disaster when resupply mechanisms may be disrupted. This stockpiling requirement applies to all materials needed for clinic operations. In the USA, the recommendation is to maintain a minimum of 3 days' worth of supplies on hand at all times, though it is widely recognized that in event of a widespread or protracted disaster, such as an influenza pandemic, this quantity is woefully inadequate.

Contingencies must be made for clinic staff absenteeism. In event of a disaster, it is probable that some support staff will be unable to perform their functions due to personal illness or injury, caring for injured or ill family members, disruption of transportation system, fear of illness or other reasons. It is important to cross-train staff to perform functions outside their usual job description to compensate for staff absenteeism. Also essential is to arrange for adequate water, food and shelter for clinic staff while at work; possibly for longer periods, as well, depending on the level of disruption of local infrastructure caused by the event. In large-scale disasters, the physician may be requested or conscripted to provide services at another site. The plan needs to include this contingency, and delineate options of when and how to provide at least limited services in the absence of a physician. This is another reason why an awareness of the disaster plan of local and regional authorities, and its intentions for local medical professionals, is vital. Consideration must be given to other issues relevant to 'business continuity' besides staffing. In the event the disaster renders the current clinical setting unusable, an alternative site must be used. The time to identify potential sites, and to explore possible arrangements for their use, is before the disaster strikes.

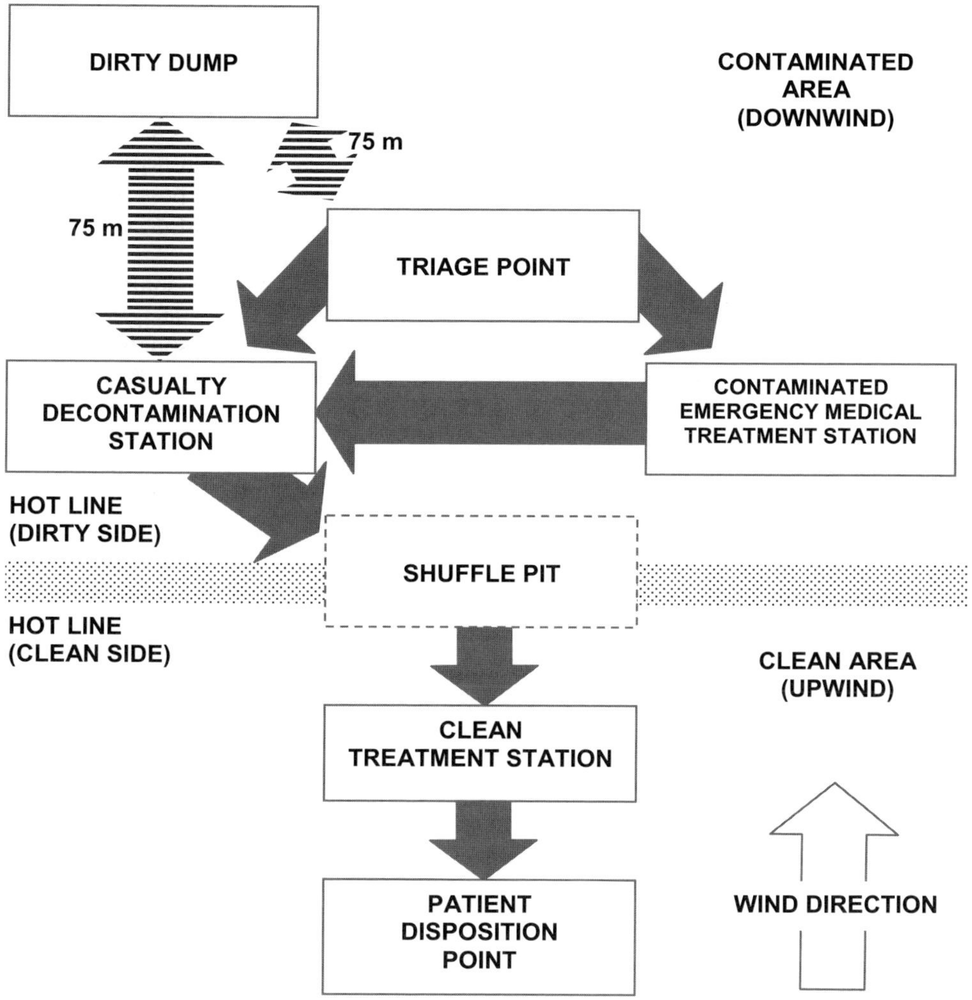

Fig. 2.2. Layout for patient decontamination, incorporating treatment areas in both the 'hot' and the 'cold' zones (from US Army, 2000).

Finally, a communications strategy should be included in the disaster plan. How will the physician communicate with his or her staff following the disaster? How will patients communicate with the clinic? How will the physician communicate with public health authorities? Alternatives need to be explored and clearly spelled out in the event local telecommunications infrastructure is damaged during the disaster. Telephone landlines, mobile telephones, two-way radios, local broadcast radio, internet and message couriers all have potential use during, and vulnerability to, the aftermath of disasters.

Preparing to volunteer

When a disaster strikes away from one's immediate locale, the humanitarian spirit in most physicians prompts them to contemplate volunteering to aid the victims. However, volunteerism requires preparation and proper integration into the response in order to be fully effective (Anonymous, 1996). The time to do this is *before* the disaster strikes. The most effective way for a physician to use their abilities to assist is to contact response agencies, whether governmental or non-governmental, to get connected into the system of training and response (Campos-Outcalt, 2006). The American College of Physicians, in response to the US Department of Health and Human Services disaster response plan, identified three critical ways in which an individual physician – not affiliated with the formal disaster response – can make a difference: (i) be a clinician and treat their patients; (ii) educate the public regarding disaster preparedness; and (iii) serve as as leader for their community (Lauer *et al.*, 2008). The first two have been discussed above; we now turn to the third.

Table 2.4. Emergency support functions.

- Transportation and infrastructure
- Communication
- Public works and engineering
- Fire service
- Emergency management
- Mass care, housing and human services
- Resource support
- Health and medical services
- Urban search and rescue
- Oil and hazardous materials response
- Agriculture, natural resources
- Energy
- Public safety and security
- Recovery and mitigation
- External affairs

Leadership role in preparedness

Disaster preparedness and response includes more than medicine (Table 2.4), but medicine is an important part and it is crucial that planners have input of a clinical and medical perspective from medical professionals. When it comes to disaster planning, as scientists, physicians are fully capable of understanding the complexities and have the public's best interests in mind (Lauer *et al.*, 2008); they are ideally suited for a role in disaster planning. However, 'physicians are busy people and it is hard for them to find time to attend more meetings' (Lauer *et al.*, 2008). There exists a conflict between need for physicians to be involved in planning and their lack of time to do so. Nevertheless, it is imperative that some make such activities a priority, and engage at the local, regional or national level to be sure that the voice of the medical providers – and their patients – be heard in the crafting of disaster response plans. This can ensure that proper prioritization of vaccine and strategic medical supplies for distribution occurs. For example, it is well documented in the literature that the willingness of community physicians to participate in disaster response and recovery drops off quickly if adequate PPE is not available (Alexander *et al.*, 2006);

conversely, with increased availability of vaccinations for medical personnel and their family members comes a substantial increase in their likelihood of working in disaster situations (Damery *et al.*, 2009). Despite this, provision of these measures not always a high priority for some disaster planners (Clawson *et al.*, 2006). Insight from physicians can aid in ensuring that steps are taken to ensure adequate healthcare providers in event of a disaster.

In addition to planning, the US National Response Framework (FEMA, 2008) includes a number of other actions essential to disaster preparedness. While specifically delineated for a North American setting, the general principles are broadly applicable in a variety of cultural and socioeconomic settings. They include training and exercises, personnel and equipment certification, mutual aid, publications management and the documentation process. There is a meaningful place for the clinical perspective a primary care physician offers in each of these.

Training and *exercises*, though related, are distinct: the former refers to development of skill sets by individuals, while the latter denotes the integration of the individual skill sets into the response as a whole through table-top simulations or full-dress field exercises. By analogy, *training* is the violinist practising her piece alone or with the violin section; an *exercise* is the rehearsal of the entire orchestra together. Individual skills are important, but the most skilled trauma surgeon is of little value if the patient transportation system fails to deliver the patients from the site of injury, or the physical plant is unable to ensure adequate lighting for a midnight operation. The individual must be competent, but the team must function together as well. That is why it is important that there be a clinical voice present during the planning and why it is important that clinical competence – under resource-limited conditions – be developed and maintained.

Ensuring adequate *quality* of both medical personnel and medical equipment is an important part of preparedness. There are situations where unqualified individuals or even imposters appear at a disaster scene and begin to work (FSMB, 2006). A mechanism to ensure credentials of individuals must be in place prior to the disaster. Confirming the validity of qualified personnel's training and credentials takes time – something that is in short supply during disaster response – and should be established during the preparedness stage. An expanded scope of practice may be necessary during disasters (Altevogt *et al.*, 2009); the extent of this should also be defined prior to the event. It is vital that primary care physicians who know the local healthcare workforce and population be involved in crafting both the definition of qualifications and the scope of practice. Similarly, ensuring that medical equipment is functional, and can remain so in adverse circumstances, is a high priority. The physicians can offer valuable insight into what is needed, what is not and how to adapt.

When a disaster strikes, local resources are often immediately overwhelmed. Neighbouring communities who are less affected by the event may be able to lend assistance; this is the meaning of *mutual aid*. This sort of assistance is greatly facilitated when a formal agreement exists prior to the event, and the involvement of the physician in reaching this agreement with a colleague, with whom a professional relationship likely already exists, can greatly facilitate medical mutual aid.

Publications management and documentation refers to the process by which the credentialing processes, mutual aid agreements and other aspects of the disaster plan discussed above are maintained, and how the activities and expenses during the disaster response are recorded. The former allows an up-to-date database of available personnel, equipment and other resources to be accessed when the need arises; the latter provides documentation for tracking the victims (allowing reunion with family) and forms a basis for reimbursement for the costs of response when aid – governmental or otherwise – arrives.

Response

When a disaster strikes, there are two ways in which primary care physicians can be involved in the response. The first is as part of the immediate, local response; the other is as the member of a disaster response organization (Table 2.5) or as part of a governmental agency. These agencies' and organizations' response is 'subacute', requiring a time lag between the disaster event and deployment to the scene. In either case, well-trained primary care physicians are ideally suited for a role in disaster response (Freedy and Simpson, 2007). As generalists, they are experienced in caring for patients without regard for their age, sex or the organ system affected. They have skills in both medical and surgical aspects of care. They have experience in both acute and chronic care, and both clinical and public health perspectives.

Table 2.5. Some examples of response organizations.

• Care International	www.care.org
• *Medicins sans Frontiers*	www.msf.org
• OXFAM	www.oxfam.org
• Red Cross/Red Crescent	www.ifrc.org
• Samaritan's Purse	www.samaritanspurse.org
and a host of others...	

Every primary care physician faces the possibility of responding to a locally occurring disaster, by default of being present at the time and place of the event's occurrence. Planning and preparation, discussed above, greatly enhance the physician's potential for being effective in a disaster situation, but the physician will be thrust into the role of responder even if he or she is unprepared. The majority of disasters occur without notice, precluding the possibility of having non-local disaster responders present at the time of the event. The local physician must actively respond until such time that outside reinforcement arrives.

Primary care physicians who serve as members of governmental or non-governmental response teams have the advantage of approaching the disaster scene with at least some degree of preparation, organization and integration; however, their response to no-notice events is delayed due to physical distance and other logistical constraints.

No matter in which capacity the primary care physician finds himself responding, certain important considerations are conserved. These include safety, triage, knowledge, evacuation and integration with other responders.

Safety

Safety is the most important consideration. While certain risks are acceptable, it is vital to recognize that an injured or ill responder is worse than no responder. When a responder is injured, the efforts of several other responders are diverted from their primary mission to the care of their injured colleague – they have become part of the problem rather than part of the solution. Disaster settings are fraught with safety hazards, ranging from collapsing buildings, downed electrical wires, hazardous weather, infectious perils and civil disorder. Responder safety and scene security must be the first consideration in a disaster response (Calland, 2006; Reissman and Howard, 2008).

Triage

Once the scene's safety is established, before care begins triage is essential. By definition, disasters are limited-resource settings. A number of triage algorithms have been developed, each geared towards a specific patient subgroup. The Simple Triage and Rapid Treatment (START) (Burstein and Hogan, 2007) and its paediatric counterpart, JumpSTART (Romig, 2002), are employed in mass casualty incidents (MCIs). Typically including a major trauma component, these algorithms divide and colour-code patients into those needing immediate care (red), those needing urgent care (yellow), those whose care may be safely delayed (green) and those who are dead or whose injuries require more resources than may be allotted to them in the current situation (black). The Seniors Without Family Team (SWiFT) (Dyer *et al.*, 2008) is applied to the geriatric population, after START or its equivalents (Bullard *et al.*, 2008; Warren *et al.*, 2008; Cone *et al.*, 2011), to address chronic medical conditions or health-related social issues.

Among the more useful strategies is a German triage system that employs five categories to denote the urgency of treatment and separates the deceased from the expectant, shown in Table 2.6 (Beck *et al.*, 2002). This scheme has the advantage over START in that it may be applied to acute and chronic medical conditions as well as trauma conditions. A Disaster Medical Acuity Scale under development is similar, with the category corresponding to T4 identifying those patients for whom current resources do not permit treatment; as new resources arrive to the disaster scene, these patients may be upgraded.

Table 2.6. Sample triage scheme.

Category	Meaning	Consequences
T1 (I)	Acute danger for life	Immediate treatment, transport as soon as possible
T2 (II)	Severe injury/illness	*Constant observation* and rapid treatment, transport as soon as practical
T3 (III)	Minor or no injury/illness	*Treatment when practical*, transport and/or discharge when possible
T4 (IV)	No or small chance of survival	Observation and if possible administration of analgesics
T5 (V)	Deceased	Collection and guarding of bodies, identification when possible

Knowledge

Following triage, physician knowledge is an important consideration in disaster medical response. Triage is only valuable in so far as it allows effective allocation of resources, most importantly, knowledgeable treatment. The most important knowledge is that which a primary care physician already possesses: good, up-to-date knowledge of clinical medicine in the care of children, adults, pregnant women and the aged. This is paramount, both during disasters and in the non-disaster setting. The primary care physician must strive to keep up with the latest literature relevant to the care of their patients. Such an investment pays high returns in improved patient outcomes; this is especially true in extraordinary circumstances such as following disasters. In addition to a solid foundation in clinical care, knowledge of some additional areas may be useful when considering the eventuality of a disaster (Table 2.7), though evidence demonstrating that training in these areas improves outcomes is difficult to acquire due to the nature of the disaster environment (Huntington and Gavagan, 2011). In the initial stages following natural and industrial disasters, an ability to manage trauma – if not definitively, at least to provide stabilizing care – is often needed. A basis of knowledge in this area may be acquired via a variety of sources, ranging from formal and informal fellowships to short courses such as Advanced Trauma Life Support (ATLS) and Comprehensive Advance Life Support (CALS). Information can be accessed at www.facs.org/trauma/atls/index.html and www.calsprogram.org, respectively. There is some evidence that short courses may be effective preparation for those who do not regularly encounter major trauma in their clinical practice (Walsh *et al.*, 1989).

Table 2.7. Disaster clinical competencies.

Triage
Emergency medical care/trauma
Chronic disease management
Maternity care
Paediatric care
Geriatric care
Psychological care
Austere environment

Another potential need in the immediate post-disaster setting is for primary care physicians to have the ability to at least recognize – and ideally provide initial care for – chemical, biological, radiological and nuclear (CBRN) exposures, whether these are accidental or intentional in origin (Noeller, 2001; Baker, 2004; Flynn and Goans, 2006; Bland, 2009). Early recognition of these events is crucial to decreasing the number of individuals exposed as well as the dose of exposure for the involved individual (Table 2.8). One online source for this information is the US Centers for Disease Control and Prevention preparedness and response website, http://emergency.cdc.gov/hazards-specific.asp. A more thorough treatment of this topic may be found in later chapters of this book. Interestingly, some studies suggest that in general, primary care physicians have more training in these topics than their subspecialist colleagues (Niska and Burt, 2007).

Following the immediate post-disaster period, other knowledge is needed. Treatment of environmental exposures, whether heat or cold, is an important part of the first few days following a disaster. The management of pre-existing chronic diseases such as diabetes, heart disease, chronic renal failure and psychological issues is often omitted from disaster planning, but is frequently the greatest need, both in terms of required resources and the amount of preventable morbidity and mortality. In every disaster, there are special needs populations such as the elderly, children and pregnant patients; knowledge of the care of these groups is important. It is in these applications that the broad training of the primary care physician has the opportunity to make a significant difference during a disaster response.

Table 2.8. Syndromes associated with CBRN events.

Agent	Intervention
Radiological (Skorga *et al.*, 2003)	
Acute radiation syndrome • Haematological syndrome (2–10 Gy): gastrointestinal symptoms and lethargy within 6–12 h, subsides within 36 h. Pancytopenia develops	Blood product replacement Colony-stimulating factors Immunosuppression precautions
• Gastrointestinal syndrome (10–50 Gy): bloody diarrhoea, bowel necrosis, bacteraemia	Antibiotics Intravenous hydration
• Central nervous system syndrome (>50 Gy): gastrointestinal symptoms and lethargy initially, progressing to tremor, convulsion, ataxia and death within hours-to-days	Supportive
Long-term physical effects • Amenorrhoea, sterility, fetal anomalies, blood dyscrasias, cataracts, premature ageing, cancer	Counsel survivors regarding their risks
Chemical (Bland, 2009)	
Nerve agents • Mild – miosis, ophthalmalgia • Moderate – increased secretions, wheezing, dyspnoea, nausea/vomiting/diarrhoea • Severe – weakness, respiratory failure	Anticholinergics, oximes, diazepam
Cyanides (onset in seconds) • Mild – nausea, dizziness, agitation • Moderate – hyperventilation, confusion • Severe – coma, seizure, respiratory arrest	Oxygen, dicobaltedtate, sodium nitrite, amyl nitrite, sodium thiosulphate
Mustard (onset in 2–4 h) • Mild – erythaema, ophthalmalgia • Moderate – bullae, airway irritation • Severe – airway burns and obstruction	No antidote available
Pulmonary agents (phosgene, chlorine) • Mild – ophthalmalgia • Moderate – airway irritation • Severe – pulmonary oedema	No antidote available
Methaemoglobinformers (nitrites, etc.) • Mild – no symptoms • Moderate – cyanosis, dyspnoea • Severe – severe cyanosis and dyspnoea, confusion	Methylene blue

Biological (Noeller, 2001)	
Anthrax • Cutaneous – swelling and oedema progressing to ulceration and necrosis • Inhalational – 'flu-like illness progressing to severe fever, dyspnoea and shock	Ciprofloxacin, doxycycline, vaccine
Smallpox • 'Flu-like illness followed by mucous membrane lesions and rash that progresses from maculae to pustules; cardiovascular collapse	Immunoglobulin, vaccine
Plague • Bubonic – 'flu-like illness, necrotic adenopathy, cardiovascular and neurological collapse • Pneumonic – 'flu-like illness, gastrointestinal symptoms, cough, haemoptysis	Streptomycin, gentamycin, doxycycline
Botulism • Descending, symmetric, flaccid paralysis, anticholinergic symptoms, cranial nerve palsies	Antitoxin

It is not just what is known, but how it is implemented that matters. In the disaster setting, it behoves the primary care physician to possess not only this broad base of medical knowledge, but also an ability to apply it in the setting of limited resources. Disaster scenes are generally austere environments, whose lack of standard technological devices and broad pharmacopeia require both outstanding clinical skills and imaginative creativity on the part of the physician. Insight into practice in austere environments may be gained via participation in Wilderness Medicine courses (WMS, 2011) or volunteer work in less-developed setting (GHEC, 2011).

Evacuation

In a disaster, two strategies exist: evacuation and shelter-in-place. A general principle favours shelter-in-place unless the immediate or long-term hazards threatening the current situation outweigh the hazards of transportation and relocation (Sorensen *et al.*, 2004; Lach *et al.*, 2005; Wein *et al.*, 2010). However, there are times when evacuation is clearly warranted. Examples of when each strategy might be appropriate are given in Table 2.9.

When evacuation of a healthcare facility is needed, triage is employed, but under a different paradigm than triage for treatment. Determining the health of potential evacuees may fall to the primary care physician. The 'walking wounded' (e.g. START green) are evacuated first, followed by the urgent, then the emergent and finally the expectant. The reversal of the order of attention to the non-expectant categories allows for the greatest number of individuals to be evacuated first, with those requiring greater assistance following, maximizing the number of individuals removed from the hazardous situation in the shortest amount of time. The primary care physician can play a critical role in determining not only the health status of the evacuees, but the destination for them. Designating who is appropriate for a regular shelter, who should go to a special-needs shelter and who needs evacuation to a hospital or other healthcare facility is a function most efficiently performed by someone familiar with the patient. Knowing their recent care, their current needs and their baseline status greatly simplifies the decision process.

Table 2.9. Situations requiring different survival strategies.

Evacuation	Shelter in place
Flood	Blizzard
Major hurricane	Nuclear blast[a]
Volcanic eruption	Riots
Wildfire	Tornado

[a]Initially, followed by informed, delayed evacuation.

Integration

Whether the primary care physician is an immediate local responder, or part of an outside response team, there is a need to know how to integrate the local response with the broader, outside response when the help finally arrives. During these transitions, it is important to be able to readily identify where authority and responsibility lie, and that clear communications – including a shared vocabulary – occur between all those involved.

One example of how this can be achieved is the Incident Command System (ICS). In the USA, disaster response has been standardized through the adoption of ICS (FEMA, 2008). This system establishes a shared organizational structure, terminology and lines of authority while preserving the autonomy of the individual agencies involved. However, to be effective all participants in the disaster response must be familiar with, and employ, the system. Online ICS training is available at no charge through the Emergency Management Institute website: http://training.fema.gov/IS/NIMS.asp. In some nations, other systems are used in lieu of ICS; non-US primary care physicians should identify what organizational scheme is used in their location, and familiarize themselves with it so that they can effectively integrate their care with the broader disaster response.

Recovery

The recovery phase of a disaster is that period of time following the acute response actions during which the community affected by the disaster begins to rebuild and rehabilitate the infrastructure, services and other aspects of community life. It is an effort to return to the pre-event norm of life. In addition to those basic aspects of life relevant to all the residents of the affected community, for the primary care physician a significant component of this is the re-establishment of the local healthcare system, continuity of care and the restoration of medical services. The ease with which this may be accomplished is dependent upon several things.

The disaster plan, discussed previously, is an important determinant of how rapidly and effectively local healthcare delivery may be re-established. If the preparedness phase resulted in preservations of adequate stock of supplies, a viable alternative temporary site of seeing patients in the event of damage or destruction of the clinic and adequate staffing, resumption of normal clinic operations will be relatively simple. If such provisions were not made in advance, or the disaster brought about challenges unforeseen by the plan, it will be more difficult. The importance of thorough planning and action in disaster preparedness cannot be overstated.

One of the most significant influences on the resilience of the local healthcare activities is the nature of the healthcare system prior to the disaster. Systems that are highly centralized and technologically dependent are much more vulnerable than those that are more broad based. For example, in the context of over a quarter of a century of war – circumstances that are disastrous by any definition – Eritrea successfully developed a healthcare system that provided effective emergency, primary care and preventative health services (Sabo and Kibirige, 1989). Decentralization and being based on local needs resulted in a more effective and resilient system than those in similar circumstances but built on systems mimicking the secondary and tertiary facilities in the West (Kloos, 1998).

Recovery is affected by the availability of financial and other forms of aid. However, in poor economies or widespread disasters, this may be limited. Mobilization of local resources and volunteers can be more effective than waiting for outside help (Bearden, 2007). As a community leader, the primary care physician can facilitate such activity on behalf of the healthcare system and the community as a whole.

Mitigation

Mitigation refers to those activities undertaken to prevent disasters or, in the event of a disaster, to minimize long-term consequences of a disaster (Haddow and Bullock, 2003). This is in contrast to the more immediate-term perspective of *response* and *recovery*. Mitigation begins during the response period and merges with the preparedness phase of the next disaster.

Disasters differ. On the one hand, there are MCIs. These result in a surge of patients that can overwhelm the healthcare infrastructure. As an isolated, single event, recovery is fairly rapid as the initial influx of patients and strain on resources resolves, and resources from nearby unaffected regions arrive. An example of this would be the '9/11' World Trade Center event. Long-term consequences include physical disability secondary to injuries sustained, and stress disorders due to the psychological trauma. At the other extreme is the 'complex humanitarian disaster', which is a more chronic situation, developing gradually over time or following an MCI, in which resources are exhausted and not replaced, generally accompanied by a total breakdown in both infrastructure and society in general. The 1984–1985 famine in Ethiopia is an example of this. Long-term consequences here include death and disability from malnutrition, spread of infectious disease, and the consequences of prolonged and on-going psychological trauma. Mitigation efforts may overlap or be unique to the specific type of disaster.

The baseline health of the population affected by the disaster influences the risk of long-term effects following the disaster. Chronic diseases, even when well managed prior to the disaster event, can lead to increased morbidity and mortality in the post-disaster period when more acute conditions garner a majority of attention (Chan and Sondorp, 2007). One way for the primary care physician to contribute to the mitigation of the effects of the disaster is to ensure that patients' chronic diseases are not neglected or 'pre-empted' during the immediate post-event time period. This may be challenging, with limited availability of medication and other health supplies in the austere setting of a disaster scene, but it is essential to decreasing long-term morbidity and mortality due to the disaster (Chan and

Sondorp, 2007; Edwards *et al.*, 2007; Fernald and Clawson, 2007; Chan and Griffiths, 2009; Chan and Kim, 2011). Immediately following the disaster event, emergency medical aid predominates, quite rightly. However, it is imperative that primary healthcare moves to the forefront shortly thereafter to mitigate the effects of that event (Van Damme *et al.*, 2002).

Table 2.10. Common disaster-associated infections. Pandemic disasters are excluded.

Infection type, by time post-event (Howard *et al.*, 1996; Noji, 2005; Gayer *et al.*, 2007)	**Reported organism, by disaster type** (Linscott, 2007)	
0–4 days Wound infections Soft tissue infections **4 days – 4 weeks** Airborne[a] infections Water-borne infections Food-borne infections **>4 weeks** Vector-borne infections Chronic infections Infections with long incubations	**Drought** *Plasmodium* St Louis encephalitis virus West Nile virus **Earthquake** *Acinetobacter* *Candida* *Coccidioides* *Enterobius* *Giardia* *Pseudomonas* *Shigella* *Staphylococcus* **Tsunami** *Aeromonas* *Apophysomyces* *Berkholderia* *Cladophialophora* *E. coli* *Klebsiella* *Mycobacterium* *Nocardia* *Proteus* *Pseudomonas* *Scedosporium* *Staphylococcus*	**Flood** *Cryptosporidium* Dengue virus *E. coli* Equine encephalitis virus (eastern and western) *Giardia* *Leptospira* *Plasmodium* St. Louis encephalitis virus Polio virus Rotavirus *S. typhi* *Vibriocholerae* West Nile virus **Hurricane** Moulds Norovirus *Plasmodium* *Vibriovulnificus* *Vibrioparahaemolyticus* *Staphylococcus* **Tornado** *Alcaligenes* *Enterococcus* *Pseudomonas* *Serratia*

[a]Aetiology of respiratory infections varies from viral and bacterial earlier to fungal (mould) later.

For the health professional, aggressive public health measures are among the most important components of mitigation. Following a disaster, there exists a high risk for disease outbreak, and steps must be taken to minimize this (Waring and Brown, 2005; Ligon, 2006; CDC, 2011). As seen in Table 2.10, the risk for infection occurs in both the immediate post-event period and subsequent weeks. The increase in infectious risk is highest *months* later, outside of the acute response phase (Bissell, 1983). Respiratory, gastrointestinal, skin and vector-borne infections are common. Adequate food and water supplies and sanitation must be facilitated. Sufficient shelter is important, minimizing crowding to the extent possible. Prevention is most important, early diagnosis and recognition of contagion are close seconds. When infectious conditions are encountered, patterns need to be identified quickly and appropriate authorities notified so that measures may be taken to limit the spread of the illness. Through vigilance by primary care physicians, lapses in sanitation or the food and water supply, and other nidi of infectious disease, may be identified and remedied.

Traumatic incidents such as a disaster have the potential to lead to long-term psychiatric problems (Nolen-Hoeksema and Morrow, 1991; Soeteman *et al*., 2007; Neria *et al*., 2010). A means by which this may be avoided is through effective psychological first aid. This is applicable to both the victims of the disaster as well as to the responders, who are at risk of becoming 'secondary victims' as the result of their experiences in the response effort.

A variety of training courses are available to equip responders to assist in this capacity, including some offered online (e.g. http://learn.nctsn.org/). It is important, however, to ensure that such aid is relevant and applicable in the local culture; care must be exercised to avoid importation of a Western model of mental illness and corresponding treatment methods into a cultural setting in which they are quite frankly irrelevant (Watters, 2010). This may not merely lack benefit, but can be harmful. Usually, local mental health expertise is better than outside 'experts' unfamiliar with the local culture. The local primary care physician is perfectly positioned to ensure that their local patient base receives appropriate care and avoids inappropriate care.

Conclusion

Disasters, both natural and anthropogenic, significantly disrupt the health of both the individual and the community. Primary care physicians are positioned to provide disaster care, by choice or by default, before outside aid arrives to beyond its departure. Preparing in advance for the contingency of a disaster greatly enhances the effectiveness of this care, and can decrease the short- and long-term adverse consequences of the disaster on their patients, community and practice. Some should step up to leadership in preparedness for their local community.

In addition to providing the local response, primary care physicians possess the foundational knowledge and skill set to effectively serve as part of the response effort to areas outside their home community. By developing these bases, primary care physicians have the potential to fill critical niches in the global disaster response systems.

References

Ablah, E., Tinius, A.M., Horn, L., Williams, C. and Gebbie, K.M. (2008) Community health centers and emergency preparedness: an assessment of competencies and training needs. *Journal of Community Health* 33, 241–247.

Alexander, G.C., Larkin, G.L. and Wynia, M.K. (2006) Physician's preparedness for bioterrorism and other public health priorities. *Academic Emergency Medicine* 13, 1238–1241.

Altevogt, B.M., Stroud, C., Hanson, S.L., Hanfling, D. and Gostin, L.O. (eds) (2009) *Guidance for Establishing Crisis Standards of Care for Use in Disaster Situations: A Letter Report*. National Academies Press, Washington, DC.

Amlot, R., Larner, J., Matar, H., Jones, D.R., Carter, H., Turner, E.A., Price, S.C. and Chilcott, R.P. (2010) Comparative analysis of showering protocols for mass-casualty decontamination. *Prehospital and Disaster Medicine* 25, 435–439.

Anonymous (1996) Emergency medical aid is not for amateurs. *Lancet* 348, 1393.

Baker, D. (2004) Civilian exposure to toxic agents: emergency medical response. *Prehospital and Disaster Medicine* 19, 174–178.

Bearden, T. (2007) Rebuilding a community health center following a natural disaster: interview in Biloxi, Mississippi. *Health Affairs* 26, w644–w650.

Beck, A., Bayeff-Filloff, M., Bischoff, M. and Schneider, B.M. (2002) Analysis of the incidence and causes of mass casualty events in a southern Germany medical rescue area. *Unfallchirurgie* 105, 968–973.

Bissell, R.A. (1983) Delayed-impact infectious disease after a natural disaster. *Journal of Emergency Medicine* 1, 59–66.

Bland, S.A. (2009) Chemical, biological and radiation casualties: critical care considerations. *Journal of the Royal Army Medical Corps* 155, 160–171.

Bullard, M.J., Unger, B., Spence, J. and Grafstein, E. (2008) Revisions to the Canadian Emergency Department Triage and Acuity Scale (CTAS) adult guidelines. *Canadian Journal of Emergency Medicine* 10, 136–151.

Burstein, J.L. and Hogan, D. (2007) *Disaster Medicine.* Wolters Kluwer Health/Lippincott Williams & Wilkins, Philadelphia, Pennsylvania.

Calland, V. (2006) A brief overview of personal safety at incident sites. *Emergency Medicine Journal* 23, 878–882.

Campos-Outcalt, D. (2006) Disaster medical response: maximizing your effectiveness. *Journal of Family Practice* 55, 113–115.

Centers for Disease Control and Prevention (CDC) (2011) Infection control after disasters[online]. Available at: www.bt.cdc.gov/disasters/infectioncontrol.asp (Accessed 24 June 2011).

Chan, E.Y. and Griffiths, S. (2009) Comparison of health needs of older people between affected rural and urban areas after the 2005 Kashmir, Pakistan earthquake. *Prehospital and Disaster Medicine* 24, 365–371.

Chan, E.Y. and Kim, J. (2011) Chronic health needs immediately after natural disasters in middle-income countries: the case of the 2008 Sichuan, China earthquake. *European Journal of Emergency Medicine* 18, 111–114.

Chan, E.Y. and Sondorp, E. (2007) Medical interventions following natural disasters: missing out on chronic medical needs. *Asia Pacific Journal of Public Health* 19 Spec No, 45–51.

Chen, A.C., Keith, V.M., Leong, K.J., Airriess, C., Li, W., Chung, K.Y. and Lee, C.C. (2007) Hurricane Katrina: prior trauma, poverty and health among Vietnamese-American survivors. *International Nursing Review* 54, 324–331.

Clawson, A., Menachemi, N., Beitsch, L. and Brooks, R.G. (2006) Are community health centers prepared for bioterrorism? *Biosecurity and Bioterrorism* 4, 55–63.

Collins, N., Litt, J., Moore, M., Winzenberg, T. and Shaw, K. (2006) General practice: professional preparation for a pandemic. *Medical Journal of Australia* 185, S66–S69.

Cone, D.C., Serra, J. and Kurland, L. (2011) Comparison of the SALT and Smart triage systems using a virtual reality simulator with paramedic students. *European Journal of Emergency Medicine* 18(6), 314–321.

Damery, S., Wilson, S., Draper, H., Gratus, C., Greenfield, S., Ives, J., Parry, J., Petts, J. and Sorell, T. (2009) Will the NHS continue to function in an influenza pandemic? A survey of healthcare workers in the West Midlands, UK. *BMC Public Health* 9, 142.

Dyer, C.B., Regev, M., Burnett, J., Festa, N. and Cloyd, B. (2008) SWiFT: a rapid triage tool for vulnerable older adults in disaster situations. *Disaster Medicine and Public Health Preparedness* 2 Suppl 1, S45–S50.

Edwards, T.D., Young, R.A. and Lowe, A.F. (2007) Caring for a surge of Hurricane Katrina evacuees in primary care clinics. *Annals of Family Medicine* 5, 170–174.

Federal Emergency Management Administration (FEMA) (2008) *National Response Framework.* FEMA, Washington, DC.

Federation of State Medical Boards (FSMB) (2006) *Responding in Times of Need: Katrina and Beyond.* FSMB, Dallas, Texas.

Fernald, J.P. and Clawson, E.A. (2007) The mobile army surgical hospital humanitarian assistance mission in Pakistan: the primary care experience. *Military Medicine* 172, 471–477.

Flynn, D.F. and Goans, R.E. (2006) Nuclear terrorism: triage and medical management of radiation and combined-injury casualties. *Surgical Clinics of North America* 86, 601–636.

Freedy, J.R. and Simpson, W.M., Jr (2007) Disaster-related physical and mental health: a role for the family physician. *American Family Physician* 75, 841–846.

Gayer, M., Legros, D., Formenty, P. and Connolly, M.A. (2007) Conflict and emerging infectious diseases. *Emerging Infectious Diseases* 13, 1625–1631.

Global Health Education Consortium (GHEC) (2011) Global Health Education Consortium [Online]. Available at: http://globalhealtheducation.org (Accessed 13 June 2011).

Greenough, P.G., Lappi, M.D., Hsu, E.B., Fink, S., Hsieh, Y.H., Vu, A., Heaton, C. and Kirsch, T.D. (2008) Burden of disease and health status among Hurricane Katrina-displaced persons in shelters: a population-based cluster sample. *Annals of Emergency Medicine* 51, 426–432.

Haddow, G.D. and Bullock, J.A. (2003) *Introduction to Emergency Management.* Butterworth-Heinemann, Amsterdam.

Howard, M.J., Brillman, J.C. and Burkle, F.M., Jr (1996) Infectious disease emergencies in disasters. *Emergency Medicine Clinics of North America* 14, 413–428.

Huntington, M.K. (1999) Comprehensive medicine. *Journal of General Internal Medicine* 14, 207.

Huntington, M.K. and Gavagan, T.F. (2011) Disaster medicine training in family medicine: a review of the evidence. *Family Medicine* 43, 13–20.

Hutton, D. (2009) Putting the puzzle together: reducing vulnerability through people-focused planning. *Radiation Protection Dosimetry* 134, 193–196.

Jepson, R.G., Harris, F.M., Platt, S. and Tannahill, C. (2010) The effectiveness of interventions to change six health behaviours: a review of reviews. *BMC Public Health* 10, 538.

Kellerman, R. and Kirk, L. (2007) Principles of the patient-centered medical home. *America Family Physician* 76, 774–775.

Kloos, H. (1998) Primary health care in Ethiopia under three political systems: community participation in a war-torn society. *Social Science and Medicine* 46, 505–522.

Lach, H.W., Langan, J.C. and James, D.C. (2005) Disaster planning: are gerontological nurses prepared? *Journal of Gerontological Nursing* 31, 21–27.

Lauer, J., Kastner, J. and Nutsch, A. (2008) Primary care physicians and pandemic influenza: an appraisal of the 1918 experience and an assessment of contemporary planning. *Journal of Public Health Management Practices* 14, 379–386.

Ligon, B.L. (2006) Infectious diseases that pose specific challenges after natural disasters: a review. *Seminars in Pediatric Infectious Diseases* 17, 36–45.

Linscott, A.J. (2007) Natural disasters – a microbe's paradise. *Clinical Microbiology Newsletter* 29, 57–62.

Neria, Y., Olfson, M., Gameroff, M.J., Digrande, L., Wickramaratne, P., Gross, R., Pilowsky, D.J., Neugebaur, R., Manetti-Cusa, J., Lewis-Fernandez, R., Lantigua, R., Shea, S. and Weissman, M.M. (2010) Long-term course of probable PTSD after the 9/11 attacks: a study in urban primary care. *Journal of Traumatic Stress* 23, 474–482.

Niska, R.W. and Burt, C.W. (2007) Terrorism preparedness: have office-based physicians been trained? *Family Medicine* 39, 357–365.

Noeller, T.P. (2001) Biological and chemical terrorism: recognition and management. *Cleveland Clinic Journal of Medicine* 68, 1001–1002, 1004–1009, 1013–1016.

Noji, E.K. (2005) Public health in the aftermath of disasters. *British Medical Journal* 330, 1379–1381.

Nolen-Hoeksema, S. and Morrow, J. (1991) A prospective study of depression and posttraumatic stress symptoms after a natural disaster: the 1989 Loma Prieta Earthquake. *Journal of Personality and Social Psychology* 61, 115–121.

Olympia, R.P., Rivera, R., Heverley, S., Anyanwu, U. and Gregorits, M. (2010) Natural disasters and mass-casualty events affecting children and families: a description of emergency preparedness and the role of the primary care physician. *Clinical Pediatrics (Philadelphia)* 49, 686–698.

Reissman, D.B. and Howard, J. (2008) Responder safety and health: preparing for future disasters. *Mt Sinai Journal of Medicine* 75, 135–141.

Romig, L.E. (2002) Pediatric triage. A system to JumpSTART your triage of young patients at MCIs. *Journal of Emergency Medical Services* 27, 52–58, 60–63.

Sabo, L.E. and Kibirige, J.S. (1989) Political violence and Eritrean health care. *Social Science and Medicine* 28, 677–684.

Shaw, K.A., Chilcott, A., Hansen, E. and Winzenberg, T. (2006) The GP's response to pandemic influenza: a qualitative study. *Family Practice* 23, 267–272.

Skorga, P., Persell, D.J., Arangie, P., Gilbert-Palmer, D., Winters, R., Stokes, E.N. and Young, C. (2003) Caring for victims of nuclear and radiological terrorism. *Nurse Practitioner* 28, 24–41; quiz 41–43.

Soeteman, R.J., Yzermans, C.J., Kerssens, J.J., Dirkzwager, A.J., Donker, G.A., Ten Veen, P.M., Vanden Bosch, W.J. and Vander Zee, J. (2007) Health problems presented to family practices in the Netherlands 1 year before and 1 year after a disaster. *Journal of the American Board of Family Medicine* 20, 548–556.

Sorensen, J.H., Shumpert, B.L. and Vogt, B.M. (2004) Planning for protective action decision making: evacuate or shelter-in-place. *Journal of Hazardous Material* 109, 1–11.

US Army (2000) Field Manual 3-5, NBC Decontamination[Online]. Available at: http://www.globalsecurity.org/wmd/library/policy/army/fm/3-5/fm3-5.pdf (Accessed 30 June 2011).

Van Damme, W.I., Van Lerberghe, W.I. and Boelaert, M. (2002) Primary health care vs. emergency medical assistance: a conceptual framework. *Health Policy and Planning* 17, 49–60.

Walsh, D.P., Lammert, G.R. and Devoll, J. (1989) The effectiveness of the advanced trauma life support system in a mass casualty situation by non-trauma-experienced physicians: Grenada 1983. *Journal of Emergency Medicine* 7, 175–180.

Waring, S.C. and Brown, B.J. (2005) The threat of communicable diseases following natural disasters: a public health response. *Disaster Management and Response* 3, 41–47.

Warren, D.W., Jarvis, A., Leblanc, L. and Gravel, J. (2008) Revisions to the Canadian Triage and Acuity Scale paediatric guidelines (PaedCTAS). *Canadian Journal of Emergency Medicine* 10, 224–243.

Watters, E. (2010) *Crazy Like Us*. Free Press, New York.

Wein, L.M., Choi, Y. and Denuit, S. (2010) Analyzing evacuation versus shelter-in-place strategies after a terrorist nuclear detonation. *Risk Analysis* 30, 1315–1327.

Wineman, N.V., Braun, B.I., Barbera, J.A. and Loeb, J.M. (2007) Assessing the integration of health center and community emergency preparedness and response planning. *Disaster Medicine and Public Health Preparedness* 1, 96–105.

Wilderness Medical Society (WMS) (2011) Wilderness Medical Society[Online]. Available at: www.wms.org (Accessed 30 June 2011).

Chapter 3

Manikin Simulation for Mass Casualty Incident Training

Dale S. Vincent and Benjamin W. Berg

Introduction

Multiple factors are increasing the likelihood of large-scale disasters in the 21st century compared to previous eras. Population growth, environmental degradation, natural and man-made contagion and sectarian violence are increasing the incidence of natural and man-made mass casualty incidents (MCIs) in ways that will require increasingly sophisticated approaches for successful management (Arnold, 2002; James *et al.*, 2008).

Medical personnel need training for MCIs (Baker, 2007). However, the training that is provided is often quite limited. In a survey of US physicians in training, surgical residents reported significantly less formal training in mass casualty triage and MCI management than residents in other specialties (Galante *et al.*, 2005).

Medical simulation using computerized manikins is established as an effective teaching methodology that complements traditional medical education (Issenberg *et al.*, 1999; McGaghie *et al.*, 2011). Simulation technology is especially well suited for outcomes-based education and competency assessment (Scalese *et al.*, 2008). Manikin simulators enable educators to create standardized educational encounters for learners who are acquiring new skills (Issenberg *et al.*, 2005). The success of educational interventions can also be facilitated using manikins as an assessment tool. In a simulated trauma scenario, educators found that surgical residents had better resuscitation skills following completion of an Advanced Trauma Life Support (ATLS) course that used Simulation-Based Medical Education (SBME) than residents who did not complete the course (Ali *et al.*, 2000). Similar findings have been reported for advanced cardiac life support (ACLS) resuscitation (Wayne *et al.*, 2008) and for performance of bedside medical procedures including central venous catheterization (Evans *et al.*, 2010).

Manikins may be positioned in groups during multi-casualty scenarios for primary triage training (Vincent *et al.*, 2009a), and have been used to replicate multi-casualty incidents in emergency department training programmes. These simulations have been thought to create a realistic training environment by replicating the stress and chaos of an MCI (Kobayashi *et al.*, 2007). The military has used multiple manikin scenarios for combat medic training (Hendrickse *et al.*, 2001; Sohn *et al.*, 2007). Manikins have been identified as a valuable adjunct for MCI training in civilian settings (Kobayashi *et al.*, 2003), and have been used to simulate victims in chemical, biological, radiological, nuclear and environmental (CBRN) disaster scenarios (Vardi *et al.*, 2002; Berkenstadt *et al.*, 2003; Subbarao *et al.*, 2006; Kobayashi *et al.*, 2007).

Manikins have the potential to be an important tool for researchers investigating the performance characteristics of triage algorithms. A recent systematic review of MCI training at the hospital level concluded that the effectiveness of disaster training needs to be proved in a scientifically rigorous manner (Hsu *et al.*, 2004). Utilizing multi-manikin simulation training scenarios may be one way to assess the performance characteristics of these algorithms. Additionally, use of multiple 'smart casualties', actors with cards, has proved to be an effective way of training for MCIs (Gofrit *et al.*, 1997), but a meta-analysis did not describe examples of manikins being used for the same purpose (Hsu *et al.*, 2004).

We describe an approach to course development for MCI training and SBME using the five phases of the ADDIE instructional design model (Miller *et al.*, 2010) for curriculum development: Analysis, Design, Development, Implementation and Evaluation.

Rationale for Simulation-based Training

A major challenge for contemporary medical educators is to engage a new generation of learners who have grown up in a state of permanent connectivity. Modern learners are often characterized by omnipresent multitasking, distractibility and the need to be entertained (Kluth, 2008).

SBME has the potential to engage and focus these learners. Several characteristics of adult learners can flourish through the use of SBME, including collegiality, collaboration and relevance (Bleakley, 2006). Adult learning is most effective when learners have a collegial relationship with their teachers in which the flow of information sharing is bidirectional, rather than unidirectional as one would see in a traditional educational setting. Adult learners like to collaborate in teams to solve problems. Moreover, they insist that the material that they are studying be relevant to their professional lives or societal roles. They simply do not want to waste time, when they have multiple competing time demands. The hands-on nature of SBME is well suited to addressing these challenges.

The ADDIE (Strickland, 2011) instructional design model is particularly well suited for course development, because it emphasizes continual, formative feedback during the creative process. Potential course directors should try to answer an ensemble of key questions early in the course development process (Table 3.1).

Table 3.1. Instructional design using the ADDIE instructional design model.

Analysis	• Learner characteristics • Learning objectives • Programme constraints • Timeline for course development and implementation	• Are learners novices, experienced providers, or a combination? • What cognitive and behavioural outcomes are desired? • How many faculty and manikins will be available? • How much training time is available for learners to complete the course?

Design	• Content • Scenario development	• Will there be pre-course requirements for learners? • What triage algorithm will be used? • What type of disaster will be modelled? • What injury patterns and syndromes will be modelled? • Will lifesaving interventions be taught? • Should triage tags be used?
Development	• Storyboard development and scenario creation • Testing and revising of scenarios	• What simulator technologies will be used? • How much scenario fidelity will be needed to achieve learner objectives? • Do the scenarios have the appropriate 'triggers', or clinical clues, to provoke a response by the learners?
Implementation	• Facilitator training • Learner orientation • Debriefing	• How will pre-course material be distributed to learners? • Who are the faculty, and do they experience using simulator-based training? • When and how will the learners be oriented to the manikins? • Who will conduct the debriefings, and when will the debriefing occur?
Evaluation	• Formative: on-going evaluation through all of the development steps • Summative: feedback from learners, faculty and institutions	• How will data be collected? • Are learners responding appropriately to the scenarios? • Were the course objectives achieved?

Analysis

What cognitive and behavioural outcomes are desired?

The Education Committee Working Group of the World Association for Disaster and Emergency Medicine (WADEM) has proposed a set of general education principles for disaster health education. These include: (i) multidisciplinary programmes; (ii) vocational focus; (iii) case- or scenario-based frameworks; (iv) themed approaches; (v) modular approaches; (vi) supervised practical experience; (vii) competency-based approaches; and (viii) competencies within a conceptual framework (Seynaeve *et al.*, 2004). SBME embodies all of these principles. Additionally, disaster experts have reached a consensus on core clinical competencies for healthcare providers in disaster settings. These include the demonstration of proficiency in the use of triage systems in disasters, and the application of clinical knowledge and skills in the management of injuries (Subbarao *et al.*, 2008). The discussion that follows will focus on the assessment of learners performing triage activities using manikin-based simulation, as well as the development of scenarios to teach and test the management of typical injuries incurred in MCIs.

Are the learners novices or experienced?

Novice learners may require substantial background information before they are able to successfully triage a set of simulated casualties. In one exercise at the University of Hawaii, we sought to train 20 medical students in principles of mass casualty triage (Vincent *et al.*, 2009b). The students were required to achieve a baseline level of triage knowledge before they could begin the hands-on part of the exercise. They listened to four podcasts (total time of 19 min 35 s) and took a 20-question test. A score of 85% correct answers was required to be able to participate in the hands-on exercise. Despite these requirements, the learners performed relatively poorly in both speed and accuracy when triaging five simulated casualties. Repeating the exercise resulted in a 42% increase in accuracy. Time to triage also improved significantly, from an average of 2 min 8 s per casualty, to 1 min 8 s per casualty. In contrast to the performance of these novice learners, experienced learners were able to triage similar simulated patients in an average of 34 s each. Thus, the experience of the learner may significantly affect the time needed to complete an exercise, as well as the necessity to repeat scenarios in order for the learners to reach a certain level of competence.

Design

Will there be pre-course requirements for learners?

Course directors should consider giving students pre-course study materials to study before beginning a hands-on simulation exercise. The material may include a short orientation to the manikin (e.g. where are the pulses located on the manikin? where are the speakers located that generate breath sounds?); principles of triage; and potential life-saving interventions (e.g. needle placement for decompression of a tension pneumothorax). A pre-course test with a specified passing score may serve as a filter to ensure that the simulation runs smoothly and that learners have the baseline knowledge to participate in the planned exercise.

What triage algorithm will be used?

What is the triage method that will be used by learners and faculty? Current primary triage algorithms have not been rigorously validated, and their reproducibility is unknown (Jenkins *et al.*, 2008). Four algorithms, CareFlight, START and modified START, and Triage Sieve have been retrospectively analysed for accuracy using trauma patients presenting to emergency room, however, this study may not be generalizable to MCI (Garner *et al.*, 2001). Additionally, some common features of triage teaching have not been validated. For example, although it is commonly taught that a palpable radial pulse correlates with a systolic BP of 80 mm Hg (Prehospital Trauma Life Support Committee of the National Association of Emergency Medical Technicians in Cooperation with the Committee on Trauma of the American College of Surgeons, 1994), this finding has not been validated (Garner *et al.*, 2001).

Manikins are unable to simulate all branch points in most current primary algorithms. For example, manikins are obviously unable to simulate 'walking wounded' adult casualties. They cannot simulate capillary refill or best motor response with a Glasgow Coma Scale score ≥ 6.

Nevertheless, by designing clever contextual clues, it may be possible to include minimally injured simulated patients in a disaster exercise even if they cannot be made ambulatory. In one training exercise for military medics, we seated a manikin on the floor and recorded an audio file that had the manikin asking questions like 'what happened?' while swearing and using a belligerent tone. The manikin had normal vital signs and was cradling a weapon. The objective of the scenario was for the medic to triage the casualty as a 'minimal' patient, recognize a possible psychological casualty and remove the weapon. In another exercise, we used a SimBaby® with a vigorous cry and normal vital signs to simulate a 'minimal' category patient.

What type of disaster will be modelled?

A course director should ask: are there any disaster scenarios that are particularly relevant to the learners? This is important because a key principle of adult learning is that the material to be taught should clearly relevant to the learners. We saw that principle in action at a military medicine conference in Sydney, Australia, during a train-the-trainer session we conducted for healthcare providers from Asia Pacific. One of our workshop exercises involved the construction of scenarios for a mass casualty exercise for earthquake victims. We were able to capitalize on the lessons learned from first responders who were on the ground for the Christchurch, New Zealand earthquake of 2010. Thus, learning objectives could be tailored to the group based on practical observations from the field. Highly relevant objectives included the prevention and management of hypothermia in trapped victims, and the management of victims with crushed limbs.

It is important to recognize that the performance characteristics of triage algorithms may vary depending on the nature of the disaster and the resources available to rescuers at different points in time. In disasters such as earthquakes, there may be widespread catastrophic damage to infrastructure and communication systems, delaying access to definitive care and necessitating frequent reassessment of victims (Benson *et al.*, 1996). This becomes a critical teaching point during the debriefing sessions.

Should life-saving interventions be taught?

Should life-saving skills be taught at the same time basic triage skills are taught? Simple interventions that open airways and stop bleeding may be life-saving when performed concomitantly with primary triage (Baker, 2007). These interventions may be broadly classified as ones that require no equipment, and ones that require some equipment. No special equipment is required to place an improvised tourniquet or pressure dressing for an exsanguinating extremity haemorrhage, or to open an airway by repositioning a patient (Benson *et al.*, 1996; Green *et al.*, 2003). The Life-Supporting First-Aid (LSFA) method emphasizes applying simple airway management techniques, controlling external bleeding, repositioning patients in the presence of shock, and calling for help (Angus *et al.*, 1993), all without the use of medical equipment. Actions that utilize simple medical equipment include administration of oxygen, applying a haemostatic dressing, decompressing a tension pneumothorax by needle thoracostomy, starting an intravenous line, immobilizing the spine and/or extremities and applying special wound dressings. The approach to triage in US combat medic training conflates primary triage and the administration of immediate life-saving interventions. Additionally, the simultaneous use of primary triage coupled with immediate life-saving measures has been advocated for disaster drills in developing countries (Green *et al.*, 2003). This is also the approach taken by the Medical Disaster Response (MDR) project (Benson *et al.*, 1996) in settings where delayed access to definitive care is anticipated.

Will triage tags be used in the training?

The use of triage tags creates a conceptual framework for discussing the categories of triage. However, when we surveyed experienced healthcare providers of the Australian Defence Force, respondents indicated that triage tags have limited usefulness in the field. Multiple reasons were cited. Because triage is dynamic and the status of the patient and available resources may change quickly, triage tags may rapidly become outdated. Tags may simply be unavailable, and the tags themselves or portions of the tags may tear off. Nevertheless, we have found that triage tags provide a potent visual and tactile frame of reference for novice learners during MCI training.

Development

Testing and revising scenarios

Scenarios must be tested to ensure that students integrate the clinical clues in ways that predictably trigger appropriate triage and intervention decisions. The following case is an illustration of the need to test scenarios before conducting a training exercise. In one course, we sought to simulate an inhalation injury with airway obstruction by applying perioral soot to the manikin, and creating wheezing sounds. During a practice session, no students were able to identify the need for airway support. However, as soon as an audible cough was integrated into the scenario, 50% of the students correctly identified the clinical problem and life-saving intervention. This demonstrates the need to create an appropriate ‘trigger’ for the scenario, a clinical ‘tipping point’ that enables successful decision-making by the learner.

What injury patterns and syndromes will be modelled?

The medical literature contains many descriptions of the types of casualties encountered in natural and man-made disasters from around the world. MCIs are likely to have unique signatures, and information about specific injury patterns provides a useful substrate for constructing an MCI exercise. We identified injuries that faculty should consider including in their exercises (Table 3.2).

Table 3.2. Injury patterns in MCI.

Type of disaster	Common injuries	References
Airplane crash	Smoke inhalation and burns	O'Hickey *et al.*, 1987
Airplane turbulence	Extremity fractures, spinal injury and traumatic brain injury	Towne, 1995
Avalanche	Asphyxia, trauma and hypothermia	Boyd *et al.*, 2009
Explosion	Burns, penetrating trauma, smoke inhalation and traumatic brain injury	Aylwin *et al.*, 2006
Earthquake	Crush injuries, fractures and traumatic brain injury	Benson *et al.*, 1996; McMillan, 2006
Fire	Smoke inhalation and burns	Hart *et al.*, 1975; Sadler, 1982; Broeze *et al.*, 2010
Terrorist bomb	Burns, fractures, soft tissue injuries and traumatic brain injury	Frykberg and Tepas, 1988; Aylwin *et al.*, 2006
Train crash	Concussions, fractures and lacerations	Kahn *et al.*, 2009

A syndrome is 'a group of signs and symptoms that occur together and characterize a particular abnormality or condition' (Merriam-Webster online dictionary). A number of syndromes (and physiological categories) reported in MCI in the medical literature may be simulated by high fidelity manikins: upper airway obstruction, lower airway obstruction, penetrating chest trauma (tension pneumothorax or haemothorax), haemorrhagic shock, burns, traumatic amputation, traumatic brain injury and psychological distress. Crush injuries, neurological injuries and abdominal trauma are more difficult for manikins to simulate, but contextual clues may provide limited opportunities to include these clinical problems.

Paediatric disaster victims pose special challenges to healthcare personnel who are performing primary triage (Phillips *et al.*, 1996a,b). Paediatric populations have different physiological norms to adults, and have the potential to introduce an emotional dimension to primary triage that may inappropriately divert resources from other immediate patients (Wallis and Carley, 2006). Paediatric manikins such as SimBaby® (2006, Laerdal Medical, Wappingers Falls, New York) may be used in MCI training exercises to add an additional element of realism and difficulty.

What simulator technologies will be used?

We have used SimMan®, SimBaby® and ALS® devices (2006, Laerdal Medical, Wappingers Falls, New York) for our exercises. These computer-enhanced manikins are able to simulate respirations, variable blood pressures, and central and peripheral pulses. They have embedded speakers capable of transmitting sounds such as speech, airway, breath and heart sounds. The ALS simulator is very portable, making it particularly easy to move if a simulated disaster scene needs to be reconfigured. Other commercially available simulators have similar operating characteristics and may also be used.

Manikin simulators have several important limitations, and course developers should keep these principles in mind. First, do not attempt to replicate circumstances that cannot be replicated by the manikin. For example, the inability to respond to simple commands, or a Glasgow Coma Scale – Motor component (GCSM) of 1–5, may be among the best predictors of mortality from serious trauma (Meredith *et al.*, 1995; Ross *et al.*, 1998);

however, it may be difficult for learners to ascertain whether a manikin is responsive or not. Second, do not assume you cannot accomplish your educational goal because of manikin limitations. For example, in adult triage algorithms, the 'minor' or 'minimal' category of patient is not modelled well by manikins, because most classify a patient based on ability to ambulate, the so-called 'walking wounded'. However, SimBaby® easily models an infant with minimal injuries. An infant with normal vital signs that is crying creates a useful scenario that is distracting, challenging and also commonly encountered in disasters, making a good teaching point for new first responders in training.

How much scenario fidelity will be needed?

How much fidelity is needed to depict the casualties to meet the learning objectives? What are the pros and cons of moulage, sound and light? Fidelity refers to the degree of 'realism' portrayed during a simulation. The aggregate realism of a simulation encompasses the four domains of fidelity: technical, physical, environmental and psychological. The ultimate goal of any simulation is to accomplish the educational goals, not to replicate a realistic situation. Incorporating increasing degrees of realism is a natural tendency during the design of simulation-based training. It is attractive to consider 'as close to real as possible' as a starting point. This degree of realism is infrequently required, rarely possible and often impractical. The degree of fidelity that is required to accomplish the educational goals should guide the degree of realism incorporated during instructional design. Considerations regarding the use of increasing fidelity include cost, time, throughput of learners, distraction from actual learning objectives and learner factors. A basic principle is to use the lowest level of fidelity that is necessary to accomplish the training objectives. If simple task training (e.g. wound dressing and detection of pulses) for inexperienced learners is required, high fidelity simulation is less important. Complex integrated task performance and decision making by experienced providers in unique environmental conditions may require higher fidelity simulations. Nevertheless, the objectives of most disaster response training exercises can be accomplished using relatively low fidelity scenarios. High fidelity simulation with realistic immersive environmental conditions (e.g. sounds, odours, *in situ* locations and confederate actors) is not required for basic triage training. Integrated assessment of triage skills with execution of immediate life-saving resuscitation for multiple victims in real time with realistic distracters would require higher levels of environmental, physical, technical and psychological fidelity. Such truly immersive high fidelity simulations are appropriate for end-of-training summative assessments, and are rarely required in routine initial and refresher training.

Moulage (the application of makeup and mock injuries) can add realism to medical simulation. Moulage overuse may, however, unnecessarily consume valuable resources without altering educational outcomes. Moulage takes time to apply and also takes time to remove. When multiple scenarios are contemplated, the use of moulage may make it difficult for course directors to quickly change the simulation. Learners may be reluctant to engage a moulaged manikin if they believe their clothes or hands will be stained. The application of moulage may require special skills that are not always available. Course directors should consider using 'dry moulage' such as towels with red paint splatters that are strategically placed on or near a manikin to simulate blood loss. In our experience, learners usually have no difficulty identifying major haemorrhage using 'dry moulage' as a contextual clue.

Do the scenarios have appropriate 'triggers'?

The design of simulation scenarios to elicit specific learner behaviours requires insertion of embedded 'triggers'. Overall scenario development includes description of case 'stems': environmental conditions, available equipment and other triggers, which may serve to establish a scene and to provide clues regarding available resources and the scope of the disaster. A simple example is the application of moulage to anatomical regions, which triggers learner attention to specific injuries. Psychological scene setting is more complex and requires embedding more unusual elements. For example, the introduction of distressed family members into an active disaster management scenario can enhance psychological and environmental realism, and can be utilized to assess the learner's ability to correctly delegate non-victim management tasks to another disaster worker. A broken radio might represent an environmental trigger for assessment of learner knowledge of alternative communication protocols. Psychological engagement is critical for optimal learning, problem solving and assessment as elaborated in the instructional design objectives. Simulation instructors may also use coaching, cueing and prompting by faculty or trained confederates as additional trigger techniques.

Implementation

How will pre-course material be distributed?

Novice learners may be unfamiliar with principles of triage in MCI, and experienced learners may possess knowledge or skills that have degraded since the most recent MCI experience or training. The distribution of pre-course material for advance study has the potential to make the course more efficient by ensuring that learners have a baseline level of knowledge at the start of the programme. Course planners may want to consider using newer methods of distributing course material to their learners. For example, we had success using podcasts to teach novice learners principles of mass casualty triage (Vincent *et al.*, 2009b). Podcasts are stored digital media files that may be distributed over the internet using syndication software (Boulos *et al.*, 2006). Podcasts usually deliver audio content to users, but they may also deliver images and video content. Playback by users is made possible using digital audio devices or computers with audio management programs such as iTunes or Windows Media Player. The podcasts may be created using software such as GarageBand (©Apple Inc.) or ProfCast (©HumbleDaisy, Ann Arbor, Michigan).

Who are the faculty?

Faculty for the programme may be broadly divided into two groups, managers and debriefers. Managers must have technical experience with the manikins. They are required to maintain the flow of learners through the MCI scenarios, reset the manikins for the next learners and record learner behaviours during the exercise. Debriefers have special expertise in MCI triage. They focus on highlighting key teaching points for learners, and providing feedback to learners when gaps in knowledge and skills are identified.

When will the learners be oriented?

Orienting learners to the equipment that is being used is an essential step that must occur before the MCI training begins. Some learners will have previously encountered manikin-based simulation in other courses, however, we recommend refresher orientation to the simulators. Important elements of the orientation include a hands-on assessment by learners of the quality and location of pulses on the manikin, the quality and location of breath sounds, and pupillary responsiveness. Learners may have to be oriented to certain triggers, such as a painted towel intended to simulate haemorrhage. Learners will also have to be apprised of available equipment to use during the MCI exercise.

Lastly, the scene needs to be set for the simulated MCI. We have used ambulance sirens and photos of incidents to inform the learners of the nature of the disaster scenario.

When and how will debriefings be conducted?

Learners may be debriefed individually or in groups, and they may be debriefed after each scenario (formative debriefing), or after all scenarios have been completed (summative debriefing). Formative debriefing is appealing to learners and faculty because it enables faculty to develop a clear understanding of whether or not the learners are 'getting the point' during the course. Immediate feedback to learners may translate into transfer of knowledge and behaviours as the learners progress through additional scenarios. We have successfully used formative debriefing for both small and large groups of learners (Vincent *et al.*, 2009a).

Triage is dynamic because the clinical status of patients changes, and available resources fluctuate. Categorizing a patient to a unique triage category challenges learners, and this becomes a valuable discussion point. The context of the scenario must be clearly established before commencing in order for students to choose an appropriate triage category. An example of the impact of context on appropriate triage is the traumatic brain injury simulation. We placed a 'bloody' cloth (a cloth painted red) underneath the manikin head, dilated a pupil and programmed agonal breathing. This simulated massive head trauma with increased intracranial pressure. If the context were a busy urban highway and a motor vehicle accident, the patient might be categorized as 'immediate' with the intention of providing resuscitation in an intensive care unit (ICU). However, if the context were an MCI in which scores of injured patients are seriously injured and critical infrastructure has been destroyed, the patient would be categorized as 'expectant'. The ability to alter the triage category of the patient based on a change in context provides an opportunity to discuss ethical decision making in resource-constrained environments.

Evaluation

How will data be collected?

Electronic polling systems are an enabling technology that not only engage adult learners and enable faculty to utilize adult learning constructs (Moredich and Moore, 2006), but also have the capability to dynamically collect data for feedback and research purposes. Known as audience response systems, the devices wirelessly poll and collate learner responses dynamically and anonymously for immediate projection as a PowerPoint (Microsoft, Inc.,

Redmond, Washington) slide. The technology we have used is the TurningPoint Audience Response System (2006, Turning Technologies LLC, Youngstown, Ohio). Teachers and learners receive immediate feedback regarding the topic being discussed: Am I keeping up with my peers? Is the pace of the course appropriate? By triggering the input device, learners develop a vested interest in the educational outcome, a type of personal accountability. Audience response systems are able to give students a 'voice', while eliminating the bandwagon effect whereby students watch to see how other students are responding before they answer. We have successfully used an audience response system during formative debriefing sessions with as few as four and as many as 30 learners (Vincent *et al.*, 2009a).

What evaluation questions may be asked?

There are several outcome measures of interest to course planners: accuracy of triage, time to triage, application of appropriate interventions, learner satisfaction and learner self-efficacy. Learners may be asked to identify the main abnormality in the simulated patient (including no abnormality), such as airway, breathing, circulation, neurological or other problem (fracture). They may be asked to assign the appropriate triage category, such as minimal, delayed, immediate or expectant. Appropriate interventions may include applying a tourniquet, using a haemostatic bandage, applying a regular bandage, performing needle decompression and inserting a nasopharyngeal airway. Self-efficacy, or learner self-confidence, may be assessed by having students respond to statements like 'I feel confident doing mass casualty triage' using a five-point Likert scale (1 = never, 5 = always). Course evaluations may assess whether learners believe that simulation-based training is valuable, and whether the use of manikins should be a regular part of MCI training.

Examples of Programmes

Programme with individual medical students

At the University of Hawaii, we trained 21 novice learners (medical students) in how to conduct mass casualty triage, and then assessed their knowledge, skills and attitudes about mass casualty triage (Vincent *et al.*, 2009b). Core concepts of mass casualty triage were taught using four brief podcasts. Learners had to pass a 20-question written test in order to advance. They then experienced three sequential mass casualty scenarios consisting of five manikin simulations each, coupled with individual feedback after each scenario. Learners were also asked to apply simple, life-saving interventions if appropriate. The simulations included four adult casualties and one baby. Each scenario consisted of three 'immediate', one 'minimal' and one 'delayed or expectant' simulated patient. Actual hands-on time for learners to complete the three scenarios was about 30 min. The learners demonstrated improved triage and intervention scores, speed and self-efficacy.

Programmes with groups of nurses, doctors and medics

We trained 182 healthcare providers from eight Asia-Pacific countries in four simulation seminars (Vincent *et al.*, 2009a). This training was conducted in Honolulu (Hawaii), Japan and Singapore. Four primary triage scenarios were created consisting of two 'immediate', one 'delayed' and one 'expectant' simulated patient. Before each scenario, a mass casualty context was established by showing a photograph of an actual disaster scene, along with information that there were scores of casualties. Learners triaged the simulated patients in groups ranging from four to eight. When only one manikin was available, a small group triaged the patient while a larger group watched and commented later. When three manikins were available, small groups triaged the simulated patients, and a single large group debriefing was performed. An audience response system was used to facilitate the debriefing. Despite the heterogeneity of the learners and the training resources, we were able to demonstrate that self-efficacy increased in many of the learners, and that experiential learning using simulation techniques was a useful way to bridge cultural barriers in disaster health education.

Programme with pairs of medics

At the University of Hawaii, we trained 19 US Navy corpsmen who were about to deploy to Iraq as first responders and healthcare providers. In a single 6-h simulation session, the corpsmen triaged and treated 16 simulated casualties while working in pairs. Each pair triaged four simulated casualties. As they moved to the next patient, another pair of corpsmen replaced them in a round-robin fashion. A group debriefing was then conducted using an audience response system and trained facilitators. This technique of iterative exposure to multiple manikin scenarios permitted the gradual escalation of complexity throughout the day. In the end, participants were successfully triaging and applying life-saving interventions to simulated casualties with complex, polytraumatic injuries and clinical situations.

Programme with individual doctors

We trained 56 doctors from eight countries at a military medicine conference in Seoul, South Korea, in two 90-min sessions (Vincent, Berg and Phrampus, 2010, unpublished data). The learners sequentially triaged five simulated patients in an MCI. The learners worked singly, and recorded a triage category (minimal, delayed, immediate or expectant) and intervention on a worksheet that was graded at the end of the exercise. The average time to triage each simulated patient was 21 s. We concluded that it was feasible to use an array of multiple manikins to train and assess large groups of learners in a simulated MCI.

Conclusions

Experiential learning using manikin-based simulation may be an effective way to train healthcare providers for MCIs. Experts have identified the applicability of simulation-based education to disaster health education. Educators who are planning an MCI training programme using manikins can use instructional design principles to guide course development. A systematic approach to the design of MCI training using manikin-based simulation may help to ensure the successful transfer of knowledge and skills to both novice and experienced learners.

Disclaimer

The views expressed in this manuscript are those of the authors and do not reflect the official policy or position of the US Department of the Army, Department of Defense or the US Government.

References

Ali, J., Gana, T.L. and Howard, M. (2000) Trauma mannequin assessment of management skills of surgical residents after advanced trauma life support training. *Journal of Surgical Research* 93, 197–200.

Angus, D.C., Pretto, E.A., Abrams, J.I. and Safar, P. (1993) Recommendations for life-supporting first-aid training of the lay public for disaster preparedness. *Prehospital Disaster Medicine* 8, 157–160.

Arnold, J.L. (2002) Disaster medicine in the 21st century: future hazards, vulnerabilities, and risk. *Prehospital Disaster Medicine* 17, 3–11.

Aylwin, C.J., Konig, T.C., Brennan, N.W., Shirley, P.J., Davies, G., Walsh, M.S. and Brohi, K. (2006) Reduction in critical mortality in urban mass casualty incidents: analysis of triage, surge, and resource use after the London bombings on July 7, 2005. *Lancet* 2219–2225.

Baker, M.S. (2007) Creating order from chaos: Part I: triage, initial care, and tactical considerations in mass casualty and disaster response. *Military Medicine* 172, 232–6.

Benson, M., Koenig, K.L. and Schultz, C.H. (1996) Disaster triage: START, then SAVE – a new method of dynamic triage for victims of a catastrophic earthquake. *Prehospital Disaster Medicine* 11, 117–124.

Berkenstadt, H., Ziv, A., Barsuk, D., Levine, I., Cohen, A. and Vardi, A. (2003) The use of advanced simulation in the training of anesthesiologists to treat chemical warfare casualties. *Anesthesia & Analgesia* 96, 1739–1742.

Bleakley, A. (2006) Broadening conceptions of learning in medical education: the message from teamworking. *Medical Education* 40, 150–157.

Boulos, M.N., Maramba, I. and Wheeler, S. (2006) Wikis, blogs and podcasts: a new generation of web-based tools for virtual collaborative clinical practice and education. *BMC Medical Education* 6, 41.

Boyd, J., Haegeli, P., Abu-Laban, R.B., Shuster, M. and Butt, J.C. (2009) Patterns of death among avalanche fatalities: a 21-year review. *Canadian Medical Association Journal* 180, 507–512.

Broeze, C.C., Falder, S., Rea, S. and Wood, F. (2010) Burn disasters – an audit of the literature. *Prehospital Disaster Medicine* 25, 555–559.

Evans, L., Dodge, K.L., Shah, T.D., Kaplan, L.J., Siegel, M.D., Moore, C.L., Hamann, C.J., Lin, Z. and D'Onofrio, G. (2010) Simulation training in central venous catheter insertion: improved performance in clinical practice. *Academic Medicine* 85, 1462–1469.

Frykberg, E.R. and Tepas, J.J. (1988) Terrorist bombings. Lessons learned from Belfast to Beirut. *Annals of Surgery* 208, 569–576.

Galante, J.M., Jacoby, R.C. and Anderson, J.T. (2005) Are surgical residents prepared for mass casualty incidents? *Journal of Surgical Research* 85–91.

Garner, A., Lee, A., Harrison, K. and Schultz, C.H. (2001) Comparative analysis of multiple-casualty incident triage algorithms. *Annals of Emergency Medicine* 38, 541–548.

Gofrit, O.N., Leibovici, D., Shemer, J., Henig, A. and Shapira, S.C. (1997) The efficacy of integrating 'smart simulated casualties' in hospital disaster drills. *Prehospital Disaster Medicine* 12, 97–101.

Green, G.B., Modi, S., Lunney, K. and Thomas, T.L. (2003) Generic evaluation methods for disaster drills in developing countries. *Annals of Emergency Medicine* 41, 689–699.

Hart, R., Lee, J.O., Boyles, D.J. and Batey, N.R. (1975) The Summerland disaster. *British Medical Journal* 1, 256–259.

Hendrickse, A.D., Ellis, A.M. and Morris, R.W. (2001) Use of simulation technology in Australian Defence Force resuscitation training. *Journal of the Royal Army Medical Corps* 147, 173–178.

Hsu, E.B., Jenckes, M.W., Catlett, C.L., Robinson, K.A., Fuerstein, C., Cosgrove, S.E., Green, G.B. and Bass, E.B. (2004) Effectiveness of hospital staff mass-casualty incident training methods: a systematic literature review. *Prehospital Disaster Medicine* 19, 191–199.

Issenberg, S.B., McGaghie, W.C., Hart, I.R., Mayer, J.W., Felner, J.M., Petrusa, E.R., Waugh, R.A., Brown, D.D., Safford, R.R., Gessner, I.H., Gordon, D.L. and Ewy, G.A. (1999) Simulation technology for health care professional skills training and assessment. *JAMA: Journal of the American Medical Association* 282, 861.

Issenberg, S.B., McGaghie, W.C., Petrusa, E.R., Lee Gordon, D. and Scalese, R. (2005) Features and uses of high-fidelity medical simulations that lead to effective learning: a BEME systematic review. *Medical Teacher* 27, 10–28.

James, J.J., Subbarao, I. and Lanier, W.L. (2008) Improving the art and science of disaster medicine and public health preparedness. *Mayo Clinic Proceedings* 83, 559–562.

Jenkins, J.L., McCarthy, M.L., Sauer, L.M., Green, G.B., Stuart, S., Thomas, T.L. and Hsue, E.B. (2008) Mass-casualty triage: time for an evidence-based approach. *Prehospital Disaster Medicine* 23, 3–8.

Kahn, C.A., Schultz, C.H., Miller, K.T. and Anderson, C.L. (2009) Does START triage work? An outcomes assessment after a disaster. *Annals of Emergency Medicine* 54, 424–430.

Kluth, A. (2008) Special Report: Mobility. Nomads at last. *The Economist*, 10 April.

Kobayashi, L., Shapiro, M.J., Suner, S. and Williams, K.A. (2003) Disaster medicine: the potential role of high fidelity medical simulation for mass casualty incident training. *Medicine & Health Rhode Island* 86, 196–200.

Kobayashi, L., Shapiro, M.J., Gutman, D.C. and Jay, G. (2007) Multiple encounter simulation for high-acuity multipatient environment training. *Academic Emergency Medicine* 14, 1141–1148.

McGaghie, W.C., Issenberg, S.B., Cohen, E.R., Barsuk, J. and Wayne, D. (2011) Does simulation-based medical education with deliberate practice yield better results than traditional clinical education? A meta-analytic comparative review of the evidence. *Academic Medicine* 86, 706–711.

McMillan, R. (2006) The South Asian earthquake: an emergency physician's perspective. *Canadian Journal of Emergency Medicine* 8, 174–176.

Meredith, W., Rutledge, R., Hanson, A.R., Oller, D.W., Thomason, M., Cunningham, P. and Baker, C. (1995) Field triage of trauma patients based upon the ability to follow commands: a study in 29,573 injured patients. *Journal of Trauma* 38, 129–135.

Miller, G.T., Motola, I., Broton, A.A. and Issenberg, S.B. (2010) Preparing for the worst: a review of the ADDIE simulation model for disaster-response training. *The Journal of Emergency Medical Services* 35, Suppl. 11–13.

Moredich, C. and Moore, E. (2006) Engaging students through the use of classroom response systems. *Nursing Education* 32, 113–116.

O'Hickey, S.P., Pickering, C.A., Jones, P.E. and Evans, J.D. (1987) Manchester air disaster. *British Medical Journal (Clin Res Ed)* 294, 1663–1667.

Phillips, S., Rond, P.C., Kelly, S.M. and Swartz, P.D. (1996a) The failure of triage criteria to identify geriatric patients with trauma: results from the Florida trauma triage study. *Journal of Trauma* 40, 278–283.

Phillips, S., Rond, P.C., Kelly, S.M. and Swartz, P.D. (1996b) The need for pediatric-specific triage criteria: results from the Florida trauma triage study. *Pediatric Emergency Care* 12, 394–399.

Prehospital Trauma Life Support Committee of the National Association of Emergency Medical Technicians in Cooperation with the Committee on Trauma of the American College of Surgeons (1994) *Prehospital Trauma Life Support: Basic and Advanced.* Mosby, St Louis, Missouri.

Ross, S.E., Leipold, C., Terregino, C. and O'Malley, K.F. (1998) Efficacy of the motor component of the Glasgow coma scale in trauma triage. *Journal of Trauma* 45, 42–44.

Sadler, C. (1982) Accident and emergency: the St. Valentine's Day disaster. *Nursing Mirror* 154, 14–16.

Scalese, R.J., Obeso, V.T. and Issenberg, S.B. (2008) Simulation technology for skills training and competency assessment in medical education. *Journal of General Internal Medicine* 23 Suppl 1, 46–49.

Seynaeve, G., Archer, F., Fisher, J., Lueger-Schuster, B., Rowlands, A., Sellwood, P., Vandevelde, K. and Zigoura, A. (2004) International standards and guidelines on education and training for the multi-disciplinary health response to major events that threaten the health status of a community. *Prehospital Disaster Medicine* 19, S17–30.

Sohn, V.Y., Miller, J.P., Koeller, C.A., Gibons, S.O., Azarow, K.S., Myers, J.B., Beekley, A.C., Sebesta, J.A., Christensen, J.B. and Rush, R.M. (2007) From the combat medic to the forward surgical team: the Madigan model for improving trauma readiness of brigade combat teams fighting the global war on terror. *Journal of Surgical Research* 138, 25–31.

Strickland, A.W. (2011) ADDIE. Idaho State University College of Education. Available at: http://ed.isu.edu/addie/index.html (Accessed 4 July 2011).

Subbarao, I., Bond, W.F., Johnson, C., Hsu, E.B. and Wasser, T.E. (2006) Using innovative simulation modalities for civilian-based, chemical, biological, radiological, nuclear, and explosive training in the acute management of terrorist victims: a pilot study. *Prehospital Disaster Medicine* 21, 272–275.

Subbarao, I., Lyzniki, J.M., Hsue, E.B., Gebbie, K.M., Markenson, D., Barzansky, B., Armstrong, J.H., Cassimatis, E.G., Coule, P.L., Dallas, C.E., King, R.V., Rubinson, L., Sattin, R., Swienton, R.E., Lillibridge, S., Burkle, F.M., Schwartz, R.B. and James J.J. (2008) A consensus-based educational framework and competency set for the discipline of disaster medicine and public health preparedness. *Disaster Medicine and Public Health Preparedness* 2, 57–68.

Towne, L.E. (1995) China eastern md-11 mass casualty – expect the unexpected: a case report. *Aviation, Space, and Environmental Medicine* 66, 998–1000.

Vardi, A., Levin, I., Berkenstadt, H., Hourvitz, A., Eisenkraft, A., Cohen, A. and Ziv, A. (2002) Simulation-based training of medical teams to manage chemical warfare casualties. *Israeli Medical Association Journal* 4, 540–544.

Vincent, D., Berg, B.W. and Ikegami, K. (2009a) Mass-casualty triage training for international healthcare workers in the Asia-Pacific region using manikin-based simulations. *Prehospital Disaster Medicine* 24, 206–213.

Vincent, D., Burgess, L., Berg, B.W. and Connolly, K. (2009b) Teaching mass casualty triage skills using iterative multimanikin simulations. *Prehospital Emergency Care* 13, 241–246.

Wallis, L.A. and Carley, S. (2006) Comparison of paediatric major incident primary triage tools. *Emergency Medicine Journal* 23, 475–478.

Wayne, D., Didwania, A., Feinglass, J., Barsuk, J. and McGaghie, W.C. (2008) Simulation-based education improves quality of care during cardiac arrest team responses at an academic teaching hospital: a case-control study. *Chest* 133, 56–61.

Section 3

Crucial Role of Communication in Disaster Management and Homeland Security

Chapter 4

The Role of Social Networking in Disaster Management

Marcia Trainer and Anju Goel

Introduction: Research on and Theoretical Background of Disaster and Risk Management for Organizational Systems

Interorganizational theory and research provides cross-relational insight to disaster and risk management policy

Part of the horror of disasters, whether natural or human-made, is the chaos and uncertainty thrust on a society and its people as they respond to the immediate destruction, then assess the damage and re-establish order. Disaster preparedness professionals are challenged to arrive at a reliable template for effective disaster management, because disasters by their very nature are 'low-probability, high consequence' events, and they happen all over the world in uniquely variable conditions. Often research in the preparedness field is helpful, but does not provide a universal 'gold standard' for application. However, a substantial body of public policy, organizational theory and research has accrued from studying the multifactorial forces at work in organizational system management of crisis and disasters. Disaster managers have found cross-relational guidance in organizational systems theory, by considering communities as complex systems. Research has shown that organizations in high-risk situations commonly encounter tensions between the hierarchical command-and-control elements that represent stasis and the processes of discovery and innovation that signify adaptation to often rapidly changing circumstances (Comfort, 1994). Theorists believe that in the dynamic, stressful interface between an organization's structural and its creative elements is where the critically vital quality of resilience lies (Comfort, 1994).

The importance of resilience in complex systems, whether organizational or community-based

The pioneering political scientist and risk theorist Aaron Wildavsky defined resilience as 'the capacity to cope with unanticipated dangers after they have become manifest, learning to bounce back' (Wildavsky, 1988, p. 224). He concluded that essential ingredients to resilience were: (i) an organization's fundamental general capacities, which were (ii) tested by trial and error, in (iii) a decentralized environment. He also identified four qualities in an organization's culture that fostered a sustainable resilience in a threatening environment: (i) an environment that encouraged creative interaction between organizational units when trying to reach a common goal; (ii) flexibility between the whole system and its parts; (iii) a policy encouraging interaction between the organization and its environment; and (iv) a recognition of the critical role of information to set the tone and tempo of the organization's success or failure (Wildavsky, 1988). Subsequent research in other regions of the world has verified the critical role that resilience plays in disaster recovery, whether it is applied to individuals, families, institutions or communities (Otobi, 2010). The concept of community resilience has received increasing research-based validation as an important goal in disaster management. It is also recognized as a fundamental building block for recovery in The Sphere Project, which focuses on setting minimum standards in world disaster response (The Sphere Project, 2007). Again, in the body of research supporting the criticality of community resilience to disaster recovery, the power of communication in its many forms and sources is uniformly considered fundamental to that resilience (Norris *et al.*, 2008; Sutton, 2010).

The 2001 anthrax attacks and the Centers for Disease Control and Prevention response as a case study on the notion that communication in building resilience goes both ways during a disaster – for both the responding organization and the community it serves

The essential significance of communication to organizational resilience in crisis applies with equal magnitude to community resilience in disaster management. Like hierarchically structured organizations, formal disaster response plans are based on their own hierarchical Incident Command System (ICS). Like the top-down communications in organizations, formal disaster response communications are one-way-driven too, from the 'producer'/command centre to the 'consumer'/public disaster victims (Keim and Noji, 2011). While there are substantial benefits to using incident command structure in chaotic situations, it is not functionally efficient in other important ways. Persistent problems from this traditional mode of communications complicate effective disaster response: information is slower moving through the hierarchical structure (Robinson and Newstetter, 2003); it needs to be translated from scientific/official vocabulary into accessible language for the public (Robinson and Newstetter, 2003); it often needs repetition due to the public's tendency to disbelieve warnings and then their need to verify with other sources (Tierney, 2001); it is more relevant and accepted if it is local and community-based (Pollard, 2003); and it must be trusted as coming from a reliable source (Pollard, 2003; Longstaff and Yang, 2008). In addition, one-way communication does not provide command and control with feedback from the public on how effective their risk communications efforts have been (Fig. 4.1). There is no system for public input on whether the information has actually been received, whether it has actually been understood, whether it tells the public what the public needs to know, whether and to what degree the public has responded to the information, whether problems have arisen in the public field that command and control is not aware of and whether command and control remains a trusted source of information (Robinson and Newstetter, 2003).

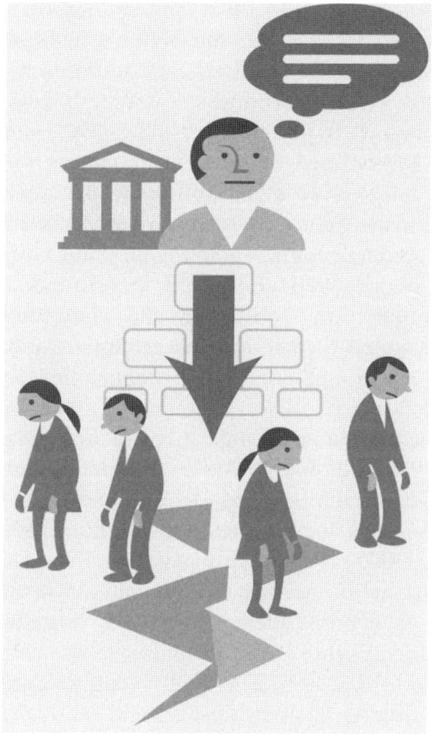

Fig. 4.1. Communication history, part a. Traditional governmental emergency communications are driven by the organization's top-down, hierarchical structure. Disaster communications are one-way driven, from the producer/command centre to the consumer/public victims. A command structure is important in chaotic situations, but problems of this traditional communications mode are: slower message delivery due to the hierarchical transmission; the need for translation from official vocabulary to accessible language, the public's need to confirm information with familiar, trusted sources and there is no way for command to receive information from 'the field' up the chain of command to find out about how the public is understanding the information given.

To be more responsive to a crisis, the hierarchical one-way message delivery system needs a reliable adaptation to also receive information from the field on its communication effectiveness. With input, command can refine its efforts. However, when public health and safety are at serious risk, this feedback information must be gained in real time during a crisis. Because the situation is fluid, a dynamic and effective response can mitigate the decline of a bad situation and save lives (Blendon *et al.*, 2003). The Centers for Disease Control and Prevention (CDC) was seriously challenged in its health and communications response during the anthrax attacks of 2001 that followed shortly after the 9/11 terrorist attacks in the USA. The scale of the biological exposure from the anthrax terrorist attacks extended from the northern Atlantic to the southern Atlantic states. The epidemiological investigation was wide-ranging, media interest was intense and the public's need to know was urgent and extensive. Within a week, the CDC realized its traditional modes of communication response were obsolete (Robinson and Newstetter, 2003). It transformed its communication operations systems in multiple ways, internally and externally. Information flow was streamlined to have headquarters work more directly with CDC field teams and also with local public health departments. CDC trained communications teams, made their jobs ready to go and dispatched them to multiple exposure sites, where epidemiologists and media staff worked together. A public inquiries team staffed phones and computers to respond to calls and to website questions from the public on confusion and mounting concerns. Specialist communicators were assigned to medical and communications teams to help shape newly developing information gathered from scientists for delivery in multiple ways that would best suit the needs of various audiences, including medical practitioners, medical responders, the media reaching different demographics and the general public (Robinson and Newstetter, 2003). Additionally, numerous 'short-duration, rapid-turnaround' surveys were polled to continuously monitor attitude and behavioural changes. Surveys were controlled for non-response bias for increased validity (Blendon *et al.*, 2003) (Fig. 4.2). In the end, the CDC's ability to adapt to a rapidly unfolding crisis with creative, fundamental, lasting changes showed a remarkable resilience. As a consequence, the CDC transformed its organizational structure and values to incorporate a robust, multi-faceted emergency communication system structure (Vanderford, 2009). The CDC recognized early the benefits of new technology in offering timely, accurate, useful and innovative ways to disseminate information to multiple stakeholders and audiences.

How the CDC has applied its 'lessons learned'

In 2001, mobile phones and the internet were proving their value to the CDC's increasingly rapid and effective communications strategies, but a mere decade has witnessed even more dramatic changes in crisis communications technology. The CDC has attended to lessons learned from the 2001 anthrax communications crisis. It assiduously monitors new technologies, assesses their value to the CDC and incorporates useful applications to innovatively further its mission of public health promotion. Additionally, the CDC has actively developed a national capacity-building programme that shares this information with state, regional and local public health agencies and other concerned organizations through content syndication, so that these partner agencies can incorporate the CDC's shared information into their own formal communications systems plans. The CDC system is designed to help coordinate and create uniform messages, and it automatically offers updates to partner agencies in real time, directly to agreed partner web pages (CDC, 2011a).

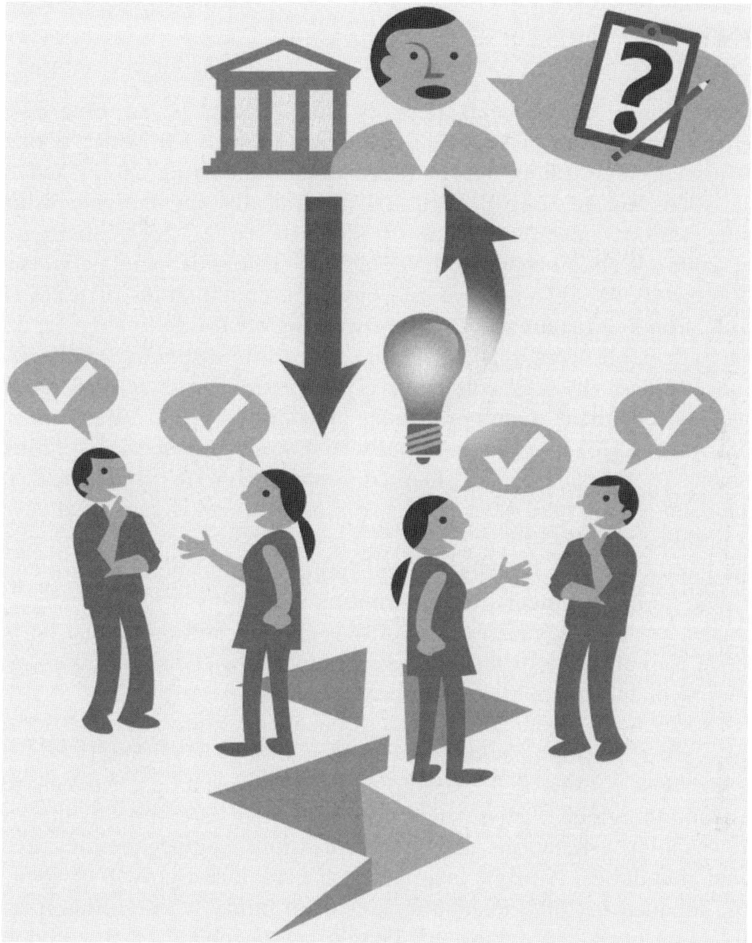

Fig. 4.2. Communication history, part b. Government emergency agencies learned from past mistakes and began trying to establish better communications by using different techniques that reached directly into the public's disaster field for feedback on messaging efficiency. Efforts included using government teams in the disaster field to communicate with and from the public back to headquarters; and using 'short-duration, rapid-turnaround' surveys, completed by the public, to help refine messaging, correct prior mistakes and develop pathways for information exchange between the public and headquarters. This resulted in relationship building and more effective communications.

What is Social Networking?

Definition and description of social networking

Social networking, or a social network site (SNS), is an outgrowth of the characteristic architecture of Web 2.0. In contrast to Web 1.0, which is one-way and producer-driven, Web 2.0 is decentralized (Keim and Noji, 2011) and interactive (Giustini, 2006; Sutton, 2010). Web 2.0 dynamically and actively brings people together in various interactive sites or applications, to freely share information (Giustini, 2006). Web 2.0 supports the democratic nature of social networking, which is peer-to-peer (P2P), collaborative and based on communities of users (Keim and Noji, 2011). The key features of social networking are the following: (i) it has broad reach that is scalable from small to global, due to its distinctive multiple points of generation and use; (ii) it is comparatively accessible to everyone, relative to the traditional closely held communications modalities used by government and traditional media; (iii) it is user friendly and needs no special training; (iv) its transmission is immediate, in marked comparison to traditional modes of communication, which take days, weeks or months; (v) it is easy to alter and edit as the need unfolds, unlike the relative permanence of communications from traditional media modalities (Wikipedia, 2011b); and (vi) communications are not controlled as they are with traditional media, thus permitting free information exchange. This final characteristic has both advantages and disadvantages, and both must be understood for effective communications through social networking (Giustini, 2006), particularly for disaster medicine and public health preparedness.

Use of social media applications such as Facebook, Short Message Service (SMS) commonly called 'texting', Twitter, YouTube and blogs have rapidly become normal conduits for both routine and extraordinary communications between people and groups around the globe. Active social networkers are as diverse as the applications they use, spanning generations, jobs and professions, socioeconomic categories and geographic boundaries. A prime example of the reach and growth of social media is Facebook, founded in 2004. Facebook is a social utility whose mission is: 'to make the world more open and connected. People use Facebook to stay connected with friends and family, to discover what's going on in the world, and to share and express what matters to them' (Facebook, 2013). Individual or group users subscribe, set up individual or group pages and share updates, photos, blogs, calendars, messages and comments (Bledsoe, 2009). It has more than 1 billion active users as of December 2012, 82% of them outside the USA (Facebook, 2013). Another global and easy-to-use application, Twitter, focuses on communications (called 'Tweets') done in real time using short bursts of 140 characters that allow updates and tracking through hash-tag identification titles (Twitter, 2011). YouTube, a utility that allows people to post their own videos online, is also global, with more than 70% of its traffic outside the USA. During 2010, over 13 million hours of video material were uploaded. YouTube has been embedded throughout 'tens of millions of websites' (YouTube, 2011). A recent Pew-Annenberg study revealed that by 2010, social network users in the USA 35 years or older had increased to 48%, from the previous 18% of a study conducted by Pew-Annenberg in November 2009 (Evangelista, 2011).

Uses of social networking in disaster response

Disaster preparedness and response fields have not kept pace with the rapid development and use of social networking, and have not routinely incorporated it into many disaster and preparedness response communications plans. Though little research has been done to systematically analyse the benefits of its use in this context, anecdotal information exists of the public's successful spontaneous use of social networking applications in multiple types of disasters. These unpremeditated, unofficial uses of social networking during disasters indicate the power of social networking to broadly and rapidly communicate essential information during disasters worldwide. In addition, social networking also has the ability to partially fill known, significant and persistent communication gaps in disaster response that sometimes lead to loss of lives.

Some professionals in public health communications have recognized the need to formally utilize social media in health communications through such applications as blogging, to disseminate general public health information; Twitter for crisis communications, particularly in remote areas during disasters; and using Google Maps as an overlay for both its visual and its cost-free benefits (Bloomberg, 2007; CDC, 2010b). Even by 2007, the CDC's research revealed that in using social media, it could potentially send its public health and safety messages to the then more than 75% of the US population that used the internet, the 75% that viewed video online and the millions who used search engines tracking more than 112 million blogs, including not just blogs but video and audio files and photos (CDC, 2010b). Use of social media has increased exponentially since then. While many of these social media applications are browsed for entertainment purposes, they are powerful means during disasters for informing people of critical information, through modalities people everywhere skilfully use daily (CDC, 2010b). The public has already used these tools during multiple types of disasters worldwide, when formal disaster communications from responders or traditional media were often lagging behind (Fig. 4.3).

Spontaneous Examples of Social Media Use in Disaster Communications

16 April 2007 Virginia Tech shootings: among the first examples noted on social media use in disasters

When officials at Virginia Tech University first learned that many students were being shot on campus by an armed individual, administrators began a series of mass alerts to the general student population by contacting them via dormitory phones, through the web and by e-mail. However, the university did not use text messaging (SMS), a form of communicating that students commonly used with their mobile phones (CDC, 2010b).

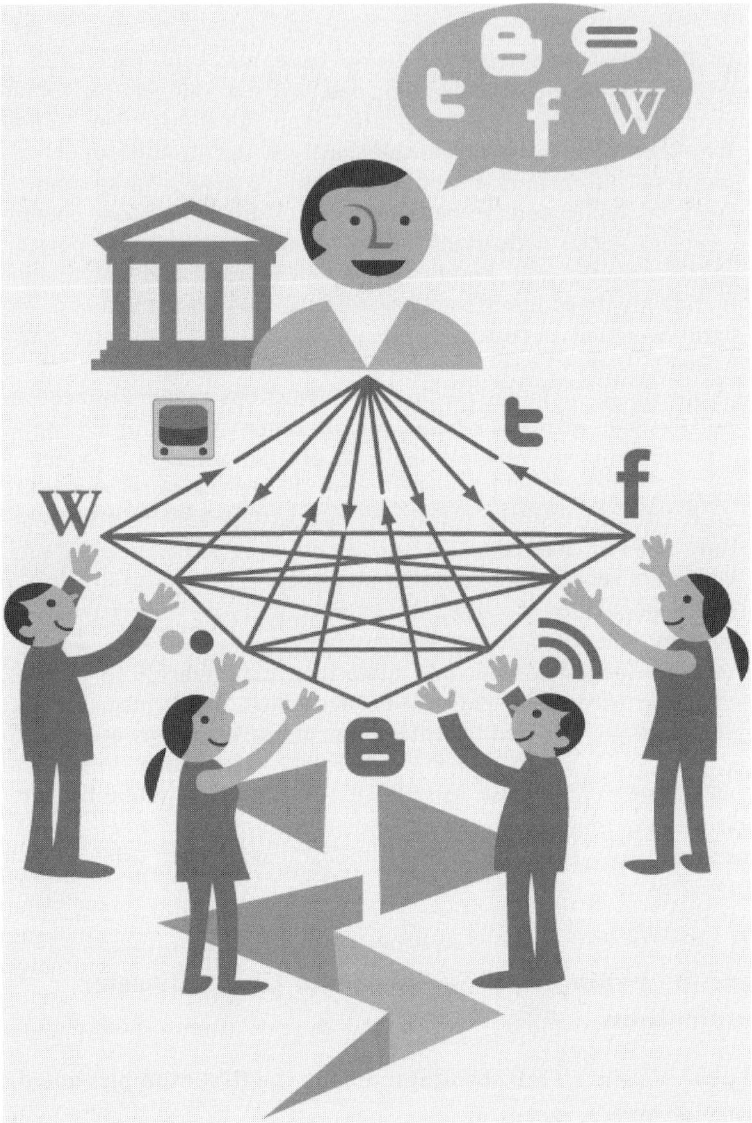

Fig. 4.3. Communication history, part c. Government emergency agencies began incorporating social networking tools that were already in place and actively used by the public on a daily basis. These tools are built on existing social networks, have trust built into the system and have spontaneously been used for years in disasters, as a method of reaching out, gaining information and effective disaster response. Used in conjunction with more traditional methods of communications, public agencies can be very effective in disaster communications and efficient disaster response.

Officials were later criticized for not formally including SMS in their disaster notification plan. Students who were not by their computers or in their dorms very often did travel with their mobile phones and would more likely have received a text message than an e-mail, a difference that could have saved lives in this situation. Students themselves widely communicated by social media and texting as the disaster unfolded. They used Flickr to upload photos minutes after the shootings had begun; they collaborated on contributing to a Wikipedia entry within 2 h, to provide an ongoing narrative and timeline of events; they blogged first-hand reports within a day on LiveJournal, an online community and social networking site (LiveJournal, 2011); they created 160 tribute groups on Facebook; and they posted 9000 videos on YouTube within a week of the shootings (Bledsoe, 2009).

2007 Southern California Wildfires: State Governor's Office, public news and citizens provide real-time coverage

California has a long history of wildfires. In 1970, there was a particularly devastating complex of wildfires that raged for 16 days, causing damage totalling US$18 million per day and involving local, regional, state and federal agencies. Subsequently, US Congress mandated that the US Forest Service design a programme to provide a systematic framework for coordinating a structured response to these disasters. The result was the hierarchical Incident Command System (ICS), which in 2004 was adopted as the entire nation's method of all-disaster response organization. It is a part of the National Incident Management System, NIMS, and is managed by the Federal Emergency Management Agency, FEMA (FEMA, 2004).

With this history, Governor Arnold Schwarzenegger quickly published 'Fire Season 2007' online through Google Maps. It offered Californians continuous visual information on fire locations, damage and fire fighting efforts (Wagner, 2007). KPBS, a public news station, maintained a Twitter feed for regular updating of fire information, too. Two citizens also spontaneously began Twitter feeds. Twitter was particularly useful to residents, because its limited-information format reduced news sharing to 'just the facts, without any "colour" or throat-clearing' (Wagner, 2007). These combined modes of rapid communication allowed endangered neighbours to closely follow the wildfire threat, make plans for evacuation of persons, pets and property, and make last-minute fireproofing defence of their homes to the degree possible.

The November 2008 terrorist attacks in Mumbai: Twitter and Flickr were first to break the news to the world

When terrorists began the Mumbai attacks, within 'mere moments' eyewitness reports were being tweeted from the region at an estimated rate of 70 tweets every 5 s (Beaumont, 2008). Included among the messages were essential disaster communications to urge blood donations as hospital reserves were depleted, information on helplines and contact numbers for those desperate to know about family and friends potentially threatened by the attacks. Metroblog, a site bloggers had previously created for general Mumbai news and local tips, rapidly transformed into a primary news wire service of events for locals as well as the greater concerned world. A Wikipedia site was quickly created, too, to offer voluminous information on the attacks, often in real time. One photographer chronicled events visually, through over 100 photos he posted to Flickr (Beaumont, 2008). The army of voluntary citizen journalists in fact worked so rapidly, thoroughly and continuously that traditional media relied on much of their work to provide mainstream coverage (Beaumont, 2008).

Winter 2008–2009 New England ice storms: the Public Service of New Hampshire, the state's largest utility, tweeted disaster communications directly 24/7 to customers suffering extended power outages

In December 2008, an ice storm caused unprecedented damage to the New England area, and left over 400,000 homes without power in the state of New Hampshire alone. Over 322,000 of those customers were serviced by the Public Service of New Hampshire (PSNH), the primary utility in the state. PSNH management used social media to meet the communications challenges of providing people the essential information they needed on outage locations, steps being taken to address the outages and repair priorities (Stambor, 2009). Twitter was the primary mode of communication, sent by managers from the field and the office in a continuous stream of information, 24/7. Throughout the 9 days of emergency tweets to consumers, PSNH's Twitter followers grew from an estimated 100 to 1900, and these diverse followers ranged from 'techies' to a rural middle-aged couple (Stambor, 2009). Twitter feeds were supplemented by the visuals that both Flickr and YouTube offered, as the utility's power restoration efforts moved forward. And when the utility reached the final stages of its investigation, results were posted on the internet and were read by over 10,000 interested viewers (Stambor, 2009).

2008 Sichuan earthquake: grassroots Twitter users tweeted news of the disaster as it was unfolding and 3 min before US Geological Service (USGS), and social networkers hastened response efforts

Grassroots-led tweets, generated during the 2008 Sichuan earthquake, were immediate notification to the world of the disaster (Gabarain, 2008). Such instantaneous notice as disaster occurs can be a help for potential victims to find safer ground. It also alerts the rest of the world to rapidly prepare an aid response for victims of a disaster, the magnitude of which, in the Sichuan earthquake case, was quickly and subsequently verified by USGS (Gabarain, 2008). Within 10 min, the Tianya forum, a popular social network community in China, posted a survey for first-person reports titled 'Did you feel it?' Thousands responded within the hour, from 22 various city locations (Qu *et al.*, 2011). This information helped quickly develop a map of affected regions to aid in accurate situation updates and refining response needs. A non-profit relief organization relied upon social networking for donations. Because it daily reported donation amount and distribution procedure updates, followers considered the foundation reliable and responded with over US$6.3 million, from more than 660,000 donors in less than 2 weeks post-quake (Qu *et al.*, 2011). The Tianya forum also served as an important outlet for people to express their feelings and offer their support. Data collected indicated more than 14% of Tianya forum's earthquake-related posts concerned personal emotions (Qu *et al.*, 2011).

2009 Fargo, North Dakota, US floods: interactive websites actively build community resilience; and public texting used to 'crowdsource' for individual aid

Wikipedia defines 'crowdsourcing' as 'the act of outsourcing tasks, traditionally performed by an employee or contractor, to an undefined, large group of people or a community (a "crowd") through an open call' (Wikipedia, 2011a). The benefits of crowdsourcing are: problems are investigated quickly and cheaply, often the job is completed free of charge, a broad range of talent is tapped and the results generate a sense of community, kinship and ownership (Wikipedia, 2011a).

Fargo, North Dakota has a deep cultural experience with flooding. The North Dakota State University at Fargo built a 'Fargo Flood' homepage on the internet in 1997 and has routinely updated it since then. It provides research- and data-driven information such as geology, flood hydrographs with daily and hourly changes in level and discharge, a 110-year plot of mean daily flow, a graphic animation of the Red River stage changes, satellite imagery of the 2011 flood and also of the last 30 days of images and a flood forecast tool that displays and visualizes the current Red River Basin status. The website also includes community-based information such as Inforum for news and information on local flooding, highway information and a Flood News and Events link (North Dakota State University, 2011). This link, in turn, offers more than a page of specific community interest and help information: how to volunteer, sandbag removal, interactive maps for residents to view not just river levels but the flood stage map of their particular property, road closures and current river conditions. The Fargo Flood Plan is placed there, too, with a simple, accessible, straightforward description of how the Plan would work for residents in each stage, from Phase I – Road Closure to Phase III – Cleanup and Recovery. The homepage ends with links for City of Fargo restoration and incentive programmes, followed by links for federal aid (City of Fargo, 2011). This website arrangement provides the essential elements for successful, empowering risk communications, telling disaster-threatened people what they need to know, what they can do and where they can go for additional information.

As structured, these internet web pages show how some community institutions use social networking tools to build community resilience. During the Fargo flood of 2009, the community itself demonstrated its own resilient use of social networking by creating a Facebook group page that served as a 'meeting place' for 4550 people within 24 h; by posting hourly river levels through Twitter posts among more than 300 field observers monitoring the event, and by responding within 3 h of an individual's text-messaged request for help (an outsource) with the arrival of 20 volunteers to help with a flooded home (Bledsoe, 2009; Wikipedia, 2011a) (Fig. 4.4).

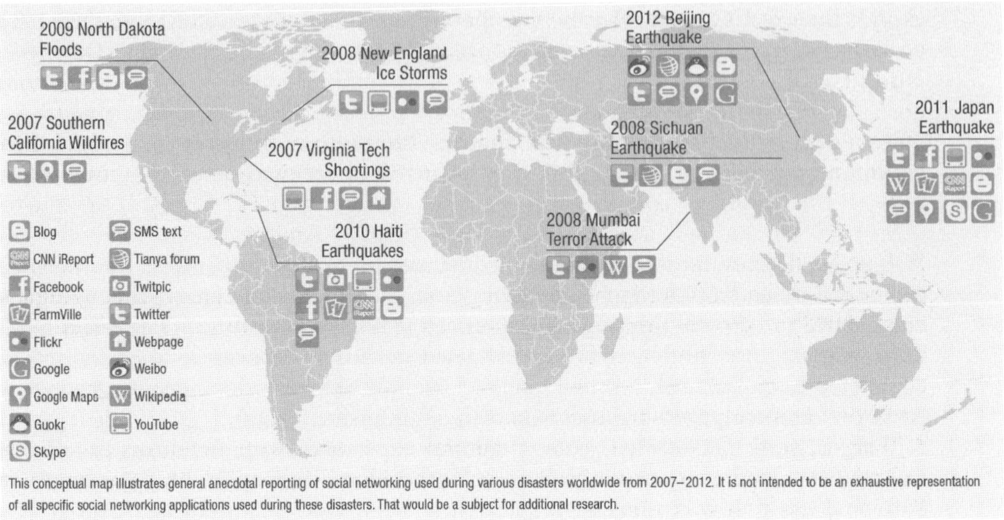

Fig. 4.4. Social networking map.

2010 Haiti earthquakes: social networking applications actively and creatively kept global interest and help alive, and CNN used iReport on its website for citizen reporting and contact information

During Haiti's powerful 2010 earthquakes, official communications were heavily damaged, but social networking substantially filled the critical information breach. Within seconds, Twitter provided information bursts as well as photos, through Twitpic (The Nation, 2010). Flickr and YouTube were sources of visual testimony as well, coming not just from citizens but from mainstream media such as the British Broadcasting Corporation (BBC) (Bunz, 2010; The Nation, 2010). The *Guardian*, another mainstream media source, set up a live blog for coverage of the rescue mission (Bunz, 2010). Cable News Network (CNN) coverage was noteworthy for its 2-year-old website section, iReport, a place where anyone could upload video reports. Verification of grassroots reports is important. CNN made efforts to verify reports, requiring contact information with the uploads. When verification was not possible, CNN clearly stated so (Bunz, 2010). In the early hours after the earthquake, CNN's iReports managed to accomplish two live interviews through its own reporters, while volunteers logged 218 quake reports in a very short time despite downed communications, and posted 212 reports of missing persons. CNN made efforts to verify these grassroots reports, and was able to confirm 17 of the quake reports and 13 missing persons reports (Bunz, 2010). Based in large part on CNN's exceptional use of social media and iReports, its viewership logged 1.4 million views, representing a 240% increase over its September–October period (Bunz, 2010).

Social networking also contributed significantly to the aid effort in Haiti when its multiple organizations served as conduits for donations and volunteer efforts. The Red Cross Twitter account grew from its usual 50–100 followers to 10,000 after the earthquake. Red Cross also reported that over US$8 million had been raised by people who donated by simply texting from their mobile phones, HAITI to 90999, which added US$10 to their mobile phone bills (The Nation, 2010). Facebook, too, provided a venue for donations through its popular FarmVille game played by millions the world over. It introduced the crop 'white corn', a special commodity that had to be purchased through real money for donation to Haiti's relief fund (The Nation, 2010). Additionally, Facebook actively posted updates on Haiti at the rate of over 1500 per minute, according to its spokesman, Andrew Noyes (The Nation, 2010). Thus, as authors Keim and Noji observed, 'social media became the new forum for collective intelligence (Vieweg *et al.*, 2008), social convergence (Hughes *et al.*, 2008), and community activism related to the Haiti disaster' (Keim and Noji, 2011, p. 49).

Japan's 11 March 2011 triple disaster of earthquake, tsunami and nuclear plant failures demolished whole coastal regions: social media organizations mobilized to assist, as did private organizations using social media, and the US government communicated through social media, too

The public's use of social media

Before its communications and other infrastructures were shattered by the multiple disasters of 2011, Japan had been known as a nation of social networkers, with an estimated 2.5 million Japanese Facebook users and 20 million Twitter users (Lee, 2011). After the earthquake struck, most communications were down, but the Japanese quickly turned to the internet and multiple social media applications to talk of the event and their direct experiences with their friends and the world (Shaw, 2011). Within the first hour, news from Japan was travelling through Twitter at the rate of 1200 tweets a minute. Tweets were arriving so rapidly that they could not actually be read in time, a 'throttle' issue and not uncommon when disasters occur (Stephens, 2011). To maintain social connections, avid Twitter users relied on applications such as HootSuite and TweetDeck to regulate Twitter feeds (Stephens, 2011) and to increase capacity for additional social networks and photos (Morris, 2010). People without a phone service were still able to use the internet's Skype and 'Facebook chat' to communicate with friends and loved ones (Shaw, 2011). One earthquake victim managed to take a video while inside a house as the earthquake occurred, and rapidly posted it on YouTube, where over 2.4 million viewers watched it in less than 24 h (Shaw, 2011). Another took a video of the on-going damage as the earth shook and posted it on to CNN's iReport. CNN requested him to participate in a live interview, which he did via Skype and wearing a headset (Owens, 2011). Because iReports was positioned to include many other first-hand reports by citizen journalists throughout the first week, its coverage outperformed competing cable news organizations that were challenged with getting reporters in the field. Consequently, CNN's ratings jumped from the bottom to the top, with more than 2 million viewers some days (Owens, 2011).

Social media organizations activate aid

As with the Haiti earthquake, social media organizations stepped forward to actively support a robust response effort. Within an hour post-quake, Google established Google Person Finder, a tool for people to post information on those they are looking for, or those they know something about who have been missing. Google also made its Person Finder easy to embed into other websites, to help spread information on the source's availability and to facilitate its use. By 15 March the site had recorded nearly 200,000 posts (Lee, 2011). Additionally, Google rapidly created the Crisis Response Information page as a resource for gathered information on blackouts, shelters, contacts, new or continuing developments, maps and whatever else was important to response efforts (Lee, 2011). Famous for its maps, Google also enhanced its Google Earth and Google Maps teams to offer response teams and the public alike a means for aiding their search efforts through satellite imagery (Lee, 2011). Facebook was a venue for multiple pages created to keep people informed, to organize aid, and to sponsor and organize donations for groups using search-and-rescue dogs (Lee, 2011). And Twitter was initially and continually instrumental as a source for keeping people informed, for reaching out and comforting, and for contact information (Lee, 2011).

Private organizations use social media to activate aid

As also with the disaster in Haiti, social media were used to inform people of various ways to donate. An example of this kind of community organizational engagement was through Telus Canada, a communications company that donated to the United Nations Children's Fund (UNICEF), the Red Cross and the Salvation Army, then matched its employees' donations, then offered a convenient way for customers to donate through their mobile phones by texting QUAKE to 45678 to donate CAN$10 to Canada's Salvation Army, or texting ASIA to 30333 to donate CAN$5 to Canada's Red Cross Society (Shaw, 2011). And also, as with Haiti's earthquake, Zynga's FarmVille, played on Facebook, was used as a vehicle for donations. The day after Japan's earthquake, virtual farmers were able to purchase a non-withering crop, 100% of which was donated to the charity, Save the Children (Gaulin, 2011).

An SOS YouTube video inspires non-profit organizational response

As weeks went by in Japan and the hazards of nuclear exposure were an increasing health issue, response efforts were challenged due to concerns about radiation exposure. Minamisoma, a small town in Japan 14 miles away from the damaged nuclear plant, had been cut off from arriving shipments of food, and everyone in town was instructed to shelter-in-place. The mayor, Katsunobu Sakurai, was desperate because his multiple appeals for aid had been ignored. A resident filmed him on his small digital camera in an 11-min video in which he pleaded for supplies and help from their isolated, untenable situation. They posted it on YouTube the next day with the title, 'SOS from Minamisoma mayor'. Instantly, interest in it 'went viral', and it gained over 200,000 viewers 2 weeks after the post, while the mayor continued to also receive calls. More important than the calls were the truckloads of food and other relief goods from responsive non-profit organizations. The Mayor felt their success was due to the YouTube video: 'Suddenly, the world was extending its hand to us' (Fackler, 2011).

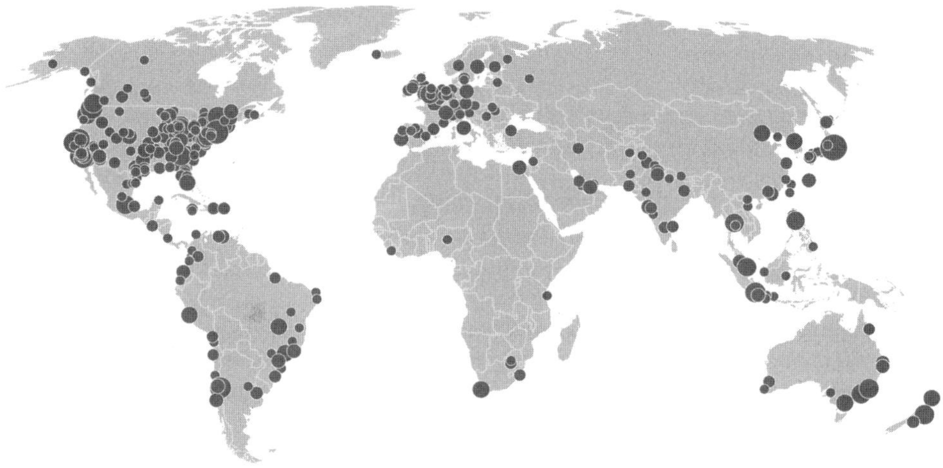

Fig. 4.5. Social networking heat map (from Sysomos.com). During and after the 2011 earthquake/tsunami, Japan's 'wired' communities initially used Twitter to tell the world of the disaster. This 'heat map' shows how people around the globe came together by tweeting the hashtags: #earthquake, #Japan, #tsunami and #prayforJapan.

US government uses social media for disaster messaging

Because it has an air base there and has an infrastructure and trained personnel particularly suited to function in austere and chaotic conditions, the US military was positioned for a rapid response to meet the desperate, multidimensional needs of post-quake/tsunami/nuclear-threatened Japan. Within a day, the US Department of Defense initiated Operation Tomodachi (Operation Friendship), a joint land–sea–air exercise bringing service people with multiple critical capabilities, including medical, civil engineering and communications, to provide aid where and as needed. Support relief operations included 'command and control, aviation and logistics', as well as basic food and shelter (Baker III, 2011). The type of boots-on-the-ground experience the military brings in disaster response is essential, and often military research and development in medical trauma has direct application in civilian disaster medicine, as is discussed later in the chapter.

The US Department of State focused immediately on disaster communications to resident and visiting US citizens. The State Department used Twitter for rapid messaging on the day the earthquake hit: '#Japan: Telephone lines disrupted; try contacting loved ones by email, text (SMS) message, or through @twitter &

facebook. #earthquake' (Stephens, 2011). This was timely, essential, concise disaster communications, and the State Department used social media for that, instantly and simply, in communications modalities the people use daily. Tellingly, social media applications were available for communications use when conventional modalities were down.

By 21 March, the US Department of Health and Human Services released a situation report on its Public Health Emergency (PHE) website, affirming its commitment 'to provide any requested public health and medical support to the government of Japan in the aftermath of the earthquake, tsunami and subsequent nuclear power plant emergency' (Public Health Emergency, 2011). Pursuant to that pledge, the Department of Health and Human Services dispatched three subject matter specialists to provide aid to the US embassy and consulates in Japan (Public Health Emergency, 2011). People in the USA were becoming concerned for their own health, from exposure to radiation in the air arriving on the westerly winds from Japan, and about radiation levels in imported goods from Japan. By 7 April, the PHE situation report addendum added information online for the US public specifically regarding the efforts of multiple agencies involved in assessing risks to public health. The Food and Drug Agency (FDA) was monitoring food and medical products from Japan; the Environmental Protection Agency (EPA) was monitoring radiation levels in the air; and the FDA was issuing warnings to consumers of drugs sold over the internet, for people to be cautious of false claims of drugs that treat or prevent radiation. The public was told to refer to the FDA's link for radiation safety, with a hyperlink included for easy reference. The bulk of the addendum to the situation report, however, focused on the CDC's efforts to keep US residents informed on how to better understand health threats and protect their health accordingly (Public Health Emergency, 2011). This is further discussed below.

2012 Beijing floods: crowdsourcing volunteers created timely, accurate flood maps of critical flood sites then widely circulated them to citizen responders who warned and rescued flood victims in advance of, then later in cooperation with, government-based efforts

In the past 1000 years Beijing has had a history of serious floods, and of those since formal record-keeping began in 1951, officials ranked the flash floods on 21 July 2012 the worst (The Economist, 2012). Damage tolls include 70 deaths, 1.5 million lives affected and US$1.6 billion in economic losses (iRevolution, 2012). The social networking site Sina Weibo reported more than 8.8 million posts by 24 July (Weiwei, 2012). Internet-savvy citizens responded rapidly with essential, wide-ranging activities that were crowd sourced to take advantage of multiple talents and availability levels. A group in the technical, science-focused social network at Guokr.com formed to rapidly create a highly accurate, user-friendly flood map of high-damage areas. The maps were broadly circulated on Weibo and served both as warnings and rescue focus areas. Further, the map was generated a day before one developed by the Beijing Water Authority, whose official map was considered by the general public to be not only late but confusing (Nedzhvetskaya, 2012). The citizen-created map worked through Google, and thus took advantage of Google Earth and features that allowed responders to plan routes, do nearby searches, and gather more information (Nedzhvetskaya, 2012).

Volunteers used texting and social networking for rescue and sheltering efforts too. Not only did they link needy victims with individual home sheltering, but volunteers also organized a free shuttle service to transport thousands of victims stranded at the airport (The Economist, 2012). Additionally, microbloggers organized essential early rescues through team efforts among themselves as well as with police by creating a rescue code with their car lights using double flashes to cue the police to come to the rescue (Weiwei, 2012). Tellingly, social netizens are quick to appreciate not just the potential immediate benefits of their effort for efficient, life-saving emergency response, but also the social benefits for building community resilience, both on- and off-line. 'The more digital volunteers engage in crisis mapping, the more they highlight the local capacity and agency of ordinary citizens to create shared awareness and help themselves – with or without the state. In doing so, volunteers build social capital, which facilitates future collective action both on *and* offline' (italics in original text) (iRevolution, 2012).

How the CDC Communicates in Public Health Preparedness and Disasters, and Includes Social Media in Risk Management

As previously discussed, the CDC had assimilated lessons learned from the 2001 anthrax attacks, and had transformed its Emergency Communication Department into teams of multi-levelled leadership with specific functions, down to branches of equivalently significant, multispecialized communications functions (Vanderford, 2009). Learning from its previous mistakes, the CDC also studied the science of disaster communications, to determine what elements are critical to effective communications when disaster strikes, and what preparations can be made to avoid early and costly mistakes. Most important is establishing trust between the response organization and the public. Trust will open up the possibility for the public to hear the message, but other critical elements must co-exist to reinforce that trust: the message must show transparency, communications must be made early, the message must show the speaker knows and understands the audience and plans must include consideration of all these elements pre-disaster, so the public's trust is warranted when disaster strikes (Vanderford, 2009).

Communications to the US public post-2011 Japanese triple disaster

In the case of the Japanese triple disaster, the CDC activated its Emergency Operations Center (EOC) in Atlanta immediately after receiving word of the 11 March 2011 earthquake, tsunami and radiation release in Japan. Its purpose was to closely monitor events and be readily available to support Japan's public health agency requests in any way the CDC could help (CDC, 2011a). In the USA, as evacuating passengers began arriving from Japan, the CDC provided a protocol to US Customs and Border Protection to aid in screening the arrivees. At the same time, the CDC gave arriving passengers alert notices, travel advisories and factsheets on health information and/or medical care. The CDC also posted these health alert documents on its radiation emergencies web page, located within the general emergency preparedness and response website. Note that the CDC followed its effective communications imperatives discussed above when it generated the following health alerts (Public Health Emergency, 2011):

- '2011 Earthquake, Tsunami, and Radiation Release in Japan'
- '2011 Earthquake and Tsunami in Japan; Health Information for Expatriates and Students Living in Japan'
- '2011 Earthquake and Tsunami in Japan: Health Information for Humanitarian Aid Workers'
- 'Potassium Iodide (KI): Frequently Asked Questions'
- 'FAQs About Iodine-131 Found in Surface Water'
- 'FAQs About Iodine-131 Found in Milk'

The CDC's use of social media in health campaigns during potential disasters

The CDC created its Social Media: 2011 Japan Earthquake and Tsunami web page (CDC, 2011a) for its partner agencies and other concerned organizations to keep the worried public informed about potential health threats related to the 2011 Japanese radiation release. The site shows various social media tools that can be used to alert and inform. The CDC also conducted a campaign during the 2009 H1N1 'flu epidemic, and it used social media based on evidence-driven strategies to protect and foster the health of its multi-faceted demographics (CDC, 2009a). Working with the Department of Health and Human Services, the CDC developed a number of social media messages and tools that its partners – such as state, regional and local health agencies – could also use to inform the public about how to protect their health, the health of their families and communities. Among social media tools used were mobile information, widgets and online videos. The objective was to take advantage of the networking, interactivity and information sharing integral to social networking (CDC, 2009a; Fig. 4.6)

The CDC's list of social media tools, with guidelines and best practices for effective use

The CDC has built a list of social media tools for its health partners to plan, develop and integrate social media in broad-reaching communications strategies. Also provided are guidelines and best practices, so other agencies and private organizations will not have to 'reinvent the wheel' to effectively implement these tools (CDC, 2011b). In its 2010 'The Health Communicator's Social Media Toolkit' download, the CDC includes button and badges, image sharing (Flickr, Facebook, Picasa), content syndication, Really Simple Syndication (RSS) feeds, podcasts, online video sharing (YouTube), widgets, e-cards, electronic games (eGames), mobile health (mHealth), microblogs (Twitter), blogs, social networking sites (Facebook, MySpace, LinkedIn) and virtual world (health-related examples are Health and Medicine in Second Life Blog from the National Library of Medicine; Why Eat in Whyville; AIDS.gov's Virtual World Page).

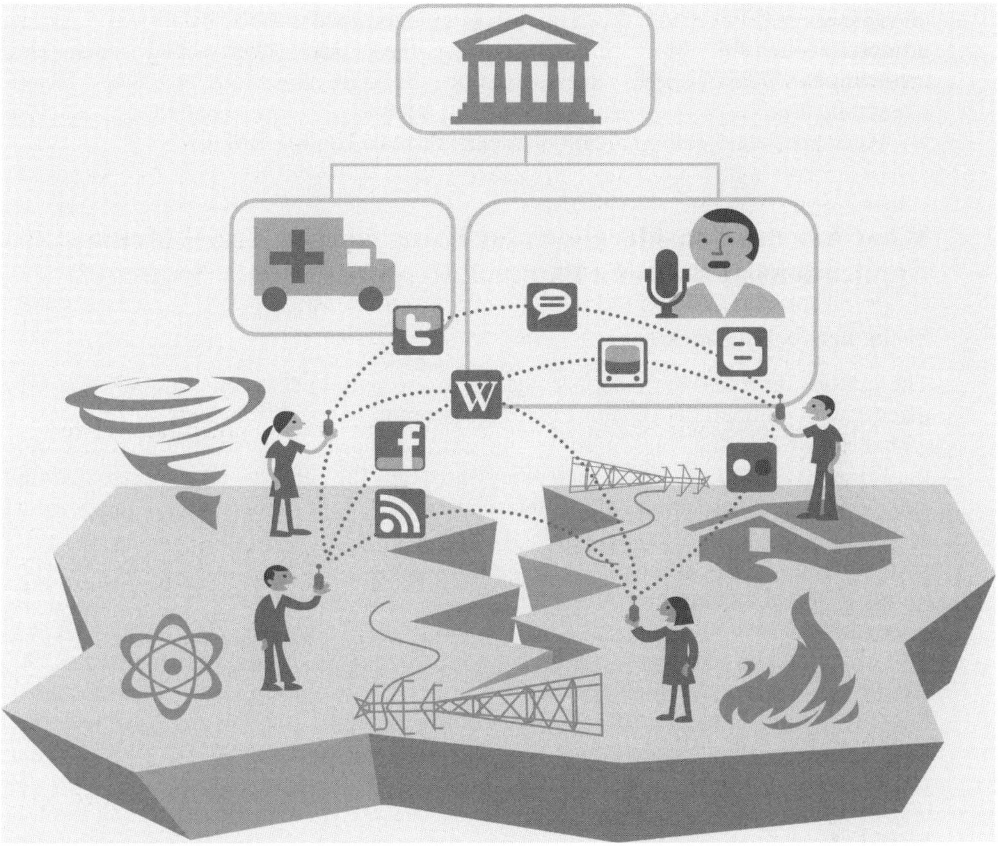

Fig. 4.6. Integrated communications concept: in the integrated communications concept, public health and disaster management agencies have already included multiple social networking modalities not just in their disaster communications plans, but into their routine communications culture on a regular basis. Over time, they have established a relationship of trust and a reputation as a reliable source of information for general good health as well as for disaster response. They have become partners with local, regional, state and federal agencies in the common cause of effective proactive health building as much as for disaster planning and management. Just as importantly, the public is included as a partner in participating in their routine health, their preparedness for disasters *and* in building their community's resilience.

These tools can variously assist in a range of health and disaster medicine communications, from generally promoting good health practices to issuing critically needed crisis messages during disasters, when standard forms of communication are down. Those social media tools that have particular pertinence to disaster preparedness and response have actually already demonstrated their spontaneous public utility in the specific disasters discussed above. A closer look at the three most used applications – social networking sites (Facebook), microblogging (Twitter) and photo sharing (Flicker and YouTube) – as planned media tools, by formal response groups, is helpful. More information on these and other social networking applications listed above are available through the CDC's 'The Health Communicator's Social Media Toolkit' at www.cdc.gov/healthcommunication/…/SocialMediaToolkit_BM.pdf.

What Are the Considerations for Using Certain Social Media Applications as Part of a Planned, Response-agency Strategy?

Social networking sites

The reasons for a disaster response agency to use social networking include that they offer a communications medium that can potentially reach hundreds of millions of global followers, they are used by an extraordinarily diverse, multinational and multilingual group of followers, they provide the ability to generate prompt situational updates, they offer interoperability with other social networking applications through links and photo sharing, they permit calendar posting and offer invitations and they allow for comments (Bledsoe, 2009). The CDC has profiled users of social networking. Of adults in the USA 18 years and older using the internet, 46% used a social networking site as of 2009 (Lenhart, 2009). The CDC has also broken down user demographics by age, income level and ethnic group (CDC, 2010a). This information is important for response agencies to know, because part of building the trust needed for effective communications is knowing your audience. Trust-building also requires that you have a credible record of presence and transparency. Agencies cannot have personal pages in social networks, but they can construct 'fan pages' or 'groups' (Bledsoe, 2009). By viewing and becoming familiar with the social networking site, an agency can construct its own page to best project its policy, current and on-going comments, posts that will engage its demographic, and other ways to promote the agency's purpose and meaning in the life and language of the public it seeks to reach (CDC, 2010a). It also provides a means for evaluating effectiveness, because 'friends', likes/dislikes and comments are quantifiably logged by viewers. This is a way to begin building, pre-disaster, the trust necessary for the effective risk communications so necessary during a disaster, and it has a built-in means for an agency to quickly evaluate its messaging success. This social networking presence can also help build and sustain a sense of community support. Results from the recent Pew-Annenberg Research Study mentioned earlier indicated social networkers were more likely to be politically engaged, more socially aware and more inclined to act collectively (Evangelista, 2011). These qualities are essential building blocks for community resilience.

Microblogging

Microblogging is defined as text messaging limited to 140 characters, which may also include interoperable links to other networking applications for photos, videos or web addresses (Bledsoe, 2009). Twitter, the most common microblog application, has demonstrated its utility in the examples of disasters with spontaneous social networking use listed above. Advantages are: it allows communication to a group in real time, feedback from the 'tweet' to the community is quick and its message can be 'retweeted' by others for maximal, even 'viral' effect (Bledsoe, 2009). Some emergency managers have found it an effective tool to disseminate information quickly, to connect rapidly with experts for advice on best practices or quick input and to listen and gather information for gauging what the community is saying regarding concerns, gossip or rumours (Bledsoe, 2009; CDC, 2010a). Microbloggers are individuals and corporations, non-governmental organizations (NGOs) and federal agencies.

Information systems specialists at the University of Buffalo, State University of New York, published a 2009 paper supporting planned use of Twitter as a potential means for emergency management to coordinate a rapid, integrated response effort. First, it is free, platform-independent and users can send their short messages by 'most internet-enabled devices capable of text messaging' (Mills *et al.*, 2009). While they concede disadvantages, it has substantial advantages. The most obvious have been discussed; it is already a popular application users select for rapid communications in challenged environments when time and information are critical. Another advantage is the 'benevolent culture' of Twitter users, who eagerly 'share, search for, and relay information on the internet and the Twitter.com network' – which lends itself to crowdsourcing for volunteering and improvising essential task completions during emergencies (Mills *et al.*, 2009). It supports a 'track' feature that facilitates connecting information updates in real time. It uses low bandwidth due to its short message, which is more reliable during disasters. Further, text messages, whether tweets or plain text messages, have the substantial advantage that they stay 'queued' until delivered, in contrast to mobile or landline phones (Mills *et al.*, 2009). Additionally, research supports the premise that short-term memory relies on visual cues, and words written are retained better than words heard (Hilton, 2001). An important disadvantage for Twitter is that it currently does not have a powerful, integrated system for geographic information that would be sufficiently streamlined for reliable emergency response management (Mills *et al.*, 2009).

Image sharing and YouTube

The CDC defines its use of image sharing as 'posting images (photos, artwork, etc.) to public websites where they can be viewed, tagged, categorized, and even used by others' (CDC, 2010c). Common sources for photo sharing are Flickr and Shutterfly, while YouTube is well known and used the world over for videos. Image sharing has vast utility for health professionals. An agency can use it to provide visuals for increasing general public health interest and awareness. Emergency medical professionals can share photos with doctors in trauma situations as diagnostic aids, or as previews to inform and prepare surgeons for the field trauma injury cases arriving for emergency treatment in the emergency department or the field equivalent.

General security concerns relating to using social network applications

The CDC has developed a download entitled Social Media Security Mitigations that lists vulnerability concerns in using social media and offers recommendations to mitigate their effects. It also provides multiple appendices for agencies to evaluate individual sites, offers sample rules of behaviour for using social media sites and explains how to conduct social media site monitoring (CDC, 2009b). Problems can include receiving web-mail that bypasses the agency filter, public comments that might be vulnerable to 'phishing' attacks, mal-attacks from 'malicious friends' who might change profiles and post inappropriate content in multiple ways and applications from malicious sources (CDC, 2009b). These concerns as well as other potential security issues should be investigated and mitigations for them planned prior to engaging in formal use of social media sites.

Disaster Medicine and Social Media

Web 2.0 and social media have not become infused into the field of disaster medicine to the same extent as they have in public health preparedness and disaster response such as that done by the CDC. One reason is the impact on patient–doctor relations. Others include concerns for the methods and tools establishing privacy and ownership, as well as methods and tools used for information accuracy (Potts *et al.*, 2008). Additionally, as Web 2.0 medical information has flourished, the medical community has increasing concerns about manipulation of information through search engines' secretive, algorithm-based ranking, and also concerns about reliability of information generally (Krimsky, 2007).

Telemedicine, a technology relying on satellite communications that was developed by the National Aeronautics and Space Administration (NASA), first became a disaster response tool in Mexico City's 1985 earthquake (Garshnek and Burkle, 1999). It has been used since then throughout the world in disaster-related situations, whether natural or human-made. Even before the 2011 triple disaster, earthquake-prone Japan had closely studied the logistical use of satellite telecommunications including how many channels might be needed for different degrees of disaster when telemedicine would be used for such purposes as case management, consultation, diagnosis and transportation coordination. Factors they considered in gauging transmission needs included uses like communications from ambulance to hospital (moving to fixed) and hospital to hospital (fixed to fixed) (Nagami *et al.*, 2008). During the Armenian earthquake of 1988, the satellite communications through both Intelsat and Comsat provided clinical consultation between multiple Armenian hospitals and four major US medical centres (fixed to fixed). Consultations among physician specialities including orthopaedics, infectious disease, general surgery, neurology and psychiatry were accomplished via two-way interactive audio and unidirectional full-motion video to transmit (Garshnek and Burkle, 1999). By the time Haiti suffered its 1994 earthquake, the US military included telemedicine equipment in its response that had improved capabilities for video teleconferencing and the ability to transmit digitized radiographic films and other digital images (Garshnek and Burkle, 1999).

Satellite-based communications are core to telemedicine during disasters, because conventional telecommunications transmissions rely upon both direct (land lines) and wireless linkages (using the entire bandwidth frequency, primarily via radio). Wireless transmissions do not rely on traditional electrical and telephone equipment, which is extremely helpful when those infrastructures are damaged in disasters. Still when disasters damage essential wireless structures too, like base stations and radio towers, wireless communications can also be disabled (Garshnek and Burkle, 1999). With satellite technology, long distance communications are still possible when direct and wireless infrastructures fail, but satellite infrastructures are quite expensive, leaving smaller governments and response organizations without effective means to communicate during disasters. Low earth orbit (LEO) nongeostationary satellite technology may be very helpful in addressing several of the current problems with satellite systems due to the satellites' ability to stay closer to the earth and therefore transmit and receive more readily. This allows for the possibility of using more portable terminals such as cell phones, a substantial advantage for disaster responders (Garshnek and Burkle, 1999).

The US Army Medical Research Institutes of Infectious Diseases and Chemical Defense have designed a prototype application for a specific type of medical disaster management that employs a mobile Apple iPod touch platform. It is particularly designed for use during a chemical, biological, radiological and nuclear (CBRN) attack (Williamson, 2011). In that type of disaster, such a device would be essential because medical responders would likely have varied levels of training, if any at all, in CBRNE symptoms and they would need assistance in creating a differential diagnosis list and treatment plan. Additionally, protocols for identification and treatment must be evidence-based. In such a chaotic, possibly austere, environment, the prototype would supplement the healthcare responder's clinical knowledge, and would also provide standardized, evidence-based algorithms and emergency protocols for CBRNE-related disaster illness and injuries (Williamson, 2011). Other features of the application include medical learning modules and animated videos (Williamson, 2011). It is currently in the evaluation stage.

Finally, Web 2.0 values of open sharing and collaboration are becoming incorporated into the general medical field, as blogs, wikis and image sharing expand and alter medicine. Updated information can be culled through an RSS reader (Bloglines), aggregated with MedWorm, and shared on blogs (Giustini, 2006). An example of an often-visited medical blog is Ves Dimov's Clinical Cases and Images, where information and images (sometimes through Flickr) have been gathered through 'presurfing' and are available for interactive sharing and discussion (Giustini, 2006). Still, as a medical doctor and an experienced blogger, Dimov warns that information gleaned from RSS feeds, Twitter and other blogs should always be checked against the original journal article source. One reason for his caution is that often the social media, secondary source, reported results are far less nuanced than those from the original source. Another significant reason is that web companies are increasingly striving to tailor information to the user, but in doing so, they are placing users in less objective 'filter bubbles' that do not include information contrary to or outside the user's 'world view' (Dimov, 2011). Still, if there is familiarity with the benefits and knowledge of the disadvantages, there is potential for these applications to be creatively and usefully adapted to fill medical disaster response needs, particularly if done with sharing and collaboration.

Conclusion

In less than a decade, social media have revolutionized traditional communications, and changed the world in the process. Where conventional communications media have been centrally controlled and hierarchically structured, social media are horizontally structured, and based on peer-to-peer information sharing in a democratic culture of collaboration that has grown to hundreds of millions of global users. Social networking media comprise several qualities essential to 21st-century communications: Web 2.0-based, mobile, one-to-many capable, integrate with geographic information systems (GIS) for visual mapping, rapidly transmit and are more reliable than traditional communications modes in challenged environments (Mills *et al.*, 2009). These communications elements are essential tools for medical and emergency managers in disaster response. Further, social media have already demonstrated their significant utility by spontaneous public and organizational use in disasters to fill important needs in response efforts. This spontaneous show of public and organizational creativity and involvement, supported through the medium of social networking, indicates an underlying community resilience to disasters' chaotic impact. Evidence substantiates that community resilience is essential to successful disaster recovery, and is so important that the fundaments of community resilience need to be cultivated before disaster strikes. The most essential building block of resilience is trusted communications between a community's preparedness organizations and its public members. Social networking has already been embraced by people around the globe. It is time for the organizations charged with protecting the health of those people to constructively and deliberately join in the sharing and collaboration necessary to build a trusted relationship by using media formats the public knows and often prefers. These communications can be cultivated with planned, informed social networking use, so when disaster strikes, a resilient community can successfully recover.

Acknowledgements

The authors are grateful to Kelly Huston of the California Emergency Management Agency (Cal EMA) for his sage advice and support. Also to Karen Minot for her professional talent, creativity and generous support. And to Sheldon Levine and Sysomos for their ready generosity in sharing their map of social media global network response to the 2011 Japan earthquake.

References

Baker III, F.W. (2011) U.S. forces provide relief aid to Japan. Available at: http://www.defense.gov/news/newsarticle.aspx?id=63144 (Accessed 19 May 2011).

Beaumont, C. (2008) Mumbai attacks: Twitter and Flickr used to break news. Telegraph.co.uk. Available at: http://www.telegraph.co.uk/news/worldnews/asia/india/3530640/Mumbai-attacks-Twitter-and-Flickr-used-to-break-news-Bombay-India.html (Accessed 7 March 2013).

Bledsoe, C. (2009) Web 2.0 & Social media: from definition to deployment. Available at: http://www.oregonemergency.com/docs/conf/presentations/bledsoe.pptx (Accessed 26 May 2011).

Blendon, R.J., Benson, J.M., Desroches, C.M. and Weldon, K.J. (2003) Using opinion surveys to track the public's response to a bioterrorist attack. *Journal of Health Communications* 8, 83–92.

Bloomberg, T. (2007) Crisis management in the year 2007 and beyond. Diva Marketing Blog. Available at: http://bloombergmarketing.blogs.com/bloomberg_marketing/2007/04/our_hearts_go_o.html (Accessed 7 March 2013).

Bunz, M. (2010) In Haiti earthquake coverage, social media gives victim a voice. guardian.co.uk. Available at: http://www.guardian.co.uk/media/pda/2010/jan/14/socialnetworking-haiti (Accessed 16 May 2011).

Centers for Disease Control and Prevention (CDC) (2009a) Social media campaigns. Available at: http://www.cdc.gov/SocialMedia/Campaigns/index.html (Accessed 3 March 2011).

CDC (2009b) Social media security mitigations. Available at: http://www.cdc.gov/SocialMedia/Tools/guidelines/pdf/securitymitigations.pdf (Accessed 28 May 2011).

CDC (2010a) The Health Communicator's Social Media Toolkit. Available at: www.cdc.gov/healthcommunication/.../SocialMediaToolkit_BM.pdf (Accessed 28 May 2011).

CDC (2010b) The Risk Communicator Newsletter. Available at: http://emergency.cdc.gov/ercn/01/rcn03.asp (Accessed 3 March 2011).

CDC (2010c) Social media at CDC: image sharing. Available at: http://www.cdc.gov/socialmedia/tools/ImageSharing.html (Accessed 16 May 2011).

CDC (2011a) Social media: 2011 Japan earthquake and tsunami. Available at: http://emergency.cdc.gov/socialmedia/japan.asp (Accessed 28 May 2011).

CDC (2011b) Social media tools, guidelines & best practices. Available at: http://www.cdc.gov/SocialMedia/Tools/guidelines/ (Accessed 3 March 2011).

City of Fargo (2011) Flood homepage: flood news and events. Available at: http://www.ndsu.edu/fargoflood/ (Accessed 7 March 2013).

Comfort, L.K. (1994) Risk and resilience: interorganizational learning following the Northridge earthquake of January 17, 1994. *Journal of Contingencies and Crisis Management* 2(3), 174–188.

Dimov, V. (2011) Beware of online 'filters' that hide the information you need. Available at: http://casesblog.blogspot.com/ (Accessed 26 May 2011).

Evangelista, B. (2011) Internet: Facebook can bring friends, trust, support. *San Francisco Chronicle*, 18 June 2011, D1, 4.

Facebook (2013) Newsroom. Available at http://newsroom.fb.com/Key-Facts (Accessed 7 March, 2013).

Fackler, M. (2011) Japanese city's desperate cry resonates around the world. *The New York Times*, 7 April 2011, A1, A10.

Federal Emergency Management Agency (FEMA) (2004) NIMS and the Incident Command System. Available at: http://www.fema.gov/txt/nims/nims_ics_position_paper.txt (Accessed 17 May 2011).

Gabarain, C. (2008) Twitter and the Sichuan earthquake: proving its value? Worldbank.org. Available at: http://blogs.worldbank.org/eastasiapacific/node/2759 (Accessed 16 May 2011).

Garshnek, V. and Burkle, F.M. (1999) Applications of telemedicine and telecommunications to disaster medicine: historical and future perspectives. *Journal of the American Medical Informatics Association.* Available at: http://jamia.bmj.com/content/6/1/26.abstract (Accessed 7 March 2013).

Gaulin, P. (2011) Social gamers of Zynga's FarmVille can donate to Japan's tsunami victims. Available at: http://voices.yahoo.com/social-gamers-zyngas-farmville-donate-japans-8065856.html (Accessed 7 March 2013).

Giustini, D. (2006) How Web 2.0 is changing medicine. BMJ.com. Available at: http://www.bmj.com/content/333/7582/1283.full (Accessed 23 January 2011).

Hilton, E. (2001) Differences in visual and auditory short-term memory. Available at: http://www.iusb.edu/~journal/static/volumes/2001/hilton.htm (Accessed 16 May 2011).

Hughes, A., Palen, L., Sutton, J., Liu, S.B. and Vieweg, S. (2008) 'Site-seeing' in disaster: an examination of on-line social convergence. Paper presentation at the fifth International ISCRAM Conference, Washington, DC. Citation accessed from Keim and Noji, 2011 article (listed below) quotation at p. 49, and included in this chapter.

iRevolution (2012) Crowdsourcing a crisis map of the Beijing Floods: volunteers vs government. iRevolution.com. Available at: http://irevolution.net/2012/08/01/crisis-map-beijing-floods/ (Accessed 29 October 2012).

Keim, M.E. and Noji, E. (2011) Emergent use of social media: a new age of opportunity for disaster resilience. *American Journal of Disaster Medicine* 6(1), 47–54.

Krimsky, S. (2007) Risk communication in the internet age: the rise of disorganized skepticism. *Environmental Hazards* 7, 157–164.

Lee, J. (2011) Search and social media responses to the Japan earthquake. Bruce Clay SEO Newsletter. Available at: http://www.bruceclay.com/newsletter/volume89/vol89print.htm (Accessed 18 March 2011).

Lenhart, A. (2009) The democratization of social networks. Available as a slide share at: http://www.slideshare.net/PewInternet/the-democratization-of-online-social-networks (Accessed 7 March 2013).

LiveJournal (2011) About LiveJournal. Available at: http://www.livejournal.com/site/about.bml (Accessed 17 May 2011).

Longstaff, P.H. and Yang, S.-U. (2008) Communication management and trust: their role in building resilience to 'surprises' such as natural disasters, pandemic flu, and terrorism. *Ecology and Society* 13(1), 3. Available at: http://www.ecologyandsociety.org/vol13/iss1/art3/ (Accessed 16 May 2011).

Mills, A., Chen, R., Lee, J. and Rao, H.R. (2009) Web 2.0 emergency applications: how useful can Twitter be for emergency response? Available at: http://denman-mills.net/web_documents/jips_mills.etal._2009.07.22_finalsubmission.pdf (Accessed 7 March 2013).

Morris, J. (2010) HootSuite or TweetDeck: which Twitter client is right for you? Available at: http://www.how-to-blog.tv/microblogging/hootsuite-or-tweetdeck/ (Accessed 7 March 2013).

Nagami, K., Juzoji, H., Nakajima, I., Igarashi, K. and Tanaka, K. (2008) In search of effective telecommunication tools for telemedicine in the aftermath of disasters. *eHealth International*, 6.

Nedzhvetskaya, N. (2012) Beijing flood mapping by volunteers beats official govt site by a day. TechPresident.com. Available at: http://techpresident.com/news/22651/beijing-flood-mapping-volunteers-beats-official-govt-site-day (Accessed 29 October 2012).

Norris, F.H., Stevens, S.P., Pfefferbaum, B., Wyche, K.F. and Pfefferbaum, R.L. (2008) Community resilience as a metaphor, theory, set of capacities, and strategy for disaster readiness. *American Journal of Community Psychology* 41, 127–150.

North Dakota State University (2011) The 'Fargo Flood' homepage. Available at: http://www.ndsu.edu/fargoflood/ (Accessed 18 May 2011).

Otobi, O.G. (2010) Untapped potential: how the sphere minimum standards for disaster response could promote human and institutional resilience in northern Uganda. *Resilience: Interdisciplinary Perspectives on Science and Humanitarianism* 1, 61–76. Available at: http://fletcher.tufts.edu/Resilience/Archive/~/media/Fletcher/Microsites/Resilience/1%20resilience/Resilience_Otobi_Untapped.pdf (accessed 7 March 2013).

Owens, S. (2011) How CNN's iReport enhanced the network's coverage of the Japan earthquake and its aftermath. Niewman Journalism Lab. Available at: http://www.niemanlab.org/2011/03/how-cnns-ireport-enhanced-the-networks-coverage-of-the-japan-earthquake-and-its-aftermath/ (Accessed 27 June 2011).

Pollard, W.E. (2003) Public perceptions of information sources concerning bioterrorism before and after anthrax attacks: an analysis of national survey data. *Journal of Health Communications* 8, 93–103.

Potts, H., Skiba, D., Paton, C., Oh, H., Hughes, B., Joshi, I. and Wareham, J. (2008) Health 2.0 and Medicine 2.0: tensions and controversies in the field. *Journal of Medical Internet Research* 10 (3). Available at: http://www.ncbi.nlm.nih.gov/pmc/articles/PMC2553249/ (Accessed 7 March 2013).

Public Health Emergency (PHE), US Department of Health and Human Services (2011) Situation report: Japanese earthquake and Pacific tsunami. Available at: http://www.phe.gov/emergency/news/sitreps/Pages/pacific-earthquake-tsunami.aspx (Accessed 19 May 2011).

Qu, Y., Huang, C., Zhang, P. and Zhang, J. (2011) Harnessing social media in response to major disasters. Available at: http://www.cs.cmu.edu/~yangwan1/cscw2011/papers/CSCW2011-workshop-DSCSC.pdf (Accessed 7 March 2013).

Robinson, S.J. and Newstetter, W.C. (2003) Uncertain science and certain deadlines: CDC responses to the media during the anthrax attacks of 2001. *Journal of Health Communication* 8, 17–34.

Shaw, G. (2011) Social media stepped into high gear covering Japan's earthquake, tsunami. *Vancouver Sun*, 11 March 2011. Available at: http://blogs.vancouversun.com/2011/03/11/social-media-stepped-into-high-gear-covering-japans-earthquake-tsunami/ (Accessed 7 March 2013).

Stambor, Z. (2009) Emergency communications in 140 characters or less. Available at: http://www.prdaily.eu/crisiscommunicationsEU/Articles/Emergency_communications_in_140_characters_or_less_3621.aspx (Accessed 16 May 2011).

Stephens, K. (2011) Social media and the Japan earthquake: what we can learn. Available at: http://idisaster.wordpress.com/2011/03/12/social-media-and-the-japan-earthquake-and-tsunami-what-we-can-learn/ (Accessed 18 March 2011).

Sutton, J. (2010) Strengthening community resiliency: new media, social networks and the critical civic infrastructure. Available at: http://jeannettesutton.com/uploads/Strengthening_Community_Resiliency.pdf (Accessed 7 March 2013).

The Economist (2012) Under water and under fire. *The Economist*. Available at: http://www.economist.com/node/21559658 (Accessed 29 October 2012).

The Nation (2010) Editorial: Tragedy in Haiti proves value of social media. *The Nation.* Available at: http://www.nationmultimedia.com/2010/01/17/opinion/opinion_30120439.php (Accessed 7 March 2013).

The Sphere Project (2007) Case study – ensuring sphere standards through disaster management programme. Available at: http://www.sphereproject.org/dmdocuments/Orrisa/Case%20Study_GRC.pdf (Accessed 17 May 2011).

Tierney, K.J., Lindell, M.K. and Perry, R.W. (2001) *Facing the Unexpected: Disaster Preparedness and Response in the United States.* Joseph Henry Press, Washington, DC.

Twitter (2011) An information network. Available at: http://twitter.com/about (Accessed 14 May 2011).

Vanderford, M.L. (2009) Planning principles: OC 2. Available at: www.paho.org/English/AD/Pan_Meeting_CDC_PresentationEng.ppt (Accessed 27 May 2011).

Vieweg, S., Palen, L. and Liu, S. (2008) Collective intelligence in disaster: an examination of the phenomenon in the aftermath of the 2007 Virginia Tech shooting. Paper presentation at the fifth International ISCRAM Conference, Washington, DC. Citation accessed from Keim and Noji, 2011 article (listed above) quotation at p. 49, and included in this chapter.

Wagner, M. (2007) Google Maps and Twitter are essential information resources. informationweek.com. Available at: http://www.informationweek.com/blog/229214645 (Accessed 16 May 2011).

Weiwei, X. (2012) Social network plays vital role in rescuing Beijing flooding victims. Morningwhistle.com. Available at: http://www.morningwhistle.com/html/2012/Chinese_twitter_0724/213203.html (Accessed 29 October 2012).

Wikipedia (2011a) Crowdsourcing. Available at: http://en.wikipedia.org/wiki/Crowdsourcing (Accessed 18 May 2011).

Wikipedia (2011b) Social media. Available at: http://en.wikipedia.org/wiki/Social_media (Accessed 4 May 2011).

Wildavsky, A. (1988) *Searching for Safety.* Transaction Press, New Brunswick, New Jersey.

Williamson, H.M. (2011) Disaster management mobile protocols: a technology that will save lives. *American Journal of Disaster Medicine* 6(1), 55–64.

YouTube (2011) Statistics. Available at: http://www.youtube.com/t/press_statistics (Accessed 16 May 2011).

Chapter 5

Regional Disaster Planning for Neonatal Intensive Care

Ronald S. Cohen

Introduction

Triage began as a means for the military to deal with large numbers of casualties. It has since carried over into the civilian world, but still is designed to deal with mass casualty incidents (MCIs) occurring outside of hospitals and affecting adults and youths mainly, and only secondarily children. There is a long list of triage systems in use, but they were all designed for MCIs, and none were designed with neonates in mind (Lerner *et al.*, 2008). This may have been appropriate in the past, since there have been no documented episodes, or plausible scenarios proposed, where large numbers of newborns have been involved in an MCI (Hardy *et al.*, 1961; Acs *et al.*, 2006; Siston *et al.*, 2010). Indeed, until rather recently, even a hospital-based disaster would not have resulted in large numbers of affected neonates, since there were not large neonatal units. However, given the increased survival of preterm infants, the growth in the number of hospitals with neonatal intensive care units (NICUs) and the increased number of neonatal beds in such units, it now is necessary to consider how to respond to a disaster that might impact significant numbers of neonates and those charged with their care. Specifically, neonatologists are likely to face one of three possible disaster scenarios: (i) the need to evacuate their own unit; (ii) the need to receive large numbers of neonates from neighbouring hospitals forced to evacuate; and (iii) the need to continue functioning in the face of marked depletion of staff. Given the special needs of NICU patients, such a response would require a regionalized, cooperative approach (Cohen *et al.*, 2010b). Neonatologists with experience from Hurricane Katrina have recognized the need for regionalization (Barkemeyer, 2011; Ginsberg, 2011). Thus, this chapter will focus on: (i) developing a resource-based triage tool acceptable to all the hospitals in a region; and (ii) developing a region-wide approach to surge capacity.

Triage for NICU Patients

Thus far, systems for categorizing severity of illness in neonates have not been designed for disaster planning or triage. They have been focused on ways to categorize neonates for such purposes as counselling parents, comparing unit outcomes, normalizing data collection, etc. Thus, methods such the Clinical Risk Index for Babies (CRIB) (The International Neonatal Network, 1993) and the Score for Neonatal Acute Physiology (SNAP-II/SNAPPE-II) (Richardson *et al.*, 2001) were never designed for use as a triage tool in a disaster. Indeed, neonatal risk assessment scores have been looked at and found to become less effective at predicting mortality over the course of the NICU stay (Lim and Rozycki, 2008; Meadow *et al.*, 2012). Attempts to have knowledgeable professionals triage neonates have also proven problematic. When studied, the results were not consistent with any known ethical framework, and showed that neonates were at a significant disadvantage compared with other age groups, despite their increased potential for total quality-of-life years (Janvier *et al.*, 2008).

Since currently available neonatal acuity scales do not appear to be applicable for NICU disaster planning, systems designed for paediatric patients must be evaluated to see if they could be applied to the NICU. Once again, the existing tools are not appropriate for use by neonatology. The Pediatric Risk Index of Mortality (PRISM) has been used for over 20 years (Pollack *et al.*, 1988) largely in the USA; the Pediatric Index of Mortality (PIM) is somewhat newer and from Australia (Shann *et al.*, 1997). Both have been updated and validated in paediatric populations, but neither would be appropriate for NICU triage for several reasons. They both were designed to use data collected on admission (Leteurtre *et al.*, 2011) and thus are not appropriate for categorizing patients who may have been in NICU for weeks. The updated PIM-2 performed well for most age groups, but dramatically over-estimated risk of mortality for premature infants (Wolfler *et al.*, 2007). A new system, the Pediatric Logistic Organ Dysfunction (PELOD) score has been proposed for repeated use over a prolonged intensive care course (Leteurtre *et al.*, 2010). When validated in several paediatric units, the patients assigned the highest risk category had only a 50% (confidence interval 33.4–66.6%) mortality rate, with the mean score of non-survivors decreasing over the hospital course. One study (Bestati *et al.*, 2010), which included neonates but not premature infants, found that PELOD had a lower ability to predict mortality for neonates than for older children, with neonates in general running higher risk scores than older children. The authors were concerned about ‘the possibility of a false association between the PELOD score and death rate in neonates’. Thus, there would be ethical concerns if used for NICU triage.

Another problem with these scoring systems is that they are very heavily based upon laboratory data. Thus, they might be useful for collecting data on intensive care patients during routine function, and may be helpful for normalizing data and quality assurance purposes. However, in the midst of a major disaster, with strained resources and stretched staff, it would be difficult and perhaps impossible technically to go about collecting laboratory specimens, running the results through complex algorithms and analysing the implications of the resulting numbers. Experience in evacuating a NICU during Hurricane Katrina pointed out that without the ability to obtain radiographs and laboratory tests, they had to rely on ‘atypical triage’ (Barkemeyer, 2006). Recognizing this problem, an attempt has been made to simplify PIM-2 by using oxygen saturation measurements instead of arterial oxygen tension (Leteurtre *et al.*, 2011). The authors noted that this would be problematic in neonates for whom the oxygen saturation is commonly kept greater than

97%, making estimates of oxygen tension inaccurate, and because the fraction of inspired oxygen is impossible to determine accurately in infants on nasal prongs, oxygen hoods, face masks, etc. Measuring hepatic enzyme levels, creatinines, bilirubins, etc., required for these scoring systems would also be difficult technically for units in a crisis. Therefore, we are unable to triage NICU patients accurately by predicted morbidity or mortality with currently available tools.

A review of the experience with Hurricane Katrina in New Orleans (Klein *et al.*, 2008) stated that 'experience clearly emphasizes that triage assessment tools should be developed … for access to definitive care and resources'. A case has been made recently for resource-based triage for hospitalized neonates (Cohen *et al.*, 2010b). Given the three likely scenarios that neonatal units might expect to face, described above, and the lack of other proven systems for predicting mortality accurately, triage based on resource need is a practical option. The crucial thing for an NICU in a disaster would be to identify resource needs and their availability. NICUs would need to work together throughout a city or region to do this. This would require the development of systems to codify both the resource needs of the patients and the resources available in the region. All the hospitals in the region would have to adopt and understand the system to facilitate communication and movement of patients and resources as possible. This point was made by the Working Group on Emergency Mass Critical Care (Rubinson *et al.*, 2005): 'Regional planning among hospitals and between hospitals and state agencies intended to share personnel, patient loads, medicines, and medical equipment'. This is commensurate with recommendations made by the Task Force for Mass Critical Care (Rubinson *et al.*, 2008): 'Every hospital with an ICU should plan and prepare … in coordination with regional hospital planning efforts'. This type of regional disaster planning has been called 'Fourth Order' triage (Bostick *et al.*, 2008). For a region-wide, resource-based triage tool to be useful in the face of a major disaster affecting one or more NICUs, several criteria had to be met.

The first criterion is that it should be readily incorporated into NICU routine. It could then be part of 'pre-planning'. A tool that could categorize patients in terms of resource needs during routine NICU operation would allow for patients to be triaged at the moment a disaster strikes, obviating the need to impose an additional work burden on the staff in the midst of dealing with a stressful, perhaps terrifying, unique event. Clearly, this would be of major importance in a situation requiring immediate evacuation, but it would still be beneficial for more deliberate patient disbursement.

The second criterion is simplicity. The tool needs to be applied to the population of a large NICU with minimal expenditure of time and effort. Luckily, resource-based tools lend themselves to this. They do not require drawing blood or running analyses, and can be designed without the need for complex algorithms. Also they can be built into an electronic medical records system, if available, since any modern one should routinely incorporate data on patient resource use.

Third, it needs to be easily communicated and understood. During disasters, communication remains one of the more crucial problems (Mattox, 2006). There would be neither the time nor the manpower available to sign out patients individually in the midst of the emergency evacuation of a large NICU. Furthermore, there probably would not be direct NICU-to-NICU communication. Under the current incident command system used in the USA, communications would be routed from the NICU to the hospital command centre. From there, requests for ambulances and equipment would be communicated to a regional command centre, where someone, certainly not a neonatologist, would be charged with arranging the appropriate transport equipment and team, and finding an appropriate receiving unit. Thus the request would pass through at least three, if not more, people, after leaving the NICU staff. Clearly, it would be advantageous to have this communication be reduced to a simple, widely understood, code.

Lastly, of course, the tool would have to be adopted by all the NICUs in the region. Thus, all would be able to speak and understand the same code. If the tool meets the above criteria, regional acceptance would likely follow readily.

At the Lucile S. Packard Children's Hospital at Stanford (LPCH), a tool was designed using these criteria, to triage neonates using resource allocation (TRAIN, Table 5.1).

Table 5.1. Triaging Resource Allocation in Neonates (TRAIN)©.

Transport	Car	BLS	Critical care	Special team	None
Color Code	Blue	Green	Yellow	Red	Black
Respiratory	Stable	Hood – Cannula	Vent – stable	Vent – unstable	DNR
Monitoring	None	CRM +/– Sat*	CRM & Sat*	CRM & Sat	DNR
Medical	NP-Peds	NP-Peds	NP-Neo	Neo	DNR
Nutrition	PO feeds	PO + NG	NG + IV	NPO on TPN	DNR
Pharmacy	PO meds	PO/IV Meds	IV Drip x×1	IV drip >2	DNR
NP = Nurse Practitioner					
Neo = Neonatologists					
Peds = Paediatrician					
Vent – stable = continuous positive airway pressure, high-flow cannula, conventional ventilation, etc.					
Vent – unstable = high frequency ventilation, nitric oxide extra-corporeal membrane oxygenation, pneumothoraces, etc.					
CRM = cardio-respiratory monitoring					
Sat = oxygen saturation monitoring					
DNT = Do Not Transport, for patients whose resources needs prevent movement					
* = monitoring may be intermittent					

It was simple to use, and could be performed by the charge nurse in a NICU during rounds, adding only about 3 min (Cohen *et al.*, 2010a). Since the original pilot, TRAIN has been used in several disaster drills. This has led to modifications to simplify TRAIN and improve its functionality. For example, the scarcity of medical personnel after Hurricane Katrina resulted in physicians working outside of their usual role (Ginsberg, 2011). Thus, TRAIN was simplified by eliminating the 'Medical' criteria from the system. It is being expanded to encompass all paediatric in-patients, and the electronic medical record is being modified to provide automated TRAIN functionality. It has already been incorporated into routine daily function at several other NICUs in our region, and in some other parts of California (A.O. Hopper, from Loma Linda at the Sixth Annual Canadian Neuroscience Meeting (CAN) Meeting in March 2012: personal communication; D.N. Carbine, from San Diego at the Seventh Annual Canadian Neuroscience (CAN) Meeting in March 2013: personal communication).

Surge Capacity for NICU Patients

Most hospitals have plans for surge capacity, but there remains a need for planned, systematic, regional cooperation. This was made very clear by the experience with Hurricane Katrina. During that disaster, those needing to evacuate paediatric patients found that 'disaster plans are not designed to accommodate such patient movement, they did not facilitate such efforts but actually impeded them' (Baldwin *et al.*, 2006). The impact of severe acute respiratory syndrome (SARS) on hospital operations in Canada did not seem to have discernible impact on NICU mortality (Stukel *et al.*, 2008). However, the impact of Hurricane Katrina on infant mortality is unclear because of the dispersion of babies to several different states and the difficulty determining the impact of the storm on the course of an already critically ill patient (Brunkard *et al.*, 2008). Clearly, the dispersion of a large number of NICU patients through multiple states was a strain on our healthcare system. Hospitals had to care for patients for several days in some cases, under far from optimum conditions. The ability to expand the number of available NICU beds in surrounding unaffected hospitals would have been helpful, particularly if this could have been accomplished and communicated to a regional command centre in a rapid fashion.

Another concern regards the location of surge capacity beds for neonates. It is plausible that the needs of some paediatric patients, particularly older teens, might be met by adult facilities. However, children with special needs would need to be moved to specialized centres (Baldwin *et al.*, 2006). Specifically, it would be inappropriate to move NICU patients to hospitals staffed and equipped for adult patients. Thus, neonatal units need to be prepared to absorb an influx of patients during a disaster, which could mean potentially altering their usual standard of care in terms of both physical plant and staffing. If this needs to be done, it would be better done according to plans and guidelines carefully thought out and tested in advance, and not done haphazardly under pressure. In making such plans, it would be wise to assume that other units (e.g. paediatric and adult units) might also be forced to handle a surge in census during the same disaster, and thus it would not be possible to 'parasitize' their space. It seems best for NICUs to plan for additional surge capacity within their own space and not rely on being able to expand into other clinical areas within their own facility.

The need for 'intra-mural' surge capacity is further underscored by the lessons of Hurricane Katrina (Mattox, 2006), specifically that 'All disaster response is local (at least for the first 48–96 hours)', and 'Most successes or failures in disaster response are determined within the first 36 hours.' Thus a damaged hospital might need to continue some operations for a period of time while arranging for evacuation. Assuming some parts of the physical plant may remain in operation, they may need to absorb patients from other areas in the same medical centre. For this, every area should be examined for potential surge capacity. Specifically, every NICU should look at how it could add space to care for neonates, not just those arriving from distal affected units, but potentially for their own patients needing to be moved for 'shelter in place' should their own facility be damaged.

It has been suggested that surge capacity plans can be based on arbitrary assumptions that units can double or even quadruple their capacity (Kanter and Moran, 2007). This seems dubious given the experience with NICUs in northern California. Though it might work in a few newer, more spacious units, it would be impossible physically for many.

In February 2010, a light plane crashed upon take-off from the airport in Palo Alto, California. It came down on the transformer providing electricity to the roughly 65,000 residents of Palo Alto and the entire campus of Stanford University, including the medical centre. Luckily, power was only out from about 8:00 to 18:00. This provided an opportunity to learn about surge capacity in a 'real world' test. From this episode, LPCH has improved plans for finding, assessing and developing NICU surge capacity.

When planning surge capacity, it is important that this be done in a regionalized fashion for several reasons. First is the obvious ethical and legal consideration; altered standards of care need to meet the basic principles of transparency and stakeholder involvement (Daniels and Sabin, 2002; Kuschner *et al.*, 2007). The community should be included in developing any altered standard of care. Second is self-interest. If forced to resort to an altered, that is, lowered, standard of care, it would be wise to know that one is still practising within defensible parameters that have been deemed acceptable to our peers. Third, it would be best if all the hospitals in a region have similar criteria for altered standards of care. Thus, once the decision is made that the response to a disaster requires resorting to altered standards of care, those in charge of assigning patients to beds would know that the beds are of roughly similar capability. If the definitions are not comparable or undefined, you either face the risk of sending a patient to a 'bad' bed when a 'good' bed was available, or have to waste valuable time and communications resources exploring the capabilities of every bed made available.

Since most countries and regions already have accepted levels of care, it seems reasonable to start with these when trying to determine acceptable altered standards. In California, there are three levels of hospital care for neonates (CCS, 1999; AAP-ACOG, 2007) that are summarized in Table 5.2.

Table 5.2. NICU surge capacity guidelines. (Modified from CCS, 1999, and AAP-ACOG, 2007.)

	NICU	IICN	Continuing	Surge
Square feet[a]	80–120	50–100	40–50 →	
Spacing (ft)[b]	6–8	4–5	4–5 →	
Electric outlets	16	8	4 →	
Oxygen	4	2	1 →	
Air	4	2	1 →	
Suction	4	2	1 →	

[a] Square feet is floor space allocated per patient.
[b] Spacing is between beds.

In our region, we have suggested taking the lowest accepted level of care, 'Continuing Care', and using that as the basis for defining the minimal standard of surge capacity for NICU patients during a major disaster. Similar standards, adjusted for local conditions, exist in other parts of the world. The local stakeholders could modify these for use in their region, thus creating a legal and ethical framework for ethically acceptable altered standards of care.

The next step in developing surge capacity is to review the floor plan or physical footprint of the NICU and all its associated support areas. Sleep rooms, conference rooms, offices, satellite labs, storage areas, etc., should all be considered in this. With the predefined and regionally accepted guidelines in hand, appropriate sized areas can be identified. Possible sites for surge beds identified by this first step can be inspected to assure that they are indeed potentially clinically useful space. For instance, if the agreed upon minimum space required is 40 ft^2 (3.72 m^2), it is still necessary to determine that the identified space has adequate access and is not an unusable shape (e.g. 4 × 10 ft (1.22 × 3.05 m) is 40 ft^2 (3.72 m^2) but would be too narrow to be useable). Spaces deemed physically adequate to serve as 'surge capacity' need to be listed in the unit's disaster plan explicitly, e.g. 'in a disaster, Room 123 can have extraneous equipment removed, and two incubators/cots brought in to provide an additional 2-bed surge capacity'.

Once a room is deemed adequate in terms of size and shape, attention must focus on access to electricity, oxygen, air and vacuum. This can be more difficult than it sounds initially. The simple thing is to explore the potential space and determine whether the number of various outlets meet the minimal standard. The tricky part is to determine that, in an area that has not been used for clinical purposes, the outlets are not only functional, but also capable of meeting patient needs without overwhelming the overall system. For example, older electrical circuits may not be able to handle the increased load created by plugging in all the new monitoring equipment, ventilators, incubators, lighting, etc. Adding unplanned-for additional ventilators to the oxygen delivery system may overwhelm the supply, resulting in a drop in wall pressure that potentially can set off alarms, impact the delivery of needed oxygen to patients throughout the unit or lower the pressure in other ventilators, and thus add further disruption to care. Our NICU is barely 20 years old, but the marked increase in electrical equipment use became very evident when we had to plug all the equipment, particularly the new computers required by our electronic medical record system, into the emergency back-up circuits after the plane crash.

Thus, one step in any unit's disaster plan should be to assess the available emergency electrical system, determine how much equipment it can support and prioritize the equipment that gets attached to that system. If the system cannot support the needed equipment, then either the system needs to be augmented, or alternative electrical sources (e.g. generators, battery packs, uninterruptable power supplies) should be arranged. Again, unit disaster plans can be updated to indicate clearly the prioritization of which piece of equipment is plugged into which emergency electrical outlet, generator, left on battery, etc.

Battery back-up commonly is relied upon to provide temporary power for life-support and monitoring equipment during a disaster. It is important to remember that advertised battery life often is overly optimistic. More importantly, battery life tends to decrease over time, so the 8-h back-up battery purchased with the equipment is unlikely to last anywhere near that long once the equipment is many years old. Merely unplugging a device and demonstrating that the battery works is not an adequate test of battery function for disaster planning. Remember, too, that recharging batteries usually takes longer than their lifespan, so that using emergency power to recharge batteries during a disaster quickly becomes a losing proposition.

Assuming the space has been found, and the support systems (electric, medical gases, vacuum) have been deemed adequate, the next step is assuring that the 'little things' are available if and when needed. There may well be spare medical gas outlets, but then you must be sure to have the proper hoses and compatible safety adaptors to connect to them. Similarly, a wall vacuum source is useless without the appropriate trap and connections. Electrical outlets may need multi-socket extension cords to support all the needed equipment. All these 'little things' – gas and vacuum connections, electrical cords, etc. – need to be available proximate to the site of their intended use, accessible and yet secured so that they won't be used unless and until a disaster strikes. So, for hypothetical surge capacity in 'Room 123', the unit disaster plan can state something like: 'Adaptors for the vacuum and necessary electric cords are stored in the plastic container sealed with red tape in the cabinet under the sink. In a disaster, open container and use to set up the additional 2-bed unit equipment.'

For a system to work, it would be best to have the potential surge capacity of NICUs throughout a region available to the regional emergency operations command centre at all times. Though this could be done on paper, a network of computers with 'cloud' back-up, which would store both the usual number of licensed beds and the potential additional surge capacity of all the NICUs in a region, would be a preferred method. In a disaster, this would facilitate rapid identification of spots available for neonates needing evacuation. The more data provided, the more useful such a site would be. Thus, not only would it be helpful to know the number of beds, but also the number of ventilators. This website could, for example, indicate that the NICU in question has 36 beds and 12 ventilators, with 32 beds and 8 ventilators in use, with the ability to surge to 42 beds in a disaster. Instantly, the incident commander would be aware that ten babies, including four on ventilators, could possibly be absorbed by this centre. If the units being evacuated are using TRAIN, the incident commander can readily determine that this unit could take four 'red' or 'yellow' patients, depending upon transport capability, and six more 'green'.

Conclusions

The risks posed to neonates in a major disaster, and their healthcare needs, differ significantly from those of adults and older children (Cohen *et al.*, 2010b). As such, it is appropriate that disaster planning for neonates takes this into account. Regional, or 'Fourth Order', disaster planning would be the preferred way to mitigate the impact of a disaster on neonatal patients. To accomplish this, regional cooperation is needed to develop acceptable tools for planning both triage and surge capacity. TRAIN, a triage system based upon resource allocation, is being developed and implemented in our region of California, USA. It can serve as a model, for regions elsewhere in the USA and other countries, for developing similar tools based upon local needs, regulations and mores. Similarly, tools for developing and sharing regional plans for surge capacity would allow the distribution of patients through a region to maximize efficient resource utilization and minimize, if not completely avoid, the need to resort to austere care. This should be the first ethical goal of any disaster plan. To deny care to patients because of lack of resource availability when those resources might be available at another hospital within the region would be a terrible, avoidable and tragic loss of life.

Acknowledgements

The author is grateful to Barbara Murphy, RN, Terence L. Ahern, MD, Alvin Hackel, MD and Brandon Bond for all their input over the years, and Aileen Cleary Cohen, MD, PhD for her support and editorial comments.

References

Acs, N., Banhidy, F., Puho, E. and Czeizel, A.E. (2006) Pregnancy complications and delivery outcomes of pregnant women with influenza. *Journal of Maternal Fetal and Neonatal Medicine* 19, 135–140.

American Academy of Pediatrics (AAP) and the American College of Obstetricians and Gynecologists (ACOG) (2007) Inpatient perinatal care services. In: Lockwood, C.J. and Lemons, J.A. (eds) *Guidelines for Perinatal Care*, 6th edn. American Academy of Pediatrics, Elk Grove Village, Illinois.

Baldwin, S., Robinson, A., Barlow, P. and Fargason, C.A. Jr (2006) Moving hospitalized children all over the southeast: interstate transfer of pediatric patients during Hurricane Katrina. *Pediatrics* 117 (Supp 4), S416–S420.

Barkemeyer, B.M. (2006) Practicing neonatology in a blackout: the University Hospital NICU in the midst of Hurricane Katrina: caring for children without power or water. *Pediatrics* 117 (Suppl 4), S369–S374.

Barkemeyer, B.M. (2011) NICU care in the aftermath of Hurricane Karina: 5 years of changes. *Pediatrics* 128 (Suppl 1), S8–S10.

Bestati, N., Leteurtre, S., Duhamel, A., Proulx, F., Grandbastien, B., Lacroix, J. and Leclerc, F. (2010) Differences in organ dysfunctions between neonates and older children: a prospective, observational, multicenter study. *Critical Care* 14, R202.

Bostick, N.A., Subbarao, I., Burkle, F.M., Hsu, E.B., Armstrong, J.H. and James, J.J. (2008) Disaster triage systems for large-scale catastrophic events. *Disaster Medicine and Public Health Preparedness* 2 (Suppl 1), S35–S39.

Brunkard, J., Namulanda, G. and Ratard, R. (2008) Hurricane Katrina deaths, Louisiana, 2005. *Disaster Medicine and Public Health Preparedness* 2, 215–223.

California Children's Services (CCS) (1999) Standards for Neonatal Intensive Care Units (NICUs). In: *Manual of Procedures*. CCS, Sacramento, California. Available at: http://www.dhcs.ca.gov/services/ccs/Documents/RegionalNICU.pdf (Accessed 21 January 2013).

Cohen, R.S., Murphy, B., Ahern, T. and Hackel, A. (2010a) Disaster planning – triaging resource allocation in neonatology. *Journal of Investigative Medicine* 58, 188 (abstract #298).

Cohen, R.S., Murphy, B., Ahern, R. and Hackel, A. (2010b) Regional disaster planning for neonatology. *Journal of Perinatology* 30, 709–711.

Daniels, N. and Sabin, J. (2002) *Setting Limits Fairly: Can We Learn to Share Scarce Resources*. Oxford University Press, Oxford.

Ginsberg, H.G. (2011) Since Katrina: neonatal and pediatric issues from both sides of the levee. *Pediatrics* 128 (Suppl 1), S15–S17.

Hardy, J.M.B., Azarowicz, E.N., Mannini, A., Medearis, D.N. Jr and Cooke, R.E. (1961) The effect of Asian influenza on the outcome of pregnancy, Baltimore, 1957–1958. *American Journal of Public Health* 51, 1182–1188.

Janvier, A., Leblanc, I. and Barrington, K.J. (2008) Nobody likes premies: the relative value of patient's lives. *Journal of Perinatology* 28(12), 821–816.

Kanter, R.K. and Moran, J.R. (2007) Pediatric hospital and intensive care unit capacity in regional disasters: expanding capacity by altering standards of care. *Pediatrics* 119, 94–100.

Klein, K.R., Pepe, P.E., Burkle, F.M. Jr, Nagel, N.E. and Swienton, R.E. (2008) Evolving need for alternative triage management in Public Health Emergencies: a Hurricane Katrina case study. *Disaster Medicine and Public Health Preparedness* 2 (Suppl 1), S40–S44.

Kuschner, W.G., Pollard, J.B. and Ezeji-Okoye, S.C. (2007) Ethical triage and scarce resource allocation during public health emergencies: tenets and procedures. *Hospital Topics* 85, 16–25.

Lerner, E.B., Schwartz, R.B., Coule, P.L., Weinstein, E.S., Cone, D.C., Hunt, R.C., Sasser, S.M., Liu, J.M., Nudell, N.G., Wedmore, I.S., Hammond, J., Bulger, E.M., Salomone, J.P., Sanddal, T.L., Lord, G.C., Markenson, D. and O'Connor, R.E. (2008) Mass casualty triage: an evaluation of the data and development of a proposed national guideline. *Disaster Medicine and Public Health Preparedness* 2 (Suppl 1), S25–S34.

Leteurtre, S., Duhamel, A., Grandbastien, B., Proulx, F., Cotting, J., Gottesman, R., Joffe, A., Wagner, B., Hubert, P., Martinot, A., Lacroix, J. and Leclerc, F. (2010) Daily estimation of the severity of multiple organ dysfunction syndrome in critically ill children. *Canadian Medical Association Journal* 182, 1181–1187.

Leteurtre, S., Dupré, M., Dorkenoo, A., Lampin, M.-E. and Leclerc, F. (2011) Assessment of the Pediatric Index of Mortality 2 with the Pao2/Fio2 ratio derived from the Spo2/Fio2 ratio: a prospective pilot study in a French pediatric intensive care unit. *Pediatric Critical Care Medicine* 12, e184–e186.

Lim, L. and Rozycki, H.J. (2008) Postnatal SNAP-II scores in neonatal intensive care unit patients: relationship to sepsis, necrotizing enterocolitis, and death. *Journal of Maternal and Fetal Neonatal Medicine* 21(6), 415–419.

Mattox, K.L. (2006) Hurricanes Katrina and Rita: role of individuals and collaborative networks in mobilizing/coordinating societal and professional resources for major disasters. *Critical Care* 10, 205.

Meadow, W., Cohen-Cutler, S., Spelke, B., Kim, A., Plesac, M., Weis, K. and Lagatta, J. (2012) The prediction and cost of futility in the NICU. *Acta Paediatrica* 101(4), 397–402.

Pollack, M.M., Ruttimann, U.E. and Getson, P.R. (1988) Pediatric risk of mortality (PRISM) score. *Critical Care Medicine* 16, 1110–1116.

Richardson, D.K., Corcoran, J.D., Escobar, G.J. and Lee, S.K. (2001) SNAP-II and SNAPPE-II: Simplified newborn illness severity and mortality risk scores. *The Journal of Pediatrics* 138, 92–100.

Rubinson, L., Nuzzo, J.B., Talmor, D.S., O'Toole, T., Kramer, B.R. and Inglesby, T.V. (2005) Augmentation of hospital critical care capacity after bioterrorist attacks or epidemics: Recommendations for the Working Group on Emergency Mass Critical Care. *Critical Care Medicine* 33 (Suppl), E2393.

Rubinson, L., Hick, J.L., Hanfling, D.G., Devereauz, A.V., Dichter, J.R., Christian, M.D., Talmor, D., Medina, J., Curtis, J.R. and Geiling, J.A. (2008) Definitive care for the critically ill during a disaster: a framework for optimizing critical care surge capacity. *Chest* 133, 18S–31S.

Shann, F., Pearson, G., Slater, A. and Wilkinson, K. (1997) Paediatric index of mortality (PIM): a mortality prediction model for children in intensive care. *Intensive Care Medicine* 23, 201–207.

Siston, A.M., Rasmussen, S.A., Honein, M.A., Fry, A.M., Seib, K., Callaghan, W.M., Louie, J., Doyle, T.J., Crockett, M., Lynfield, R., Moore, Z., Wiedeman, C., Anand, M., Tabony, L., Nielsen, C.F., Waller, K., Page, S., Thompson, J.M., Avery, C., Springs, C.B., Jones, T., Williams, J.L., Newsome, K., Finelli, L. and Jamieson, D.L. (2010) Pandemic 2009 influenza A (H1N1) virus illness among pregnant women in the United States. *Journal of the American Medical Association* 303, 1517–1525.

Stukel, T.A., Schull, M.J., Gurrmann, A., Alter, D.A., Ping, L., Vermeulen, M.J., Manuel, D.G. and Zwarenstein, M. (2008) Health impact of hospital restrictions on seriously ill hospitalized patients: lessons from the Toronto SARS outbreak. *Medical Care* 46, 991–997.

The International Neonatal Network (1993) The CRIB (Clinical Risk Index for Babies) score: a tool for assessing initial neonatal risk and comparing performance of neonatal intensive care units. *Lancet* 342, 193–198.

Wolfler, A., Silvani, P., Musicco, M. and Salvo, I.; Italian Pediatric Sepsis Study (SISPe) Group (2007) Pediatric Index of Mortality 2 score in Italy: a multicenter, prospective, observational study. *Intensive Care Medicine* 33(8), 1407–1413.

Chapter 6

Application of Mobile Grids for Disaster Management

Monideepa Roy and Nandini Mukherjee

If sufficient numbers of management layers are superimposed on top of each other, it can be assured that disaster is not left to chance. – Norman Augustine

The Need for a Disaster Management System

All countries face the risk of being struck by disaster in its various forms leading to widely adverse effects on its inhabitants and the environment. In spite of the best efforts of governments and associated non-governmental organizations (NGOs), the overwhelming nature of these hazards cannot always reduce the number of the casualties to the desired low levels. Although technological advancements are growing by leaps and bounds, vulnerability to either natural or man-made disasters has not subsequently reduced to such a commensurate degree. Disaster can strike at any moment and in any place. It may strike in the form of natural calamities, terrorist attacks and accidents. Thus an efficient disaster management system that will work in such adverse conditions should be a priority for any country. The need for an efficient disaster management system becomes imperative in public places, residential areas and even in business establishments and important commercial operations where people are generally expected to move around in large numbers. Such an efficient system would be instrumental in diverting or reducing extensive loss and damage to life or property.

The entire process of disaster management can broadly be divided into four fields: these four fields normally deal with: (i) mitigation or risk reduction; (ii) preparedness, i.e. preparing resources to respond to the hazard; (iii) response, i.e. responding to the actual damage caused by the hazard; and (iv) recovery, which is limiting further damage and returning as close as possible to normalcy at the earliest possible time span. Among these four phases, the response phase consists of the mobilization of the necessary emergency services and first responders to the disaster area. The disaster management crew must be well trained and equipped with the best appliances to help them to communicate the condition they are in and the status of the calamity in the region they work for. These well-organized responses to emergency situations, e.g. earthquakes, floods, terror incidents, etc. involve efficient coordination and collaboration among public safety/medical organizations and sharing of emergency alerts and incident-related data between disparate systems. Efficient management of rescue work in disaster-hit areas can be crucial in saving the lives of the survivors there. This, however, depends to a large extent on the effectiveness of communication for the exchange of information between the rescue teams and the victims. So the enforced communication system should be reliable and in working order at all times. But during such situations, it is quite common to experience disruptions in the static infrastructure of wired communication. The disruption of most infrastructure-based communication systems becomes unavoidable under such conditions. Hence if rescue groups from different locations and medical departments come together to implement their respective rescue operations it is important that these groups quickly establish networks among themselves, and exchange data, so as to complete their missions speedily and efficiently. Under such circumstances, Mobile Ad hoc Networks (MANETs) are increasingly being perceived as the preferred types of networks because they require no central nodes and because of their unique characteristics of independent network organization, dynamic topology and ease of deployment. A mobile grid environment for a disaster management system based on MANETs is presented. But before moving on to the description of our proposed system, a brief discussion follows on why having a ready and systematic response approach is so crucial from a medical perspective.

Response to Disaster Management from a Medical Perspective

The process of disaster management, as mentioned in the previous section, consists of four phases: mitigation, preparedness, response and recovery. Out of all the four phases, the response phase is the one phase where instant action is needed and speed and time are of primary importance, as compared with the other three phases, which are basically long-term action plans. The response phase includes the mobilization of the necessary emergency services and first responders to the disaster area to provide relief. This phase usually includes a first wave of core emergency services, such as doctors, firefighters, police and ambulance crews. These teams may also be supported by a number of secondary emergency services, such as specialist rescue teams. So to have a shorter response time, it is necessary that communication with that place remains good and uninterrupted at all times. The main objective of a response to a disaster from a medical perspective is to reduce the loss of lives of the victims of such an event. So, although the process of successfully handling a disaster scenario is a culmination of several processes, the role of the medical department is probably the most crucial, as it is directly related to saving human lives. Other objectives include assuaging the pain and suffering of the victims, restoring the health status in the area to the pre-disaster level and establishing a recovery process for those affected by the disaster (Roy and Mukherjee, 2008). But for this a very well-organized and prepared medical system needs to be in place.

However, no matter how well prepared and organized a medical system claims to be, its effectiveness depends on how successful it is in its practical implementation.

The primary hindrances that are faced by rescue teams are as follows:

- Since the relief teams consist of people from different organizations, and hospitals, whether government-based or private, they have different types of equipment and software set-up with which they have been instructed to tackle these situations. So interaction among these teams and along with a standardized software support is helpful in such situations.
- The teams may come from different areas and may not have prior knowledge of the area or may not have interacted with the local administration there.

- When the teams first reach the area, if they know the type of help that is primarily required, then they can prioritize the work and accordingly allocate it among themselves.
- Information pertaining to missing people or the search for victims needs to be locally accessible, as base stations or wired lines may become affected during such times.

So, creating a standardized and uniform set of applications with user friendly Graphical User Interfaces (GUIs) that can be used by all the medical teams and disaster workers is therefore a good idea for people involved in the rescue process or any other person or organization involved at any stage of the disaster management handling process. This would result in uniformity of the system and it could be adapted to various types of disaster scenarios. The GUIs described later on are an attempt to standardize and refine the work of medical response teams in disaster management. They can be further homogenized to adapt to a wider range of disaster situations. Moreover, to ensure that communication between the various rescue groups remains unaffected, using MANETs to set up the communication framework is cheaper and faster than conventional wired or infrastructure-based communication systems, and no pre-deployed infrastructure is necessary.

The Proposed Disaster Management System

There are at present a number of existing disaster management systems that provide solutions to the problems caused by disasters, two of which are mentioned below in order to provide a comparative illustration of the advantage of our proposed system.

MyDisasterDroid

A mobile disaster management system using Android Technology (Fajardo and Oppus, 2009) has been developed, which has been implemented as a smartphone application called MyDisasterDroid (MDD). It determines the optimum route along different geographical locations that the volunteers and rescue workers need to take in order to serve the greatest number of people and give maximum coverage of the area in the shortest possible time. MDD was implemented using the travelling salesman problem (TSP) (entails that given a list of cities and the distances between each pair of cities, an individual has to find the shortest possible route to visit each city exactly once and return to the city of origin. The problem was first formulated in 1930 and is one of the most intensively studied problems in optimization) as a basis and using generic algorithms to generate a solution. Here the geographic locations of people in need are set by either using the application installed in MDD or sending location via text or short message service (SMS) to MDD. Geographic locations or geo-locations are described in terms of latitude and longitude. The distances between these locations are calculated based on the travelling salesman problem, as previously mentioned. Although this is an application that addresses the response phase in disaster situations, this system requires the support of the base stations of the service operators/carriers, which are basically static infrastructure for interacting with each other and finding locations.

SAHANA

The SAHANA software foundation has developed a disaster management system that provides information management solutions for tracking disaster victims and helps organizations to respond to disasters (www.sahanafoundation.org). It is open-source software and has the following features:

- It has a facility for registering missing and found persons, and helps families of victims to get information about them.
- It also offers help for tracking and managing requests for help from individuals and organizations.
- It tracks organizations and programmes who respond to the disaster, which includes the coverage and balance in the distribution of aid, providing transparency in the donations and response effort.
- It enables the relevant sharing of information across organizations, connecting donors, volunteers, NGOs and government organizations, enabling them to operate in synchronization.

The rescue workers collect the relevant data and send them via Global Systems for Mobile Communications (GSM)/General Packet Radio Service (GPRS) to the central servers, which in turn send the information to the main relief coordinating authority SAHANA server to publicly publish the consolidated statistical data for the disaster. The victim's family or friends can then access these data though a web browser.

The systems described above are based on centralized servers and rely on a functioning internet and cellular network backbone. In such circumstances, the application of MANETs to act as mobile grids has the advantage in that it assumes no infrastructure support and is suitable for enabling swifter and more effective management of rescue work in a disaster management scenario.

The proposed system

The sample application described here is for seeking out survivors or helping rescue operations as part of a disaster management system. When an area is struck by an earthquake, flood, etc. essential communication is one of the first things to be affected, which is caused by the breakdown or disruption of infrastructure support. During such times even the prevalent mobile network services may not work due to damage sustained to the static infrastructure of the base stations. So even if medical teams or relatives of victims physically reach the vicinity of the disaster-hit area, it may not be feasible for them to visit each and every point to ascertain the damage or the nature of help to be dispatched. Moreover, searching for or locating survivors also becomes difficult and time-consuming under such circumstances. In such cases communication among the various teams is crucial for the rescue operations to be fast and effective. So if the teams can somehow know the nature of help to be disbursed, the positions of the survivors or other such vital information, then it helps in gaining precious time. Mobile rescue team units carrying laptops, personal digital assistants (PDAs), mobile phones or other mobile devices can spread out in groups at the affected areas, acting as leader nodes. Applications running on the stranded victims' mobile phones (or other devices) at various locations can search for, discover and register on the nearest leader nodes with their location information and other vital data, e.g. name, age, blood group, etc. In case the victim is able to communicate, he or she can also use a GUI to provide information regarding location and type of aid needed, etc. Other relief teams can then share this information as clients to disburse the necessary help to the respective areas. Similarly, relatives of victims can use this service network to retrieve information about their family members. The teams can send a response to the survivors stating the approximate time they may reach them or any other such important information such as relevant advice on first aid until a team reaches them. The system presented here also incorporates a search mechanism for faster matching of results. Eventually it is planned to upgrade this application to a more exhaustive system to include several additional features and modules for a wider applicability and acceptance.

A brief introduction to grids and MANETs is given in the next section as the concept of the mobile grid is based on them.

A Brief Introduction to the Grid and MANETs

Grid computing

'Grid computing is a technology for coordinated large scale resource sharing and problem solving among many autonomous groups (referred to as VOs, virtual organizations), with the potential to completely change the process of computing and data access' (Foster, 2001). With the introduction of the grid computing concept, the concept of *on demand* computing was brought forward and the resources that were otherwise lying un-utilized or under-utilized in locations other than where the researchers were physically located could be put to use. For example, when we turn on a light switch, we do not know exactly from which power grid source the power comes that is being drawn to that switch. In the same way that electricity is available on demand, the aim of the grid was to make computational power (and other such services) available on demand. When a user wants to avail him or herself of a service, they make a request for the service through a GUI in the grid, although the user does not know the availability or the location of the resources on the grid. A resource manager on the grid is responsible for balancing the utilization of the resources, executing the service and sending the result back to the user. Furthermore, grid computing has the option of adding a large amount of computational power, storage space and other devices *dynamically* into any grid environment, thereby adding to the capacity of the environment as and when required.

Some of the features of the grid that have made it such a useful technology are as follows:

- Exploiting under-utilized resources – when a machine is temporarily not able to run an application because its own resources are being used to peak capacity, then that application can be run on another machine that is idle on the grid. However, from the users' point of view the whole grid is seen as a single entity with appropriate software, hiding all the technical details related to physical locations, middleware, operating system, etc. Once a request for a service has been made by a user, the grid has a resource manager who is responsible for the searching and resource allocation and management of resources on the grid on behalf of the user. The user of the grid does not need to have any information about the individual location or availability of the resources on the grid.

- Access to additional resources – suppose a device needs to process an application that is beyond its individual resource capabilities. If it joins a grid where the participating devices share their resources on the network, the device has the advantage of getting access to additional resources as per its requirements. Another instance is, suppose a device wants a particular application that is not available to it, e.g. a printing service. If there are other devices on the grid that offer that printing service, then by accessing a grid, the device can use that printing service.
- Heterogeneity – it consists of multiple heterogeneous resources at various physical locations working together as a single entity.

Moreover grids can be of various types, i.e. computational grids, data grids, application grids, information grids and knowledge grids, etc. A device can join any type of grid depending on the type of service it wishes to access and thus have additional access to a wide variety of applications or resources, which cannot be accessed on a standalone machine.

However, since the setting up of a grid requires infrastructure set-up and its participating devices are essentially static, utilizing grids during a disaster may not be possible. Since such situations warrant that the rescue teams set up communication among themselves quickly and with little or no infrastructure support, MANETs have been found to be very useful in such circumstances.

MANETs

A wireless mobile environment is one where the users can freely move with heterogeneous mobile devices, and where this wireless communication is used mainly to access information, not to compute the information. A MANET, sometimes also called a mobile mesh network, is a self-configuring network of mobile devices connected by wireless links. Often the devices in a MANET suffer from resource constraints that prevent them from performing complex functions on their own. However, an environment where the nodes share their resources in a cooperative manner enables thin nodes to overcome these constraints and perform complex functions.

The mobile nodes in a MANET can communicate with each other via radio waves. Mobile nodes that are within radio range of each other can directly communicate, whereas others need the aid of intermediate nodes to route their packets. These networks are fully distributed, and can work anywhere without the help of any infrastructure. This property makes these networks highly robust. They are the preferred choice for use in disaster areas owing to the following properties:

- They provide access to information and services regardless of geographic position.
- These networks can be set up at any place and at any time.
- These networks work without any pre-existing infrastructure.

Since the availability of wirelessly connected mobile devices has also grown considerably in recent years, it has created an enormous collective unexploited potential for resource utilization. However, mobile devices do not always satisfy user requests effectively, because they suffer from a small display, low speed central processing unit (CPU) and low capacity memory. So, the resource-sharing potential of grid computing opens up the possibilities of new applications that involve the integration of the mobile technologies with grid technology and lead to the concept of the mobile grid.

The next section introduces the concept of mobile grids, which are the basis for the proposed disaster management system.

The Mobile Grid Concept

Since mobile and nomadic devices are everywhere today, the question that arises is why they cannot share resources to overcome their individual resource constraints. While considering the technological and functional constraints of mobile devices, a method to process the individual user requests of each mobile device is proposed based on mobile grid computing and extending traditional grid computing, to efficiently solve these issues. A group of mobile devices could set up an ad hoc network and collectively work to function as a mobile grid. It could also harness the services of other devices that are in the area and come within the range of the mobile grid.

Thus the concept of wireless/mobile grids, which will have the power of grids and the mobility of mobile devices, has been coined. A synergy of the resource-sharing potential of grid computing with the flexible, ubiquitous availability of MANETs can be used to create a mobile grid environment.

Mobile grids provide us with the following novel elements:

- Mobile devices usually have constrained resource limitations such as storage space and battery and computation power. A mobile grid would allow the networked mobile devices to accomplish a specific mission that may be beyond the computing or communication capacity of an individual device due to its inherent constraints in terms of processing power, node life or low resources, etc.
- Since they do not require any static infrastructure support, these networks can be used to set up Virtual Organizations (VO), at short notice in any place, and information accessibility can be accelerated by delivering availability to relevant information anytime and anywhere.
- Mobile devices provide connections in places where wired connections are not feasible, e.g. in underground mines, elevator shafts, remote areas, etc.

Mobile grids could be deployed in disaster recovery, outdoor empirical studies and for research in environments where computers are inaccessible or wired links have broken down or are not feasible. The reach of wireless grids can be to any geographical setting where computers have not yet penetrated or where the carrying of wired computers may not be feasible.

A detailed example of a disaster management system that has been based on mobile grids is now given to provide a clear idea of the applicability of the system.

Implementation of the System

Here a disaster management service is implemented using Jini over MANETs (Roy *et al.*, 2010). The system consists of several mobile nodes building a MANET with peer-to-peer connection, where the nodes are classified as service provider nodes, client nodes and leader nodes based on the types of roles they perform in the network.

A *service provider* is a node that is capable of providing (and is willing to provide) a service. A service can be a computation, storage, a search, hardware, etc.

A *client* is a thin node that wants to execute a particular job but does not have the necessary resources to do so.

A *leader node* is a node that hosts a lookup service. A *lookup service* acts as repository of services, where each registered service is stored with a set of attributes describing the service.

This system was implemented in a MANET. In this network the mobile nodes communicate with each other via peer-to-peer connections. The operating system of each node needs to be configured in such a manner that the nodes can establish peer-to-peer connections between them.

The system is based on the Jini framework (Edwards, 2000). Jini (Fig. 6.1) is a service-oriented framework where the devices in a distributed environment can define, discover and advertise their services in an ad hoc manner. It provides a self-healing environment where services and service consumers can enter and leave a network seamlessly. The Jini technology consists of three protocols: *discover*, *join* and *lookup*. The discovery protocol is used when a new service provider joins a Jini federation and wants to register with a lookup service, and the service provider uses either unicast or multicast discovery to find a lookup service. The lookup service is the Jini service repository. The join protocol consists of the service provider uploading a service object to the lookup service. As a result of the discovery protocol, the service is now ready to be discovered. Accordingly the client also searches for a lookup service and its desired service. In the final stage the client communicates directly with the service provider via the proxy object (Hashman and Knudsen, 2001).

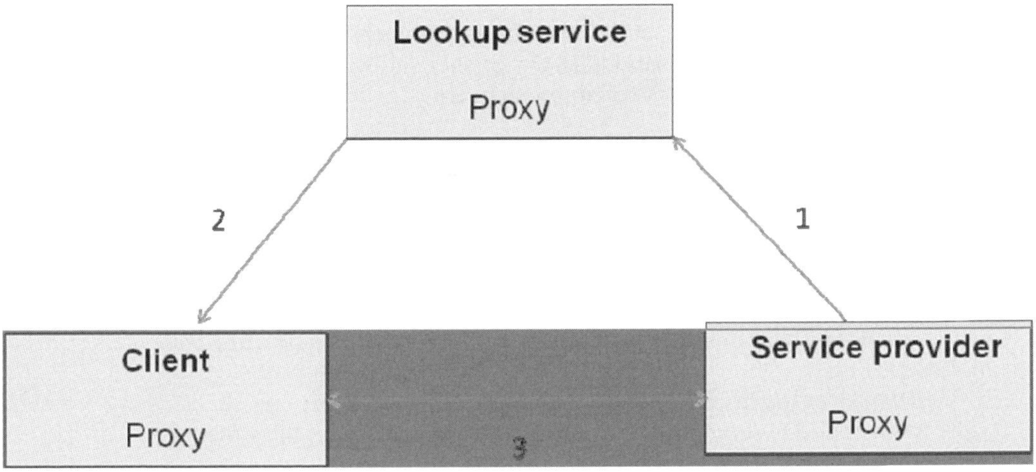

Fig. 6.1. The Jini framework.

The entire process of implementation is divided into the following sub-steps based on the nodes they are performed on.

Service provider process

To make a service available to the clients on a MANET, a service provider has to register it on a lookup service. For this, the service provider performs multicast discovery to search for nearby leader nodes in a network. When it finds one or more leader nodes, the choice is made based on a selection algorithm; otherwise there is a chance that a leader node that has better signal strength than the others will be discovered by most service providers and its resources will be drained. If the request is approved, then the service provider registers its services on that node along with its service attributes for some duration of time decided by the leader node, which is called the lease time. The service attributes are stored within a copy of the service proxy on the lookup service. If the allocated lease time expires but the service provider wishes to continue, then it requests a renewal of the lease from the lookup server. If at any time the service provider wants to exit before its lease time is over, a notification is sent to the lookup server. For this particular application the service provider's details are the information about the victims or the survivors. The service attributes for this application are given in Table 6.1. The entire process of discovery and registration by the service provider is carried out through a GUI.

Table 6.1. Attributes of the service.

Name of attribute	Description of attribute
String service name	This attribute is the name of the service
String name	This attribute is the name of the victim
Integer age	This attribute specifies the age of the victim
String sex	This attribute gives the gender of the victim
String blood group	This attribute gives the blood type of the victim
String location victim	This attribute specifies the approximate location of the victim
String aid type	This attribute specifies the type of aid the victim needs

Client-side process

Subsequently the client nodes also search for nearby leader nodes and register with them to place their service requests. The clients enter their service requests through another GUI and the details are sent to the lookup server. Here the rescue workers or doctors are denoted as the clients since they enter their queries or search criteria through a client-side GUI. Figure 6.3 shows the GUI to be filled by the rescue workers or doctors to search for victims or find out what type of help they require. The search can be done on all or some of the parameters as per the choice of the client, but should include the service name attribute.

Figure 6.2 shows the GUI to be filled in with the victim's details.

Leader node process

The lookup service is the crucial part of the Jini network technology. The lookup service runs on the leader node. There may be more than one leader node in the Jini federation.

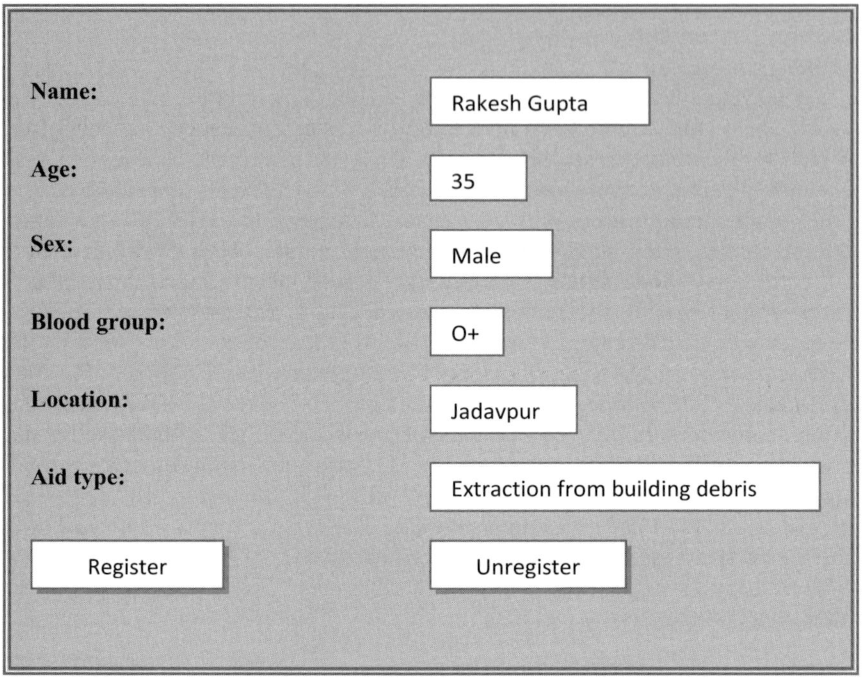

Fig. 6.2. The Survivor Registration Form (service provider form).

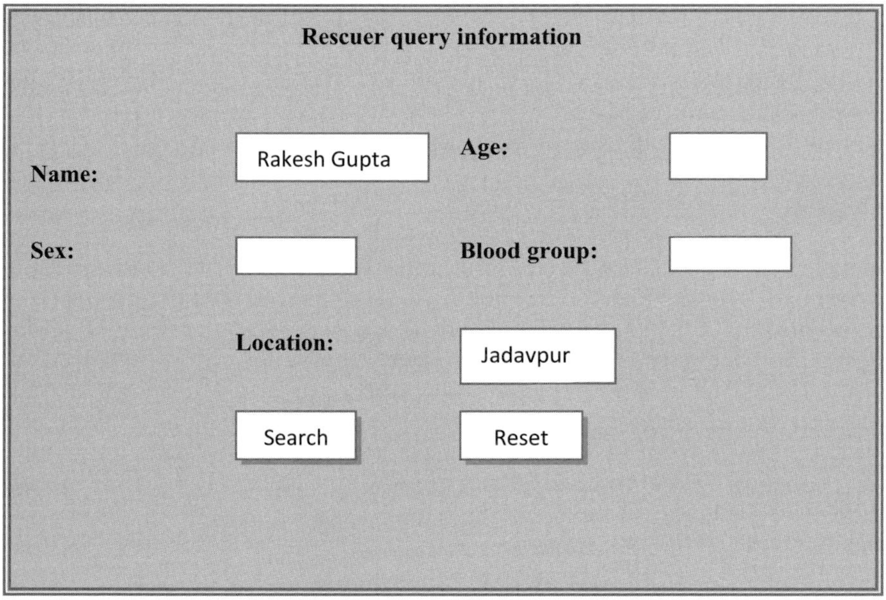

Fig. 6.3. The Rescue Worker Query Form (client form).

The lookup service hosts the service proxies of the registered service providers and filters and delivers responses to the clients within the range of communication of the lookup service. Each service proxy stores the information of one service as service attributes. This framework allows multiple leader nodes to be accommodated within the network with overlapping ranges. Therefore if a service provider or client is within the range of multiple leader nodes, an algorithm is applied to select the most suitable leader node based on a parameter called the threshold value. The threshold value t is calculated for each leader node in the network, based on battery life b, number of nodes n registered with it and the distance d from a registered node, as $t = f(b, n, d)$. The leader node with the minimum threshold value is chosen. Each leader stores its threshold value, which is recalculated and updated every time a new node registers with it. Once the lookup service is selected, the service providers and clients can register themselves with the lookup service.

The registration process is implemented using the join protocol in a Jini federation. The registration consists of acquiring a lease from the lookup service and letting the lookup service know what services they have to offer (if any). Once the lease expires, the proxies are flushed out by the lookup service. The leasing procedure makes Jini a self-healing technology, i.e. it basically allows the lookup service to clean up services that have left the federation.

Once the survivors start registering their details, the rescue workers can begin their search queries also. But if the number of casualties is high then this search process can take a long time. To ensure a faster search and quicker response time, a two-phase searching algorithm has been devised.

Two-phase service matching

The lookup service in the leader node performs a first phase filtering of the services it hosts as well as those hosted on nearby lookup servers, based on the service name parameter only, to find matches, which are sent to the client (Fig. 6.4). The client now unmarshalls the rest of the attributes of the selected services and performs a more detailed service matching based on them. It then receives the necessary information that it asked for (Fig. 6.5). If no matching service is found, a regret message is displayed.

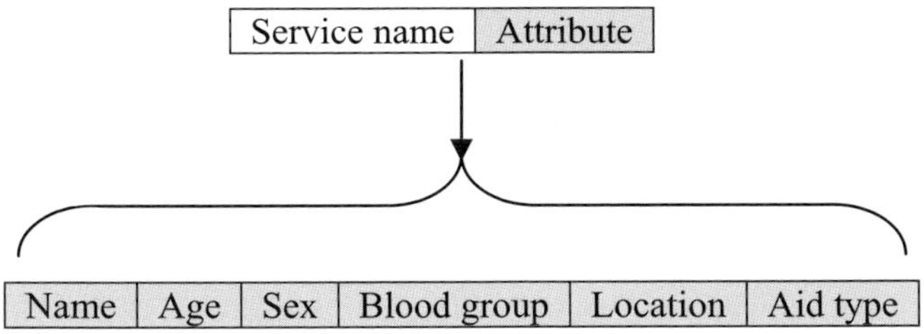

Fig. 6.4. Attribute parsing.

A sample application

As an example we illustrate a sample scenario. Suppose in an affected area, different groups of rescue workers, doctors, etc. take their mobile devices and laptops and spread out over the area. The mobile devices function as service provider or client devices. The laptops are of higher configuration and so function as the leader nodes, which host the lookup service. The rescue workers search for survivors or victims in the area and fill out the survivor details and send the service provider form through a GUI on their mobile devices on behalf of the victim. If the victim is capable, he or she can also use an autofill option to send his or her details through a mobile device. The service provider devices search for laptops with a lookup service on them and their details are registered and stored on the leader node. In this way, the details of the survivors and victims are registered on the leader nodes in the area. Now the other rescue teams or families of the victims who need to query or retrieve this information are the clients and enter their queries though a client-side GUI on their mobile devices. These queries are sent to the leader nodes and the clients then receive the matching results.

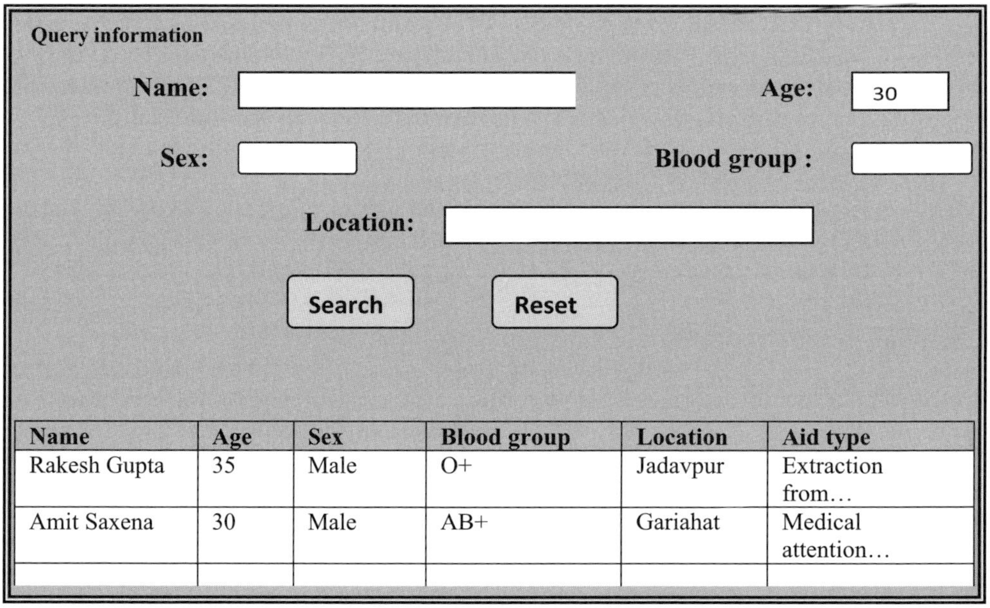
Query information

Name:

Age: 30

Sex:

Blood group :

Location:

Search

Reset

Name	Age	Sex	Blood group	Location	Aid type
Rakesh Gupta	35	Male	O+	Jadavpur	Extraction from…
Amit Saxena	30	Male	AB+	Gariahat	Medical attention…

Fig. 6.5. The results of the two-phase matching.

Conclusion

Thus by incorporating grid functionalities into MANETs, we can synergize the resource-sharing potential of grid computing with the flexible, ubiquitous availability of MANETs to create mobile grids. Although this framework has been implemented for a disaster management system, a generalized version can also be made to adapt to a wider variety of applications, with a few modifications. If various organizations come forward and get together to standardize a design template for a centralized national disaster management system, it will ensure that uniformity is maintained in the system. This will save valuable time wasted in the briefing and assembling of the participating rescue organizations every time a new disaster occurs.

References

Edwards, W.K. (2000) The Jini Model. In: *Core* Jini, 2nd edn. The Sun Microsystems Press, Java Series, Prentice Hall, New York, pp. 61–88.

Fajardo, J.T.B. and Oppus, C.M. (2009) A mobile disaster management system using the Android Technology. *International Journal of Communications* 3, 77–86.

Foster, I. (2001) The anatomy of the grid: enabling scalable virtual organizations. Euro-Par '01 *Proceedings of the 7th International Euro-Par Conference Manchester on Parallel Processing*. Springer-Verlag, London, pp. 1–4.

Hashman, S. and Knudsen, S. (2001) The application of Jini™ technology to enhance the delivery of mobile services. Available at: http://www/psinaptic.com/ (Accessed 21 January 2013).

Roy, M. and Mukherjee, N. (2008) Mobile nomadic healthcare in rural areas. *11th National Conference on e-Governance*, Haryana, India, 7–8 February, pp. 85–90.

Roy, M., Kar, P. and Mukherjee, N. (2010) An enhanced service framework in MANETs for application in emergency services. *Proceedings of International Conference on Intelligent Network and Computing 2010* (IEEE), Kuala Lumpur, Malaysia, 26–28 November, pp. V1 191–198.

Section 4

Disasters and Mass Casualty Incidents:
Incident Site Command and Control, Point-of-Care Testing

Chapter 7

Disaster Point-of-Care Testing: Fundamental Concepts and New Technologies

Gerald J. Kost, Corbin Curtis, Richard Louie and Ann Sakaguchi

Introduction

The objective of this chapter is to provide a conceptual basis for use of point-of-care (POC) testing, defined as medical testing at or near the site of care (Kost, 2002), in emergencies and disasters with the ultimate goal of *improving crises standards of care worldwide* (Kost *et al.*, 2011c).

Typically, communities lack adequate POC testing resources and trained personnel to effectively handle disaster situations that may arise, and individuals who respond to sudden crises and emergencies may be unfamiliar with the evidence-based advantages that test results at the point of need can yield. Conversely, newdemics, defined as unexpected and disruptive problems that affect the health of large numbers of individuals in a crowded world (Kost, 2006), highlight the potential for POC testing to enhance preparedness, disaster response, crisis management and outcomes and also to positively impact everyday emergency medicine and urgent care.

In view of the rapid expansion of proven technologies, in the next decade healthcare personnel increasingly will use POC instruments on a daily basis as testing moves to the distributed hybrid laboratory (Kost, 1992) of personalized medicine. Well prepared responders will carry reliable POC devices and test kits wherever disaster and emergency situations arise. To capture the essence of this transformation, the chapter concludes with four illustrative value propositions and a summary of the important role of the POC Coordinator, who provides oversight.

Thus, in this chapter we lay the fundamental groundwork for transitioning to a new evidence-based approach where POC testing will be used outside the hospital environment for screening, diagnosis, treatment and monitoring in emergency and disaster medicine. We present six fundamental principles, then illustrate 'how to' use POC testing in a practical and cost-effective manner not only for preparedness, but also for efficient and cost-effective emergency and urgent care in small-world networks (Kost *et al.*, 2010) worldwide.

Principles

Principle 1 – solution

Past disasters demonstrate the feasibility and role of POC testing, while future POC testing will bring high impact

Feasibility

The 2004 tsunami in South-east Asia and Hurricane Katrina in 2005 in the USA proved not only the need for, but also the feasibility of deploying POC testing (Kost *et al.*, 2006), and while the disaster response was extensive, follow-up studies showed rescue was slow and inadequate. Table 7.1 lists the sites, organizations, instruments and test clusters that were available from about before the middle of the first week after Hurricane Katrina reached New Orleans until as much as a month or more later during which time manufacturers donated large numbers of glucose meters to patients with diabetes for chronic disease management. Flooding disabled most traditional clinical laboratories in civilian hospitals in the New Orleans area, and POC testing filled the gap, but not at all completely. In fact, several of the tests listed in Table 7.1 were available in association with military fixed resources in the area or moved there.

POC instruments carried by US Disaster Medical Assistance Teams (DMATs) enable testing for blood gases (with i-STAT EC8+/CG8+ cartridges), electrolytes/metabolites, haematocrit/haemoglobin, coagulopathy with Prothrmobin Time/International Normalized Ratio (PT/INR), blood glucose, non-invasive monitoring (e.g. O_2 saturation, capnography, electrocardiography and vital signs), and sometimes imaging by ultrasound (e.g. SonoSite MicroMaxx). However, interviews with Hurricane Katrina responders revealed the need for POC cardiac biomarker field testing to triage victims with complaints of chest pain. Generally, such testing is not part of the typical DMAT repertoire, but instead was provided on hospital ships in nearby locations like other military assets close to New Orleans, but not exactly at the point of need in the field. Local emergency medical services' POC testing capabilities generally are much more limited than those of DMATs, but usually include at least handheld glucose meters of various brands.

Role

Now in retrospect, we know that POC testing could have played a much larger role in Hurricane Katrina and follow-up care. For example, the incidences of chest pain in shelters (Greenough *et al.*, 2008) and the occurrence downstream of acute myocardial infarct (Gautam *et al.*, 2009) were significant. To plan an appropriate POC armamentarium, one can assess the need for vital functions and diagnostic pivots in the 'crisis care profile', an innovation that appeared as an early derivative of the merging of biosensor, conductivity and other measurement principles on to single transportable, portable or handheld POC platforms (Table 7.2) capable of whole-blood analysis of electrolytes, blood gases, haematocrit and metabolites (Kost, 1993). Please note that in the USA testing in the field may be limited to only so-called 'CLIA-waived' tests indicated by the grey shading in Table 7.2, because these tests, which are not moderate or high complexity, do not require licensed medical technologists or rigorous quality control to be performed.

Table 7.1. Use of POC testing in Hurricane Katrina in 2005.

Used by Used where Time of arrival	Device Manufacturer Website	Test menu
US Army 14th Combat Support Hospital Day 24	ID-Micro Typing System™ Gel Test™ Ortho-Clinical Diagnostics www.orthoclinical.com	Antibody screening and identification, ABO grouping/Rh phenotyping, compatibility testing, direct antiglobulin testing, reverse serum grouping and antigen typing
US Navy Unknown Days 1, 4 and 9	Nexus Dx Cardiac STATus® www.nexus-dx.com	CK-MB, cTnI and myoglobin
US Army 14th Combat Support Hospital Day 24	Rapidpoint Coag® Bayer Diagnostics No longer available	aPTT, HMT and PT
US military Local surveyed hospital -	i-STAT® Abbott Diagnostics www.abbottpointofcare.com	ACT Celite®, ACT Kaolin, BNP, BUN, Ca^{2+}, CK-MB, Cl^-, creatinine, cTnI, glucose, Hb, HCO_3, Hct, K^+, lactate, Na^+, pCO_2, pH pO_2, PT/INR, sO_2 and tCO_2
Local Red Cross - -	Acsensia Bayer Healthcare No longer available	Glucose
US Army, Navy, Marine Corps - -	Piccolo Abaxis No longer available	Albumin, ALP, ALT, amylase, AST, BUN, Ca^{2+}, cholesterol, CK, Cl^-, creatinine, dBil, GGT, glucose, HDL, K^+, LD, LDL, Mg, Na^+, phosphorus, triglycerides, tBil, tCO_2, TP and uric acid

Table 7.1. Use of POC testing in Hurricane Katrina in 2005 (continued).

Used by **Used where** **Time of arrival**	**Device** **Manufacturer** **Website**	**Test menu**
US Air Force - -	Triage Biosite www.biosite.com	BNP, CK-MB, cTnI and myoglobin

ACT, activated clotting time; ALP, alkaline phosphatase; ALT, alanine aminotransferase; aPTT, activated partial thromboplastin time; AST, aspartate aminotransferase; BNP, B-type natriuretic peptide; BUN, blood urea nitrogen; Ca^{2+}, calcium; CK, creatine kinase; CK-MB, creatine kinase MB; Cl^-, chloride; cTnI, cardiac troponin I; dBil, direct bilirubin; GGT, gamma glutamyltransferase; Hb, haemoglobin; HCO_3^-, bicarbonate; Hct, haematocrit; HDL, high-density lipoprotein cholesterol; HMT, Heparin Management Test; K^+, potassium; LD, lactate dehydrogenase; LDL, low-density lipoprotein cholesterol; Mg, magnesium; Na^+, sodium; pCO_2, partial carbon dioxide; pH, potential hydrogen; pO_2, partial oxygen; PT, prothrombin time; PT/INR, prothrombin time/international normalized ratio; sO_2, oxygen saturation; tBil, total bilirubin; tCO_2, total carbon dioxide; TP, total protein.

Table 7.2. Crisis care profile: vital functions, diagnostic pivots and waived tests (from Kost *et al.*, 2011c.)

Function/target	Point-of-care pivot(s) or rationale
Energy	Glucose, β-hydroxybutyrate Haemoglobin pO_2, O_2 saturation
Conduction	Potassium Sodium Ionized calcium (free calcium, Ca^{2+}), ionized magnesium (Mg^{2+})
Contraction	Ionized calcium, ionized magnesium
Perfusion	Lactate
Acid-Base	pH CO_2 content (TCO_2), pCO_2 End-tidal CO_2 tension Bicarbonate (calculated HCO_3^-)[a]
Osmolality	Measured osmolality Calculated osmolality
Hemostasis	Haematocrit, haemoglobin Prothrombin time (PT), international normalized ratio (INR) Activated partial thromboplastin time (aPTT) Activated clotting time (ACT) D-dimer Platelet count and function (e.g. thromboelastogram)
Homeostasis	Creatinine, urea nitrogen B-type natriuretic peptide (BNP) Chloride, inorganic phosphate White blood cell count, haemoglobin E, fragility (e.g. thalasaemia) Co-oximetry variables
Biomarker	Cardiovascular risk (cholesterol, HDL, LDL, triglycerides; hs-CRP) Bone formation (bone-specific Alk Phos)[a] and resorption (NTx)[a] Cancer (prostate-specific antigen, urine NMP22 – bladder cancer) Cardiac injury (myoglobin, CK-MB mass/isoforms, troponin I/T) Endocrine (intraoperative parathyroid hormone) Trauma (S100 (brain injury marker))
Sepsis	Lactate, procalcitonin,[a] C-reactive protein[a]
Birthing	Prenatal testing (glucose, urine protein, sexually transmitted disease) Antenatal screening (genetic disorders) Delivery monitoring (e.g. fetal heart rate and *Group B Streptococcus*) and transcutaneous neonatal bilirubin

Table 7.2. Crisis care profile: vital functions, diagnostic pivots and waived tests (continued).

Function/target	Point-of-care pivot(s) or rationale
Women's health	Fertility (FSH) Pregnancy (β-hCG) Bone resorption (NTx)[a] Human papillomavirus[a] Cervical cancer[a]
Emergency blood donor screening	HIV-1/2, hepatitis B, hepatitis C
Transfusion	ABO blood typing, Rh class
Infectious disease	HIV-1/2, *H. pylori*, Dengue, others – rapid Dx-Rx with multiplex assays Primary care, public health, surveillance – prevention, control
Influenza pandemic	Influenza A, influenza B, subtypes: H1N1, 2009 H1N1, H3, H5N1 Drug resistance: oseltamivir, zanamivir, amantadine, rimantadine
Epidemic	Cholera (stool test, rectal swab) Tuberculosis (PPD skin test) Avian influenza[a] (EUA)
Newdemic	Diabetes: glucose, haemoglobin A1c, AGE, urine AGR, fructosamine[a]
Biothreat	Anthrax, botulism, plague, tularaemia, Ebola, west Nile

[a]A POC test is needed or in development. CLIA-waived tests are indicated by the grey highlight.

Impact

Most manufactures seek CLIA-waived status and must demonstrate to the US Food and Drug Administration that results are accurate, precise and interpretable regardless of who performs the testing. None the less, personnel who operate POC devices and use test kits should be well trained and perform quality control because, fundamentally, POC testing is not an excuse for inaccuracy irrespective of where it is performed or by whom. Outside the USA, the waiver concept becomes vague, hence, more extensive test clusters are becoming available worldwide, as illustrated in Fig. 7.1.

For example, Fig 7.1B and H shows handheld POC devices, and D and G portable instruments, all of which offer essential tests, including cardiac troponin I or T, other cardiac biomarkers and moderately complex assays, which are vital to field triage, diagnosis and therapy. However, the instruments in Fig 7.1G and H are not available currently in the USA or Western Europe. The other instruments, which are available for use in the USA, must comply with federal and state regulations. As more POC formats emerge

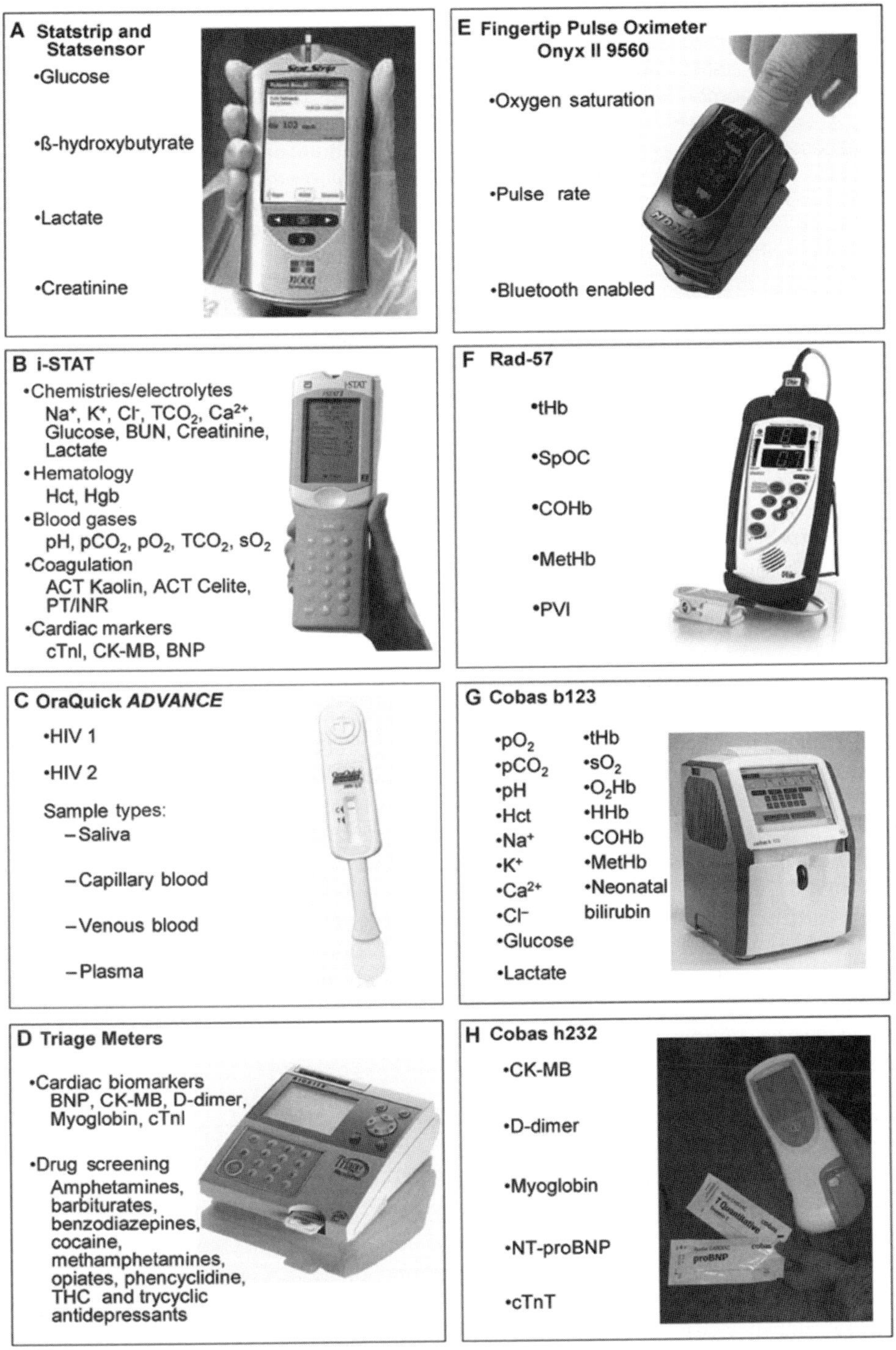

Fig. 7.1. POC instruments of high value in emergencies and disasters (from Kost *et al.*, 2011c). POC devices cover several of the multifaceted testing and monitoring needs of first

responders. The device in (A) is US CLIA-waived for glucose; in (B) for haematology and chemistries/electrolytes except lactate; in (C), for saliva and capillary and venous blood; and in (D), for B-type natriuretic peptide (BNP). (E and F) show monitoring devices useful for O_2 saturating and haemoglobin trend following. Devices in (G and H), which are not available in the USA or Western Europe, provide valuable test results for blood gases, electrolytes, metabolites, co-oximetry, cardiac biomarkers and coagulation status. Manufacturers and websites are: (A) StatStrip, www.novabiomedical.com; (B) i-STAT, www.abbottpointofcare.com; (C) OraQuick ADVANCE, www.orasure.com; (D) Triage, www.biosite.com; (E) Onyx II, www.nonin.com; (F) Rad-57, www.masimo.com; (G) Cobas b123, www.roche.com; and (H) Cobas h232, www.roche.com.

worldwide, so will extensive testing capability, built-in quality control, robustness and relaxed constraints on device operators. Hence, the impact of POC testing is increasing in emergency and disaster medicine, and we should plan ahead for that bright future.

Principle 2 – balance

Needs assessment guides POC invention, innovation and technology development

Historical roots

POC testing, per se, arose out of spontaneous and original clinical discovery in three main areas: (i) critical care (e.g. early use of ionized calcium (Ca^{2+}) measurements performed directly by whole-blood biosensor in the operating room for efficient management of liver transplant patients receiving massive transfusions during surgery (Kost *et al.*, 1986)); (ii) glucose monitoring (e.g. self-monitoring with glucose meters by patients with diabetes); and (iii) coagulation testing (e.g. trend following of prothrombin time (PT), then later the International Normalized Ratio (INR), in patients receiving anticoagulation therapy).

The definition of POC testing and this new field were codified by a group of clinicians and laboratorians as a result of the 'Cape Cod Project' and published in *Chest* (Kost *et al.*, 1999). Formal needs assessment now is used to guide POC invention, innovation and technology development, and in the area of pathogen detection for urgent, emergency and disaster care, the reader is referred to papers by Brock *et al.* (2010), Kost *et al.* (2009, 2010) and Mecozzi *et al.* (2010) for details. Table 7.3 summarizes research results that have been generated in the past 3 years by these authors. In general, survey respondents agree regarding key factors, such as the need for rapid whole-blood detection of methicillin-resistant *Staphylococcus aureus* (MRSA) and for screening emergency blood donors to rule out viral infections.

Guidance and access

Henry Ford once said, 'If I had asked people what they wanted, they would have said a faster horse!' In fact, results from recent needs assessment surveys are partly obvious and intuitive, but also at times somewhat unexpected. For example, respondents stated that biohazards should be confined (obvious), detection of MRSA was paramount (intuitive) and, rather than direct sampling from venipucture, in some cases use of a Vacutainer was preferred (unexpected) (Kost *et al.*, 2012). Possibly, they did not consider fully the potential for contamination during specimen transfer for pathogen detection by nucleic acid testing.

Table 7.3. Needs assessment survey results.

Survey question	Answers
Top three disaster pathogen priorities	(i) MRSA,[a] (ii) *Vibrio cholera*, [a] (iii) *Salmonella typhi*[a]
Top blood stream pathogen priority	MRSA (unanimous)[a]
Top three blood donor screening priorities	(i) HIV 1/2 (unanimous),[a] (ii) hepatitis B[a] and C,[a] (iii) hepatitis C[a] and B[a]
Top pandemic screening priorities	Influenza A/B,[a] SARS,[a] 2009 H1N1,[a] avian H5N1[a]
Test cassette versus vacutainer with hub for sample collection in disaster setting	Test cassette (unanimous)[a]
Direct versus coupled direct sample collection in disaster setting	Direct[a]
Biohazard waste disposal in disaster setting	Stores all in test cassette (unanimous)[a]
Most desirable testing location outside hospital	Patient-side (unanimous)
Device performance characteristics	Predictors of respondent device selection: high clinical sensitivity,[a] time to result,[a] clinical specificity[a] and battery operation[a]
Top four settings for pandemic infectious disease	Emergency room, disaster setting, outpatient testing clinics and urgent care clinics
Top three preferred sample types for pandemic infectious disease testing	Sputum, blood and swabs
Device design in disaster settings	Handheld

[a] $P < 0.05$ or less.

MRSA, methicillin-resistant *Staphylococcus aureus*; SARS, severe acute respiratory syndrome.

Table 7.4. New POC technologies with potential application in emergencies and disasters.

Author/ year	Invention/ innovation	Variable measured	Method	Potential in emergencies and disasters
Barfield *et al.*, 2011	PATH-Lemos ICS-based POC Chagas test	Antibodies to *T. cruzi*	Test strip	Rapid detection of Chagas disease
Bearinger *et al.*, 2011	POC device for infectious disease	MRSA	LAMP	Rapid detection of bloodstream pathogens
Brozik *et al.*, 2010	POC device for blood pathogens	HIV 1 and 2, hepatitis B and C	Acoustic wave biosensing	Rapid detection of important pathogens for blood donor screening
Clayden, 2011	Burnet Institute CD4 counter	CD4 T cells	Immuno-chromatography	Rapid detection of HIV
	Daktari CD4 counter	CD4 T cells	Microfluidic cell chromatography and lysate impedance spectroscopy	Rapid detection of HIV
	Liat™ Analyzer	DNA/RNA of bacteria and viruses	PCR	Rapid detection of 2009 H1N1
	M Bio CD4 Counter	CD4 T cells	Fluorescence using LightDeck technology	Rapid detection of HIV

	NWGF rapid test strip	p24 antigen	Lateral flow assay	Rapid detection of HIV in infants
	SAMBA	HIV RNA or influenza	Isothermal amplification and visual detection by dipstick	Rapid detection of HIV
	Zyomyx CD4 Counter	CD4 T cells	Disposable cartridge	Rapid detection of HIV
D'Arcy *et al.*, 2011	Halifax Consciousness Scan	Neural activity	EEG	Rapid diagnosis of brain damage
Jung *et al.*, 2011	Handheld scanner	Cross-sectional imaging of eye, skin and oral cavity	Optical coherence tomography	Rapid diagnosis and monitoring capabilities of eye, skin and mouth problems
Lee and Chon, 2011	Filtering algorithm	Breathing frequency	COPS-MPF algorithm	Add breathing frequency to existing pulse oximeters
Mandal *et al.*, 2011	POC heart care and patient monitoring system	Heart sound	Device that uses a mixed signal sound processer interfaced with a computer	Rapid diagnosis of heart problems, and rapid spot-check monitoring
Barker *et al.*, 2006	Rad-57™	Total Hb, oxygen content, carboxyHb, metHb, pulse rate, perfusion index and PVI	Masimo SET® technology	Handheld pulse oximeter for monitoring the measured variables

Table 7.4. New POC technologies with potential application in emergencies and disasters (continued).

Author/ Year	Invention/ innovation	Variable measured	Method	Potential in emergencies and disasters
Yi *et al.*, 2011	CMOS/CCD imaging sensor	OxyHb and DeoxyHb concentrations	Multispectral imaging	Tool to assess and monitor impending metabolic shock

CMOS/CCD, complementary metal oxide semiconductor/charge coupled device; COPS-MPF, combined TV and TIVOPS-based multiple modes particle filter; EEG, electroencephalography; Hb, haemoglobin; HIV, human immunodeficiency virus; ICS, immunochromatographic strip; LAMP, loop-mediated isothermal amplification; OCT, optical coherence tomography; POC, point-of-care; TIVOPS, time-invariant optimal parameter search; TV, time-varying.

In any case, four POC Technologies Centers (Kost *et al.*, 2008) funded from 2007 to 2012 by the National Institute for Biomedical Imaging and Bioengineering (NIBIB) at the National Institutes of Health (NIH) have produced a needs assessment knowledge base that helps guide future investment in POC testing and its commercialization, with the objective of making inventions and innovations more accessible and successful, including in crises. The direct implication of needs assessment is to match POC test clusters to the purpose of the user and response.

Principle 3 – efficiency

POC test clusters allow 'mission matching' – one can select instruments and tests for triage, diagnosis, treatment and/or monitoring, but devices and reagents must be operated within environmental tolerances and legal constraints specified by the manufacturer

New technologies and test clusters

One of the most exciting developments in the POC testing field is the rapid emergence of numerous new technologies potentially useful in emergencies, disasters and public health crises (Table 7.4). Some new technologies target specific problems, such as neurological emergencies (Table 7.5) and biothreats (not shown), for which diagnosis is particularly challenging. However, as noted above, testing in sites outside accredited hospitals and clinics may be constrained to so-called 'CLIA-waived' tests (see Table 7.2), with attendant sacrifice of screening, diagnostic and monitoring capabilities.

For example, in disasters physicians could benefit from POC cardiac biomarker testing, but may be prevented from carrying this out if not in compliance with local, state and federal regulations in the USA or with governing authorities in other nations. Hence, whatever the setting or country, responders are obligated to consider the legal ramifications of the types of POC tests that they perform, and to prepare in advance by working with relevant authorities to establish suitability.

Thus far in the USA, non-invasive continuous monitoring devices are not regulated as tightly as *in vitro* diagnostics. Pulse oximeters (O_2 saturation monitors) and non-invasive continuous haemoglobin monitoring (Table 7.6) now are used extensively in critical care (Kost and Tran, 2011) and disaster response (Kost *et al.*, 2013). Cost-effective oxygen saturation monitoring derives from reduced O_2 consumption during ambulance transport, especially long distances and durations (Macnab *et al.*, 1999; Howes *et al.*, 2000) and then, from efficient triage (Summers *et al.*, 1998) and monitoring (Jones *et al.*, 1988) in the emergency department. New designs work well during ambulance transport (Weber *et al.*, 2011) and can screen patients for carbon monoxide exposure (Nilson *et al.*, 2010).

Continuous haemoglobin monitoring (Frasca *et al.*, 2011; Kost and Tran, 2011) should be explored for decision-making during the care of critically ill patients, such as those with Dengue haemorrhagic fever, when hospitalized and in need of frequent haematocrit (haemoglobin) determinations and blood transfusions to keep up with haemolysis. Pathogen detection by biosensor-, nuclear magnetic resonance (NMR) and polymerase chain reaction (PCR)-based assays for bacteria, viruses and fungi increasingly will play an important role as larger format instruments currently available shrink in size and move into the pipeline. For example, a small POC surface acoustic wave sensor that detects HIV-1/2 and hepatitis B/C now is in commercial development (Brozik *et al.*, 2010).

Table 7.5. Neurotechnologies potentially useful at the point of need.

Major problem/ challenge	How often it appears	Current and emerging technologies
Traumatic brain injury	With addition of spinal cord injuries accounted for 57% of deaths in 1999 Athens, Greece earthquake (Mateen, 2010)	Ahead™ EU-100 InfraScan: mobile imaging device SFC Fluidics TBI device Banyan Biomarkers TBI assay
Spinal cord injury	650–750 cases in 2005 northern Pakistan earthquake with 600 cases of paraplegia (Mateen, 2010) 240 cases in 2003 Bam, Iran earthquake (Mateen, 2010)	–
Peripheral nerve injury	Cases were reported in 1999 following the Marmara earthquake in Turkey (Mateen, 2010)	–
Stroke	The incidence of haemorrhagic stroke increased for 1 month following the Noto Peninsula, Japan earthquake (Mateen, 2010) Relative risk of stroke increased for 1 year following 1995 Hashin-Awaji earthquake (Sokejima *et al.*, 2004)	Biosite Triage Stroke Panel (Sibon *et al.*, 2009) Ischiban: Stroke Assessment Headband Jan Medical: Portable Brain Sensing System

Environmental robustness

POC testing devices typically encounter harsh environmental conditions, temperature extremes and high humidity. Despite substantial improvements, large gaps still exist between current POC technologies and 'real-world' demands. Inability of POC instruments and reagents to withstand harsh conditions present at emergency and disaster sites can compromise performance (Louie *et al.*, 2009, 2012). For example, glucose test strips and blood gas cartridges may not provide accurate measurements at disaster sites because thermal stresses adversely and inconsistently affect performance (Fig. 7.2).

In Hurricane Katrina flooded hospitals, roads and communication breakdowns hindered rescue efforts by responders that carried limited POC devices such as oxygen saturation monitors (pulse oximeters), blood glucose meters and other small handhelds (Kost *et al.*, 2006). Instruments failed to operate effectively under adverse environmental conditions at respective disaster locations, where temperatures reached 110°F (43.3°C) or higher in hospitals (Anonymous, 2007; Diiulio, 2007).

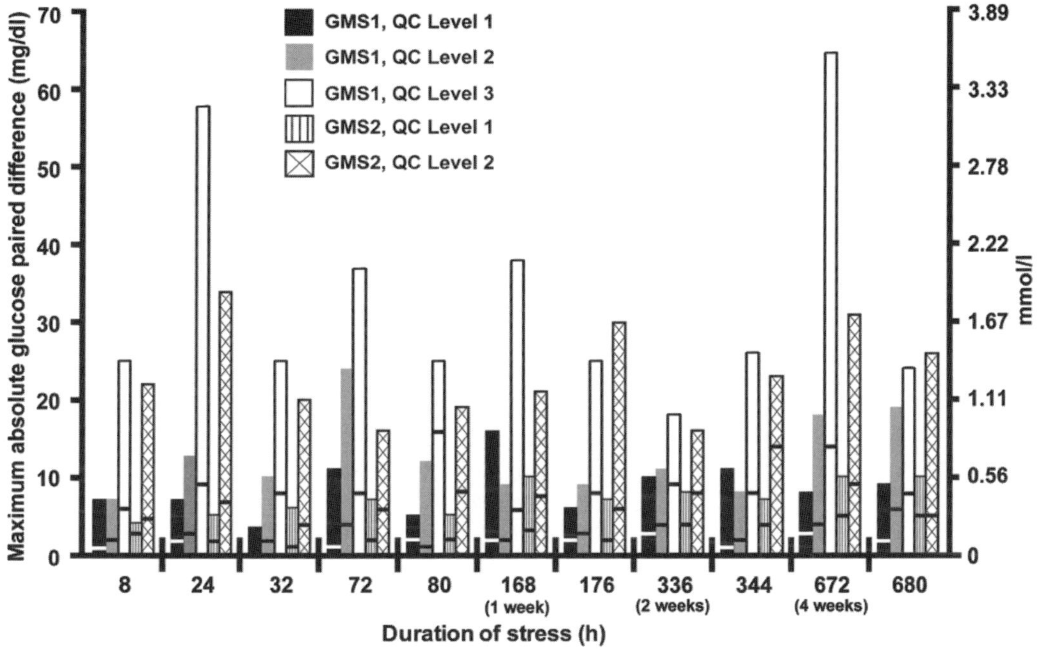

Fig. 7.2. Maximum absolute differences resulting from environmental stress (From Louie *et al.*, 2012).

Cold weather in Japan impeded rescue following the recent devastating earthquake and tsunami and, as such, these newdemics (Kost, 2006) lead to sequentially magnified setbacks, including radioisotope exposure. Thus, thermoregulated (Fig. 7.3) POC devices may be of use in such settings, because generally, they perform measurements at body temperature or another fixed temperature (Table 7.7) and may be able to compensate for, and operate in, cold environments. However, this hypothesis must be proven prior to full-scale deployment.

The heights of the columns in Fig. 7.2 represent the maximum absolute differences in paired glucose observations between thermally stressed and control strips. Glucose median absolute paired differences are displayed as horizontal lines across the vertical bars. Two glucose meter systems (GMS) were evaluated over more than 4 weeks. Temperature varied dynamically from 20°C to 45°C in a profile that simulated disaster conditions. Humidity varied from 30% to 90%. Environmental stress clearly affected handheld glucose meter performance.

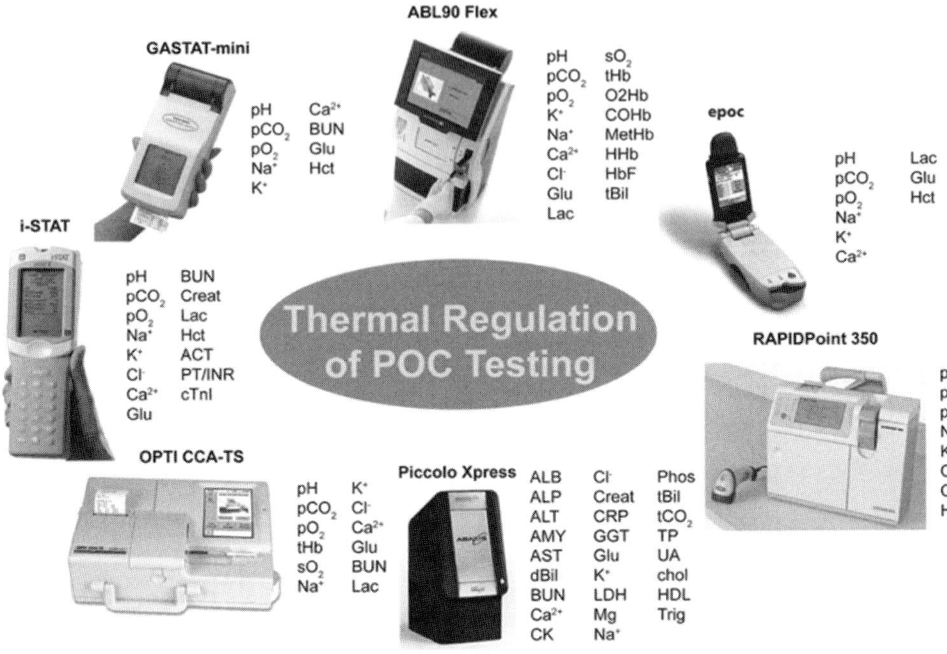

Fig. 7.3. Instruments with thermal regulation of POC testing. POC instruments designed to measure blood gases and pH typically have built-in thermal regulation that may allow them to be used in disaster settings where environmental conditions are cold. However, this hypothesis must be tested and, until proven, manufacturer requirements and limitations regarding temperature should be observed.

Requirements for current use

In view of these types of current limitations and the obvious technical gaps in POC devices as we know them today, the USA and other countries *are not prepared for disasters*! If POC devices and test kits are used, then they should *be operated within environmental tolerances and legal constraints specified by the manufacturer and licensing body*. Additionally, substantial funding will be needed to improve environmental robustness for civilian uses of POC testing in crises. This type of research and development will improve not only the usefulness and flexibility of POC devices, reagents and test kits, but also once they are deployed, the standard of care in emergencies and disasters (Kost *et al.*, 2011c).

Table 7.6. Oxygen saturation and haemoglobin monitoring POC devices.

Manufacturer	Device name (format)	Continuous measurements	Methodology	SpO_2 analytical measurement range	Hb analytical measurement range	Manufacturer's product claims	FDA approved intended use
Biosense www.biosense.in	ToucHb[a] (portable)	THb	In development	N/A	In development	In development	Not applicable
Hutchison Technologies www.htch.com	InSpectra Model 325	Tissue Hb,[a] StO_2	3 wavelengths spectro-photometry (Myers *et al.*, 2009)	N/A	Tissue Hb sensor In development	In development	Not applicable
Masimo www.masimo.com	Pronto[b] (handheld)	THb, SpO_2, pulse	8-wavelength spectro-photometry	70–100%[c,d] (adults and paediatrics)	8–17 g/dl, ±1 g/dl[c,d] (adults and paediatrics) (FDA, 2010a)	THb spot checking	THb spot checking in clinical and non-clinical settings (FDA, 2010a)
	Pronto-7[b] (handheld)	THb, SpO_2, pulse, PI[f]	"	70–100%[c,d] (adults and paediatrics >30 kg)	6–18 g/dl, ±1 g/dl[c,d] (adults and paediatrics >30 kg) (FDA, 2010a)	"	THb spot checking in clinical and non-clinical settings (FDA, 2010b)
	Rad-57 (portable)	THb, SpO_2, COHb, MetHb, pulse, PVI[e,g]	≤8 wavelengths spectro-photometry (Barker *et al.*, 2006)	70–100%[c,d] (adults and paediatrics)	7–17 g/dl, ±1 g/dl[c,d] (adults and paediatrics) (FDA, 2008)	Continuous monitoring of THb	Continuous THb monitoring (FDA, 2008)
	Rad-87 (handheld)	THb, SpO_2, COHb, MetHb, pulse, PVI[e,g], RR	"	"	"	Continuous THb monitoring with wire-less connectivity	"
	Radical-7 (portable)	THb, SpO_2, COHb, MetHb, PI[f], PVI[e,g], total O_2	≤12 wavelengths spectrophotometry	"	"	Continuous and trend monitoring of THb	"

Table 7.6. Oxygen saturation and haemoglobin monitoring POC devices (continued).

Manufacturer	Device name (format)	Continuous measurements	Methodology	SpO_2 analytical measurement range	Hb analytical measurement range	Manufacturer's product claims	FDA approved intended use
MBR Optical Systems www.mbr-optical-system.com	Mediscan 2000[a] (portable)	THb	Wavelength ranging from 350 to 1020 nm (Rabe *et al.*, 2005)	N/A	In development	In development	Not applicable
Nonin www.nonin.com	Onyx II 9550/ 9560 (fingertip)	SpO_2, pulse	2-wavelength spectro-photometry	70–100%[c,d] (adults and paediatrics)	N/A	SpO_2 spot checking	Spot checking on fingers, not thumbs (FDA, 2008)
Nellcor www.nellcor.com	OxiMax N-600x (portable)	SpO_2, pulse, PR	2-wavelength spectro-photometry	70–100%[c, d] (adults, paediatrics and neonatal)	N/A	Continuous monitoring	Continuous monitoring (FDA, 2009)
OrSense www.orsense.com	NBM-200MP[a] (portable)	THb, SpO_2, pulse, pleth	4-wavelength spectro-photometry	In development	THb sensor in development	In development	N/A
Sysmex www.sysmex.com	Astrim[a] (portable)	THb	In development	N/A	Evaluated with Hb from 6.7–18.4 g/dl (Saigo *et al.*, 2004)	In development	N/A

[a] Not FDA-approved.
[b] CLIA-waived.
[c] Accuracy claim from 510k FDA-approval.
[d] Determined during conditions of non-motion and good perfusion.
[e] Calculated parameter.
[f] PI = (variable amount of absorbed light/constant amount of absorbed light) × 100%.
[g] $PVI = [(PI_{max} - PI_{min})/(PI_{max})] \times 100\%$.
COHb, carboxyhaemoglobin; Hb, haemoglobin; MetHb, methaemoglobin; PI, perfusion index; PR, perfusion range; pleth, plethymographic waveform; PVI, plethymographic waveform variability index; RR, respiratory rate; SpO_2, oxygen saturation; StO_2, tissue oxygen saturation; THb, total haemoglobin.

Table 7.7. Mechanisms of POC devices with thermal regulation.

Device Manufacturer Website	Handheld/portable tests	Temperature control method	Temperature set point
ABL90 Flex Radiometer www.radiometeramerica.com	Portable blood gases, electrolytes, metabolites and oximetry	Heating block	37°C
epoc® Alere www.alere.co.uk	Handheld blood gases and electrolytes	Heating blocks located above and below the test card	37°C
GASTAT-mini Techno Medica www.technomedica.co.jp/English	Handheld blood gases and electrolytes	Pre-heater	Not available
i-STAT® Abbott Point of Care Inc. www.abbottpointofcare.com	Handheld blood gases, electrolytes, haematology, coagulation and cardiac markers	Thermistors and heating contact wires in test card	37°C
OPTI® CCA-TS OPTI Medical www.optimedical.com	Portable blood gases and electrolytes	Heating block located below sample	37°C
Piccolo Xpress® Abaxis www.abaxis.com	Portable chemistry analyser	Heating plates located above and below test disc	37°C
RAPIDPoint® 340/350 Siemens Healthcare Diagnostics www.medical.siemens.com	Portable blood gases	Heating block	37°C

Principle 4 – evidence

POC technologies enable evidence-based decision-making at the point of need, and also can transfer ownership for personalized medicine there!

Evidence-based medicine

POC testing helps transform empirical judgement into evidence-based decision-making at the point of need by supplying critical test results quickly where they are needed the most. Test results can be of value not only to disaster victims and patients, but also to volunteers working in the field. For example, during rescue efforts following the 2011 earthquake in Haiti, volunteers subject to accidental needle sticks could not properly ascertain thc IIIV status of the blood sources. Thus, in order to protect themselves, responders should be equipped with HIV-1/2 test kits suitable for field conditions.

Fortunately, some HIV-1/2 tests are CLIA-waived (see Table 7.2), but environmental robustness has not been evaluated fully, so test kits should be transported, stored and used as specified on the product insert provided by the manufacturer. Another common example involves cardiac biomarker testing. In low-resource settings, community hospital physicians often need fast POC cardiac troponin I or T test results to determine the disposition of patients with chest pain, rather than waiting for the EKG to evolve and delaying transfer (Fig. 7.1).

Ownership and empowerment

The instruments shown in Fig. 7.1 B, D and H perform cardiac biomarker tests, and the instrument in H has been implemented extensively in community hospitals throughout Thailand since early introduction in settings along the Mekong River near the Laos border and provinces in Isaan (Kost *et al.*, 2010) for evidence-based care of patients with acute coronary syndromes. Repeatedly, where POC testing has been rolled out to rural settings, local practitioners take ownership of instrument operation, maintenance and results reporting. Next, they recognize the value of immediate test results in patient management.

Examples of distributed ownership include: (i) POC testing in 'mobile medical units', which are truck-based roving clinics with diagnostics tests and professional personnel that cover several districts in Phitsanulok Province, Thailand (Boonlert *et al.*, 2006); (ii) haemoglobin A1c testing for care of Aboriginal diabetic patients in remote Australia (Shephard and Gill, 2003; Martin *et al.*, 2005; Shephard *et al.*, 2005, 2009); and (iii) village rotational POC testing performed directly in low-resource Primary Care Units of Amphur Khumuang in Buriram, Isaan (Kost *et al.*, 2011a). Thus, with POC ownership comes empowerment for heathcare teams and patients to manage changes in therapy and other interventions directly and efficiently.

Principle 5 – integration

Strategic planning optimizes small-world networks; healthcare teams and patients become experienced with POC testing through education, training and everyday use

Small-world networks

Small-world networks (Kost, 2006) are 'like your family and friends ... you have fun and work with them every day, and in times of need, you call on them for assistance!' Examples include six degrees of separation between people, social influence networks, food chains, electric power grids, airline flight patterns and road maps. Usually, most small-world network nodes are connected by several paths, there is an over-abundance of 'hubs' with high numbers of connections, common connections mediate short path lengths between edges and emergency medical system personnel learn to navigate optimal routes that are efficient and spare transit time.

Historically derived features generally found in small-world networks include demographic roots (e.g. transportation routes), geographic and topographic congruity (e.g. ambulance short cuts), regional interconnections with neighbouring networks and patterns reflecting health resource disparities (Kost *et al*., 2011b). Hence, small-world networks can be used quite effectively to guide POC resource allocations with the counsel of local emergency medical system personnel, because they provide ambulance services through the network every day and know the transportation and strategic bottlenecks where decision-making needs to be accelerated.

Strategic planning

Figure 7.4 characterizes successful 'hub' applications of POC testing in a small-world network modelled after healthcare delivery in rural provinces of Thailand. Once empowered with immediate test results, healthcare practitioners come to realize the utility and importance of testing at the point of need and quickly learn to take advantage of the efficient small-world network design as cost-effective infrastructure for delivery of everyday urgent and emergency care, as well as primary care and community preparedness for major crises. Hence, POC testing instruments, test clusters and monitors should be selected for prevailing conditions, anticipated disease threats, points of distribution and triage/referral to regional centres with graduated levels of medical, surgical and trauma expertise that exist and are available within the small-world network and nearby referral resources, such as specialty, university and national centres.

Principle 6 – synthesis

Value propositions generate tactics for placing POC testing appropriately in physical, demographic and geographic settings; however (the 'corollary'), if POC testing does not change decision making or add value, then do not use it!

Next, we review examples of four value propositions, which are presented as practical recommendations.

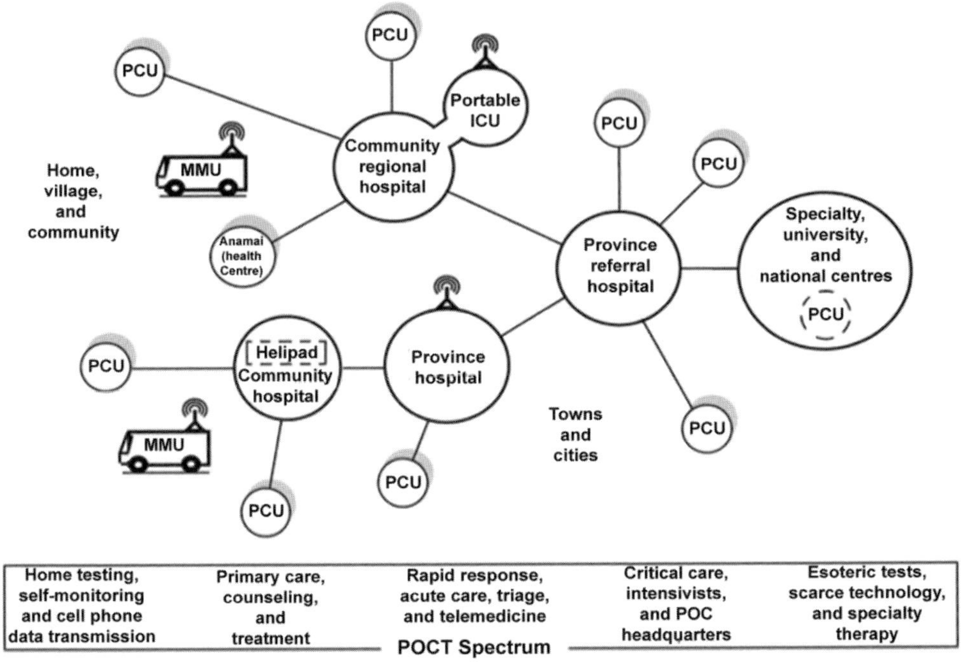

Fig. 7.4. Small-world network as a suitable infrastructure for preparedness. The 'POC testing spectrum' (bottom band) covers a broad range of needs in the infrastructure and for the healthcare team in small-world networks. 'Mobile medical units' (MMUs), portable intensive care units (ICUs) and deployable hospitals bridge gaps and have been used in several situations, including disasters. However, any of the locations, including primary care units (PCUs), can become isolated. Therefore, POC testing should be planned carefully to meet simultaneously the complex needs of daily healthcare operations, such as urgent and emergency care, as well as of preparedness.

The first value proposition: reduce Therapeutic Turnaround Time (TTAT) to speed critical paths

Evidence-based research shows that POC testing decreases TTAT and improves satisfaction, which correlates with improved patient care, labour conservation, timeliness and convenience (Kilgore *et al.*, 1998; Kost, 2002). Fast TTAT enhances emergency room patient triage, treatment and transfer, all of which observers deemed important, for example, during the 2004 tsunami response in South-east Asia (Kost *et al.*, 2006). Figure 7.5 illustrates the placement of POC testing in the receiving area of a typical rural community hospital in a small-world network, with POC testing integral to services provided by the emergency room ('bedside testing'), small clinical laboratory ('near-patient testing') and other adjacent units.

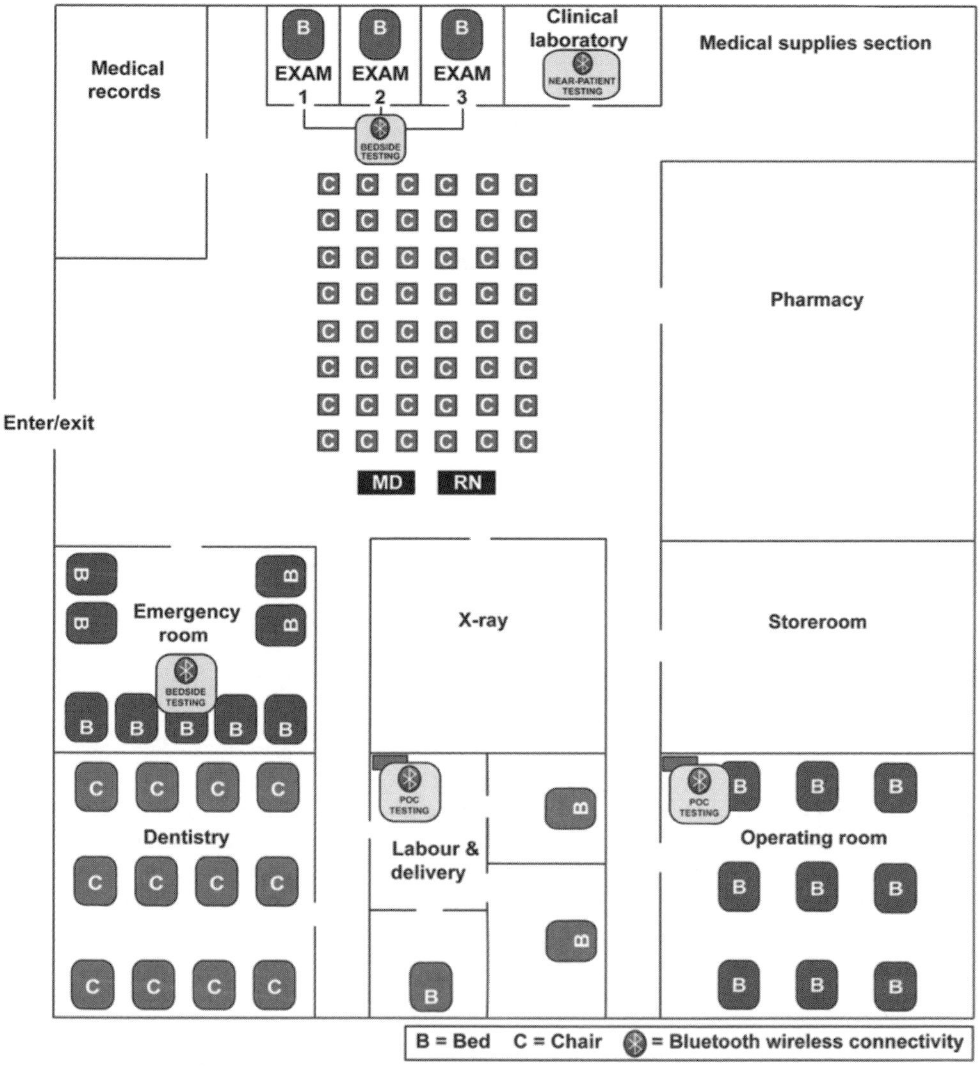

Fig. 7.5. Access, emergency support and POC value in the community hospital. (From Kost *et al.*, 2011c.) Access to POC testing typically is immediate in the relatively small intake area of a rural community hospital and for all practical purposes, close proximity of the clinical laboratory is equivalent to 'near-patient testing', so hours of coverage should be addressed. That is, if laboratory staff do not work nights or weekends, then POC testing fills voids in diagnostic testing and monitoring, especially in the emergency room, and hence, adds value by continuously assuring rapid TTAT.

Low-resource community hospitals often lack whole-blood analysers capable of performing *in vitro* blood gas (pO_2, pCO_2), pH and electrolyte (e.g. Na^+, K^+ and Ca^{2+}) measurements, so instead in the past few years, particularly nurses have adopted extensive use of pulse oximeters, inexpensive POC oxygen saturation monitoring devices that now can be purchased in the USA for a few dollars and operate long-term on one set of two AA batteries. These *in vivo* POC technologies reduce TTAT while fulfilling the need for acute monitoring of key pivots in the crisis care profile (see Table 7.2).

The second value proposition: use POC testing in high impact sites during emergencies and disasters

These sites include: (i) *physical locations:* shelters, community hospitals and alternate care facilities (Lam *et al.*, 2006; Cantrill *et al.*, 2009; Altegovt *et al.*, 2010; Glassman and Parrillo, 2010); (ii) *demographic settings:* rural areas, primary care and regions with poor health resource scores (Kost *et al.*, 2011b); and (iii) *geographic terrain:* healthcare systems with challenging regional topographies at high risk of isolation. For example, Fig. 7.6 illustrates a theoretical alternate care facility design with placement of near-patient testing in the mini-laboratory and bedside testing in the procedure room. The impact of POC testing in this case is that it brings evidence-based decision-making into the facility itself, and there are no delays waiting for results. Therefore, the use of POC testing provides an opportunity to enhance the standard of care for victims, not to mention quicker triage, isolation and referral, without over-burdening local emergency rooms during patient surges.

The third value proposition: Optimize practitioner experience with POC testing

Tactical POC testing should: (i) complement healthcare delivery resources; (ii) fulfil needs for simultaneous emergency care and disaster preparedness; and (iii) compensate for geographic isolation, current or anticipated. Therefore, routine daily use of POC testing assures the high quality of trained operators, who serve as 'POC Coordinators' by integrating POC testing within small-world networks. Excellent courses have emerged to train medical technologists and nurses in POC testing, and these courses also can be used to train emergency medical system personnel and disaster responders.

In fact, some programmes, such as one developed by the American Association for Clinical Chemistry in 2011, are web-based and therefore accessible worldwide. In particular, a session in this web-based course supplements this chapter (Kost, 2011). Others developed by the authors and colleagues are online at: http://www.youtube.com/user/POCTCTR. Table 7.8 summarizes key attributes of the role of the POC Coordinator. Emergency and disaster response teams should call on, or have as part of their membership, a POC Coordinator. Small community hospitals (up to 100 beds) may have just one Coordinator, who covers the entirety of the hospital practice and its primary care network referral system, while larger regional hospitals (up to 500 beds) typically have two or more Coordinators, who cover numerous sites and oversee many POC tests.

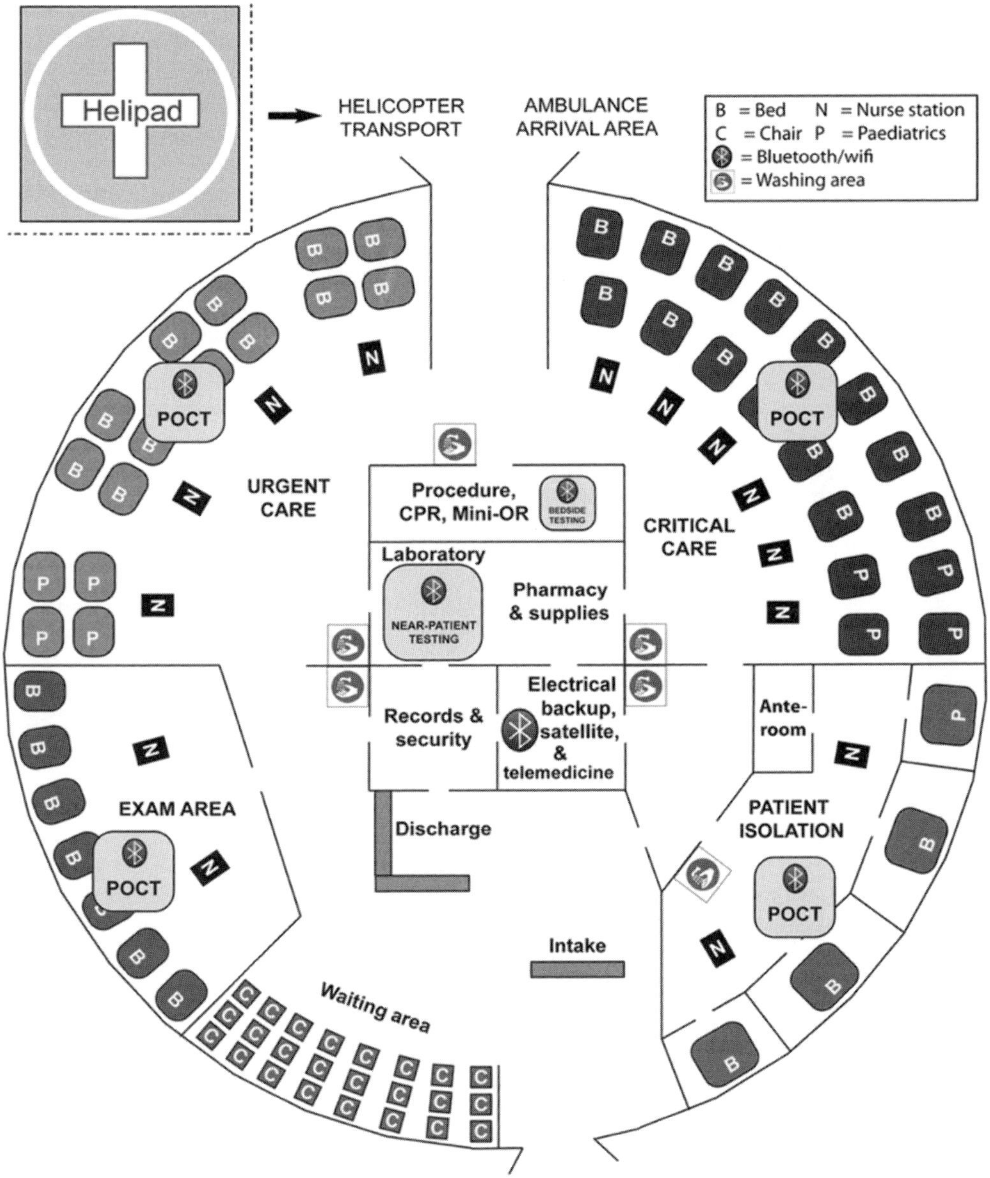

Fig. 7.6. Alternate Care Facility (CAF) and the usefulness of POC testing. (From Kost *et al.*, 2011c.) This ACF could be implemented in a temporary structure, a pre-planned facility or a community building, such as a high school gymnasium. A rigid structure is not implied, but instead, a design for flexible functional units to which POC testing brings evidence-based decision-making medicine without delays in results.

Table 7.8. The essential role of POC Coordinators.

• Provide oversight for the POC programme in the hospital, including the emergency room, operating room, intensive care units and clinics, and for networked primary care.
• Take responsibility for proper quality assurance, test performance, proficiency testing, accreditation, training and education, irrespective of where POC testing is performed.
• Help select new tests and instruments, and validate them before implementation.
• Communicate with physicians, nurses, laboratory personnel and administration to solve problems and assist the POC Director and Committee in setting the mission, goals and objectives.
• Integrate POC testing properly within the hospital disaster preparedness plan and its policies.
• Train first responders in emergency and disaster POC, or alternatively, help develop the educational programmes that are used.
• Perform strategic planning to assure that the small-world network is resilient to the challenges of crises and that community hospitals (see Fig. 7.4) and emergency access 'hubs' (see Fig. 7.5) are properly equipped to deal with sudden victim surges.
• Participate in the planning of POC testing for placement in alternate care facilities (see Fig. 7.6).
• Work to integrate community preparedness, emergency medicine and disaster response by assuring the consistency of POC instrumentation and the competency of operators.
• Guarantee that the POC programme is delivering fast decision making in the hospital, efficient urgent emergency care and cost-effective disaster preparedness in the small-world network.

The fourth value proposition: assess POC testing in context

Critical information has value exceeding the costs of tests. Physicians assign high value because test results impact decisions. Nurses assign higher value than laboratory technicians. Speed has value, and often is life-saving. Patient self-care and responder welfare garner value as well! Total value depends on the sum of benefits minus costs – *Value* = *Σ [Benefits – Costs]* when assessed in context.

As an example, capillary glucose meter monitoring (for self-monitoring of blood glucose, or 'SMBG'), POC HbA1c testing (to gauge the efficacy of therapy) and urinary albumin to creatinine ratio (ACR) screening (to detect nephropathy) can be implemented (Kost *et al.*, 2011b) to facilitate the care of patients with diabetes during and after disasters, since chronic illnesses should not be ignored.

In essence, POC testing represents a 'bridging' technology, for both time and space, and as the number of devices and tests available mushrooms in the future, there will be many bridges to cross! Figure 7.7 sums up the viewpoint. Community preparedness, disaster response and emergency medicine can be optimized through the use of POC testing in the small-world network, and if the POC devices include appropriate wireless connectivity (Yu *et al.*, 2010), the common thread of evidence-based medicine will become ubiquitous, which ultimately, is the goal.

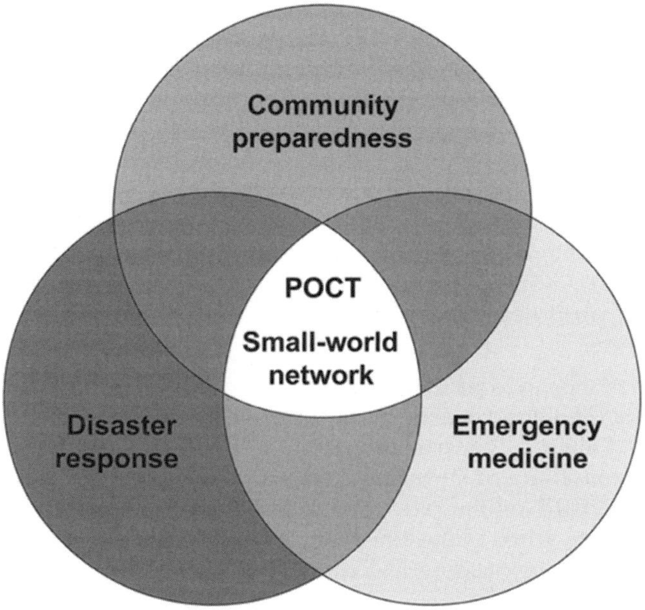

Fig. 7.7. Synthesis and integration: POC testing and the small-world network (SWN). (From Kost *et al.*, 2011c.) Tactical integration, synthesis and optimization help improve crisis standards of care. The advantage of the holistic SWN-POC approach is that local community and regional healthcare leaders can blend preparedness synergistically with routine daily use of POC testing to attain operator competency, meet disaster needs and achieve emergency medicine goals.

Conclusions and Recommendations

As a new field, POC testing has matured to the point where several devices, both *in vitro* discrete sampling instruments and *in vivo* non-invasive continuous monitors, now are available with the mobility necessary to strategize, unify and problem solve at the point of need in emergency, disaster and public health crises.

With numerous innovative technologies in a rapid growth phase, POC devices will enable: (i) the healthcare team to enhance evidence-based practice regardless of location; (ii) the patient to empower for personalized medicine; and (iii) responders to encourage POC coordinators among them to take responsibility for proper training, quality assurance and test performance.

Ongoing research: (i) reveals which POC devices and reagents can be used subject to limitations in and adaptations for different climates; (ii) identifies how and what to design to improve robustness in emergency and disaster settings; (iii) describes test clusters necessary for critical decision-making that matches field responses and medical conditions; and (iv) provides practical approaches for implementing POC testing cost-effectively.

Practical roadmaps for expedient POC testing readiness spring from, and reside in, small-world networks and their regional interconnections and thus, by establishing flexibly equipped network hubs, POC testing can be managed cost-effectively for disaster preparedness and simultaneously for efficient daily urgent-emergency care.

The conceptual framework in this chapter represents the 'compass' to navigate individual 'maps', that is, the reader's specific physical settings and small-world networks, in order to improve crisis standards of care, including in situations of low-resource community hospitals and the associated primary care units at the village level.

Acknowledgements

This study was supported primarily by the Point-of-Care Testing Center for Teaching and Research (POCT•CTR) and in part by a NIBIB Point-of-Care Technologies Center grant (Dr Kost, Principal Investigator, NIH U54 EB007959). The content is solely the responsibility of the authors and does not necessarily represent the official views of the NIBIB or the NIH. The authors thank the staff and students who contributed to this work at the University of California, Davis. Figures and tables were provided with permission and courtesy of Knowledge Optimization®, Davis, California, USA.

References

Altegovt, B.M., Stroud, C., Nadig, L. and Hougan, M. (2010) *Institute of Medicine (US) Forum on Medical and Public Health Preparedness for Catastrophic Events. Medical Surge Capacity: Workshop Summary.* National Academies Press, Washington, DC.

Anonymous (2007) Katrina's death: who's to blame? *The Economist* 13, 35.

Barfield, C.A., Barney, R.S., Crudder, C.H., Wilmoth, J.L., Stevens, D.S., Mora-Garcia, S., Yanovsky, M.J., Weigl, B.H. and Yanovsky, J. (2011) A highly sensitive rapid diagnostic test for Chagas disease that utilizes a recombinant *Trypanosoma cruzi* antigen. *IEEE Transactions on Biomedical Engineering* 58, 814–817.

Barker, S.J., Curry, J., Redford, D. and Morgan, S. (2006) Measurement of carboxyhemoglobin and methemoglobin by pulse oximetry: a human volunteer study. *Anesthesiology* 105, 892–897.

Bearinger, J.P., Dugan, L.C., Baker, B.R., Hall, S.B., Ebert, K., Mioulet, V., Madi, M. and King, D.P. (2011) Development and initial results of a low cost, disposable, point-of-care testing device for pathogen detection. *IEEE Transactions on Biomedical Engineering* 58, 805–808.

Boonlert, W., Kost, G.J., Jiraviriyakul, A. and Tangvarasittichai, S. (2006) Point-of-care testing on a Mobile Medical Unit in Northern Thailand: screening for hyperglycemia, hyperlipidemia, and Thalassemia trait. *Point of Care* 5, 164–167.

Brock, T.K., Mecozzi, D.M., Sumner, S.L. and Kost, G.J. (2010) Evidence-based point-of-care test cluster and device design for disaster preparedness. *American Journal of Disaster Medicine* 5, 285–294.

Brozik, S., Branch, D., Wheeler, D., Edwards, T., Larson, R., Hjelle, B., Brown, D., Hall, P. and Bisoffi, M. (2010) *Acoustic Wave Biosensors: Rapid Point-of-Care Medical Diagnostics – R&D 100 Entry.* Sandia National Laboratories, Albuquerque, New Mexico.

Cantrill, S.V., Pons, P.T., Bonnett, C.J., Eisert, S. and Moore, S. (2009) *Disaster Alternate Care Facilities: Selection and Operation.* Agency for Healthcare Research and Quality, Rockville, Maryland.

Clayden, P. (2011) HIV point of care diagnostics pipeline. In: Clayden, P. (ed.) *HIV, Hepatitis C Virus (HCV), and Tuberculosis Drugs, Diagnostics, Vaccines, and Preventive Technologies in Development: 2011 Pipeline Report.* i-base/Treatment Action Group, New York, pp. 53–58.

D'Arcy, R.C.N., Hajra, S.G., Liu, C., Sculthorpe, L.D. and Weaver, D.F. (2011) Towards brain first-aid: a diagnostic device for conscious awareness. *IEEE Transactions on Biomedical Engineering* 58, 750–754.

Diiulio, R.A. (2007) New Orleans hospital weathers the storm. *Medical Laboratory Observer* 39, 18–20.

Food and Drug Administration (FDA) (2008) Masimo Rainbow SET 7, Rad-57, and Rad-87 co-oximeters, K080238. Available at: http://www.accessdata.fda.gov/cdrh_docs/pdf8/K080238.pdf (Accessed 9 October 2011).

FDA (2009) OxiMax N-600x pulse oximeter with SPD, K083325. Available at: www.accessdata.fda.gov/cdrh_docs/pdf8/K083325.pdf (Accessed 9 October 2011).

FDA (2010a) Masimo Rainbow Pronto pulse oximeter, K080403. Available at: www.accessdata.fda.gov/cdrh_docs/pdf9/K091057.pdf (Accessed 9 October 2011).

FDA (2010b) Masimo Rainbow Pronto-7 pulse co-oximeter, K100403. Available at: www.accessdata.fda.gov/cdrh_docs/pdf10/K100403.pdf (Accessed 9 October 2011).

Frasca, D., Dahyot-Fizelier, C., Catherine, K., Levrat, Q., Debaene, B. and Mimoz, O. (2011) Accuracy of a continuous noninvasive hemoglobin monitor in intensive care unit patients. *Critical Care Medicine* 39(10), 2277–2282.

Gautam, S., Menachem, J., Srivastav, S.K., Delafontaine, P. and Irimpen, A. (2009) Effect of Hurricane Katrina on the incidence of acute coronary syndrome at a primary angioplasty center in New Orleans. *Disaster Medicine and Public Health Preparedness* 3, 144–150.

Glassman, E.S. and Parrillo, S.J. (2010) Use of alternate healthcare facilities as alternate transport destinations during a mass-casualty incident. *Prehospital and Disaster Medicine* 25, 178–182.

Greenough, P.G., Lappi, M.D., Hsu, E.B., Fink, S., Hsieh, Y.H., Vu, A., Heaton, C. and Kirsch, T.D. (2008) Burden of disease and health status among Hurricane Katrina-displaced persons in shelters: a population-based cluster sample. *Annals of Emergency Medicine* 51, 426–432.

Howes, D.W., Field, B., Leary, T., Jones, G.R. and Brison, R.J. (2000) Justification of pulse oximeter costs for parametric prehospital providers. *Prehospital Emergency Care* 4, 151–155.

Jones, J., Heiselman, D., Cannon, L. and Gradisek, R. (1988) Continuous emergency department monitoring of arterial saturation in adult patients with respiratory distress. *Annals of Emergency Medicine* 17, 463–468.

Jung, W., Kim, J., Jeon, M., Chaney, E.J., Stewart, C.N. and Boppart, S.A. (2011) Handheld optical coherence tomography scanner for primary care diagnostics. *IEEE Transactions on Biomedical Engineering* 58, 741–744.

Kilgore, M.L., Steindel, S.J. and Smith, J.A. (1998) Evaluating stat testing options in an academic health center: therapeutic turnaround time and staff satisfaction. *Clinical Chemistry* 44, 1597–1603.

Kost, G.J. (1992) The hybrid laboratory: shifting the focus to the point of care. *Medical Laboratory Observer* 24(9 Supplement), 17–28.

Kost, G.J. (1993) New whole blood analyzers and their impact on cardiac and critical care. *Critical Reviews in Clinical Laboratory Sciences* 30, 153–202.

Kost, G.J. (2002) The hybrid laboratory, therapeutic turnaround time, critical limits, performance maps, and Knowledge Optimization. In: Kost, G.J. (ed.) *Principles and*

Practice of Point-of-Care Testing. Lippincott Williams and Wilkins, Philadelphia, Pennsylvania, pp. 13–25.

Kost, G.J. (2006) Newdemics, public health, small-world networks, and point-of-care testing. *Point of Care* 5, 138–144.

Kost, G.J. (2011) *Improving the Standard of Care for Disaster Medicine.* American Association for Clinical Chemistry (www.aacc.org), Washington, DC, Point-of-Care Coordinator Course, Online Lecture. Available at: http://www.aacc.org/members/divisions/cpoct/newsletter/archives2011/december/Pages/CertificateProgram.aspx# (Accessed 15 March 2013).

Kost, G.J. and Tran, N.K. (2011) Continuous noninvasive hemoglobin monitoring: the standard of care and future impact. *Critical Care Medicine* 39(10), 2369–2371.

Kost, G.J., Jammal, M.A., Ward, R.E. and Safwat, A.M. (1986) Monitoring of ionized calcium during human hepatic transplantation: critical values and their relevance to cardiac and hemodynamic management. *American Journal of Clinical Pathology* 86, 61–70.

Kost, G.J., Ehrmeyer, S.S., Chernow, B., Winkelman, J.W., Zaloga, G.P., Dellinger, R.P. and Shirey, T. (1999) The laboratory-clinical interface: point-of-care testing. [multicentre paper] *Chest* 115, 1140–1154.

Kost, G.J., Tran, N.K., Tuntideelert, M., Kulrattanamaneeporn, S. and Peungposop, N. (2006) Katrina, the tsunami, and point-of-care testing: optimizing rapid response diagnosis in disasters. *American Journal of Clinical Pathology* 126, 513–520.

Kost, G.J., Korte, B., Beyette, F.R., Gaydos, C. and Weigl, B. (2008) The NIBIB Point of Care Technologies Research Network: Center themes and opportunities for exploratory POC projects. *Point of Care* 7, 41.

Kost, G.J., Hale, K.N., Brock, T.K., Louie, R.F., Gentile, N.L., Kitano, T.K. and Tran, N.K. (2009) Point-of-care testing for disasters: needs assessment, strategic planning, and future design. *Clinics in Laboratory Medicine* 29, 583–605.

Kost, G.J., Kost, L.E., Suwanyangyuen, A., Cheema, S.K., Curtis, C., Sumner, S., Yu, J. and Louie, R. (2010) Emergency cardiac biomarkers and point-of-care testing: optimizing acute coronary syndrome care using small-world networks in rural settings. *Point of Care* 9, 53–64.

Kost, G.J., Kanoksilp, A., Mecozzi, D.M., Sonu, R., Curtis, C. and Yu, J.N. (2011a) Point-of-need hemoglobin A1c for evidence-based diabetes care in rural small-world networks: Khumuang Community Hospital, Buriram, Thailand. *Point of Care* 10, 28–33.

Kost, G.K., Katip, P., Kanoksilp, A. and Mecozzi, D.M. (2011b) New demographic strategy for point-of-need medical testing: linking health resource scores, poverty levels, and care paths. *Journal of Demography* [Chulalongkorn University, Bangkok] 27, 1–31.

Kost, G.J., Sakaguchi, A., Curtis, C., Tran, N.K., Katip, P. and Louie, R.F. (2011c) Enhancing crisis standards of care using innovative point-of-care testing. *American Journal of Disaster Medicine* 6, 351–368.

Kost, G.J., Mecozzi, D.M., Brock, T.K. and Curtis, C.M. (2012) Assessing needs for point-of-care pathogen detection in emergencies and disasters. *Point of Care* 11, 119–125.

Kost, G.J., Katip, P., Kulrattanamaneeporn, S. and Gentile, N. (2013) Point-of-care testing value proposition for disaster preparedness in small-world networks: post-tsunami Phang Nga Province, coastal Thailand. *Point of Care* 12, 9–22.

Lam, C., Waldhorn, R., Toner. E., Inglesby, T.V. and O'Toole, T. (2006) The prospect of using alternative medical care facilities in an influenza pandemic. *Biosecurity and Bioterrorism* 4, 384–905.

Lee, J. and Chon, K.H. (2011) Time-varying autoregressive model-based multiple modes particle filtering algorithm for respiratory rate extraction from pulse oximeter. *IEEE Transactions on Biomedical Engineering* 58, 790–794.

Louie, R.F., Sumner, S.L., Belcher, S., Mathew, R., Tran, N.K. and Kost, G.J. (2009) Thermal stress and point-of-care testing performance: suitability of glucose test strips and blood

gas cartridges for disaster response. *Disaster Medicine and Public Health Preparedness* 3, 13–17.
Louie, R.F., Ferguson, W.J., Sumner, S.L., Yu, J.N., Curtis, C.M. and Kost, G.J. (2012) Effects of dynamic temperature and humidity stresses on point-of-care glucose testing for disaster care. *Disaster Medicine and Public Health Preparedness* 6, 232–240.
Macnab, A.J., Susak, L., Gagnon, F.A., Alred, J. and Sun, C. (1999) The cost-benefit of pulse-oximeter use in the prehospital environment. *Prehospital and Disaster Medicine* 14, 245–250.
Mandal, S., Basak, K., Mandana, K.M., Ray, A.K., Chatterjee, J. and Mahadevappa, M. (2011) Development of cardiac prescreening device for rural population using ultralow-power embedded system. *IEEE Transactions on Biomedical Engineering* 58, 745–749.
Martin, D.D., Shephard, M.D., Freeman, H., Bulsara, M.K., Jones, T.W., Davis, E.A. and Maguire, G.P. (2005) Point-of-care testing of HbA1c and blood glucose in a remote Aboriginal Australian community. *Medical Journal of Australia* 182, 524–527.
Mateen, F.J. (2010) Neurological disorders in complex humanitarian emergencies and natural disasters. *Annals of Neurology* 68, 282–294.
Mecozzi, D.M., Brock, T.K., Tran, N.K., Hale, K.N. and Kost, G.J. (2010) Evidence-based point-of-care device design for emergency and disaster care. *Point of Care* 9, 65–69.
Myers, D., McGraw, M., George, M., Mulier, K. and Beilman, G. (2009) Tissue hemoglobin index: a non-invasive optical method of total tissue hemoglobin. *Critical Care* 13, S2.
Nilson, D., Partridge, R., Suner, S. and Jay, G. (2010) Non-invasive carboxyhemoglobin monitoring: screening emergency medical services patients for carbon monoxide exposure. *Prehospital and Disaster Medicine* 25, 253–256.
Rabe, H., Stupp, N., Ozgun, M., Harms, E. and Jungmann, H. (2005) Measurement of transcutaneous hemoglobin concentration by noninvasive white-light spectroscopy in infants. *Pediatrics* 116, 841–843.
Saigo, K., Imoto, S., Hashimoto, M., Mito, H., Moriya, J., Chinzei, T., Kubota, Y., Numada, S., Ozawa, T. and Kumagai, S. (2004) Non-invasive monitoring of hemoglobin. The effects of WBC counts on measurement. *American Journal of Clinical Pathology* 121, 51–55.
Shephard, M.D. and Gill, J.P. (2003) Results of an innovative education, training and quality assurance program for point-of-care HbA1c testing using the Bayer DCA 2000 in Australian Aboriginal Community Controlled Health Services. *Clinical Biochemistry Review* 24, 123–130.
Shephard, M.D., Mazzachi, B.C., Shephard, A.K., McLaughlin, K.J., Denner, B. and Barnes, G. (2005) The impact of point of care testing on diabetes services along Victoria's Mallee Track: results of a community-based diabetes risk assessment and management program. *Rural Remote Health* 5, 371.
Shephard, M.D., Mazzachi, B.C., Watkinson, L., Shephard, A.K., Laurence, C., Gialamas, A. and Bubner, T. (2009) Evaluation of a training program for device operators in the Australian Government's Point of Care Testing in General Practice Trial: issues and implications for rural and remote practices. *Rural Remote Health* 9, 1189.
Sibon, I., Rouanet, F., Meissner, W. and Orgogozo, J.M. (2009) Use of the Triage Stroke Panel in a neurologic emergency service. *American Journal of Emergency Medicine* 27, 558–562.
Sokejima, S., Nakatani, Y., Kario, K., Kayaba, K., Minowa, M. and Kagamimori, S. (2004) Seismic intensity and risk of cerebrovascular stroke: 1995 Hanshin-Awaji earthquake. *Prehospital and Disaster Medicine* 19, 297–306.
Summers, R.L., Anders, R.M., Woodward, L.H., Jenkins, A.K. and Galli, R.L. (1998) Effect of routine pulse oximetry measurements on ED triage classification. *American Journal of Emergency Medicine* 16, 5–7.

Weber, U., Tomschik, E., Resch, I., Adelmann, K., Hasun, M., Mora, B., Malzer, R. and Kober, A. (2011) Comparison of two new generation pulse oximeters during emergency ambulance transportation. *European Journal of Anaesthesiology* 28, 92–96.

Yi, D., Wang, C., Qi, H., Kong, L., Wang, F. and Adibi, A. (2011) Real-time multispectral imager for home-based health care. *IEEE Transactions on Biomedical Engineering* 58, 736–740.

Yu, J.N., Brock, T.K., Mecozzi, D.M., Tran, N.K. and Kost, G.J. (2010) Future connectivity for disaster and emergency point of care. *Point of Care* 9, 185–192.

Chapter 8

Incident Command Systems

Steve Parrillo and Jean Bail

Historical Background

The western US state of California is plagued with wildfires. Many are large enough that firefighters from several jurisdictions respond. The Standardized Emergency Management System (SEMS) was developed in the 1970s to clarify the chain of command and address a general lack of accountability. Not only did responders have problems communicating because of poor interoperability, they often used codes and terminology that were confusing to others. Planning during the event was less than optimal. Well-meaning 'freelancers' often arrived and could not effectively be used because there was no common organizational structure. Finally, there was no clearly defined way to coordinate the many agencies who responded. SEMS promoted standardized language, roles and responsibilities and a clear reporting structure for the many firefighters. It quickly became apparent that firefighting was a more efficient and effective operation under the Incident Command System (ICS). Its use then spread to law enforcement, emergency medical services and medical care. The term ICS replaced SEMS. The National Incident Management System (NIMS) became the national version of ICS. The first Hospital Emergency Incident Command System (HEICS) was released in the late 1980s. It is now in its fourth version as the Hospital Incident Command System – HICS.

Overview

NIMS originated from Homeland Security Presidential Directive 5 in 2004 as a system to meet a major national need. It is essentially a national ICS, so the combined term ICS/NIMS is commonly used when discussing the US version of incident command. The term NIMS is used in this chapter.

The long-term goal of NIMS is to provide a consistent framework for all aspects of emergency management and incident response including prevention, protection, mitigation, response and recovery. This framework is sustainable, flexible and scalable to meet changing incident needs, and allows for integration of other resources from various partners through mutual aid agreements and/or assistance agreements. This model applies to all types of disciplines and levels of government and non-governmental agencies, including private and public organizations. Being scalable, it applies to all sizes of events, from the single unit response to a major nationally significant event.

The system is intended to serve as the tool by which an emergency operations plan (EOP) is carried out. This standardized model offers many advantages over non-standardized ones. Terminology is common to all users. That is, all users speak the same language. A word or phrase used in one area of the country means the same thing to a user elsewhere. Procedures are also standardized, allowing diverse response entities to work together as efficiently and effectively as possible.

Measurable objectives are established and monitored to ensure that incident goals are met.

In terms of management, ICS uses proven modalities (FEMA 501, March 2004, pp. 9–12; NIMS, 2008):

- The common terminology mentioned above is an important part of effective event management. NIMS includes consistent terms in areas of organizational functions, resource descriptions (personnel, facilities, equipment, supplies) and incident facilities.
- The organization is modular and flexible and is organized from 'the top down'. While overall responsibility rests with the Incident Commander (IC), depending on the incident's complexity, any section can be mobilized to meet the need and demobilized when no longer needed. Conversely, a section or branch that is not needed at the time can stay closed, yet remain available. Only the position of IC is filled in every event.
- Before ICS, disaster management was often reactive rather than proactive. The standard is now to develop an incident action plan (IAP) and manage by objectives. The result is a well thought-out, organized approach to a difficult situation.
- The span of control for any leader is three to eight subordinates. Unity of command refers to the fact that each person with a job to do knows the one person to whom he or she must report. Branch directors, for example, cannot report to the IC, only to the Section Chief. Command is clearly established and transferred as needed in an organized, clearly defined and documented process. The chain of command is orderly and clearly defined.
- A unified command is established in those events in which there are multiple jurisdictions, a single jurisdiction with involvement from multiple agencies or multiple jurisdictions with multiagency involvement. This allows for a single set of objectives, a coordinated approach to a complicated problem, uniform flow of information to all involved agencies and a single IAP. In most cases there is a single IC, though scene decisions are often left to jurisdictional authorities. Trust among agencies is key to the success of a unified command.
- All resources are categorized, ordered, dispatched, tracked and recovered in a comprehensive, organized fashion.
- Communications are integrated to allow for a common plan and interoperability. This is the link between operations and support.
- Accountability is defined in the areas of personnel check-in, IAP response operations, unity of command assignments, span of control and resource tracking.

Command Staff Positions and Duties

Overall responsibility under ICS falls to the IC. The person in this position develops incident objectives to maintain the priorities of safety, stabilization of the incident and strategies to manage the event. The IC stays in the Command Centre along with the other members of the command staff, monitoring the situation and incident organization. Other command staff includes the Public Information Office (PIO), the Liaison Officer (LNO), Safety/Security Officer (SO) and the Technical/Medical Specialist. Any staff person can have an assistant. Staff report only to the IC.

The LNO serves as the IC's 'right-hand man', interfacing with outside agencies. In both single and unified command situations, all representatives from governmental, non-governmental and private entities coordinate through this officer.

The PIO is the specially trained person who interacts with the public and the media. He prepares factual information to be released after approval by the IC. One person handles this responsibility even in the setting of unified command.

The SO has two primary duties. First, he monitors incident operations. He also advises the IC regarding operational safety. The latter includes emergency responder health and safety-related issues. This officer coordinates closely with Section Chiefs from Planning and Operations.

The position of Technical/Medical Specialist is dependent on the event. This office position could be filled by a radiation safety officer, infectious disease specialist, hazmat expert, an attorney, ethicist, public health official or paediatrician.

General Staff Positions and Duties

There are four sections in the ICS hierarchy, with all Section Chiefs serving on the general staff. Each Chief reports to the IC or unified command. General staff members are responsible for all functional aspects of the ICS.

The Operations Section 'is responsible for all activities focused on reduction of the immediate hazard, saving lives and property, establishing situational control, and restoration of normal operations' (National Incident Management System, 2008). Team members are the people at the scene. Branches, Divisions and Groups complete the section. Resources – personnel and equipment – are then divided into three groups. Single resources are just that. A Task Force is a combination of any type of resources assigned to a specific mission or operation. A Strike Team has a set number of resources of the same type and has an established minimum number of personnel. Both task forces and strike teams have designated leaders.

The Planning Section collects, evaluates, prepares and disseminates the tactical, event specific information regarding the incident (National Incident Management System, 2008). This occurs by creating an incident action plan (IAP), briefings, maps and status updates. The IAP, when approved by the IC, serves as the guide for the next operational period focusing staff on the objectives, resources and personnel needed to accomplish the IC's priorities and objectives.

The Logistics Section acquires the necessary infrastructure to support the response. This includes facilities, transportation, communications, supplies, equipment, fuel and food and medical support for responders. All off-site equipment and resource needs are coordinated and arranged by logistics (National Incident Management System, 2008).

The Finance/Administration Section handles all financial aspects, including cost analysis of all resources utilized and compensation. Contract administration, time-keeping and detailed records are essential for accurate payment of bills.

The ICS organizational chart then adds Branches, Divisions, Groups and Units, each with a specific job and headed by a leader with a clearly defined role (Fig. 8.1). For more information, please visit www.fema.gov/emergency/nims/.

Overview of HICS

Once it became apparent that the ICS made the approach to mass casualty incidents (MCIs) and disasters more efficient and effective, the ICS originators in California developed a version applicable to hospitals. The initial version was called HEICS – Hospital Emergency Incident Command System – but the name was changed to HICS in the third edition (California Emergency Medical Services Authority, 2007).

Similar to what the ICS does in other settings, HICS allows a healthcare entity to establish command and general staffs that are appropriate for the particular facility. The concept is well enough established that The Joint Commission (TJC) – the agency that evaluates and accredits most US hospitals – has mandated that it be used. FEMA did heavily promote the use of NIMS for hospitals (Federal Emergency Management Agency, 2008). The federal government attached a financial incentive in that hospitals could only receive Hospital Resource Service Administration (HRSA) emergency preparedness grant funds if they were 'NIMS-compliant' by 2008.

The IC has overall responsibility for activation and use of the emergency operations plan. Most often the IC is an administrator or other non-clinical person. Realistically, a clinician will probably be in the emergency operations centre to assist with medical issues. The IC depends on the usual command staff, but the organization chart has a position for a technical/medical specialist. Depending on the event, that person may be a toxicologist, radiation physicist, infectious disease person, etc.

Section Chiefs are appointed in Operations, Logistics, Planning and Finance/Administration. Most hospitals name positions (e.g. VP of Nursing) rather than individuals for each position.

Job Action Sheets are available for 46 HICS positions and can be customized to the needs of the hospital, although nomenclature must remain standardized. Like all ICS Job Action Sheets, each one lists the mission, contact information, reporting structure and duties. Duties are divided into immediate, intermediate and long-term.

HICS is available for download from http://www.emsa.ca.gov/hics/default.asp.

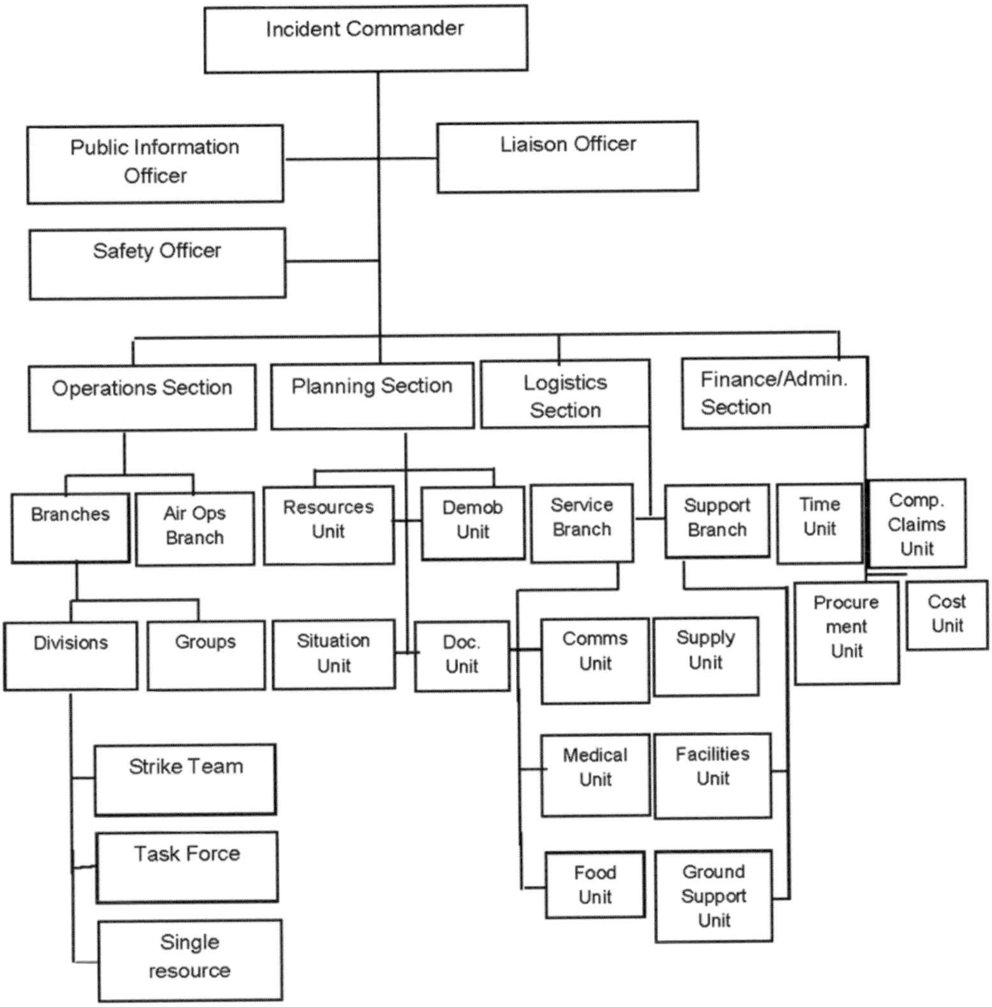

Fig. 8.1. Example of ICS design (http://www.training.fema.gov/EMIWeb/IS/ICSResource/assets/reviewMaterials.pdf).

Overview of Other Systems

Canada

Geographically contiguous with the USA and the second largest nation in the world, Canada is adapting many of the international concepts for emergency management to fit its municipal, provincial and federal design. The emergency management process that began decades ago is slowly being refined with the focus now on public safety and the implementation of the Emergency Management Act in 2007, the release of the Federal Emergency Response Plan in March 2010, and the revisions to the National Emergency Response System in January 2011. According to Lindsay (2009) Canada has not sustained forward momentum due to many interruptions in its development including multiple identity changes, fluctuations in governmental support and changes in organizational structures. The report from the Senate Standing Committee on National Security and Defence (2008) asked direct questions regarding the government's progress and accountability in disaster preparedness and response. It found that over a 4-year period there had been some progress in military capabilities and communications to support response needs but this capability needs to be increased. Additionally, there has been insufficient progress on inter-governmental emergency planning and departmental business continuity. Fiscal cuts to planned military growth and inadequate first responder equipment and training have also hampered development. An increase in collaboration on emergency management is needed from the smallest unit of government through to the largest.

Public Safety Canada, created in 2003, functions as the coordinating body for all federal departments dealing with public safety. Similar to the US Department of Homeland Security, this agency serves to create national policy, response systems and standards while housing the governmental emergency operations centre. Federal agencies are mandated to create internal emergency management plans to address each specific component's risk and to ensure continuity of operations. It is undocumented presently if these internal emergency management plans have been created and tested. Each of the ten provinces and three territories is required to address all aspects of emergency preparedness and response to be able to respond in support of municipal needs.

Tension exists between the provincial and federal levels dealing with financial support, integration and mission. Authority and responsibility for disaster response comes from jurisdictional mandates, placing the elected municipal and regional district officials at the centre of each local response (Kuban *et al.*, 2001). Each province and territory has approached this in its own manner, leading to variations in legislation, system design, training and communications capabilities. There is a disconnect in inclusion and communication of military, municipal and federal governmental resources (Senate Standing Committee on National Security and Defence, 2008).

It appears Canada is moving into a phase of development and realignment in spite of budgetary cuts from the government. Although the recent push for development has come from political pressure, international and US events, lessons have been learned through incidents such as the 2003 severe acute respiratory syndrome (SARS) outbreak, forest fires in British Columbia and the Winter Olympics in 2010. Since emergency management is decentralized, lessons learned and best practices are not easily disseminated. Many agencies participate in disaster management, including Public Safety Canada, Canadian Standards Association, Centre for Excellence in Emergency Preparedness, Canadian Emergency Management College and Public Health Agency of Canada. Coordination and integration of these and the many private and public resources, including critical infrastructure partners will be essential as Canada continues its evolution.

Growing out of the wildfire experiences and models developed by the US FIRESCOPE project and Canada's own wildfire experiences, the fire service has refined its use of incident command and created an effective forest fire management system. The Canadian Interagency Forest Fire Centre, Inc. (CIFFC) provides a resource allocation system for equipment, personnel and aircraft, including cross-provincial and cross-border agreements with the USA. Preparedness activities such as planning for resource sharing, finance and cost reimbursement, and communications networks have reached a level of sophistication. Based on an ICS model there are many commonalities that provide similar terminology and function for cross-jurisdictional responses, adopted by most Canadian police, fire and emergency medical services responders.

The main principles of unity of command, scalability, span of control and the four phases of emergency management – prevention/mitigation, preparedness, response and recovery all need to be operationalized. Respecting the unique needs of the Canadian governmental design, support needs to be increased to bring to fruition a cohesive system. In the meantime, various interpretations of incident command will continue to be found based on use, tradition and interpretation across the first responder communities. Kuban *et al.* (2001) discuss three basic versions of Incident Command in use – the traditional model coming from the Fire Service, the British Columbia Emergency Response Management System (BCERMS) and Emergency Site Management (ESM). All of these incorporate a foundation in incident command while addressing various municipal and provincial needs.

Health Canada is the federal agency charged with maintaining and improving the health status of all Canadians. The Emergency Preparedness and Occupational Health Directorate houses the bureau that plans and responds to federal requests for assistance to suspected or actual terrorist events. Focused on chemical, biological, radiological and nuclear events, the agency has refined its ability to support first responders and investigative needs. The Public Health Agency of Canada (an agency within Health Canada) takes an active role in developing and evaluating its ability to respond to a national health emergency or disaster. Through its surveillance and quarantine mission, information is exchanged with international health organizations. Through the Office of Emergency Response Services it funds and manages the National Emergency Stockpile System (NESS). This resource includes 165 field or mobile 200-bed hospitals with all necessary equipment and pharmaceuticals. Issues revolve around the implementation of NESS when needed with concern for the antiquated equipment not congruent with the current level of materials available, the lack of knowledge of what is in the stockpile and the need for inventorying and replacement of outdated medications and supplies (Senate Standing Committee on National Security and Defence, 2008).

In support of the National Emergency Response System, Health Canada, working with Public Safety and Emergency Preparedness Canada is aligning its internal emergency response plan using an ICS framework. This alignment will continue its growth to be interoperable with the first responder communities, municipalities, provinces and the federal government. Of note, epidemiological surveillance methods and data gathering for use in immediate trending and case recognition are being refined with the international pandemic planning initiatives.

Hospital preparedness in Canada has suffered from a lack of evidence-based risk and readiness assessment according to Kollek (2010), even though validated assessment tools exist. This is reinforced by Gomez *et al.* (2011), who found that trauma centre directors have not uniformly been included in disaster planning activities. Affecting all first receivers is a lack of all-hazards planning, training and exercises, preplanning for surge and leadership. The hospital community needs to engage in building relationships with those community partners and regional assets that will need to work together when an MCI occurs.

Canadian provinces and territories are addressing the local community needs for emergency management. Although uneven in progress, work is being done with incident command as a foundation for response and the four-phase model of disaster preparedness. At the federal level, it appears to be more fragmented with concern over a lack of momentum and steady progress.

United Kingdom

Incident command is done very differently in the UK. Only the fire and rescue services use a model similar to the US one.

Emergency management is done according to 'The Central Government Arrangements for Responding to an Emergency – Concept of Operations' (The United Kingdom Concept of Operations, 2005). This 2005 document outlines the centralized approach in use in England, Northern Ireland, Scotland and Wales. Although there are a few minor differences in the way each country manages an event, this section will only discuss the overall command system.

The UK Response Framework Civil Contingencies Act defines an emergency (or disruptive challenge) as 'a situation or series of events that threatens or causes serious damage to human welfare, the environment or security of the United Kingdom' (The United Kingdom Concept of Operations, 2005). The Concept of Operations then further stratifies emergencies into three categories. Emergency management response varies according to level and will be discussed later. Level 3 events are catastrophic and require 'immediate central government direction and support'. Level 2 are serious and require 'sustained central government co-ordination and support from many departments and agencies'. Both levels 3 and 2 would be led from the Cabinet Office Briefing Room (COBR). Level 1 events are significant but would not normally require COBR activation (Kapucu, 2008).

Local emergencies fall outside the three levels and are managed by local authorities. Most often, law enforcement is the Lead Government Department (LGD). In that setting, the Police Gold Commander takes the operational lead, often enlisting the help of the Strategic Co-ordination Group (SCG) to coordinate the response of other agencies. In some cases, the SCG may involve a relevant Regional Resilience Team (RRT). That team serves as interface or liaison between local responders and the central government.

The concept of Lead Government Department is key to the UK central government response. If the LGD is not clear, the Cabinet Office appoints one. The COBR is activated to support the LGD for all level 3 and 2 events. Members of the COBR include the Prime Minister, the Home Secretary (who chairs the group), representatives from relevant departments and agencies, and a Government Liaison Officer who interfaces with the Gold Commander's SCG. The Home Office serves as the LGD when the event is related to terrorism. The COBR serves then, as the emergency operations centre. It stays active until the emergency has passed.

A News Coordination Centre serves to handle media and public information.

Local command begins with the Police Gold Commander who chairs a multi-agency Strategic Coordination Group manned by representatives of key local organizations. A separate Recovery Working Group focuses on recovery efforts. A Government Liaison Officer coordinates group activity with the COBR.

When the emergency is large or complex enough to require direct central government coordination or support, a LGD takes command of overall central government response. The government maintains a pre-designated list of LGDs and maintains the list at the UK resilience website – www.ukresilience.gov.uk. When the LGD is not clear, the COBR appoints one. Once again, a Government Liaison Officer coordinates activities between the COBR and the SCG. For terrorism (or potential terrorism) events, the Government Liaison Officer is a senior Home Office official.

The UK response and recovery framework also designates three tiers, differing from each other in function (Kapucu, 2008). The bronze level is operational at the site of the event. The silver level is tactical and seeks to ensure that bronze level actions are coordinated and integrated. Silver leaders are staged at command posts close to the scene. The gold level is strategic. SCG Golden Commanders from appropriate agencies establish the framework within which the silver tier works.

Israel

Israel has adopted an approach to emergency management that is based primarily on the need to prepare for and respond to attacks against the nation. Rozdilsky (2009) calls this a 'military-centric' model. Christiansen and Blake noted that, 'Emergency management in Israel can be considered an outgrowth of the concept of defense of the rear area' (Christiansen and Blake, 1990). That is, after each attack changes were made to emergency management to better prepare for the next attack. For most of its history emergency management was the purview of the Israel Defense Force (IDF). That changed in 1992 with the creation of the Home Front Command (HFC) section of the IDF (Home Front Command, 2009). This fourth IDF command is a senior operational echelon. Each command fulfils the same charge, but with a focus unique to that command. The mission of the HFC is stated here:

> The Command constitutes a national branch responsible for preparing the country, its citizens, its institutions, its infrastructures, and its operational formations in confronting different emergency situations. The Command constitutes a national branch responsible for the integration and assimilation of the operational blueprint and combined doctrine used to confront emergency situations in conjunction with all search and rescue organizations, civilian as well as military establishments (Israel Defense Forces, 2009).

There are five specialized units within the HFC to deal with unique emergency management related activities: Atomic, Biological, Chemical Warfare Battalions, Extrication Battalions, National Search and Rescue Unit, Search and Rescue Companies, and a Casualty and Wounded Identification Unit (Israel Defense Forces, 2009). The HFC is the primary supplier of disaster-related plans, products, equipment and social-psychological services to the citizens of Israel (Kirschenbaum, 2004).

In addition, the HFC focuses on three issues: legal, operational and organizational (Home Front Command, 2009). For the first time since the passage of the 1951 Civil Defence Act there was an entity with autonomy for emergency management combined with 'on the ground' authority. Operationally, one Command assumed control of emergency management. From the perspective of organization, the HFC allows for better coordination of military and civilian emergency entities.

Kirschenbaum (2004) described the HFC as 'a National organization staffed by military personnel, whose specific goals are designed to protect the civilian population from natural, technological, and non-conventional war-related acts'.

While the HFC remains the primary Israeli agency for emergency management, the government created the National Emergency Authority or Reshut Heyrum Le'umit (RACHEL for short) in 2007. This agency serves to help balance military and civilian aspects of emergency management. Elran (2007) called this a significant step in Israeli emergency management because it implied official recognition of the centrality of the civilian home front along with the military front.

Comparing the Israeli approach to incident command with the US and UK models is difficult. As a primarily military system, the Israeli model relies heavily on the day-to-day way the Israel Defense Forces operate in purely military affairs. The hierarchy of command, then, is entirely military, even within the HFC. Incident command within RACHEL is still a work in progress.

Additionally, in most situations, local law enforcement serves as the command and control agency.

Summary

Incident command serves as the modality that allows for effective and efficient management during small and large incidents. It is an evolving system ideally practised on small local events so it is familiar to the users who are then better able to operationalize the system in large incidents. Although national systems vary, each allows leadership to establish and maintain command and control through guidance and structure. The most effective ones share the features of standardization and flexibility.

References

California Emergency Medical Services Authority (2007) Disaster medical services division – Hospital incident command system. Available at: http://www.emsa.ca.gov/HICS/default.asp (Accessed 24 May 2011).

Christiansen, J.R. and Blake, R.H. (1990) Israeli Civil Defense: historical background. *Journal of Civil Defense* April, 6–8.

Elran, M. (2007) Strategic assessment – the National Emergency Authority: New prospects or more of the same? A publication of the Institute for Strategic Studies, Tel Aviv University. 10 (3). Available at: http://www.inss.org.il/publications.php?cat=21&incat=&read=1380 (Accessed 17 May 2011).

Federal Emergency Management Agency (2008) ICS Review Document. Incident Command System Resource Center. Available at: http://www.training.fema.gov/EMIWeb/IS/ICSResource/assets/reviewMaterials.pdf (Accessed 18 July 2011).

Gomez, D., Haas, B., Ahmed, N., Tien, H. and Nathens, A. (2011) Disaster preparedness of Canadian trauma centres: the perspective of medical directors of trauma. *Canadian Journal of Surgery* 54(1), 9–16.

Home Front Command (Israel) (2009) The Home Front through time. Available at: http://www.oref.org.il/82-en/PAKAR.aspx (Accessed 23 January 2013).

Israel Defense Forces (2009) Home Front Command history. Available at: http://dover.idf.il/IDF/English/units/pikudim/homefront/History/default.htm (Accessed 10 May 2011).

Kapucu, N. (2008) Emergency and crisis management in the United Kingdom: disasters experienced, lessons learned, and recommendations for the future. Available at: http://www.training.fema.gov/EMIWeb/edu/CompEmMgmtBookProject.asp (Accessed 23 January 2013).

Kirschenbaum, A. (2004) Measuring the effectiveness of disaster management organizations. *International Journal of Mass Emergencies and Disasters* 22(1), 75–102.

Kollek, D. (2010) Hospital disaster readiness: why are we unprepared? Available at: http://www.ceep.ca/publications/HospitalDisasterReadinessWhyAreWeUnprepared.pdf (Accessed 1 June 2011).

Kuban, R., MacKenzie-Carey, H. and Gagnon, A.P. (2001) Disaster response systems in Canada. Institute for Catastrophic Loss Reduction, Toronto. Available at: www.iclr.org/images/Disaster_response_in_Canada.pdf (Accessed 31 May 2011).

Lindsay, J. (June 2009) Emergency management in Canada: near misses and moving targets. Available at: http://www.training.fema.gov/EMIWeb/edu/CompEmMgmtBookProject.asp (Accessed 31 May 2011).

National Incident Management System (2008) National Incident Management System, US Department of Homeland Security, Washington, DC. Available at: http://www.fema.gov/pdf/emergency/nims/NIMS_core.pdf (Accessed 18 July 2013).

Rozdilsky, J.L. (2009) Emergency management in Israel: context and characteristics. Available at: http://www.training.fema.gov/EMIWeb/edu/CompEmMgmtBookProject.asp (Accessed 23 January 2013).

Senate Standing Committee on National Security and Defence (2008) Emergency Preparedness in Canada: How the fine arts of bafflegab and procrastination hobble the people who will be trying to save you when things get really bad… Available at: http://www.parl.gc.ca/Content/SEN/Committee/392/defe/rep/rep13aug08vol1-e.pdf (Accessed 15 June 2011).

United Kingdom Concept of Operations (2005) Responding to emergencies: the UK Central Government Response Concept of Operations 2005. Available at: http://interim.cabinetoffice.gov.uk/media/349120/conops-2010.pdf (Accessed 5 July 2011).

Chapter 9

Incident Site Command and Control

Anders Rüter

Introduction

Command and control is originally a military term that is described as the process where the exercise of authority and direction by a properly designated commanding officer over assigned and attached forces in the accomplishment of the mission, is carried out (Builder *et al.*, 1999). In civilian management command and control refers more generally to the maintenance of authority with somewhat more distributed decision-making. These two definitions, which are basically the same, can also be used in the context of disaster management. Let's start by looking into the meaning of the two words command and control. Should they always be used together? Or do they represent different aspects of management in disasters and major incidents? In this chapter disaster and major incidents will be discussed under the term mass casualty incidents (MCIs).

Before exploring this issue of definition it is imperative that one is aware of the different legislation involved in command and control. Several different agencies will always be involved in the response and management of an MCI. And, they all have different laws and regulations to follow. In these regulations responsibility of the agency or authority in question is often stated, e.g. fire service, healthcare system, police, etc. In a civilian society different responsibilities as described in the different laws are usually linked to the authority and responsibility to exercise command. This means that decisions made have to be obeyed within the organization and that the decisions made are linked to the responsibilities for the consequences.

So let's explore the meaning of the two words *command* and *control* and look into whether the words should be placed together or whether they have separate meanings. According to the Webster's dictionary the word *command* means 'to direct authoritatively' or 'to exercise dominating influence over' (Webster Online Dictionary, 2011). This implies that the command is closely linked to a process where somebody expresses their will and/or intention and that this has to be obeyed. With this definition the receiver of the order is left with little or no choice other than to do or perform whatever is requested. The commander (person that gave the order) must also be prepared to assume the responsibility for the consequences assuming that the order is carried out correctly.

If this is put into a disaster situation where healthcare is involved, orders given will have an influence on the outcome for the patients (victims). And, by law it is always the healthcare professionals who have the responsibility for the patients. So, does this mean that agencies not regulated by healthcare legislation cannot exercise command over healthcare professionals? In one respect it could be argued that this is the case, but on the other hand there are several issues involved in disaster response where the healthcare system does not have enough knowledge and where direction is needed. Examples of this are most issues regarding safety on scene and also access to the victims in the case of a hazardous situation. These hazardous situations could be fires and chemical spills or risk of violence. There may be numerous other situations where the healthcare system does not possess adequate knowledge and authority and it is important that agencies trained to deal with these have the possibility to put restraints on others.

When the word *control* is addressed you may find different definitions that can be applied in a disaster context. The best is probably 'to exercise restraining or directing influence over' or 'to regulate' (Merriam-Webster, 2011). This is not the same meaning as the definition of command, which makes it necessary to debate whether these two words should be used together as 'command and control', or whether they have separate meanings and therefore it is possible (and sometimes necessary) to use them separately. With the definition as stated above this means that control is a different process to command. The word control means having the authority (often regulated by law) to limit other agencies to act. These limitations or restraints should not be considered as direct command. Examples of these limitations are whether different areas of an incident scene could be accessed, or what protective gear should be used. Another example is if there is an on-going threat that results in only the police being able to access the incident site. Whatever agency is in control must have the restraints they put on others respected although the legal responsibility always remains within each agency. In other words: the healthcare system is always responsible for healthcare, and thereby the patients, even if we (temporarily) cannot reach them for one reason or another.

Using the two words command and control separately would probably make the understanding of the processes involved easier. However, it is crucial that each organization closely look into their own legislation, as well as other involved agencies regarding this issue. It is also imperative that there is a mutual understanding on these issues and that all agreements are made in advance. When an MCI strikes there is definitely not time or room for a discussion on definitions and who should decide on what issue. It should be the responsibility of each agency or organization to discuss and decide on these important issues together with others involved and the results of these discussions should be put into disaster plans and action cards.

However, it must be recognized that many organizations prefer to use the same meaning for the words command and control. This must of course be respected, but in order to understand the processes involved it may be easier to use them separately as described above.

Coordination is also a process that is often mentioned whenever command and control are discussed. Coordination comes from the prefix 'co-' meaning 'with' and the Latin word 'ordinate', which means 'arrange'. Coordination is defined according to Webster's dictionary as harmonious functioning for effective results. In this context coordinate means arranging the different agencies (functions) to give effective results (Webster Online Dictionary, 2011). Coordination is therefore not so closely related to command but is more the act of ensuring that the agencies involved in a response are working towards a common goal and that actions taken are harmonized. In an MCI, coordination is often carried out in liaison, i.e. decisions that are more general guidelines for response are made by different agencies together.

One way of describing the relationship between the different terms ‘command’, ‘control’ and ‘coordination’ is shown in Table 9.1 and Fig. 9.1.

The term management system will also be used in this chapter as a general term when describing the command and control system within an agency.

Table 9.1. Command, control and coordination.

Term	Means	Directed to
Command	Orders	Within own organization/agency and legislation
Control	Setting limits	All involved agencies
Coordination	Arranging for communications	All involved agencies between involved agencies

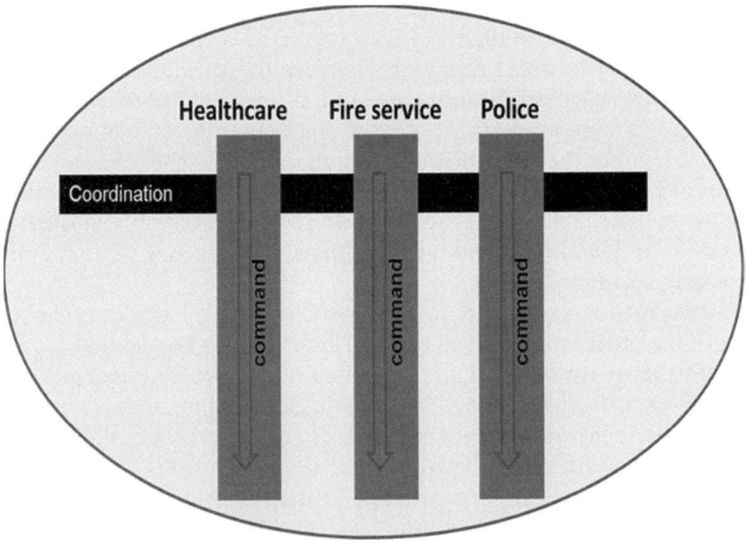

Fig. 9.1. The relation between different agencies in a management system. Healthcare, fire service and police are used as examples.

Command and Control: A Problem Area

In after action reports from incidents, command and control is often reported as an area where problems have been identified. In a study from 13 incidents performed in 2004, areas where problems had been identified were categorized (Rüter *et al.*, 2004a). In this study it was substantiated that the most common problems reported emanate from shortcomings regarding command and control. And, as a consequence of this there were suggestions in several reports on how to be better next time. But still, in reports from MCIs occurring later, the same problems were described again. In this context it must be mentioned that there are no widely accepted report forms to use after MCIs so conclusions from the study mentioned above must be drawn with caution.

One reason for identifying, and in general terms describing command and control as a problem area could be the difficulty in evaluating results. Research in this field is often carried out using qualitative methods and often by performing interviews with involved persons. This inductive way of creating evidence is important, but often leads to new questions being asked (theories) and not to conclusions as to which method is most effective. For this purpose you *also* need quantitative evaluation methods, or even more interesting, a combination of qualitative and quantitative research.

Current Situation

Command and control are almost always put into focus after an incident. A lot of 'why' questions are usually asked. Why was *this* or *that* not done differently? Why wasn't all the information present? Why did *this* or *that* order take so long to carry out? These are only a few of the questions that are usually raised after an MCI. These are not only important issues to be clarified but also reflecting the fact that we do not know how to evaluate an MCI. Quality indicators should be developed for quantitative data together with qualitative tools. As well as defining data that should be registered it should also decide on performance standards for the standard operating procedures (SOP).

The development of validated evaluation tools for MCI is one of the most important areas for future disaster medicine projects. Whenever possible, a common terminology should be implemented, and standards and benchmarks must be set. Unless this is done, in the future we will probably be asking ourselves the same questions after an MCI. And the answers are likely to be the same. Later in this chapter suggestions on how to use quality indicators will be discussed.

Aim of a Command and Control System in the Healthcare System

Aims are important. The aim of something should answer the 'why question'. Why do we do this? This is also true for a command and control/management system. The answer is easy: it is *for the patients*. It seems natural and impossible to misinterpret that the aim of a management system should be for the good of the patients (victims/casualties). But still this must be emphasized. There will be occasions during an MCI response when you must ask yourself: is this the best solution for the patients? Unexpected situations may occur that require rules or SOP to be bent or bypassed in order to do the best for the patients. This is not wrong, and should, in my opinion, not be considered as 'malpractice'. We must, however, document all actions taken and reasons behind the decisions. This quite delicate issue is something that needs to be discussed within all involved healthcare organizations before an MCI occurs. If not, this may lead to an evaluation after the MCI having the wrong focus.

Structure

A command and control system must have a structure. This structure should be as close as possible to the structure used in the daily routine of work and it should be easy to understand. Therefore the terminology should also resemble what is used in daily work. Structure is one of the three types of indicators used for evaluation of a system.

Activation

A command and control system must be able to function at all times. There should be no delay in the start-up phase and there must be a preparedness to make important decisions very early during the response, sometimes within minutes of an alarm being raised. It is also crucial for management to be established early in order to seek and gain important information and knowledge. If decisions are delayed this can lead to units not being alerted in adequate time. In most incidents there will often be technical communication problems and sometimes even breakdowns. If the response is operative very early this will decrease the risk of being affected by technical problems. Even small delays in the early phase can lead to important information not reaching the intended recipients in time or maybe not at all.

There are several solutions in order to make a command system operational within a very short timeframe. One is to have people on active duty who have as part of their job to handle alarms and alerts. An alarm and dispatch centre is an example of this. However, the alarm and dispatch centre very seldom has knowledge of the situation in the different referral hospitals. Sending victims to a hospital that is already overcrowded for one or another reason may even worsen the whole situation both for the victims and for the whole system. However, the possibility of this happening in spite of good management must be taken into account in the disaster plans. Situations may occur where no other option is available than to send all patients to one, usually the closest, hospital.

Another solution to the activation of incident management is to have a designated duty officer (DDO) who has an updated knowledge of the situation at the hospital/s and is only alerted when there is a possible MCI. This function could have other duties depending on how often he/she is alerted and also depending on the resources in the area.

A third solution is to have a doctor and/or nurse at the closest hospital trained to take the necessary initial decisions. No matter what solution is preferred it is important that the preparedness of the organization is not based on persons but on functions. By this it is meant that the function in question should always be manned. This means at all times – 24/7! The alerting of a management system should of course also include alerting individuals with special training, knowledge and/or experience, but in the initial phase the system must not be based on this.

Hierarchy

In a command system there is a need for hierarchy. Ultimately, there must be one function (role) that makes decisions, and takes the responsibility for decisions made. This does not mean that this function, or role, must make all the decisions by him- or herself. This would be an almost impossible task and possibly also counterproductive. In any case a person who tries to make all decisions by themselves during a complex situation like an MCI is likely to wear him/herself down very fast. What is recommended is that decisions made should be done in the spirit of guidelines presented by the chief (leading function/role). The Incident Commander should, however, establish guidelines for the work and revise them whenever necessary. This does not differ from other management situations.

Roles

In a staff there must be different roles with the mandate to make decisions within their own speciality, field or area of competence. But, if in doubt, decisions must be approved by the Incident Commander. Within each area there can only be one responsible role. Due to legislation and/or regulations and guidelines the number of different roles may vary. It must also be clear in advance what persons (names of individuals) can assume the different roles. The difficulty and challenge is how to make a hierarchy with very qualified leaders operational at very short notice. A lot of important decisions must be made at a very early phase and the highest level of the hierarchy must be engaged already at this time. There are different ways to achieve this. One way is to have direct access to qualified persons who are expected to stop whatever they are doing and assume command directly. If this can work this is perhaps the best solution. But, very often important people are not that easy to reach, and it is even more difficult to make them assume command immediately.

Another solution is to use people who are working with command and control and emergency medicine on a daily basis but at a very low level in the healthcare system. These persons can, after training, be mandated to have the authority to make decisions that normally should be made at the highest levels of the hierarchy. Decisions that these persons should/must make can easily be predefined. At the same time as this, the more qualified competencies are alerted and can take over within a reasonable timeframe. This is a way of alerting the system that minimizes the risk of initial important decisions being postponed or sometimes even missed. What these decisions are may vary, and should of course be defined as process indicators, which will be discussed in a later paragraph. However, in most MCIs these decisions include how to support the incident site and deciding on the referring hospitals. It also includes alerting the closest hospitals and sometimes even making a brief press statement. As discussed above this may and will vary, but can easily be included in the disaster plan. It is a good solution to alert the command system by using healthcare functions that already are on call or on duty, doctors and nurses. It must be emphasized that in this context is discussed how to alert the highest levels in the hierarchy of a command system, and not how to alert dispatch or alarm-call centres. The table below (Table 9.2) contains a list of important decisions that have to be made at an early phase of a response. There are also suggested timeframes that the decisions have to be made within. Please note that this is just an example; other timeframes may be suitable in other settings. It only stresses the importance of making decision on a 'high' level at a very early phase where available information often is sparse.

The time stamps should be considered as suggestions and will vary in different organizations. They can also be used as indicators that can be used for evaluation purposes (see paragraph on 'Indicators for Command and Control').

Table 9.2. Examples of actions for the initial command on a strategic level, including time stamps.

Declare major incident	Within 1 min
Decide level of preparedness for the strategic management	Within 5 min
Decide what additional resources to be sent to scene	Within 5 min
Decide which hospitals should be alerted	Within 5 min
Establish contact with on-scene Incident Commander	Within 5 min
Decide on guidelines for the referral of casualties	Within 10 min
Brief information to media	Within 15 min
Begin the process of making definitive referrals	Within 20 min
First evaluation of the capacity and endurance of healthcare system	Within 30 min
Notify results of the referring of the casualties to all involved hospitals	Within 40 min

Levels of hierarchy

There is no general knowledge regarding what levels of hierarchy must, or should be present in a management system. Each different agency must decide on this in accordance with expected need and available resources. There are, however, results from research within this field that suggest that there should be at least a few defined hierarchal levels in a management system (Lindell *et al.*, 2005; FitzGerald *et al.*, 2010; Advanced Life Support Group, 2011).

The reason for this is that different levels have different tasks to perform and different considerations to be made and also different responsibilities. There is also a general opinion that the time scales for different hierarchy levels are different. This makes it difficult or even impossible for organizations to successfully have only one function/role that is responsible for all levels. Unfortunately this is often seen – one person/function that is working both with regional issues (usually strategic decisions) and at the same time operational on a local level. The reason for this may be that often the organization only has access to a limited number of highly qualified persons during an MCI. Nevertheless, one person functioning on more than one hierarchical level should be avoided as much as possible.

What are the levels of management that should be included in an MCI response? The most uncontroversial is that there must be an operational level. On this level of management is where actions are performed. This is where orders are transferred into actions. The operational level is almost always close to the site of the incident. Another kind of operational management can also be present at a hospital, depending on how the organization is built.

The level above in the system is usually the tactical level. On this level is where tactics are worked out and decided upon. By this it is meant that decisions made on a higher level in the system are made into operational guidelines for the staff on the operational level.

The level above the tactical level is usually called the strategic level. This level will also ‘do’ things, and in this sense is operative although this is still a higher level of management. It will also make guidelines while considering different issues on the tactical level. Decisions on this level often concern resources, both the acquisition and the distribution of them. It can sometimes be argued that the name strategic may not an adequate label and this level of management is better named in relation to the geographical area the management has its jurisdiction within. Another name could therefore be local or regional command or even state or national command. The name may not be important, but it is important that names and levels of command are not mixed.

Figure 9.2 shows how a hierarchical system management could look. In this figure you can also note that the highest level of management is often called normative management. It should be emphasized that there is a risk that decisions made high up may take a long time (sometimes too long) to reach the operational level where they are to be carried out. Unforeseen things may take place and, although general guidelines are present, new decisions may have to be taken at the highest level. There must be preparedness for this and also higher levels in the management system must at all times follow up the effect of the decisions made as well as the situation as a whole.

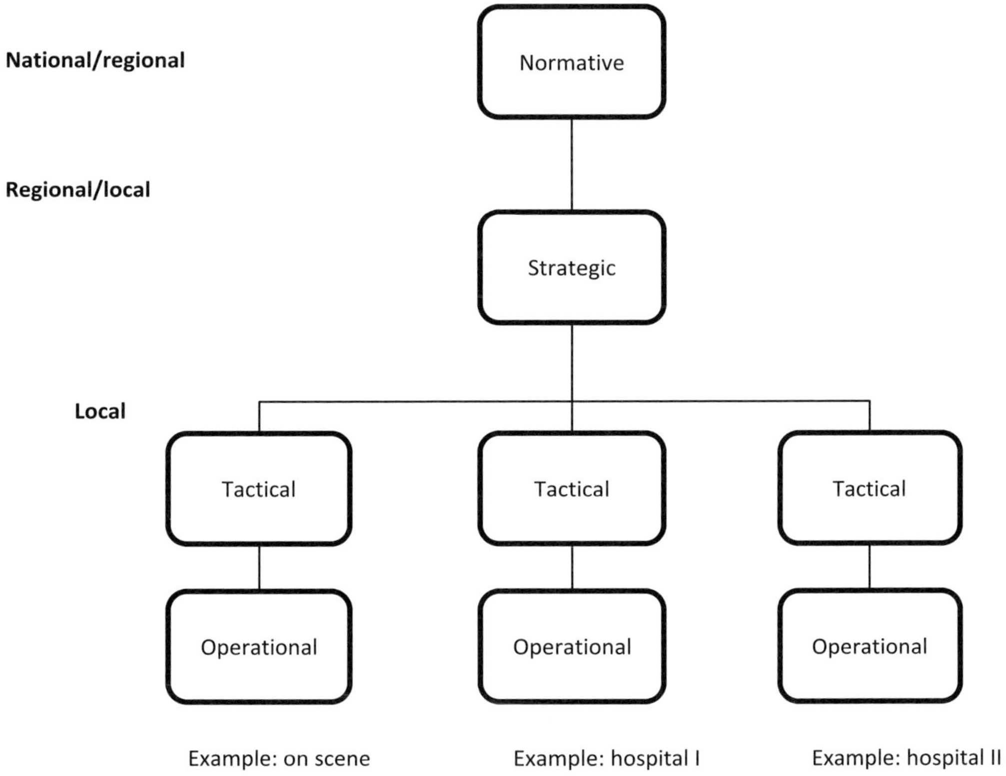

Fig. 9.2. Example of hierarchy levels in a management system.

Indicators for Command and Control

Indicators are important for determining what is to be considered as a standard or good quality. Indicators in this context are therefore also called quality indicators. There are in principle three different kinds of indicators: structure indicators, outcome indicators and performance indicators. A *structure indicator* describes physical, organizational and other characteristics of the system, for example, the staff, the level of education and the equipment of the department (Donabedian, 1980). In command and control systems this is how the structure is built, who (what function) is in charge of the different levels in the system, how the system is alerted, evaluated, etc. Structure indicators are easiest described in algorithms. An *outcome indicator* is the result of something. Outcome is what is achieved that is an important improvement, usually in health, but also in attitudes and knowledge (Donabedian, 1986). Outcome indicators are more difficult to define in a command and control system. Patient outcome is the most important outcome indicator in the healthcare system. In disasters and major incidents this could be defined as mortality and morbidity for the victims. Another outcome indicator could be the impact a disaster or a major incident has on patients who are not primarily affected by the incident but because of its occurrence their treatment, operation or other procedure is postponed or delayed. This is an area that needs to have more attention so that we will know whether in the case of an incident we are transferring the 'lack of resources' from one category of patients (disaster victims) to another (normal patients). It is also something that must be considered for management and therefore it is important that the highest level of the command hierarchy also has the mandate to make decisions regarding daily healthcare.

So far in research outcome indicators are very seldom linked to command and control in a validated way. There are, however, educational models that have addressed this issue but more research is needed (Emergo Train System®; MACSIM®; e-semble®). Although difficult, linking the decision making to outcome for the victims must be considered as one of the most important areas for future development and research. In this context it should also be mentioned that since the healthcare system is not an isolated area, there may be outcome indicators important for the command system as a whole that may affect healthcare. This must be considered and therefore indicator development should be done together with other involved agencies.

The third type of quality indicator, which sometimes can be used as a proxy for outcome indicators, is the *process indicator* (Joint Commission on the Accreditation of Healthcare Organizations, 1989). Process indicators generally measures discrete steps in the patient care process that are important and often linked to patient outcome. In order to find the process indicators you must have a good knowledge of how your system works, or is intended to work and also what is to be considered as important. There must also be a clear understanding of the order processes should be carried out in and how to set standards for these. An example of how an action card can be used as a template for process indicators has previously been demonstrated in Table 9.2.

So far research in this area has mostly focused on educational models (Rüter *et al.*, 2004b, 2007). The reason for this is the difficulty in obtaining data from 'real' incidents. However, there are now systems for capturing data in real time during MCIs under development, and future results from analysing data may lead to important knowledge and understanding of the important processes (Nilsson *et al.*, 2011). There are also international initiatives that in consensus have defined what data should be recorded regarding all three types of indicators (Debacker *et al.*, 2012).

Liaison

Liaison is the process where different agencies or authorities meet to coordinate efforts and to decide on issues that are of interest for all involved. The responsibilities for the decisions always lie within the different agencies and therefore decisions made in liaison are from a legal perspective more like strict recommendations. The healthcare organizations will always be responsible for medical decisions, if steering documents or laws do not state otherwise. However, it is important to be aware that during an MCI there is no single agency or authority that by themselves can manage the situation. Liaison is necessary and decisions made in liaison must be respected. If the command system has one single function with the overall responsibility, the person holding this position should of course be able to make and enforce all overall decisions. This function must then also assume the responsibility for decisions made and actions taken.

Issues that are usually brought up in liaison differ depending on what level (hierarchy) of the management system is involved. Usually the liaison takes place during meetings where all, or at least most, involved agencies meet. Issues that are brought up include updates on the situation within each agency, current and expected problems, how and when to inform the media, etc. Decisions on the coordination of the response can also be brought up if these have been prepared properly within each agency. Since there is usually a lack of time during MCI response, liaison meetings have to be well planned and well structured. Otherwise there is a risk that these meetings take up so much time and effort that the liaison process infringes on other management issues to the extent that the liaison may be given a lower priority. This should of course be avoided. Usually the person responsible for liaison is called a Liaison Officer (O'Neill, 2005; Born *et al.*, 2007).

It should also be mentioned that liaison meetings usually require that most participants have to be transported to the meeting place. This is also time-consuming and efforts should be made to make the liaison process as effective as possible. One solution is to have video-conference equipment in the staff room. Like all technical solutions, this equipment should be installed and tested before the incident occurs. The staff must, of course, also be familiar with its use.

Staff Room

Is there a need for a staff room, sometimes called a situation room, to be used during MCIs and equipped in a special way? The answer to this is both yes and no. On an operational level, at the incident site the 'staff room' is usually in a predesigned and pre-equipped vehicle, but can of course also be indoors in whatever building is available. A staff room at the incident site is more correctly named a staff place and should be located after liaison on the most suitable place. The important thing is that the operational work can be directed from this point and this is where the communications are best. And, the staff place should also be a safe and secure place.

On a higher level in the management hierarchy there are more demands on how a staff room should be placed and equipped. The reason is that the tasks are different as well as the responsibilities. Space is important. There must be enough space so that each staff member can work without being (too) disturbed. At the same time the staff room must not be so big that this makes it difficult to communicate with other staff members. The Incident Commander should, if possible, have a separate room (Heck, 1990).

There must be possibilities for good and robust communication. Mostly this means telephones (including mobile phones) but also radio communication systems. There are several systems nowadays that uses digital techniques that minimize the risks of others (who are not involved) overhearing. This is usually a minor problem for healthcare, but can be an issue for other agencies such as the police.

There should be computers and printers available and if possible a projector to use during staff briefings. Whiteboard tables are also good to have. One important factor to consider is that the more advanced a technique you use, the more training your staff needs. During an MCI there is no time for training or learning new systems. The pen-and-paper (PAP system) should therefore never be underestimated!

Whatever space or room is intended for staff work during an MCI, this must be tested and all involved staff members should be familiar with the equipment. And, of course, all staff members must know where the staff room is located and how to access it. Considering that for various reasons it may not be possible to use the intended staff room, there must be a reserve room. Examples of this are when there is a power breakdown at a hospital or even a fire.

Working as Staff

Staff skills

All persons working as staff should be trained, not only for the tasks that they are expected to perform, but also in how you work as a staff member. These skills are called staff procedure skills. In an incident staff, there are rules and procedures that are not usually practised in the daily routine of work. Also, the terminology used by staff members is often not practised routinely. Normal staff members are usually familiar with this but healthcare professionals like doctors and nurses usually are not. And furthermore, when working as management staff, you should always be prepared to work within a sector that you are not familiar with, at least during the initial phase of an MCI response. This will, of course, put demands not only on training, but also on the disaster plans as well as the action cards, which at all times must be immediately available.

Another issue to be considered is that the order of the arrivals of the different roles and functions can seldom be determined in advance. The staff members will, after being called, arrive as soon as they can. However, it is important to understand that during the initial response important decisions have to be made regardless of whether the 'specialist' has arrived or not. If using a model, as suggested in the previous paragraph, with a 'representative' from the daily work as a temporary commander, this will ensure that initial decisions and actions are taken within the desired timeframes. It should be emphasized that these decisions and actions are not usually very sophisticated or difficult to make. But they require subject matter (healthcare) knowledge as well as disaster management training – and, of course staff procedure knowledge and training. There are studies from training situations that indicate that good staff skills may lead to better decision making (Rüter *et al.*, 2009). More studies on this are necessary to demonstrate whether this relationship can be demonstrated during a real MCI response. It is important to understand that results from training may or may not be 100% valid for a real disaster response.

How you should organize the different roles and functions in a staff may vary. Military-trained persons are often used to having numbers assigned to different functions representing special areas, such as analysis, logistics, human resources, etc. There are obvious advantages with this approach, since staff from other agencies can easily adopt (or maybe have already adopted) the same system and therefore the liaison and sometimes even the direct command are more easily executed. Different functions and roles usually have no problems getting in contact with the correct function in another staff. The disadvantage is that this requires extra training for all staff members, which may be a problem for healthcare professionals who are more familiar working within their own speciality such as emergency medicine, surgery, intensive care, internal medicine, etc. When an incident has occurred, it may be difficult to assume a role as an analyst or in logistics, instead of being responsible for the operating theatres, the emergency ward, etc. In order to find the best solution for the organization, issues like these must be considered when disaster plans are written and must be discussed with all involved persons. During a situation when an incident has occurred there is definitely no time for starting a debate on this. And there usually is no time to start training the staff.

Staff Commander

A Staff Commander is a person responsible for the different procedures carried out during the staff work. The function of Staff Commander is not the same as that of Incident Commander. This is very important to be aware of. The *Incident Commander* is commanding *the response to the incident*, and the *Staff Commander* is responsible for the *administrative processes within the staff.* The Incident Commander should be presented with the problems, questions and issues that he/she has to decide on. And whatever is presented must be well prepared. The responsibility for this lies with the Staff Commander, sometimes also called the Chief of Staff. Examples of different tasks for this important staff role are presented in Table 9.3. These tasks can also serve as a basis for developing performance indicators.

Table 9.3. Example of tasks (responsibilities) for a Staff Commander (Staff Chief) during the response to an MCI. It should be noted that having the responsibility is equivalent to ensuring that different tasks are performed.

- Introducing new staff members
- Assigning staff members to different roles/functions
- Preparing and conducting staff briefings
- Documentation
- Incoming and outgoing correspondence
- Liaison
- Meals and relief for the staff members
- Time schedules for staff meetings
- Follow-up of decisions made
- Communication structure within the staff
- Reporting of staff work to the Incident Commander

Communications

It is not controversial to state that communications are an essential part of command and control. This is true, no matter if you are on the scene of incident or in a staff room on a strategic level of command. Different technical solutions have previously been discussed. However, when addressing the issue of communications it is much too easy to focus on the technical equipment. Failures in communication are often attributed to technical mishaps. Although there is not enough evidence on this, it is the author's opinion that communication problems often spring from SOP issues; that is, who should say what, to whom, and at what time, more than actual technical failures. To be clear: how, when and what we communicate. If SOPs for MCI management do not state how the communications should be carried out, the problems may become two-fold. First, the correct information may not be sent or received by the intended receiver within the correct timeframe. Second, this will lead to increased efforts for different staffs, commanders and even the media in using their communication equipment to seek information. This will eventually overload the communications systems and is likely to contribute to a communication breakdown. The solution to this problem is easy: structured templates of: (i) what is to be reported; (ii) to whom it should be reported; and (iii) at what time. These templates should be included in the SOPs and should be well known within an organization. Training should be given in the use of these templates. The SBAR way of communication is another technique for improving the structure of communications in the healthcare system (Dunn *et al.*, 2007). The acronym means Situation Background Assessment and Recommendation. It is also used as a daily routine in several countries.

Results are good and there are good reasons to believe that this also could work well during an MCI response. More research in this field needs to be done, and maybe there are techniques of communications other than the SBAR that are equally good. The important issue is that this is addressed in advance and that training has been carried out on ways of communicating. It is probably easy to develop indicators that will allow evaluation of the chosen communication technique.

After deciding on SOPs regarding communications and what technique you want to use you will probably not have problems when deciding on the most suitable technical equipment. If you work the other way around, there is a greater risk of problems and perhaps even failure.

Information

Having access to correct and timely information is crucial for the management of and response to an MCI. This should not be mixed up with having access to complete information, more on this later. Let's start by pointing out the differences between data and information. The term data is defined as known facts, things or observations, while information is a collection of facts or data (Kleinelder, 2002; Sundnes and Birnbaum, 2003). Decisions are made based on information that is derived from the data available (Birnbaum, 2007). Information received is almost always filtered or interpreted by the sender. This may sometimes be done on purpose and sometimes not. The implication of this is that during an MCI response the management on different levels must have resources for seeking, and be prepared to seek for a lot of information and information from more than one source. And, at the same time this information must be analysed before actions may be taken. And this process of analysing information must be done under time pressure, at least during the beginning of a response. Command and control staff must be trained for this. There must, however, be awareness that within a staff may be members who can analyse and interpret information and data better than others. It must also be recognized that in order to be good at this, these persons must also have subject matter knowledge (healthcare and disaster medicine) as well as being familiar with staff skills and how to present their findings and results. It is the author's opinion that media training only is not enough for staff members with the responsibility for obtaining, analysing and interpreting information.

Measures can be carried out beforehand to ensure that information is correct and timely, and one example is the different kinds of report from incident scenes. There are many different report forms but one that has been frequently used and proven very good during training and exercises is the 'METHANE' report introduced by the Major Incident Medical Management System (MIMMS) concept (Advanced Life Support Group, 2011).

It is important when deciding on report forms that they are well-known on all levels of the management system. This will possibly ensure not only that the function/role sending the report knows what should be included, but also that the receiver knows what to expect. And maybe more importantly, the receiver knows what not to expect. Also when developing report forms it must be clear to whom the different reports should be sent, and when.

This leads into the discussion of completeness of information. It must be stated clearly that information during an MCI will never be 100% complete during the response, and sometimes not even afterwards. Reports, being one kind of information, must be interpreted by the receiver. And this requires subject matter knowledge, as discussed earlier. However, the more structured the report forms that are used, the less interpretation will be necessary.

Education and Training

Education and training are probably more important when it comes to MCI management than most other activities for the healthcare system. The reason for this statement is that MCI occurrences are infrequent; the chance of a healthcare professional being involved in an MCI response is, in most organizations, quite small. But, when an MCI occurs, all staff members are expected to manage the situation properly and lack of training should never be an acceptable excuse. And, we must always be aware that the media will follow MCI responses, scrutinize the results and ask the 'what', 'how' and 'why' questions. In other words, situations that we are least likely to have the experience of will be the ones that draw the most public and media attention. And, in the eye of the public, the healthcare system sometimes will be 'evaluated' on the basis of how it copes with MCIs.

Basic education could, and should be part of the training all staff should be offered when employed in an organization potentially involved in MCI response. Reading and understanding the disaster plan is basic training and should be done by all personnel at least before the first time of being on call. Being aware of all things new hospital employees must pay attention to, we must put the need for more advanced MCI response training on a realistic level, but of course, the goal must be that all involved staff should have all necessary education and should train on a regular basis. In Sweden it is regulated that all staff should train as a minimum once a year (The Swedish National Board of Health and Welfare, 2005).

If possible training should be performed as exercises. These could be simulation- or table top exercises or now computer training. No matter what type of exercise is chosen, they must be evaluated using the same indicators that will be used during real MCIs. There are several systems for training available and the price for training a whole hospital management staff may be considered by some as high. It is the author's belief that the price will be higher if you do not have the training. The difference is that the price for training is paid by the organization, the price for not training will be paid by our patients. This is perhaps expressed a little dramatically but there are reports suggesting this (Hersche and Wenker, 2000).

Full-scale exercises are often popular and are conducted on a regular basis. If not well-prepared, including a good system for evaluation, the effectiveness of these full-scale exercises tends to be overestimated in relation to the results that are achieved. The total costs for these exercises are seldom presented, and full-scale exercises should mostly be used for testing the organization whenever other testing is not possible. One example is conduction of full-scale exercises together with other agencies where many different aspects of MCI management can be evaluated (Gryth *et al.*, 2010).

Research

Command and control and management of MCIs are topics that need, and deserve more attention from the academic world. More research is needed and perhaps one reason for the sparse number of published papers in this area of disaster medicine is the lack of valid and reliable indicators. There needs to be established consensus on indicators, at least to the extent to make research possible. Another reason may be the lack of validated research methods where patient outcome can be related to the decision-making process. So far development has mainly focused on educational models, but it is now time to take the next step. Both quantitative and qualitative methodology is needed in order to establish knowledge of the 'what' issues as well as the 'whys'. Qualitative methodology can also be used for the identification of new areas for research.

The key issue for research, also regarding command and control, is to find funding. Disaster medicine is a young research area and very little is evidence-based. This makes it difficult to find funding, since research groups often must compete with disciplines within the healthcare system that maybe have hundreds of years of research tradition and results. There is no quick-fix solution to this problem. The only way forward is to start with whatever funding you can find and follow your ideas. As a final remark I would like to wish you all good luck and, if you document and publish your results, it would be interesting to read and learn from them.

References

Advanced Life Support Group (2011) *Major Incident Medical Management and Support: The Practical Approach at the Scene*. Wiley-Blackwell, Oxford, UK.

Birnbaum, M. (2007) Data, information, and indicators. Editor's corner. *Prehospital and Disaster Medicine* 22(6), 471.

Born, C.T., Briggs, S., Ciraulo, D., Frykberg, E., Hammond, J., Hirshberg, A., Lhowe, D.W. and O'Neill, P.A. (2007) Disasters and mass casualties: I. General principles of response and management. *Journal of the American Academy of Orthopedic Surgeons* 15(7), 388–396.

Builder, C.H., Bankes, S.C. and Nordin, R. (1999) *Command Concepts. A Theory Derived from the Practice of Command and Control*. National Defense Research Institute RAND, Santa Monica, California, 144 pp.

Debacker, M., Hubloue, I., Dhondt, E., Rockenschaub, G., Rüter, A., Codreanu, T., Koenig, K., Schultz, C., Peleg, K., Halpern, P., Stratton, S., Della Corte, F., Delooz, H., Ingrassia, P.L., Colombo, D. and Castrèn, M. (2012) Utstein-style template for uniform data reporting of acute medical response in disasters. *PLoS Currents Disasters*. doi: 10.1371/4f704f93f3807.

Donabedian, A. (1980) *Explorations in Quality Assessment and Monitoring Vol. 1. The Definition of Quality and Approaches to its Management*. Health Administration Press, Ann Arbor, Michigan.

Donabedian, A. (1986) Criteria and standards for quality assessment and monitoring. *Quality Review Bulletin* 12(3), 99–108.

Dunn, E.J., Mills, P.D., Neili, J., Crittenden, M.D., Carmack, A.L. and Bagian, J.P. (2007) Medical team training: applying crew resource management in the veterans health administration. *The Joint Commission Journal on Quality and Patient Safety* 33(6), 317–325.

Emergo Train System® (n.d.) Available at: www.emergotrain.com (Accessed 22 September 2011).

e-semble® (n.d.) ISEE simulation software for crises-management training and assessment. Available at: www.e-semble.com (Accessed 22 September 2011).

FitzGerald, G., Aitken, P., Arbon, P., Archer, F., Cooper, D., Leggat, P., Myers, C., Robertson, A., Tarrant, M. and Davis, E.R. (2010) A national framework for disaster health education in Australia. *Prehospital and Disaster Medicine* 25(1), 4–11.

Gryth, D., Rådestad, M., Nilsson, H., Nerf, O., Castrén, M. and Rüter, A. (2010) Evaluation of medical management by performance indicators in a full scale major aircraft accident exercise. *Prehospital and Disaster Medicine* 25(2), 118–123.

Heck, J.P. (1990) Comments on 'The Zeebrugge ferry disaster'. *Crime, Law and Social Change* 14(4), 351–355.

Hersche, B. and Wenker, O. (2000) Case report: Lassing Mining Accident. *The Internet Journal of Rescue and Disaster Medicine* 2(1) DOI: 10.5580/2213.

Joint Commission on the Accreditation of Healthcare Organizations (1989) Characteristics of clinical indicators. *Quality Review Bulletin* 15(11), 330–339.

Kleinelder, S.R. (Senior ed.) (2002) *American Heritage College Dictionary*, 4th edn. Houghton Mifflin Co., New York, p. 712.

Lindell, M.K., Perry, R.W. and Prater, C.S. (2005) Organizing response to disasters with the Incident Command System/Incident Management System (ICS/IMS), International Workshop on Emergency Response and Rescue, 31 October–1 November, 2005.

MACSIM® (n.d.) Available at: www.macsim.se (Accessed 22 September 2011).

Merriam-Webster (n.d.) Available at: www.merriam-webster.com (Accessed 18 September 2011).

Nilsson, H., Lundin, R., Bengtsson, E., Gustafsson, L., Jonsson, C. and Vikström, T. (2011) Support system for medical command and control at major incidents. *Prehospital and Disaster Medicine* 26(supplement 1), 148.

O'Neill, P.A. (2005) The ABCs of disaster response. *Journal of Surgery* 94, 259–266.

Rüter, A., Örtenwall, P. and Wikström, T. (2004a) Performance indicators for major incident medical management – a possible tool for quality control? *International Journal of Disaster Medicine* 2(1–2), 52–55.

Rüter, A., Örtenwall, P. and Wikström T. (2004b) Performance indicators for prehospital command and control in training of medical first responders. *International Journal of Disaster Medicine* 2, 89–92.

Rüter, A., Örtenwall, P. and Vikström, T. (2007) Staff procedure skills in management groups during exercise in disaster medicine. *Prehospital Disaster Medicine* 22, 318–321.

Rüter, A., Örtenwall, P. and Vikström, T. (2009) Improved staff procedure skills lead to improved management skills, a study in an educational setting. *Prehospital and Disaster Medicine* 24(5), 376–379.

Sundnes, K.O., Birnbaum, M.L. (eds) and the Task Force for Quality Control of Disaster Management: Health disaster management (2003) Guidelines for evaluation and research in the Utstein style. *Prehospital and Disaster Medicine* 17(Suppl 2), 148.

The Swedish National Board of Health and Welfare (2005) The national board of health and welfare regulations on peacetime disaster medicine preparedness. *SOSFS* 13(M). Available at: www.socialstyrelsen.se (Accessed 26 September 2011).

Webster Online Dictionary (2011) Available at: www.websters-online-dictionary.org (Accessed 18 September 2011).

Chapter 10

Disasters in Medical Care Contexts: Planning for Resilience in Incident Command Personnel and Systems in Hospitals

Douglas Paton and David Allen

Introduction

Hospitals and healthcare workers play key roles in both the initial response to a disaster and the longer term recovery (Smith, 2007). How they can do so effectively is the subject of this chapter. This chapter discusses the systems, procedures and competencies required to respond to disaster. This raises a question. Why is it necessary, given that hospitals regularly deal with crises and emergencies, to devote attention to preparing for disaster? To appreciate why, it is necessary to understand what a disaster is.

A disaster is an event whose demands exceed the capacity of the available resources to respond (Auf der Heide, 1989). A summary of how Auf der Heide distinguished between accidents and emergencies is presented in Table 10.1. Disasters can result in hospitals being overwhelmed by the sheer number of casualties (Benson *et al*., 1996; McCaughrin, 2003; Hick *et al*., 2004; Banks *et al*., 2006) or they may be unable to function at all. Disasters such as Hurricane Katrina and the Japanese tsunami illustrated how hospitals could be destroyed or so badly damaged as to render them unusable during a disaster and after the hazard threat had subsided. Hospitals and medical staff may thus be forced to establish and work from ad hoc facilities. Even if they remain intact, hospitals will have to operate at considerably reduced capacity as a result of infrastructure losses (e.g. damage to buildings and equipment, loss of utilities) that results in, for example, the closure of critical care facilities. Disasters can result in staff being unable (e.g. owing to impassable roads) or unwilling (e.g. owing to concerns for their safety) to work. When working in disaster contexts, staff will have to contend with working longer hours than normal, being deployed to other locations or functions, and dealing with personal loss, confusion or grief. These demands can come from several sources.

Table 10.1. Differences between emergency and disaster operating contexts (Adapted from Auf der Heide, 1989).

Routine emergencies	**Disasters**
Interaction with familiar people	Interaction with unfamiliar people (different departments and agencies)
Familiar roles, tasks and procedures	Unfamiliar roles, tasks and procedures
Intra-organizational coordination needed	Intra- *and* inter-organizational coordination needed
Environment and infrastructure (roads, telephones and facilities, etc.) intact and useable	Environment and infrastructure damaged and possible unusable (e.g. roads blocked/jammed, telephones overloaded or non-functional, facilities damaged)
Communication adequate	Communication infrastructure lost or damaged and communication inadequate
Communication and decision making primarily intra-organizational	Need for inter-organizational communication, information sharing and decision making
Use of familiar terminology and procedures	Working with others and using unfamiliar terminology and procedures
Management structures and response capacity adequate to coordinate resources and respond	Management and response capacity exceeded and hospital infrastructure may be destroyed or unusable

Hospitals and healthcare staff must be prepared for disasters arising from hazards ranging from earthquakes to pandemics to acts of bioterrorism. Meteorological and geological hazard activity can injure staff or they may be infected or contaminated by pandemic or biohazard events. Hazards also differ in their response implications. Earthquakes create a period of acute demand that can subside over a period of days but may require a longer period of caring for those sick or injured. Pandemic influenza hazards, on the other hand, can create steadily escalating demands as more people become infected. At the same time, increasing rates of staff infection reduce staff availability. These problems can persist for several weeks or months. The task facing hospitals is complex and they must accommodate a range of events, circumstances and consequences in disaster response planning.

Being able to respond is a function of the degree to which medical facilities and staff develop the beliefs, competencies, processes and procedures required to respond to the large-scale, complex, evolving and unpredictable circumstances and consequences that arise when disaster strikes. An ability to respond effectively derives from developing planning and preparedness processes that culminate in different ways of thinking and novel ways of acting.

Planning and preparing occur prior to disaster. To increase the applicability and effectiveness of plans and preparedness, it is important to ensure that the contexts and scenarios used to frame and develop these processes are as representative of what hospitals and staff will have to contend with as possible. One way of doing so involves using worst case scenarios.

The importance of using worst case scenarios derives from their capacity to accommodate most of the circumstances and consequences that planning and response management would have to cater for (Auf der Heide, 1989). By considering the worst that could happen, plans, response procedures and training will be able to accommodate lesser events. In contrast, planning based on smaller scale events or assumptions that existing capabilities will suffice does not readily scale upwards. This heightens the risk of medical facilities overestimating their capacities (Auf der Heide, 1989; Benson *et al.*, 1996) and increases the likelihood of staff having to react to events rather than being able to respond. Planning for worst cases facilitates identifying areas for developing response capability or accommodating factors beyond the control of the hospital but which will affect or constrain response. This chapter commences with an outline of the context in which disaster response planning occurs. Then it discusses the systems, procedures and competencies that facilitate the ability of hospitals and medical staff to adapt to the circumstances and consequences encountered when responding to a disaster.

The Disaster Context

When conceptualizing disaster response, it is pertinent to distinguish between resilience and adaptive capacity (Paton and Auld, 2006). Resilience defines the ability of hospitals and their staff to accommodate crisis events. Adaptive capacity describes the capability to anticipate, cope with, adapt to and recover from events that impose excessive demands on healthcare resources. Developing adaptive capacity starts with using worst case scenarios to identify what hospitals and staff would have to contend with when disaster strikes.

Disasters pose excessive and unique environmental and response demands on hospitals and medical staff (Hick *et al.*, 2004; Dara *et al.*, 2005; Farmer and Carlton, 2005; Paton and Auld, 2006). For example, systems and staff will have to respond to large scale hazard impacts whose consequences can escalate and evolve (increasing numbers of people injured or infected, reducing numbers of staff, loss of resources), and that create dynamic conditions and shifting and competing goals and tasks. Staff members have to make decisions under conditions of uncertainty and ambiguity because reliable information is difficult to obtain. Medical professionals can find themselves functioning in multi-jurisdictional and multi-agency contexts (e.g. interaction between medical staff and police when treating people in what is a crime scene or working with representatives of diverse religious ordinations attending to the needs of the dead and the critically injured). From a planning perspective, the context in which healthcare will be applied will include:

- Hospitals being overwhelmed to the point of actual functional collapse;
- Staff working in ad hoc, remote treatment centres;
- Staff working with representatives of several departments, agencies and jurisdictions;
- Infrastructure/service failure or intermittent access to services and utilities;
- Reconciling inpatient and survivor medical needs;
- High levels of public risk and multiple deaths;
- Distressed publics seeking guidance, information and services;
- Dealing with the worried well;
- Staff shortages as a result of lack of availability, exhaustion or sickness that can increase over time;
- Staff concerns for workplace and family safety;
- Public searching for friends and relatives in hospitals;
- Blood shortages;
- Integrity of information channels being overwhelmed, disrupted or lost;

- Medical supply and personal protection equipment inadequacies, shortages and losses;
- Managing current inpatients;
- GPs seeking advice;
- Private hospitals and rest homes seeking advice and/or being overwhelmed;
- Mass evacuations into or away from a city;
- Large numbers of patients and staff requiring decontamination;
- Resource limitations that can be increasing over time.

Central to adaptive capacity is anticipation. One issue that has to be anticipated is the point where the surge in demand will reach disastrous proportions. Contemporary hospitals often function at or near maximal system capacity on a daily basis (Farmer and Carlton, 2005). Hospital, health boards or districts need to anticipate when this will happen and develop response plans and capabilities required to optimize functioning under extraordinary conditions (Hick *et al.*, 2004). This process is depicted in Fig. 10.1. Identifying where this occurs signals the point of transition from crisis response (resilient response to a crisis) to disaster response management (adapting to extraordinary events). The remainder of this chapter explores what this means in practice.

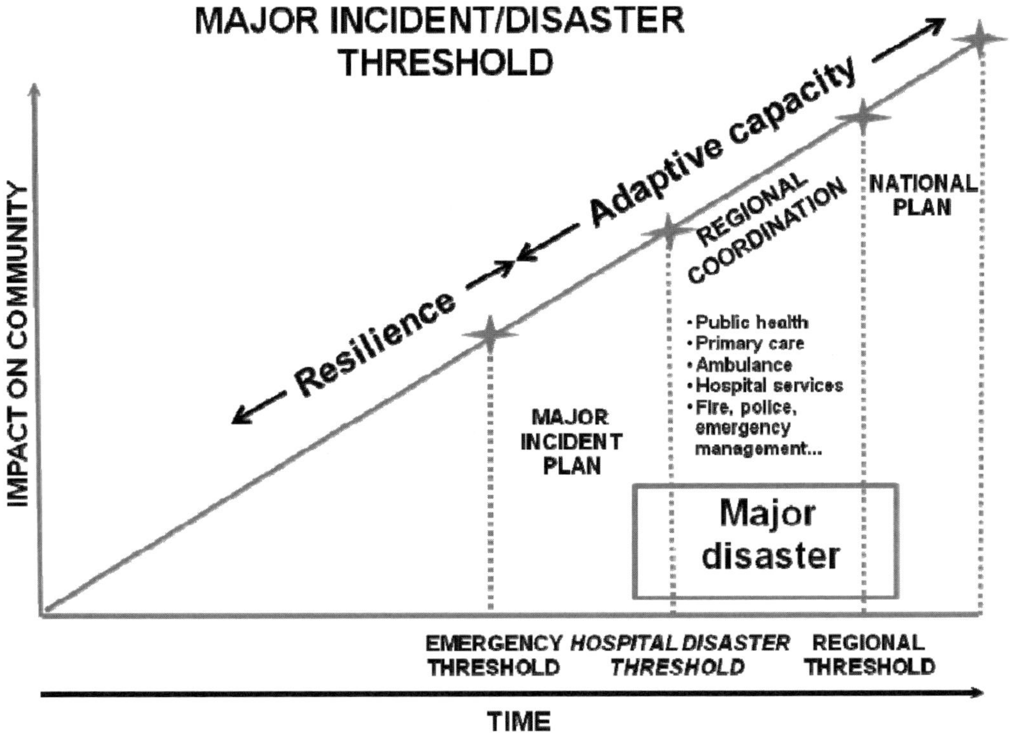

Fig. 10.1. Transitioning between major incident (resilient) and disaster (adaptive) response.

Developing disaster management capability starts with identifying the systems and procedures required to facilitate a capacity to adapt to disastrous circumstances (Hick *et al.*, 2004; Paton and Hannan, 2004; Markenson *et al.*, 2005; Hope *et al.*, 2010). This provides the foundation for developing comprehensive, integrated disaster planning (Banks *et al.*, 2006; Farmer and Carlton, 2005). One important issue that arises in this context concerns the need for new management structures and competencies.

The atypical nature of the demands posed by disasters and the fact that these demands exceed normal response capacities introduces a need for the development of super-ordinate response management practices at three interdependent levels: strategic planning, coordinating or tactical incident management and operational response (Flin and Arbuthnot, 2002). An appreciation of the need for this approach can be illustrated by discussing what happens from the bottom up.

When disaster strikes the operational demands are such that there will be too few staff members available and those who are available will be presented with an event whose scale makes it impossible to treat everyone. When this circumstance prevails, decisions have to be made regarding the use and deployment of limited staff members and other resources to the most pressing issues or neediest patients. Nufer and Wilson-Ramirez (2004) have discussed about patient needs following two hurricanes. Such crucial decisions are made at a tactical or coordinating level of response management. Finally, in a context in which demands may be experienced over a period of weeks or months, a third level of management, strategic management, is introduced to manage, for example, securing the resources required to sustain response over the longer term (e.g. conduct a residual risk assessment to accommodate the implications of any shortfall in resources) and to plan for recovery. The integration of these different levels of management optimizes the response to complex disasters (Flin and Arbuthnot, 2002).

The strategic level is also primarily responsible for planning. This includes developing integrated disaster management capability, how this capability will be activated and used, and the procedures and practices required for effective functioning. It is to a discussion of issues that must be accommodated in this process that this chapter now turns.

Strategic Response Planning and Management

Events such as the 9/11 terrorist attacks, Hurricane Katrina, and the Indian Ocean and Japanese tsunamis and recognition of the threat that large-scale pandemic influenza outbreaks pose have revealed potentially large gaps in the ability of healthcare systems to cope with disasters that severely injure or infect a large number of victims (Hick *et al.*, 2004). Developing incident management systems to expedite response is essential for effective medical disaster response (Banks *et al.*, 2006). Developing this capacity is a strategic function.

Consistent with its membership being drawn from senior management levels, the strategic level of disaster management has a significant role in developing disaster response policy and ensuring that plans can be implemented promptly should the need arise. During a disaster event, the strategic level focus is on future resource needs and recovery planning. The time frame for such activities is approximately 1–7 days (for resource procurement) to months (for recovery planning). Before planning can occur it may be necessary to develop different ways of thinking about the events that are being planned for.

Disaster preparedness and organizational learning

Disasters are an enduring element in the environment in which hospitals and their staff will operate. Developing a capability to adapt to this circumstance calls for a new approach to organizational learning (Berkes *et al.*, 2003). The natural, human and technological events that have occurred over recent years have provided several opportunities for hospitals to learn lessons and develop their capabilities. However, a capability to learn from experience should not be taken for granted (Mitroff and Anagnos, 2001; Berkes *et al.*, 2003). For example, bureaucratic inertia, underestimating consequences or assuming that their size and existing resources will safeguard them from significant disruption and allow prompt recovery can increase risk, resulting in hospitals underestimating or overlooking problems or initiating inadequate actions. This will reduce their capacity to plan for disasters and increase the likelihood of their having to react to disaster rather than being able to respond in a planned and systematic way. To enhance adaptive capacity to respond to disasters, hospitals must learn from past events, learn to think 'outside the box' and develop their risk management culture in ways that extend to large-scale disasters.

According to Berkes *et al.* (2003) this involves, first, ensuring that lessons from prior disasters are incorporated into planning. Second, realistic risk estimates should be derived from comprehensive reviews of potential events and realistic audits of competence (Jackson *et al.*, 2003). These risk estimates will form the basis for developing and implementing response systems and identifying staff training needs. Finally, disaster management must be consolidated in the policies, procedures, practices and attitudes required to facilitate a capacity for adaptive response to uncertain future events (Paton and Jackson, 2002; Berkes *et al.*, 2003; Jackson *et al.*, 2003; Kendra and Wachtendorf, 2003; FEMA, 2004).

An important part of this process is ensuring that planning extends beyond identifying the structural (e.g. identifying an organizational structure and chart) characteristics anticipated to be activated during a disaster (Flin and Arbuthnot, 2002). All too often organizations become over-reliant on structural planning and equate this with response knowledge and assume that the structure on paper will convert into an integrated response process. It is important to differentiate the structural elements that arise from planning (e.g. organizational charts and plans) from the interpretive elements and competencies (e.g. knowing how to work out what to do when) that need to be developed to implement plans. Planning should thus culminate in the development of capability across all hospital functions. What does thinking outside the box mean in practice? What kinds of novel issues need to be considered? These include multi-agency response, staff roles, remote treatment needs, and staff ability and willingness to report to work.

Multi-agency response

Planning should extend beyond a given hospital to encompass regional and multi-agency levels of response in order to develop a tiered, scalable and flexible surge capacity to provide care for prolonged mass casualty events (Hick *et al.*, 2004). Strategic planning should take place within an incident management system that involves key stakeholders (e.g. EMS, emergency management, public health, public safety/law enforcement, health-care systems, hospitals and hospital associations, Red Cross, mental health, jurisdictional legal authorities, professional associations (pharmacy, medical, nursing, mental health) and health professional training institutions). This is necessary to ensure that, as far as possible, all professional, jurisdictional and regional stakeholder groups likely to have roles and responsibilities are identified and included in the planning process. This can be facilitated using a functional health incident management system such as the Medical and Health Incident Management System (Hick *et al.*, 2004). It is also important to consider likely public actions and behaviour (Lasker, 2004). For example, Lasker reported on public reluctance to turn up to inoculation centres in the event of a bioterrorist event and points out how lack of understanding of likely public behaviour could result in resources being wasted by planners' inappropriate assumptions about public response.

Staff roles and deployment

Healthcare system planning must anticipate increased needs over prolonged periods of time. Planning must consider how pre-existing staff roles and functions may change and how staff may have to be deployed in novel ways in threatening circumstances for periods that may range from days to months. For example, Banks *et al.* (2006) discuss how employees without on-going duties could be re-deployed and given temporary jobs (e.g. removing debris from hospital grounds, assisting with repair work). To expedite this, it is necessary to conduct comprehensive staff audits to identify all staff members (include those from satellite functions) and to think about staff deployment in relation to disaster demands and needs and not in terms of normal staff roles and patterns of deployment.

Disaster response plans should accommodate the following: identify the roles and type of staff required; identify the threats to staff and their families from the disaster and from staff fulfilling their role across different hazards; provide basic education on disaster preparedness, response and support; develop strategies to ensure staff confidence in their role and to mitigate risk in the workplace (e.g. risk management protocols, personal protective equipment (PPE), antivirals); involve all staff in planning and identify how medical and medical staff play key roles in response management; and develop strategies to maintain knowledge and engagement of health workforce (Paton and Hannan, 2004; Barnett *et al.*, 2005). These preparedness plans should be accompanied by exercises and simulations (Crego and Spinks, 1997). Proper planning and drilling for multiple contingencies are important and will help drive changes in response, equipment and training (Hope *et al.*, 2010).

Remote treatment centres

Mechanisms for the integrated management of healthcare facilities distributed over a wide geographical area will be required. Large numbers of victims can be anticipated, many of whom will not have immediate access to hospital care. Consequently, systems must be developed to treat survivors *in situ* and to plan their systematic access to hospitals over time. The scale of disaster means that remote facilities will be required to compensate for overwhelmed, damaged or destroyed hospitals.

Remote settings for establishing temporary hospital facilities (e.g. in churches, community/recreation centres, government buildings, hotels/motels, meeting halls, medical clinics and surgeries, sports facilities/stadiums and warehouses) should be identified (Hick *et al.*, 2004). Hick and colleagues suggest that planning should be modular, in 50-patient increments, to facilitate estimating staffing, resourcing and administrative needs. This information can be available to tactical managers to reconcile with available resources during response. Plans should also address transportation to and from the site, how healthcare workers from other agencies or special teams will be deployed and integrated into these locations, and how communications will be established to coordinate implementation. In these settings, mechanisms to communicate with, and provide support for, the public need to be considered. Good communication with the public may reduce the need for patient care surge capacity by preventing the healthcare system from being submerged under a deluge of patients who may not be ill but have concerns and seek further information or evaluation (Hick *et al.*, 2004).

Staffing issues

While hospitals are familiar with staffing problems during periods of peak demand, the question of staff availability during disaster requires specific consideration. When disaster occurs, hospital planners and the public may assume that healthcare staff will be willing to work. The reality is that some staff members may be unable to work (e.g. transportation problems) or unwilling to work due to concerns about their own safety and health, or that of their families (DiMaggio *et al.*, 2005; Qureshi *et al.*, 2005; Smith, 2007). Accommodating this issue is important both to ensure that plans do not over-estimate staff availability and to plan ways of increasing staff intention to turn up and to stay involved to increase the capacity of the healthcare system to cope with the surge of demand associated with disasters (Koh *et al.*, 2005). Staff inability or unwillingness to work can stem from both hazard and staff perceptions of risk and capability issues.

Hope *et al.* (2010) found that hazard type influenced reporting intentions. Some 78% of staff would be willing to report to work during a weather-related event. This number dropped to 67% for an influenza pandemic, and to 52% for a bioterrorism scenario. Reasons why reporting to work may be higher for conventional (e.g. weather or geological) hazards may relate to familiarity with local natural disasters (Cretikos *et al.*, 2007). The validity of staff concerns about health hazards is borne out by findings that the infectiousness of severe acute respiratory syndrome (SARS) was substantially higher among healthcare workers than the general population (Maunder, 2004) and resulted in heightened staff concerns about their own health and that of their family (Koh *et al.*, 2005).

During a catastrophic event, employers must recognize that their staff are, as a result of their greater understanding of the associated risks, likely to be as or even more concerned than the average citizen and this can influence staff willingness to present for work (Qureshi *et al.*, 2005; Smith *et al.*, 2009; Hope *et al.*, 2010). Reasons for this include:

- Fear and concern for the safety of their families, themselves and their pets;
- Childcare and eldercare responsibilities;
- Personal health concerns;
- Ability to communicate with public;
- Confidence in personal safety while at work and confidence in ability to perform duties;
- Transportation issues and being able to safely get to work;
- Being able to get to and work safely in a different location;
- Confidence in the Area Health Service preparedness;
- Trust in employers and the credibility of the information and their risk management practices;
- Access to vaccines and antivirals;
- Second job obligations.

Knowledge of these factors can inform planning (Qureshi *et al.*, 2005). They identify a need for training, transparent protocols for the provision of vaccinations and/or antivirals (for health workers and their immediate family) and the provision of adequate protective equipment to all staff (DiMaggio *et al.*, 2005; Cretikos *et al.*, 2007). Strategies must address the need for staff education and training to promote better understanding of risk and to enhance perceived knowledge and the ability to function safely and effectively in threatening disaster contexts (Lanzilotti *et al.*, 2002; Paton and Hannan, 2004).

Transportation barriers can be addressed by having pools of employees with four-wheel-drive vehicles, with pick-up points situated along major roads and arranging with emergency management officials to provide transportation for essential personnel. Hospitals can pre-plan emergency childcare and eldercare facilities by establishing childcare/eldercare 'pools', where healthcare workers can leave their family members with people who they already know and trust (Qureshi *et al.*, 2005). Personal health issues can be mitigated by encouraging staff to maintain an emergency supply of medication at work. Staff can be encouraged to engage in household preparedness, and workplace personal emergency planning (e.g. emergency contact information, identification of caregivers for children, elders and pets and how to contact them, personal medication list, and how the family will operate during an emergency event), prior to disaster occurring (Qureshi *et al.*, 2005). Training can equip staff with the skills to discuss such events with their family members, develop their own family plan and also be assured of reliable communication links and the welfare of family (Barnett *et al.*, 2005; Dalton *et al.*, 2008). Planning should also develop communication channels dedicated to informing family members of developments during an event, and the opportunity for voluntary isolation and quarantine should be incorporated into emergency preparedness plans.

Staff ability or willingness to work provides a good illustration of one way in which disaster can affect resource availability over time. It introduces the need for a tactical level of management to accommodate resource constraints and to make decisions about how to deploy limited resources to confront demands.

Coordinating/Tactical Incident Management Teams

At the coordinating or tactical level of disaster management, the key activity involves adapting plans and actions by balancing healthcare objectives and operational realities (e.g. standards of patient care against the number of staff members available to provide that care). The time frame of their activities can be measured in hours to days. A need for multidisciplinary and multiagency team composition is necessitated by a need to balance medical, public health, transportation and public order in response management. These diverse inputs ensure more representative situational awareness, definitions of response problems (which can change rapidly as events escalate and resources get depleted) and they facilitate the ability of the incident management team (IMT) to prioritize problems and needs and plan the allocation of limited resources (Endsley and Garland, 2000; Paton and Hannan, 2004).

The major challenge is deciding how to best deploy limited resources in a context in which demands exceed resources by a large margin and making decisions about optimizing response (Flin and Arbuthnot, 2002). Because they have to anticipate factors such as the nature and distribution of demands, key competencies in tactical decision making include anticipating/predicting problems and needs under conditions of high uncertainty, in which there are typically incomplete, ambiguous and missing data. Central to adaptive capacity at this level of management is the quality of information and decision management. That is, the degree to which incident management staff can access, interpret, collate and use information to manage complex events (Jackson *et al.*, 2003; Paton and Hannan, 2004).

For it to work effectively, IMT members need training in multidisciplinary team skills, and extensive joint planning and team development activity involving agency representatives prior to a disaster occurring (Brannick *et al.*, 1997; Salas *et al.*, 1999; Pollock *et al.*, 2003; Farmer and Carlton, 2005; Banks *et al.*, 2006). Team work affords several benefits, including providing opportunities for tactics to be discussed and agreed, second opinions sought and tasks delegated. Realizing these benefits requires attending to team development and maintenance of team roles and training in team skills (Pollock *et al.*, 2003).

Incident management team development and management

Team selection is informed by the functional expertise required, but the team development process must accommodate diversity (e.g. professional roles, procedures, terminology, personality etc.). The goal is to facilitate cohesion in multidisciplinary and agency-operating contexts. This involves training that covers, for example, developing consensus on goals and roles, language and terminology and team structures and procedures.

With regard to structures and procedures, several team management models are appropriate for disaster response. These include the collaborative team management model in which members work as equals and contribute different perspectives that inform understanding of complex scenarios and making decisions. An alternative, and one that is particularly appropriate for complex multiagency environments in which teams and groups have to interact in ad hoc ways, is the consultation model. This model advocates the direction of team activities by a well-trained team manager. By having this person playing a superordinate team management role (i.e. coordinate team activities but not contribute to content), this model is more appropriate for accommodating the political, resource allocation and policy issues that permeate the response environment.

The need to function in contexts that are dynamic and which can present evolving and novel problems calls for the development of several decision-making competencies. Incident management team members need to be proficient in creative (Jackson *et al.*, 2003; Kendra and Wachtendorf, 2003) and naturalistic decision making (Flin, 1996). Naturalistic decision making, where a person recognizes the type of situation encountered and, from previous experience, selects an appropriate course of action, is highly adaptive when having to respond to events characterized by substantial time pressure and high risk (Flin *et al.*, 1997).

Team and inter-agency operations

Tactical management entails functioning in multiagency and multijurisdictional contexts (Jackson *et al.*, 2003; Kendra and Wachtendorf, 2003; FEMA, 2004). The capacity for inter-agency communication and decision-making operations must be specifically targeted within planning and training processes (Farmer and Carlton, 2005; Banks *et al.*, 2006; Hope *et al.*, 2010).

However, simply bringing together representatives of departments and agencies who have little contact with one another under normal circumstances will not guarantee a coordinated response. Rather, such ad hoc arrangements are more likely to increase conflict, result in a blurring of roles and responsibilities. Thus, and irrespective of the quality of the planning that precedes it, a capacity for cohesive response should not be assumed. It can be developed using liaison mechanisms, and the integration of respective agency roles through inter-agency team development (Flin and Arbuthnott, 2002). A key factor underpinning the benefits that can accrue from these collaborative activities concerns good information sharing (Pollock *et al.*, 2003).

In effective teams, members provide more unprompted information, increasing a capability for proactive response management through better decision making and resource allocation when responding to complex acts of disaster (Entin and Serfaty, 1999). Effective incident management team performance is a function of the degree to which members share a ‘team mental model’ specifically relating to the goal-related information required by decision-makers at critical periods (Cooke *et al.*, 2000) and contributes to members being able to share understanding of evolving events and coordinating inputs to develop a capacity to work on the same plan towards common goals. It is a capacity that is developed through team exercises and simulations (Paton and Hannan, 2004; Hope *et al.*, 2010).

As the level of team work and planning activity increases, members will develop progressively more similar mental models of response environments and the roles and tasks to be performed within them. This, in turn, increases implicit information-sharing during high workload periods, enhancing team performance and adaptive capacity (Stout *et al.*, 1999; Paton and Jackson, 2002). In effective teams, the provision of unprompted information between members facilitates a capability for proactive response management through better tactical decision making and resource allocation (Entin and Serfaty, 1999).

The coordinating IMT have to be able to operate in an environment in which information required for decision making could be coming from diverse sources (Jackson *et al.*, 2003; Kendra and Wachtendorf, 2003). For example, information could be coming from medical, public health, emergency response teams, biological and radiological experts, emergency management officials, municipal agencies and private organizations responsible for transportation, communications, medical services, disaster assistance and public works construction (Carafano, 2003).

Given that the IMT is activated for large-scale disasters, the input to situation assessment can come from diverse professions and from people who may be spread over a large geographical area. The concept of distributed decision making recognizes the need for contributions from people who differ with respect to their profession, functions, roles and expertise, and who may be in different locations or involved at different levels (e.g. operational versus tactical) of decision making (Paton and Flin, 1999; FEMA, 2004). The quality of shared understanding and procedural integration thus determines the capability of the multiagency team to utilize its collective expertise, even if dispersed or contributing different perspectives, to manage the response. It also increases the likelihood of their operating with a shared mental model of the situation that facilitates the effective and efficient allocation and use of limited resources.

The object of coordinating or tactical management is to make decisions about the deployment of operation resources: the doctors, nurses and paramedics who are actively dealing with the medical consequences of disasters. The IMT makes the decisions about how medical resources are deployed and the roles they will perform. This should not be done in an autocratic manner. The degree to which management and the systems used to facilitate disaster response empower operational staff has an important bearing on the effectiveness of the response and the well-being of those operating on the front line (Johnston and Paton, 2003). The trust that operational staff have in management is crucial to effective performance of medical roles (Hope *et al.*, 2010).

Johnston and Paton (2003) described how empowerment mediated the relationship between the above predictors and resilience (job satisfaction) in hospital staff dealing with critical incidents. Consistent with the issues identified by Hope and colleagues, the model developed by Johnston and Paton (Fig. 10.2) illustrates how trust in management and perceptions of the quality of the information (e.g. regarding risk, training) and resources (e.g. antivirals, equipment) influenced staff ability to perform in their role (task assessment) and, importantly, in their capacity to adapt and respond to novel circumstances (global assessments). The link with satisfaction illustrates how the quality of the relationships between the healthcare organization (management and systems) influenced both the performance and well-being of operational staff.

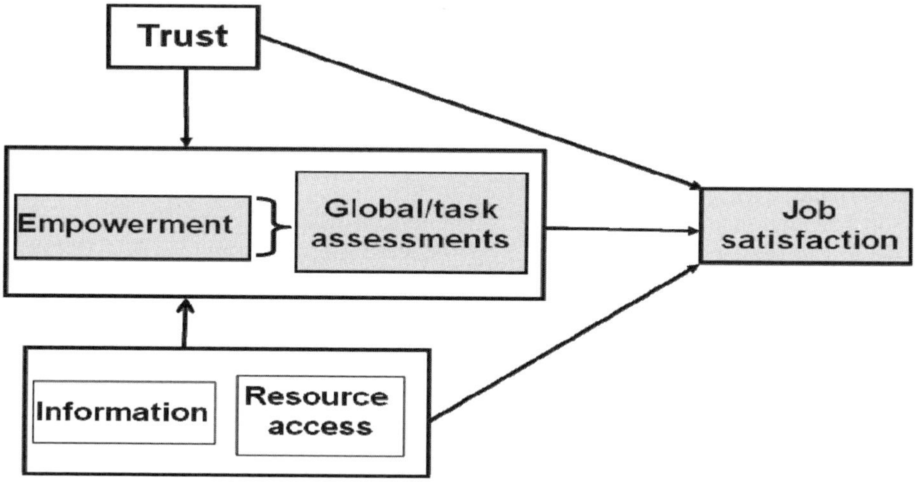

Fig. 10.2. The relationship between strategic/IMT management and effective operational response. (Adapted from Johnston and Paton, 2003.)

Operational Response

Operational response involves the execution of the tactical plan based on exercising professional, technical or scientific skills, but in atypical, challenging and threatening circumstances. Operational staff (e.g. doctors, nurses, emergency medical technicians (EMTs)) may be functioning in a hospital environment or they may be working in remote locations with varying degrees of access to resources and facilities (e.g. remote, temporary hospital facilities set up in a town hall). They may be performing their normal roles or they may be reassigned to non-routine roles such as communicating with the public, disaster triage or assisting with body identification (Benson *et al.*, 1996; Simpson and Stehr, 2003).

Disaster triage provides a good example of how working in disaster contexts can result in familiar tasks taking on an unfamiliar guise.

Triage during a disaster differs from triage performed in routine pre-hospital and hospital settings (Benson *et al.*, 1996). The number of people to be treated increases substantially and the availability of medical resources to treat them is limited severely and may be absent. Consequently, patients may remain in situ for prolonged periods of time during which they will need to have their status reassessed frequently. Furthermore, Benson and colleagues point out that triage will be decentralized and possibly occurring in several locations spread over a large geographical area simultaneously. Under these circumstances, patients who might recover may experience deterioration in their condition as a result of delays in getting hospital care.

In the absence of specific disaster training, medical staff members are likely to present to the triage site with triage experience derived from situations in which definitive care is immediately available and triage required only once. Benson *et al.* (1996) discuss a method of disaster triage that staff can be trained in and which is suited for making treatment decisions when access to definitive care is problematic. This includes estimating delay before definitive care will be available or accessible and thus the time patients will require care before being evacuated to hospital. Including these additional time and assessment issues is important. The longer staff members will be required to treat survivors in isolation, the more frugal they must become in the use of supplies and in the selection of patients to treat (Benson *et al.*, 1996). This conflict between their role expectations and the demands of disaster work can be a significant source of stress. Because it can have a profound impact on staff performance and well-being, managing psychological stress in frontline staff is an important component in an effective operational response.

Medical staff members involved in a disaster are at risk for experiencing stress and traumatic stress reactions from their direct experience of the disaster and from working in stressful roles in challenging (e.g. too few staff members, non-routine roles) and threatening (e.g. risk of infection or contamination) circumstances. There are several ways stress can be managed, including management practices, support and training.

Management practices

Organizational processes influence staff performance and well-being. Effective disaster response is a function of the degree to which a culture supports autonomous response systems, a flexible, consultative leadership style, and practices that ensure that role and task assignments reflect incident demands (Paton and Hannan, 2004). Managers also have important roles to play in staff recovery following the termination of the disaster by assisting staff members to appreciate that they performed to the best of their ability, and reducing performance guilt by realistically reviewing how situational factors constrained performance (Paton and Hannan, 2004). Managers can also maintain trust and facilitate positive resolution by assisting staff to identify the strengths that helped them deal with the disaster and building on this to plan how future events can be dealt with more effectively (Gist and Woodall, 2000; Hope *et al.*, 2010).

Support

Operational performance and stress resilience can be enhanced by ensuring that staff members work in teams. Cohesive teams can constitute a natural protective resource and increase stress resilience (Park, 1998). Lyons *et al.* (1998) describe team resilience as a function of their ability to engage in 'communal coping'. This is characterized by members' collective acceptance of responsibility for event-related problems and the existence of mechanisms by which they can cooperate to resolve problems. Acknowledging and building on effective collaboration during the disaster and working together afterwards, to develop understanding and enhance future preparedness has an important role to play in mitigating stress and in developing future stress resilience.

Individuals can also differ in their resilience characteristics. Traits such as understanding the meaning of one's role as a helper and hardiness can constitute resilience factors (Paton and Hannan, 2004; Hope *et al.*, 2010). Other factors such as emotional stability, decisiveness, controlled risk-taking, self-awareness, tolerance for ambiguity and self-efficacy also facilitate resilience (Flin, 1996; Paton and Hannan, 2004). Knowledge of these factors can be used to select people for high-demand operational tasks (e.g. managing inoculation or triage centres) and to plan for monitoring and support and counselling needs (Paton and Stephens, 1996; Banks *et al.*, 2006).

Staff members can be affected by transient factors such as health status (e.g. colds, 'flu), fatigue (e.g. if called to manage a disaster at the end of the working day) and psychological fitness (e.g. occupational stress, personal concerns) and pre-existing health and mental health issues. Pre-existing health issues can reduce the likelihood of staff turning up for work (Qureshi *et al.*, 2005; Hope *et al.*, 2010). Staff members must understand how such transient factors can affect their performance and their well-being and should increase their utilization of support resources. This can be accomplished through training.

Training

Education of healthcare professionals who will provide disaster care is currently inadequate in many or most hospitals, falling short in disaster-specific content and issues arising from performing clinical roles under atypical circumstances (Hick *et al.*, 2004; Markenson *et al.*, 2005; Banks *et al.*, 2006). Hope *et al.* (2010) identified a lack of specific disaster training as a significant predictor of staff members not reporting to work in the event during a disaster. Markenson and colleagues identified several core competencies that should be targeted in disaster training for medical workers. This includes issues associated with surveillance, diagnosis, reporting and patient care as well as emergency (e.g. hazards risk assessment and planning, response roles, incident command, integration with emergency management and communication) and public health emergency preparedness.

Training can enhance performance capability and reduce vulnerability to negative stress effects (Driskell and Salas, 1996; Paton and Stephens, 1996). In addition to knowledge and skill development in relation to anticipated role, training should address how the disaster context (e.g. hospital closure, treating people in situ with limited resources) influences performance and well-being (Paton, 1994).

Disasters are, fortunately, rare in any one area. This has implications for training designed to prepare people for the unexpected. Realizing the full benefits of training, and facilitating its transfer to response contexts, requires the use of simulations and exercises that challenge assumptions and push boundaries (Paton and Auld, 2006). Simulations afford opportunities for individuals to review plans, develop technical and management skills, construct realistic performance expectations, practise their use under realistic circumstances, receive feedback on their performance, increase awareness of stress reactions and facilitate rehearsal of strategies to minimize stress reactions.

To be effective, simulations should integrate the systematic analysis of emergency roles, tasks, responsibilities, skills and knowledge required for effective all-hazards management with the disaster characteristics and response demands (e.g. scale of damage, multiagency operations, rapid role change) likely to be encountered (Paton and Jackson, 2002; Paton and Auld, 2006). At a practical level, simulations should be designed to facilitate competence in, for example, identifying risk factors and their consequences for disaster stress; the translation of plans into action and their adaptation to cater for events differing in type, scale or complexity. They should also cover team processes and management; delegation of authority and responsibility; information management and communication, creative problem-solving, multiagency response management, and decision making under conditions of uncertainty (Endsley and Garland, 2000; Pollock *et al.*, 2003; Paton and Auld, 2006).

Conclusions

To enhance their capacity to respond effectively to disasters, hospitals need to develop both disaster response plans, systems and procedures and staff competencies to implement them in the context of the atypical, challenging and threatening circumstances posed by disaster. Learning and development is required at all levels. Hospitals need new ways of thinking about risk and the conditions under which they will operate. Healthcare staff members need to know how to apply their specialist and technical skills in non-routine settings and acknowledge that they may have to perform new roles in remote treatment locations. The effectiveness of the response to disaster is a function of the ability to respond by activating specially developed crisis management systems that require the integrated actions of operational, coordinating and strategic levels functions and response management.

References

Auf der Heide, E. (1989) *Disaster Response: Principles of Preparation and Coordination.* C.V. Mosby Company, St Louis, Missouri.

Banks, L.L., Richards, M.E. and Shah, M.B. (2006) An assessment of the personal and emotional barriers to effective disaster response on the part of healthcare professionals. *Quick Response Report*, 188. Natural Hazards Center, University of Colorado, Boulder, Colorado.

Barnett, D., Balicer, R. and Blodgett, D. (2005) Applying risk perception theory to public health workforce preparedness training. *Journal of Public Health Management* Supp. 4, s33–s37.

Benson, F., Koenig, K.L. and Schultz, C.H. (1996) Disaster triage: START, then SAVE – a new method of dynamic triage for victims of a catastrophic earthquake. *Prehospital and Disaster Medicine* 11, 117–124.

Berkes, F., Colding, J. and Folke, C. (2003) *Navigating Social-ecological Systems: Building Resilience for Complexity and Change*. Cambridge University Press, Cambridge, UK.

Brannick, M., Salas, E. and Prince, C. (1997) *Team Performance, Assessment and Measurement.* Lawrence Erlbaum, Mahwah, New Jersey.

Carafano, J.J. (2003) Preparing responders to respond: The challenges to emergency preparedness in the 21st century. *Heritage Lectures* #812. The Heritage Foundation, Washington, DC.

Cooke, N.J., Salas, E., Cannon-Bowers, J.A. and Stout, R.J. (2000) Measuring team knowledge. *Human Factors* 42, 151–173.

Crego, J. and Spinks, T. (1997) Critical incident management simulation. In: Flin, R., Salas, E., Strub, M. and Martin, L. (eds) *Decision Making Under Stress*. Ashgate, Aldershot, UK, pp. 85–94.

Cretikos, M.A., Merritt, T.D. and Main, K. (2007) Mitigating the health impacts of a natural disaster – the June 2007 long-weekend storm in the Hunter region of New South Wales. *Medical Journal of Australia* 187, 670–673.

Dalton, C.B., Durrheim, D.N. and Conroy M.A. (2008) Likely impact of school and childcare closures on public health workforce during an influenza pandemic: a survey. *Communicable Disease Intelligence* 32, 261–262.

Dara, S.I., Ashton, R.W. and Farmer, J.C. (2005) Engendering enthusiasm for sustainable disaster critical care response: why this is of consequence to critical care professionals? *Critical Care* 9, 125–128.

DiMaggio, C., Markeson, D., Loo, G.T. and Redlener, I. (2005) The willingness of U.S. emergency medical technicians to respond to terrorist incidents. *Biosecurity and Bioterrorism: Biodefense Strategy, Practice and Science* 3, 331–337.

Driskell, J. and Salas, E. (1996) *Stress and Human Performance*. Lawrence Erlbaum, Hillsdale, New Jersey.

Endsley, M. and Garland, D. (2000) *Situation Awareness. Analysis and Measurement*. Lawrence Erlbaum, Mahwah, New Jersey.

Entin, E.E. and Serfaty, D. (1999) Adaptive team coordination. *Human Factors* 41, 312–325.

Farmer, J.C. and Carlton, P.K. (2005) Hospital disaster medical response: aligning everyday requirements with emergency casualty care. *World Hospitals and Health Services* 41, 21–24.

Federal Emergency Management Agency (FEMA) (2004) *Responding to Incidents of National Consequence*. FEMA, Washington, DC.

Flin, R. (1996) *Sitting in the Hot Seat. Leaders and Teams for Critical Incident Management*. Wiley, Chichester, UK.

Flin, R. and Arbuthnot, K. (2002) *Incident Command: Tales from the Hot Seat*. Ashgate, Aldershot.

Flin, R., Salas, E., Strub, M. and Martin, L. (1997) *Decision Making under Stress*. Ashgate, Aldershot.

Gist, R. and Woodall, J. (2000) There are no simple solutions to complex problems. In: Violanti, J.M., Paton, D. and Dunning, C. (eds) *Posttraumatic Stress Intervention: Challenges, Issues and Perspectives*. Charles C. Thomas, Springfield, Illinois.

Hick, J.L., Hanfling, D., Burstein, J.L., DeAtley, C., Barbisch, D., Bogdan, G.M. and Cantrill, S. (2004) Health care facility and community strategies for patient care surge capacity. *Annals of Emergency Medicine* 44, 253–261.

Hope, K., Durrheim, D., Barnett, D., D'Este, C., Kewley, C., Dalton, C., Manager, N.W., Kohlhagen, J. and Links, J. (2010) Willingness of frontline health care workers to work during a public health emergency. *Australian Journal of Emergency Management* 25, 39–47.

Jackson, B.A., Baker, J.C., Ridgely, M.S., Bartis, J.T. and Linn, H.I. (2003) *Protecting Emergency Responders Volume 3: Safety Management in Disasters and Terrorism Response*. National Institute for Occupational Safety and Health, Cincinatti, Ohio.

Johnston, P. and Paton, D. (2003) Environmental resilience: psychological empowerment in high-risk professions. In: Paton, D., Violanti, J. and Smith, L. (eds) *Promoting Capabilities to Manage Posttraumatic Stress: Perspectives on Resilience*. Charles C. Thomas, Springfield, Illinois, pp. 136–151.

Kendra, J. and Wachtendorf, T. (2003) Creativity in emergency response to the World Trade Center disaster. In: Monday, J.L. (ed.) *Beyond September 11: An Account of Post Disaster Research*. Special Publication #39. Institute of Behavioral Science, Natural Hazards Research and Applications Information Centre, University of Colorado, Boulder, Colorado.

Koh, D., Lim, M.K. and Chia, S.E. (2005) Risk perception and impact of SARS on work and personal lives of healthcare workers in Singapore – what can we learn? *Medical Care* 43, 676–682.

Lanzilotti, S., Galanais, D. and Leoni, N. (2002) Hawaii medical professionals assessment. *Hawaii Medical Journal* 61, 162–173.

Lasker, R.D. (2004) *Redefining Readiness: Terrorism Planning Through the Eyes of the Public*. The New York Academy of Medicine, New York.

Lyons, R.F., Mickelson, K.D., Sullivan, M.J.L. and Coyne, J.C. (1998) Coping as a communal process. *Journal of Social and Personal Relationships* 15, 579–605.

Markenson, D., DiMaggio, C. and Redlener, I. (2005) Preparing health professions students for terrorism, disaster, and public health emergencies: core competencies. *Academic Medicine* 80, 517–526.

Maunder, R. (2004) The experience of the 2003 SARS outbreak as a traumatic stress among frontline healthcare workers in Toronto: lessons learned. *Philosophical Transactions of the Royal Society of London* 359, 1117–1125.

McCaughrin, W. (2003) Perfect storm: organizational management of patient care under natural disaster conditions. *Journal of Healthcare Management* 48, 295–308.

Mitroff, I.I. and Anagnos, G. (2001) *Managing Crises Before They Happen*. AMACOM, New York.

Nufer, K.E. and Wilson-Ramirez, G. (2004) A comparison of patient needs following two hurricanes. *Prehospital and Disaster Medicine* 19, 146–149.

Park, C.L. (1998) Stress-related growth and thriving through coping: the roles of personality and cognitive processes. *Journal of Social Issues* 54, 267–277.

Paton, D. (1994) Disaster relief work: an assessment of training effectiveness. *Journal of Traumatic Stress* 7, 275–288.

Paton, D. and Flin, R. (1999) Disaster Stress: An emergency management perspective. *Disaster Prevention and Management* 8, 261–267

Paton, D. and Auld, T. (2006) Resilience in emergency management: managing the flood. In: Paton, D. and Johnston, D. (eds) *Disaster Resilience: An Integrated Approach*. Charles C. Thomas, Springfield, Illinois, pp. 267–287.

Paton, D. and Hannan, G. (2004) Risk factors in emergency responders. In: Paton, D., Violanti, J. and Smith, L. (eds) *Promoting Capabilities to Manage Posttraumatic Stress: Perspectives on Resilience*. Charles C. Thomas, Springfield, Illinois, pp. 111–128.

Paton, D. and Jackson, D. (2002) developing disaster management capability: an assessment centre approach. *Disaster Prevention and Management* 11, 115–122.

Paton, D. and Stephens, C. (1996) Training and support for emergency responders. In: Paton, D., Violanti, J. and Smith, L. (eds) *Promoting Capabilities to Manage Posttraumatic Stress: Perspectives on Resilience*. Charles C. Thomas, Springfield, Illinois, pp. 173–205.

Pollock, C., Paton, D., Smith, L. and Violanti, J. (2003) Team resilience. In: Paton, D., Violanti, J. and Smith, L. (eds) *Promoting Capabilities to Manage Posttraumatic Stress: Perspectives on Resilience*. Charles C. Thomas, Springfield, Illinois, pp. 74–88.

Qureshi, K., Gershon, R.R.M., Sherman, M.F., Straub, T., Gebbie, E., McCollum, M., Erwin, M.J. and Morse, S.S. (2005) Health care workers' ability and willingness to report to duty during catastrophic disasters. *Journal of Urban Health: Bulletin of the New York Academy of Medicine* 82, 378–388.

Salas, E., Fowlkes, J.E., Stout, R.J., Milanovich, D.M. and Prince, C. (1999) Does CRM training improve teamwork skills in the cockpit? Two evaluation studies. *Human Factors* 41, 326–343.

Simpson, D.M. and Stehr, S. (2003) *Victim Management and Identification after the World Trade Center Collapse*. Special Publication #39. Institute of Behavioral Science, Natural Hazards Research and Applications Information Centre, University of Colorado, Boulder, Colorado.

Smith, E. (2007) Emergency health care workers' willingness to work during major emergencies and disasters. *Australian Journal of Emergency Management* 22, 21–24.

Smith, E., Morgans, A., Qureshi, K., Burkle, F. and Archer, F. (2009) Paramedics' perceptions of risk and willingness to work during disasters. *Australian Journal of Emergency Management* 24, 21–27.

Stout, R.J., Cannon-Bowers, J.A., Salas, E. and Milanovich, D.M. (1999) Planning, shared mental models and coordinated performance: an empirical link is established. *Human Factors* 41, 61–71.

Chapter 11

Information Management during the Disaster Medical Support Planning and Execution Phases

Rostislav Stefanov Kostadinov

Introduction

Almost every day somewhere in the world a disaster occurs. Regardless of its origin, natural or man-made, a disaster event always requires rapid mobilization of all community resources to meet the demand for delivery of proper assistance to the devastated area (Kostadinov, 2010c). In the majority of disasters people's lives, health and well-being are endangered, therefore, urgent provision of medical care is of the utmost importance. Retrospective analyses of previous disasters highlight the severe discrepancy between the needed and available medical assistance. The ultimate objective of medical support during disasters is to decrease mortality, morbidity and disability among the affected population. In order to achieve this objective, Disaster Medical Support Management (DMSM) has to best utilize the available medical resources and in a very limited time frame to direct their efforts and activities towards providing medical care to the maximum number of people in need. The decision-making process requires information about the current situation, desired end state, as well as available and required resources for mission accomplishment. During a disaster, medical managers have to make their decisions in a constantly changing situation and under time constraints – time is a crucial factor in life-saving actions (Kostadinov, 2010d). Therefore, providing DMSM with accurate and up-to-date information is a prerequisite for efficient and adequate medical response to the disaster. Collecting relevant data and providing required information to the Disaster Medical Support (DMS) planners and executive officers are core requirements for effective and efficient DMSM. All processes for gathering, processing and transferring information have to be properly managed, in the order requested by DMSM, information needs to arrive on time and needs to be of sufficient quantity and quality to enable planners and managers to execute prompt and appropriate DMS.

Information Flow and Disaster Medical Support Management

Why is there a need for information during the planning and execution of DMSM? Before describing the significance of information management throughout the DMSM cycle, it is necessary to define the terms data, information, information flow and information management. Therefore, the chapter will begin with some definitions.

There is still no consensus on the definition of information. A lot of studies have been dedicated to defining what information is. The very broad meaning of the word information has been, and still is, an object for analyses from different sciences. For the purposes of DMSM I am using a modified variant of the so-called general definition of information defining information as well-formed and meaningful data. Data are defined as a collection of facts from which conclusions may be drawn (Thesaurus, 2011). Information and data are closely related to knowledge, defined as an organized body of information, or the comprehension and understanding subsequent to having acquired and organized a body of facts (Thesaurus, 2011). But as with the definition of information, the definition of knowledge is a matter of on-going debate among philosophers, researchers and scientists. From the above-presented definition it could be construed that information is, and always has been, everywhere around us saturating the universe. The term flow means moving a substance between two or more points. Information flow could be defined as a directed (managed) movement of well-formed and meaningful data from the source to the recipient. As information surrounds us, to execute information flow (transmission), a specific piece of information has to be selected from that available and then moved; therefore the definition of information flow includes the prerequisite for deriving some information from another (analysis) in accordance with some requirements or references, a prerequisite for management. By extracting the appropriate piece of information and transmitting it to a particular recipient the raw data have been transformed into knowledge – an organized body of information. As a sequence, the information flow converts raw data into knowledge. Information management is defined as application of management techniques to collect information, communicate it within and outside an organization, and process it to enable managers to make quicker and better decisions (Business Dictionary, 2011).

This brief overview of the meaning of information, data, knowledge and information management leads to the conclusion that effective and efficient management of any environment is impossible without appropriate information flow.

When disaster strikes, DMSM requires information flow to be not only appropriate, but also as fast as possible, because disaster victims' life and health are time-dependent. Therefore, the establishment of comprehensive and clear medical information management procedures is mandatory to fulfil the ultimate objective of DMSM – preserving the life and health and preventing residual disability of the maximum possible number of people injured and harmed by the disaster event. These procedures have to be standardized prior to the disaster and implemented into the DMSM contingency plans (CONOPS) for every possible disaster event foreseen in the particular area – country, province, district or municipality (Kostadinov *et al.*, 2009). By implementing standard operating procedures (SOPs), disaster medicine information flow management (DMIFM) provides specific, up-to-date, comprehensive information to all engaged in the disaster medical relief – affected population, medical care providers and national and international organizations. In order to meet the requirements for timely provision of concise, specific, comprehensive pieces of information to a variety of different recipients, a particular algorithm for DMIFM has to be implemented in practice. A great number of tools concerning information management in different areas of business and science have been created and published recently. In the course of this chapter the intent is to draw your attention to an information management algorithm modified for DMSM purposes. The algorithm is described in a sequence of seven steps. These seven steps are the cornerstones of the DMIMF. There is no attempt to present an argument for them. Rather, their practical implementation is illustrated.

All the steps of the algorithm are closely linked to the presented definitions. For information flow to occur at least the following conditions must be fulfilled:

1. Availability of two or more distinguished, divided groups that could be separated by different causes – status, space, tasks, etc. An obvious example of such groups in DMSM is the presence of medical care providers and the affected and non-affected population in the area of damage. Both of the groups are source and recipients of the DMSM information required in order to plan their activities in the austere disaster background;
2. Presence of a structure that extracts and directs the pieces of the available information significant for DMSM. Good examples are the medical specialists performing medical reconnaissance, intelligence and surveillance, as well as the disaster medicine planning and executive officers (Kostadinov and Kanev, 2009);
3. Presence of doctrinal and operational requirements for information analyses and directions. The disaster medicine SOPs guide the above-mentioned processes (Kostadinov, 2010b);
4. Implementation of management techniques to collect and disseminate information are illustrated in the preparing of DMSM CONOPS, as well as in the planning and execution of training activities and implementation of the lessons learned.

The steps of the DMIFM algorithm are:

1. Setting the DMSM information requirements;
2. Allocating target groups to the information requirements;
3. Establishing appropriate structure for managing the information flow;
4. Preparing questionnaires for each of the target groups and SOPs;
5. Planning the DMIFM activities;
6. Target group training;
7. Lessons Learned (LL) implementation.

Setting the DMSM information requirements

As stated above the differences between information and data are related to the organization and content of the data. Therefore, the first step in the process of management is to convert the raw data into information. The most important activity within this step is to separate the data containing information valuable for DMSM, from the great variety of available information. It is reasonable to ask how this division could be made. As the meaningfulness of the information during the planning and execution of DMSM is closely and exclusively related to the role of the medical manager he or she is the person who has to set the requirements regarding information needed. Moreover the medical manager in the course of DMSM is not only the recipient, but also has to generate information, directed to a spectrum of organizations, groups and individuals affected by the disaster or involved in the disaster consequences management.

Retrospective analysis of DMSM activities performed over the past 50 years has highlighted the significance of timely provision of reliable and up-to-date information for the decision-making process. Countless errors have been made owing to insufficient or wrong information. On-going development of communications means and technologies is a powerful tool for decreasing the number of inappropriate decisions related to information flow. In the course of this first step every designated disaster medicine manager has to set up his information requirements. From our experience (Kostadinov, 2010a) the following areas of incoming information could be a useful template for disaster medicine managers:

1. Type of disaster – What has happened?
2. Location – Where it has happened?
3. Time of onset – When did it happen?
4. What are the damaging factors?
5. What are the health threats?
6. Scope of disaster – What is the extent of the damage?
7. Heath consequences – How many casualties are there?
8. Where they are concentrated?
9. Medical situation on the ground – Who is providing medical assistance to the affected population, with what capabilities?
10. What are the available medical means and capabilities in the affected area?
11. Consequences regarding medical care provision – What is the damage to the medical infrastructure?
12. What are the routes for ingress and egress?
13. Medical evacuation – available and required means and capabilities – routes and destinations?
14. Requirements for additional medical means, capabilities and resources?
15. Medical strength in the vicinity of the affected area – Available medical means and capabilities for deployment, as reinforcement?
16. Planning information – CONOPS for the area in case of this type of disaster occurrence.
17. Possible courses of actions (COAs) with the available resources in the given situation.

As stated above the assigned disaster medical manager is to distribute information as a part of the information flow management. The main areas that have to be covered by this outgoing information are:

1. Information still needed for the decision-making process – for directed medical information collection and processing;
2. The most appropriate COA – for converting the CONOPS into an operational plan (OPLAN);
3. Medical advice to the affected population and rescue teams and services – to minimize the number of victims and enable better protection of the survivors and rescuers;
4. Selected medical evacuation (MEDEVAC) routes and destinations – for medical facilities preparedness;
5. Request for assistance with manpower, equipment, means and capabilities, in order to faster deploy required medical reinforcements.

Allocating target groups to the information requirements

By drafting requirements for incoming and outgoing information the first step of an effective DMIFM plan is accomplished. Reading the definition of information flow, logically, the points of information flow have to be described. The role of the disaster medicine manager is two-fold – as a recipient and as a source of information. Acting as a recipient the manager has to allocate the available sources of information. The main ones are listed:

1. Affected population;
2. Healthcare providers in the affected region;
3. Media – all types of media could be used as a source of information – TV, radio broadcasts, newspapers, online news sites, etc.;
4. Rescue teams active in the area of damage;
5. Medical intelligence and reconnaissance teams;
6. Governmental and non-governmental organizations (NGOs) participating in the disaster's relief operations – the specialized structures for rapid reaction in case of disaster of the Ministry of Internal Affairs, the Ministry of Emergency Situations, the Ministry of Defence – civil protection, fire brigades, police, gendarmerie, etc.;
7. International organizations (IOs) – United Nations (UN) and its Office for Coordination of Humanitarian Affairs (OCHA) in particular, the World Health Organization (WHO), The International Committee of the Red Cross and Red Crescent (ICRCC) and non-governmental organizations (NGOs);
8. Disaster medicine chairs, teams and detachments, as well as expert panels, related to the Disaster Medical Support (DMS), on the national and international level;
9. National and international systems for early warning, control and management of disasters – e.g. the Global Disaster Alert and Coordination System, the Monitoring and Information Centre (MIC), operated by the European Commission, Euro-Atlantic Disaster Response Coordination Centre (EADRCC) and so on;
10. National and international databases related to the DMS – for example, as created by the US National Library of Medicine, Disaster Information Management Research Centre (DIMRC) and the related Hazardous Substances Databank (HSDB), Wireless Information System for Emergency Responders (WISER) and so on. These databases provide health information in preparation for and in response to all types of disasters, and some of them have developed a number of tools and advanced information services designed for emergency manager and responder use.

Only a few of the potential sources for information for DMS planning are listed. Every designated DMS manager should make a list of those available in their particular region in accordance with the directives given in the higher level DMS CONOPS. The main sources of information aiding the decision-making process for the DMS manager are the DMS planners. They are the focal point of the incoming information. During crisis response planning, the pre-planned activities described by the CONOPS are compared with the medical situation's requirements, thus highlighting the areas of medical support that have to be enhanced, modified or even substituted for something more appropriate, with regards to the rapidly changing general and medical situation in the affected region. Adjusting the CONOPS with medical planners, the DMS manager prepares the OPLAN for the particular event. In addition to outlining the required medical activities for minimizing the impact of the disaster on health and health-threatening environmental consequences, the plan should deal with information flow during DMSM. The recipients of the medical information have to be clearly stated. The main groups that have to be addressed are:

1. Medical healthcare providers. All the elements of the medical support teams should receive clear directives, guidance and orders on what they have to do, where, when and with whom they have to do it. Every particular medical team (triage, evacuation, treatment, etc.), every hospital or other medical facility involved in DMSM should be informed about the part of the OPLAN they have to execute. Health hazards, health risk and the required preventive measures should be highlighted and expressed in a comprehensive manner.
2. Medical planners and medical intelligence, reconnaissance and surveillance teams are part of the DMSM team receiving the DMS manager's critical information requirements for information, as well as his directions and guidance on what is needed to be modified into the OPLAN for better disaster relief operation execution (Tonev *et al.*, 2008).
3. Higher level DMS manager, or National Disaster Coordination Centre, when DMSM is on Ministry of Health level.
4. Affected population. Addressing the affected population with information about the health threat and hazards, related to the disaster event, as well as giving advice on preventive measures and descriptions of the healthcare providers' location, and safely routes for movement, have proven to reduce in a timely manner the number of fatalities and residual disability.
5. Media – all available. Reliable media sources have to be briefed at the very beginning of the DMS. The requirement for this activity is based on the media's power for information distribution. Advice given to the population can reach a greater number of the population when delivered via media broadcasting. The rationality of addressing the media at the earliest possible time is to stop growing panic within the population, based on the fear that they have been left alone to overcome their own misfortune. By providing timely media coverage on on-going medical activities and the coordinating efforts between all relief services, confidence in the rescue teams, as well as mobilization of the population, is achieved. Clear and factual media communication also aims towards preventing all possible speculation for gaining some political, financial or other benefits from the disaster and population suffering. All the steps and means for the best communication and coordination with media outlets should be described in the OPLAN.
6. All non-medical structures taking part in the disaster relief. As mentioned above, disaster relief-dedicated structures and formations from different ministries should join together to provide the affected population and region with rapid and appropriate measures in order to minimize the impact and consequences of the disaster. As healthcare providers are part of the disaster relief team, it is of the utmost importance that communication between the rescue teams and relief management is obtained at the earliest stage of the planning and executing of disaster relief operations, in order to achieve the best possible coordination. Moreover, the rescue teams have to be aware of the specific health hazards in the area of damage and the required personal protective measures, thus ensuring the safety of the rescuers.

7. IOs and NGOs. All disaster relief operations depend on the type, severity, location of the disaster and extent of the damages. When the national resources are assessed to be insufficient for execution of the appropriate disaster relief and/or there is risk of a neighbouring country/countries being affected, the National Disaster Management Coordination Centre should address IOs and NGOs appealing for disaster relief assistance – an essential part of which is the medical overview of the situation. Purely on a medical basis, IOs must be informed about any foreseen or on-going disease outbreak or health-threatening deterioration in the health status of the population (hygiene, nutrition, water availability and safety, etc.).
8. National and international systems for early warning, control and management of disasters should be constantly informed about any threat to the affected population's health and well-being.

Depending on the region, disaster event and national regulations, the DMS manager should add other groups to his information delivery list as appropriate.

DMIFM structure and organization establishment

When the required information, sources for gathering it and the destination for its direction are set, DMSM could carry out a DMIFM. As has been highlighted repeatedly, time is a critical factor in the decision-making process when conducting disaster relief operations. In order to speed up the decision-making process and to minimize the possibility of errors all the 'tracks' of the information flow chain (providers and recipients) have to be prepared and trained for information collection and utilization. The main goal of the preparatory process is to minimize the time required for information processing, as well as avoidance of the errors recorded during previous disaster relief operations. What are the steps for speeding up the information flow? Once again we have to look at the definition – information is well formed and meaningful data, therefore, DMSM has to establish a structure for extracting the appropriate data from the multitude of available information and for organizing, processing and directing the data to the recipients. From a medical point of view one possible structure for a DMIFM consists of:

1. Medical intelligence, reconnaissance and surveillance team (MIRST). The objectives of this team are collection of all available medically significant information. This information could be gathered by exploring all available sources of information – databanks, media reports, governmental statements, witness reports, awareness signals, etc. Reconnaissance is gaining information by direct, on-the-spot observations and information gathering, while surveillance is information-gathering through monitoring the development of the medical situation. As a result of these three activities the team produces the medical intelligence product, where the health hazards in the affected and surrounding regions are identified, the level of health risk related to the hazards is assessed and measures for minimizing, or in an ideal situation eradicating, the health risk are recommended. This team is the main source of medical information for DMSM. This team is one of the primary recipients of information during the process of the DMIFM, because the process of information collection is directed mainly by the DMS manager's directions and guidance.
2. Medical support planning team (MSPT). The main aim of the team is to convert the CONOPS into OPLAN in accordance with the intent of the DMS manager and

the disaster event impact. In order to fulfil their task the planning team must be continuously provided with information on all changes to the medical background, both with the manager's intent of utilization of the available medical capabilities on the spot, and with the DMS manager's design for manoeuvre with the reserve medical resources.

3. Decision-making team (DMT). This team is led by the DMS manager and is in constant communication with the higher level of DMSM. The team takes the decisions on type, time and coordination of all medical activities, for provision of the DMS. The DMS has to be appropriate and adequate to the disaster's health consequences given the scarcity of available medical means and capabilities in the affected area and its vicinity, within the shortest possible time frame. All the decisions made by the DMT are based on the information and products received by the TMIRS and MSPT regarding the medical situation development. The team issues the medical SOPs to be used in the disaster relief operation. The DMT also analyses the feedback received through the lessons identified (LI) process, and evaluates the DMS results and recorded shortfalls, thus transforming the incoming LI into lessons learned (LL). LL are transferred to MSPT to be taken into consideration during the planning process.
4. Information dissemination team (IDT). The main goal of this team is to distribute the DMS manager-approved information and medical intelligence products to the target groups. The team is responsible for providing the processed medical information to the target audience in a comprehensible format. The directed information has to be tailored to the outcome every group has to achieve in order to support DMSM.
5. Communication and Information Systems Technical Team (CISTT). The team is responsible for providing DMSM with operational means of communication and sustainment of information flow during DMS execution. Communication systems have to be compatible with the systems of all the structures involved in the disaster relief operation.

DMIFM questionnaires preparation

The next requirement for data to become information is for it to be meaningful. As previously mentioned the DMS manager is the one who sets the requirements for incoming data. To save time and effort in the time-constrained DMSM process, all the elements in the DMIFM have to be aware of what kind information they are required to provide and disseminate. The fourth step in DMIFM is providing all target groups with sample questionnaires. The questionnaires consist of a number of questions that have to be answered during information collection, processing, direction and dissemination. A set of templates for general questionnaires to be used in DMIFM planning is listed below.

MIRST questionnaire

1. Type of disaster;
2. Time of onset and duration;
3. Grid location of the disaster;
4. Disaster's primary and secondary damaging factors;
5. Area of damage – the region exposed to the impact of the disaster's damaging factors;

6. Identified health hazards and assessed health risk;
7. Current number and type of casualties;
8. Provisional number and severity of casualties;
9. Location of the casualties;
10. Damage to medical infrastructures in the affected region;
11. Operating medical facilities in the area of damage – location, residual medical means and capabilities;
12. Required medical means and capabilities for provision of prompt, adequate and efficient DMS;
13. Critical infrastructure damage – roads, electricity and water distribution systems, etc.;
14. Routes for ingress and egress into the area of damage;
15. Recommended locations for establishment of triage, treatment and evacuation areas;
16. Operating airports, helipads, ports and highways;
17. Medical facilities operating in the area of damage and in the vicinity – capabilities and readiness for DMS activities;
18. Rescue teams operating in the area of damage;
19. Established incident command organization;
20. Established medical command, control, communication, coordination and intelligence (C4I);
21. Recommended personal protective equipment and preventive measures in order to minimize the health risk level.

MSPT questionnaire

1. The impact of the disaster, with regards to its type, location and severity, on pre-planned DMS activities;
2. Comparison between available and expected/foreseen damaging factors – the impact on medical mission execution;
3. The impact of medical infrastructure damage;
4. Significance of the critical infrastructure damage for DMS execution;
5. Comparison between the available and required medical means and capabilities – requirements for medical support enhancement;
6. Assessment of the readiness and capabilities of the medical facilities available in the vicinity for provision of DMS assistance or as a medical evacuation (MEDEVAC) destination;
7. Availability and readiness of MEDEVAC teams and means;
8. Provisional times for MEDEVAC in accordance with the available means and infrastructure damages;
9. Possible routes and destinations for MEDEVAC – recommended plan for MEDEVAC execution;
10. DMS courses of action (COAs), based on casualty number, severity, location and available medical capabilities. COA describes the type of medical activity, the time frame for their execution, desired outcomes, etc.;
11. Recommended medical COA;
12. Recommendations for COA changes in view of the development of a foreseen medical situation;
13. Required medical command and control (C2);

14. Required medical reporting format and timing – required medical communication;
15. POCs for medical communications;
16. Coordination with the other rescue teams involved in the disaster relief – POCs;
17. Required medical reports to the incident command – template and timing for the communication.

DMT questionnaire

The DMT has to take decisions on and inform the respective recipients about:

1. DMS manager responsible for DMS tasks and execution;
2. Medical COA;
3. Medical C2;
4. Medical SOPs;
5. DMS manager critical information requirements;
6. Medical reports and returns – timing, format;
7. Medical communication with the others rescue teams – established incident command – the role and subordination of the medical incident commander;
8. Feedback expected.

The IDT should prepare and distribute the DMS manager-approved information to all target groups in a comprehensive format. The most important groups for the IDT to communicate with are the affected population, the media and medical care providers. MIRST and MSPT, as well as higher level DMS managers, or the National Disaster Coordination Centre are usually addressed directly by the DMT.

Healthcare providers are the most important recipient target group, because they are responsible for executing the DMS activities. IDT is expected to inform the medical community involved in the relief operation with data about:

1. Type of disaster;
2. Time of onset and duration;
3. Grid location of the disaster;
4. Disaster's primary and secondary damaging factors;
5. Area of damage;
6. Identified health hazards and assessed health risk;
7. Required personal protective equipment and preventive measures in order to minimize the health risk level (Kostadinov and Sapundzhiev, 2010);
8. Current number and type of casualties;
9. Location of the casualties;
10. Operating medical facilities in the area of damage – location, residual medical means and capabilities;
11. Critical infrastructure damages – roads, electricity and water distribution systems, etc.;
12. Routes of ingress and egress for the damaged area;
13. Established, or to-be-established triage, treatment and evacuation areas;
14. Operating airports, helipads, ports and highways;
15. Medical C2;
16. Medical COA;
17. Medical SOPs;

18. Established incident command organization;
19. Reports and returns;
20. Established medical (C4I);
21. Means of communication to be used;
22. MEDEVAC organization – means, capabilities, SOPs;
23. Locations and POCs of the medical facilities involved in the DMS;
24. DMSM POCs.

The main information the affected population expects to receive is related to four areas:

1. What is the threat to my life and health?
2. Do I have to evacuate myself and my family?
3. How can I protect myself and my family?
4. Who and where is supposed to help me?

The countless records of these questions serve as a basis for drafting the IDT sample questionnaire aimed at improving medical communication with the affected population. It consists of:

1. Type of disaster;
2. Damaging factors;
3. Health risks related to the damaging factors;
4. Areas exposed to the damaging factors' impact;
5. Preventive measures to be taken – explained in plain, non-medical language;
6. Requirement for evacuation – if needed, time, direction to points of recall, points for collections;
7. Medical activities performed and on-going;
8. Advice for safe behaviour;
9. Location of established temporary medical stations;
10. Water safety and points for safe water distribution;
11. Food safety and points for food distribution;
12. Environmental pollution;
13. Foreseen diseases outbreak and means for prevention and protection;
14. Duration of medical-related limitation – e.g. quarantine;
15. POCs for additional medical information.

In the contemporary world the media is often recognized as the fourth power, because of its capabilities to modulate people's thoughts, activities and behaviour. When disaster strikes the media's capabilities to influence the population are powerful tools for DMSM. With proper media communication and coordination efforts, both healthcare providers and media managers can attain their objectives. The needs of the media include breaking news, novelty and profound analyses. All these could be provided by the DMS managers. By using the media, medical information will reach audiences far beyond the capabilities of medical information channels. Therefore, media communication is of utmost importance for the success of the DMS and DMIFM. All media outlets are very cautious when dealing with information; all sources are carefully examined prior to being labelled as reliable. This is the rationality behind advising DMS managers to begin their cooperation with selected media during the preparatory phase of the DMS. By providing reporters with data regarding medical preparedness for disaster relief operations and inviting media to cover disaster medical response training, two objectives can be easily achieved – becoming a favourite and reliable source for the media and informing the population of the medical community's readiness for confronting disaster challenges. Some of the topics to be highlighted by the IDT are listed in this sample questionnaire:

1. Type and scope of disaster;
2. Affected regions, medical and critical infrastructure;
3. Damaging factors and related health risk;
4. Number and severity of the casualties;
5. Water safety;
6. Food safety;
7. Environmental pollution;
8. Location of safe water and food distribution;
9. Required preventive measures to be taken by the affected population;
10. Required medical activities for DMS;
11. Performed medical activities;
12. Medical means and capabilities involved in the disaster relief;
13. Expected outcome of the medical activities;
14. Shortfalls in the disaster relief and their mitigation;
15. Requirement for evacuation – details – where, when, how, etc.;
16. Location of the established temporary medical stations;
17. MEDEVAC activities performed;
18. MEDEVAC areas;
19. Medical C2;
20. Disaster relief coordination between the rescue structures involved;
21. Medical POCs.

IDT should address national (depending on the level) and international NGOs, as well as IOs with the following information:

1. The disaster's health-damaging factors and related health risk level;
2. Performed medical activities;
3. DMS shortfalls – means, capabilities;
4. Foreseen disease outbreak;
5. Urgent critical medical requirements – water, food, sanitation, decontamination, transport means, medical consumables, technical and medical equipment, communication support, general and specialized medical teams, MEDEVAC capabilities, medical treatment facilities – field or stationary, etc.;
6. Information and financial support;
7. Safety and security.

Planning DMIFM activities

Every sequence of activities, if it is to be executed properly, has to be planned in order for the flow of events to follow the design and the desired outcome to be achieved. As the DMIFM is a process of simultaneously performed activities, the need for planning is indisputable. What should a DMIFM plan consist of? The answer to the question can be found, once again, in the definition of the term information flow: transfer of well-formed and meaningful data between at least two separate points. The first part of the plan has to deal with the process of data transfer. Several items and activities have to be clarified:

1. Time – Starting point of the movement – when the data transfer has to start. In DMSM most of the activities are constant; others are performed only when there is an imminent threat or disaster event. Examples of activities that are performed during all the phases of DMSM are medical intelligence, disease surveillance, planning and training activities. The reconnaissance, on the other hand is a perfect example of an activity performed immediately after the disaster occurrence.
2. Location – Starting point and destination of the information. In the plan all the sources of information have to be listed with their respective POCs. The types of information required by every source are described, together with the respective recipient.
3. How – Means of data movement. The communications means available and ready for use are listed with the particulars of the utilized equipment, and the time window dedicated for medical information exchange.
4. What – Templates for every single report and required classification should be part of the DMIFM plan.

The second part of the plan should describe the information hierarchy. All DMS managers should maintain a database of hazardous sites in their respective area of responsibility. This database should consist of information regarding the location of the hazardous site, the type of health hazard – e.g. chemical production with processing of highly toxic materials, expected consequences in case of process failure, preventive measures required, available protective equipment, available medical healthcare in the vicinity, population at risk, environmental factors with potential to increase or decrease the hazard impact, etc. All these medical intelligence data have to be constantly updated and stored as a basis for proper DMS planning. The second layer of information building consists of the operational links with national and international disaster medicine databanks and think tanks. Critical DMS manager information requirements in case of disaster form the third level of the information pyramid. These three levels are constantly filled with relevant data during the preparation phase of DMSM. The fourth level consists of the different CONOPS, where DMIFM scenarios during disaster events that could occur in the region/municipality country are described. The fifth level consists of the incoming information during the disaster – the basis for the creation of the OPLAN for information medical flow, concerning the on-going DMSM.

During a disaster, the medical situation is unsteady, with the possibility of dramatic changes in a narrow time frame. Therefore, the collected and stored information has to be available for immediate access and updating. A good example of utilization of information technologies in the planning and execution process is the North Atlantic Treaty Organization (NATO)-created operational level medical command wise page for quick reference to the stored information, with possibilities for quick amendment and adjustment in accordance with the situation's development. The wise page is constructed according to the above-described information layer hierarchy with restrictions on the validating and inserting of information, but accessible as read only to every medical officer assigned to the operational medical support team.

POCs responsible for the management of every layer of information should be listed in the DMIFM plan.

Target groups training

There are many challenges for DMSM, but the main, decisive one is time. Time has been recorded in all disaster medical responses as a crucial element in saving casualties' lives, limbs and abilities, as well as in affected population health protection. In order to minimize the time required to provide the DMS manager with relevant and reliable information regarding the changing medical situation during and after disaster, all participants in the information flow chain have to be familiar with their responsibilities and trained on SOPs implementation. The main objectives of the training process are:

1. Establishing the information flow chain. This objective is met by establishing the teams for collecting, analysing, processing and distributing information. All the team members have to be acquainted with their role and responsibilities with regards to information flow. Every member is to know from what source (POCs), when and what kind of information they are required to collect, as well as when, in what format, quantity and quality, to send it to the respective POC (recipient).
2. Training information flow. The team members are expected to be trained in using the appropriate means for information collection – technical equipment, questionnaires, etc. Teams are trained in order to be able to rapidly process the obtained raw data into medically meaningful information, the process described in the respective SOPs.
3. Training teams in coordination and DMIFM comprehension by applying different disaster scenarios in computer-based or live exercises. Introducing the prepared CONOPS for the particular disaster and exercising medical information flow management.
4. Training the population to provide medical significant data, look for medical information and understand the provided medical advice.
5. Training in coordination and cooperation with the media to enable sharing of medical information during disaster relief operations.
6. Individual training with questionnaires for collection or/and dissemination of medical information.
7. Individual training for assessing the performed activities and preparing daily summary reports (DSRs). The report is a tool designed to provide higher level managers with an overview of developments in the medical situation in a timely manner. The DSR sample in use is:
    - **a.** Name, position of the originator;
    - **b.** Date;
    - **c.** Summary of the performed activities;
    - **d.** Current highlights – presenting the difficulties in DMS execution;
    - **e.** OPLAN required activities and performed ones;
    - **f.** Proposals for OPLAN modification;
    - **g.** Medical infrastructure update;
    - **h.** Medical means and capabilities update;
    - **i.** MEDEVAC issues;
    - **j.** Rescue teams' health protection and preventive medicine issues;
    - **k.** Humanitarian situation;
    - **l.** Medical situation assessment with regards to the possibility of DMS execution.

The expected outcome of the training is that all target groups from medical teams to the media and the population at large are prepared for providing, receiving and understanding medical information during a disaster event and disaster relief operation. One frequently underestimated outcome of the training process is LI data collection and processing, which is in close connection with the seventh step of DMIFM. LI are reports on all observed shortfalls in manning, organization, C4I, as well as difficulties in implementing the CONOPS/OPLAN and all other factors that have hampered the execution of DMS.

LL implementation

The LL process is of utmost importance for management. During this process the LI during the trainings or executions are analysed, validated and transformed into LL. What distinguishes LI from LL? In LI the observed obstacles, shortfalls and deficiencies are presented from the originator's point of view and with his/her own perception of how this issue could be solved. All the LI are the object of thorough analysis and their impact on the success of the DMS is assessed. With regards to their significance LI are prioritized in different categories – impact on entire DMS execution, partial impact on a phase, minimal impact on the outcome, significant only for the particular event, with negligible impact. The next step in the process is linking validated LI, in accordance with their significance, with measures for reducing their impact, thus transforming them into LL.

All medical personnel involved in DMMS should be familiar with the requirements for provision of observations on the execution of DMS activities and LI approved templates. One possible template for an observation form consists of:

1. Name, position and contact details of the originator;
2. Date;
3. References – CONOPS, OPLAN, SOPs for the training or DMS execution;
4. Title of the observation – stating the main shortfall, concern, etc.;
5. Observation – describing the facts – what was planned and what happened;
6. Discussion – analysis of the described above facts and their impact on DMS outcome;
7. Conclusion – statement about the significance of the observation;
8. Recommendation and proposed action body – what has to be done and by whom for improvement of DMS execution;
9. Supervisor comments.

When LL are validated and approved by the DMT they are sent to DMPT for implementing the prescribed measures into the CONOPS, so as not to face the same obstacles and deficiencies again. The amendments to the CONOPS have to be considered when revising the SOPs and then should be implemented into the ensuing data collection, processing and dissemination process.

Conclusion

Information flow management is one of the greatest challenges DMSM faces during DMS execution. On the one hand the austere environment, damaged communication, and infrastructure jeopardize information movement from the sources to the recipients. On the other hand, panic spreading within the affected population and media coverage of the disaster consequences can hamper reliable data collection. Moreover, the imperative of saving casualties' lives reduces the time frame for information gathering, processing and implementation into the decision-making process. Therefore, all the providers and recipients of medical information during the DMS execution have to be aware of what, when and to whom they are expected to provide. Failure to meet this objective could result in errors during the planning and execution of DMS or in delays in provision of medical assistance to the injured and population in need. In order to minimize the possibility of delayed or insufficient DMS provision, the DMS manager has to plan adequate DMIFM and to train all the elements of the information flow chain in the implementation of this plan. The author's humble opinion is that the described algorithm and provided templates will facilitate proper information flow management during the planning and execution of DMS.

Acknowledgements

First I would like to record my gratitude to Professor Kamen Kanev, MD, DSc for his advice, supervision and crucial contribution to the research from the very beginning. I gratefully acknowledge the President of the Military Medical Academy, Sofia Major General Professor Stoyan Tonev, MD, PhD for his directives and guidance. It is a pleasure to pay tribute to all colleagues from Chair 'Disaster Medicine and Toxicology', and the Educational and Scientific Department of the Military Medical Academy, Sofia, Bulgaria for supporting my research. I would also like to acknowledge Colonel Dr Renzo Mattei, MD (NATO Joint Force Command Head Quarters Naples Medical Advisor) and Commander Roy Henderson for their advice and willingness to implement the above-described algorithm in practice.

References

Business Dictionary (2011) Available at: http://BusinessDictionary.com (Accessed 26 June 2011).

Kostadinov, R. (2010a) Medical Teams' theoretical preparation for major incident medical support. In: Hristov, J., Kyriopoulos, J., Konstantinidis, T. and Shipkovenska, E. (eds) *Public Health and Health Care in Greece and Bulgaria.* Papazissis Publishers, Athens, pp. 223–229.

Kostadinov, R. (2010b) Major incident management and support – Bulgarian Policy. In: Hristov, J., Kyriopoulos, J., Konstantinidis, T. and Shipkovenska, E. (eds) *Public Health and Health Care in Greece and Bulgaria.* Papazissis Publishers, Athens, Greece, pp. 691–696.

Kostadinov, R. (2010c) Population protection and medical support organization in case of disasters. In: Hristov, J. (ed.) *Disaster Medical Support Management Manual.* VAK Publishing House, Plovdiv, Bulgaria, pp. 18–31.

Kostadinov, R. (2010d) Population disaster medical support. In: Hristov, J. (ed.) *Disaster Medical Support Management Manual.* VAK Publishing House, Plovdiv, Bulgaria, pp. 31–37.

Kostadinov, R. and Kanev, K. (2009) MED in Bulgaria. *CBRNe World* Winter, 57–58.

Kostadinov, R. and Sapundzhiev, K. (2010) Medical teams' protection: crucial step in disaster medical management and support. In: Hristov, J., Kyriopoulos, J., Konstantinidis, T. and Shipkovenska, E. (eds) *Public Health and Health Care in Greece and Bulgaria.* Papazissis Publishers, Athens, pp. 197–202.

Kostadinov, R., Dimitrov, A. and Kanev, K. (2009) Military medical readiness for chemical and biological terrorists' attacks. In: Tonev, S., Kanev, K. and Dishovsky, C. (eds) *Medical Management of Chemical and Biological Casualties*. Irita Publishing House, Sofia, Bulgaria, pp. 44–49.

Tonev, S., Kanev, K., Kostadinov, R. and Gulubova, A. (2008) Medical assessment state of Kuwait. In: Tonev, S. (ed.) *Medical Support Principles and Current Military Missions Medical Assessment*. Irita Publishing House, Sofia, Bulgaria, pp. 253–358.

Thesaurus (2011) Available at: http://thesaurus.com/ (Accessed 26 June 2011).

Section 5

Medical Management of Complex Disasters and MCI Victims in Hospitals

Chapter 12

Potential Application of Established Pre-hospital and Hospital Synergy in Disaster Management

Jameel Ali

Introduction

Disaster, by nature, most often occurs in an environment of unpreparedness and unpredictability. By definition, disaster is associated with inadequate resources. Ideally, as awareness increases and planning becomes proactive most medical institutions would be prepared to deal with disasters in an organized fashion by having formal training (Waeckerle, 1991; Briggs and Brinsfield, 2003; Bazerman and Watkins, 2004; Frykberg *et al*., 2010; Disaster Management and Emergency Preparedness Course, 2010) on the nature of and approaches to disaster management, which involves pre-empted planning, identification of resources, communication systems and a prepared disaster management document with command system. Until this situation of disaster preparedness becomes reality, disasters will continue to occur in an atmosphere of unpreparedness. The phases of the disaster response have been characterized by the initial phase of 'chaos' (panic, fear, disorganization), followed by the organization crisis management stage where there is establishment of a command post, needs assessment, establishing security and safety procedures and casualty evacuation to the casualty collection areas (Klein and Weigelt, 1991; Waeckerle, 1991; Briggs and Brinsfield, 2003). At some point, a triage process that may or may not be properly organized takes place when immediately life-threatening injuries are identified and attended to and a categorization of injuries into immediate, delayed, minimal, expectant and dead would occur. In many circumstances the location of the disaster is such that this organized approach is not common knowledge or within the experience of the personnel involved and a disaster structure established well in advance is frequently non-existent. Whether planned or not there is frequently a primary triage at the scene and in the process patients will be categorized according to life threat.

In the absence of a coordinated pre-planned approach to disaster management, systems that involve the utilization of well-established synergism between the pre-hospital and hospital setting should be explored. This requires consideration of the resources in the vicinity of the disaster area including the capabilities of different levels of institutions and established levels of communication within the medical care system.

In this chapter the presumption is that the ideal preparation for disaster management does not exist in the environment where the disaster has occurred. Because of its very nature disaster occurs in unpredictable locations with variable availability of resources. Examination of already established systems of medical care in this environment allows adaptation in order to meet the needs of the disaster victims. This type of adaptation is similar to the change that occurs in an institution that is forced to make changes within its structure and function as a result of disaster victims being brought in large numbers to the institution. In the disaster situation sheer numbers of victims within a very short period of time is frequently the factor that overwhelms the institution's capabilities thus satisfying disaster categorization. In these situations adaptations such as converting ambulatory facilities into triage areas, emptying the operating rooms, intensive care unit (ICU) and emergency rooms to the extent feasible are examples of adaptation within already established systems within an institution.

Reference will be made to already established protocols of management each having the possibility of adaptation to accommodate the needs of disaster management. These well-documented areas of management include emergency treatment of strokes and cardiac emergencies, the establishment of trauma systems and trauma centres, Advanced Trauma Life Support Course (ATLS® – American College of Surgeons, Chicago, 2008), Pre-hospital Trauma Life Support Course (PHTLS 6th Edition, National Association of Emergency Medical Technicians and the Committee on Trauma, American College of Surgeons, 2007), as well as the establishment of programmes such as the Rural Trauma Team Development course (RTTDC – American College of Surgeons, Committee on Trauma, 2011) and training and treatment programmes involving telemedicine technology (Latifi *et al.*, 2007; Todder *et al.*, 2007; Duchesne *et al.*, 2008). The programmes described are not meant to be all-inclusive because many others also qualify. However, all of these could be accessed and modified in order to meet the unpredictable needs of disaster occurring within a community. In situations where a formal disaster management protocol exists, these programmes may also prove useful in meeting the needs of disaster management.

Adapting Protocols for Management of Stroke and Cardiac Emergencies to Disaster Management

Many centres have established protocols for dealing with strokes and cardiac emergencies that involve hospital staff training and 24-h availability of hospital staff linked by a communication system for managing urgent problems relating to strokes and cardiac emergencies such as ST Elevation Myocardial Infarction (STEMI) (Charbonneau, 2009; Daudelin *et al.*, 2010; Herlitz *et al.*, 2010). In these types of emergencies, as it is in the category of disasters where immediate life threat occurs, timely intervention is a key element. In the stroke victim there is a finite initial period within which thrombolytic therapy is effective and beyond which time this therapy could even be dangerous. In institutions where these stroke protocols have been instituted there is a built-in system of communication between the pre-hospital personnel and the 24-h in-hospital staff that allows direct communication and timely intervention prior to the patient arriving in the hospital. This type of system can be utilized in a disaster situation using the structure in place for stroke and adapting to immediate management of victims within a disaster. The key element common to the management of stroke and disaster management, particularly trauma, is timely intervention.

Similarly, in patients with cardiac emergencies, intervention in the form of thrombolytics or prompt transfer to the receiving institution for percutaneous vascular intervention have proven to be key elements in survival and early management. This system can be of immense use when adapted and applied on an urgent basis in the presence of a disaster by facilitating the management of the 'immediate' category of patients in the triage process of disasters. The action required is the cooperation of involved personnel to allow a communication system devised for other programmes to be adapted in order to meet the disaster management requirements.

Trauma-related Management Relationships

A major part of most disasters involves trauma of different types and many institutions and communities have in place systems established for dealing with trauma.

The establishment of trauma centres for definitive care of trauma patients has been shown to improve survival (Demetriades *et al.*, 2005). Designation of levels of trauma centres has been necessary to ensure that patients are taken from the injury scene to the appropriate trauma centre. This designation of level of trauma centres is a key element in the establishment of trauma systems. This system ensures that the trauma centres are not overwhelmed by patients who do not require their resources and who can be managed at lower levels of trauma centres (Shackford *et al.*, 1986; Mullins *et al.*, 1996; Jacobs *et al.*, 2003; MacKenzie *et al.*, 2006; Rehn *et al.*, 2009). The process of triage is also in place in many institutions and is practised by many pre-hospital personnel with avoidance of over-triage (which will unnecessarily burden the higher level trauma centres) and under-triage (which will bring severely injured patients to centres incapable of meeting their needs). Whereas many trauma systems incorporate formal disaster management protocols with appropriate training and infrastructure, there are many areas where formal disaster management programmes are not yet available as part of their trauma system. In a disaster situation, adherence to the established trauma system and recognition of capabilities of different levels of institution within the system would allow a distribution of patients after secondary triage to the appropriate institution. Since one of the main parameters that categorizes an incident as a disaster is the sheer numbers of casualties involved, distribution of those casualties to different institutions that are capable of dealing with the problems of the individual patients would lessen the burden on one particular institution. Thus the adherence to already established trauma systems and how they function in a community would allow appropriate management in the disaster situation.

With regards to pre-hospital management and triage, many communities have pre-hospital personnel trained in courses such as the Pre-hospital Trauma Life Support programme. In a study from Trinidad and Tobago it has been demonstrated that trauma patients arriving at the institution where physicians were trained in ATLS had improved outcomes (Ali *et al.*, 1993). However, after the introduction of the ATLS programme widespread improvement in trauma outcome in that country as a whole was not evident (Ariyanayagam *et al.*, 1992). Their study allowed the identification of many patients who arrived at the hospital dead or in very poor condition after ordinarily survivable anatomical injuries. The level of pre-hospital resuscitation made some of these patients non-salvageable. Indeed, many of these patients died at the scene of the motor vehicle collision from lack of pre-hospital care. This identified the need for improvement in pre-hospital trauma care and was the stimulus for introducing the Pre-hospital Trauma Life Support course in that country. Follow-up data showed that after the Pre-hospital Trauma Life Support course was instituted there was an overall improvement in trauma outcome (Ali *et al.*, 1997a). This impact of the Pre-hospital Trauma Life Support programme could indirectly decrease the burden on the major trauma centres that receive victims from disaster areas. This results in not only better outcomes, but less time and resources spent in continuing management of these patients in the trauma centre because of their improved status on arrival at the referral centre. Better resuscitation by the pre-hospital personnel may also result in triage and transfer to institutions at a lower level of trauma designation thus impacting on the overall distribution of trauma volume to the different institutions in a particular community. Involvement of the Pre-hospital Trauma Life Support programme existing in a particular community would thus impact significantly on disaster management.

Training in Under-resourced Institutions – a Role in Disaster Management

The American College of Surgeons has established a Rural Trauma Team Development course (RTTDC) aimed at improving the level of trauma resuscitation in institutions where patients are frequently seen immediately after major trauma. Because of distance, traffic and density of population it is frequently not possible for these patients to be taken to the trauma centre in a timely fashion. Part of this Rural Trauma Team Development course involves establishment of a method of communication with the trauma centres, and it also focuses on simple techniques aimed at resuscitating the trauma victim. Communication links between the rural institution and the trauma centre are established through the RTTDC training programme and this can also be employed in disaster management in a particular community. Thus patients who are severely injured could be taken to the nearest rural hospital rather than the trauma centre initially for immediate resuscitation because it is not feasible to transport them safely to the trauma centre. At the rural institution, patients are resuscitated and the chances of survival are improved by having a more appropriately resuscitated patient transported to the trauma centre. The care is enhanced also by the communication system between the trauma centre and the rural institution. Utilizing such communication systems as telemedicine has also been shown to be effective in implementing even complex life-saving procedures at a distant setting through communication between trauma centres and personnel at the rural hospital (Latifi *et al.*, 2007; Todder *et al.*, 2007; Duchesne *et al.*, 2008).

Apart from distribution of victims to different institutions, distribution of trained personnel among institutions could prove beneficial in disaster management.

In many instances the disaster population at a particular trauma centre may not be manageable because the capacity of the institution is overwhelmed and not because of the lack of personnel. This differentiates capacity and capability. Capability may be there but the capacity is overwhelmed. In these situations it is possible for appropriately trained personnel to leave the trauma centre where they may not be immediately needed in order to assist with management of victims in a distant rural under-resourced centre. This more rational distribution of manpower could conceivably lead to better outcome in disaster management. This is totally different from the dangerous alternative of having personnel leave their institution to go to the disaster site, a practice that is more likely to create chaos at the disaster site. At the disaster site, resuscitation by pre-hospital personnel and organization of triage and decision making with regard to transferring victims are more essential than having extremely skilled personnel available on-site.

Role of ATLS® Trained Personnel in International Disaster Management

Tsunamis, earthquakes and hurricanes are among the well-known international disasters leading to situations that outstrip the medical capabilities of the countries involved. Part of the response of the international community in such disasters is the mobilization of resources and personnel from different parts of the world to assist in the resuscitative efforts. Although personnel at many different levels play important roles in this effort, ATLS® trained physicians figure significantly among the medical personnel assisting in these catastrophes. Thus, tapping into an already established system of training through the ATLS® programme is an effective way of responding to these disasters. Many ATLS® trained physicians are themselves part of established disaster management systems in their own communities. Their expertise can be very helpful in disaster management in other countries. The potential for a positive worldwide influence on disaster management through the ATLS® programme is immense. Since its inception in the late 1970s in the USA, more than 1 million physicians have been trained worldwide in ATLS® and more than 50% of these physicians are from countries outside North America (Ali, 2008; American College of Surgeons, Committee on Trauma ATLS® Manual Chicago, 2008). Although the programme was initially transmitted in the English language, the course has been translated into many other languages such as Spanish, Portuguese and French. Ideally, the programme should be taught in the language of the participants. However, even in situations where the participants do not speak any of the languages in which the course is already translated, these courses can be taught through the use of interpreters. This was successfully accomplished when physicians from the Baltic Nations completed ATLS® training in Landstuhl, Germany through interpreters in preparation for United Nations-sponsored missions during the Bosnian conflict (Ali *et al.*, 1997b).

Conclusion

Disaster management, ideally, should follow protocols involving well-established programmes that are dedicated for disaster management with appropriately trained personnel and infrastructure. However, in situations where this is not possible, which may be a frequent occurrence because of the unpredictable nature of disasters, utilization with minor modification of already existing synergistic relationships between pre-hospital and hospital systems could lead to improvement in disaster management. Existing communication systems designed for emergency, time-sensitive, non-disaster situations and trauma training programmes including trauma systems could be modified to meet disaster management needs. These programmes can also complement already established formal disaster management protocols.

References

Advanced Trauma Life Support (2008) American College of Surgeons, Chicago, Illinois.

Ali, J. (2008) The Advanced Trauma Life Support program: historical perspectives and future directions. *Journal of Trauma* 64(5), 1149–1158.

Ali, J., Adam, R., Butler, A.K., Chang, H., Howard, M., Gonsalves, D., Pitt-Miller, P., Stedman, M., Winn, J. and Williams, J. (1993) Trauma outcome improves following the advanced trauma life support program in a developing country. *Journal of Trauma* 34(6), 890–899.

Ali, J., Adam, R.U., Gana, T.J. and Williams, J.I. (1997a) Trauma Patient outcome after the Prehospital Trauma Life Support Program. *Journal of Trauma* 42(1), 1018–1022.

Ali, J., Freyfogle, E.B., Parker, R.J., Bell, R.M., Maimaris, C., Krantz, B. and Hughes, I. (1997b) Overcoming language barriers when teaching the Advanced Trauma Life Support Course. *European Journal of Surgery* 163, 483–486.

Ariyanayagam, D.C., Naraynsingh, V. and Maraj, I. (1992) The impact of the ATLS course on traffic accident mortality in Trinidad and Tobago. *West Indian Medical Journal* 41, 73–74.

Bazerman, M.H. and Watkins, M.D. (2004) *Predictable Surprises: The Disasters You Should Have Seen Coming and How to Prevent Them.* Harvard Business School Press, Cambridge, Massachusetts.

Briggs, S.M. and Brinsfield, K.H. (2003) *Advanced Disaster Medical Response.* Harvard Medical International Trauma and Disaster Institute, Boston, Massachusetts.

Charbonneau, F. (2009) Creating synergy in our health system: the challenges of primary angioplasty. *Canadian Journal of Cardiology* 25(11), 387–388.

Daudelin, D.H., Sayah, A.J., Kwong, M., Restuccia, M., Porcaro, W., Rutnazer, R., Goetz, J., Lane, W., Beshansky, J. and Selker, H. (2010) Improving use of prehospital 12-lead electrocardiogram for early identification and treatment of acute coronary syndrome and ST-elevation myocardial infarction. *Circulation Cardiovascular Qualitative Outcomes* 3(3), 316–323.

Demetriades, D., Martin, M., Salim, A., Rhee, P., Brown, C. and Chan, L. (2005) The effect of trauma centre designation and trauma volume on outcome in specific severe injuries. *Annals of Surgery* 242(4), 512–519.

Disaster Management and Emergency Preparedness Course (2010) Disaster Subcommittee, Committee on Trauma, American College of Surgeons, Chicago, Illinois.

Duchesne, J.C., Kyle, A., Simmons, J., Islam, S., Schmeig, R.E. Jr, Olivier, J. and McSwaine, N.E. (2008) Impact of telemedicine upon rural trauma care. *Journal of Trauma* 64, 92–97.

Frykberg, E., Weireter, L. and Flint, L. (2010) 10 questions and answers about disasters and disaster response. *Bulletin of the American College of Surgeons* 95 (3), 6–13.

Herlitz, J., Wireklin Sundstrom, B., Bang, A., Berglund, A., Svensson, L. and Blomstrand, C. (2010) Early identification and delay to treatment in myocardial infarction and stroke. *Scandinavian Journal of Trauma Resuscitation and Emergency Medicine* 18, 48. Available at: http://www.sjtrem.com/content/18/1/48 (Accessed 28 January 2013).

Jacobs, L.M., Burns, K.J. and Gross, R.I. (2003) Terrorism: a public health threat with a trauma system response. *Journal of Trauma* 55, 1014–1021.

Klein, J.S. and Weigelt, J.A. (1991) Disaster management: lessons learned. *Surgical Clinics of North America* 71, 257–266.

Latifi, R., Weinstein, R.S., Porter, J.M., Ziemba, M., Judkins, D., Ridings, D., Nassi, R., Valenzuela, T., Holcomb, M. and Leyva, E. (2007) Telemedicine and telepresence for trauma and emergency care management. *Scandinavian Journal of Surgery* 96, 281–289.

MacKenzie, E.J., Rivara, F.P., Jurkovich, G.J., Nathens, A.B., Frey, K., Egleston, B., Salkever, D. and Scharfstein, D. (2006) A national evaluation of the effect of trauma-center care on mortality. *New England Journal of Medicine* 354, 366–378.

Mullins, R.J., Veum-Stone, J., Hedges, J.R., Zimmer-Gembeck, M.J., Mann, N., Southard, P., Helfand, M., Gaines, J. and Trunkey, D. (1996) Influence of a statewide trauma system on location of hospitalization and outcome of injured patients. *Journal of Trauma–Injury Infection and Critical Care* 40, 536–545.

Prehospital Trauma Life Support Program (2007) National Association of Emergency Medical Technicians, American College of Surgeons, Chicago, Illinois.

Rehn, M., Eken, T., Kruger, J., Steen, P., Skaga, N. and Lossious, H. (2009) Precision of field triage in patients brought to a trauma centre after introducing trauma team activation guidelines. *Scandinavian Journal of Trauma Resuscitation and Emergency Medicine* 17, 1–10.

Rural Trauma Team Development Course (2011) American College of Surgeons, Committee on Trauma, Chicago, Illinois.

Shackford, S.R., Hollingworth-Fridlund, P., Cooper, G.F. and Eastman, A.B. (1986) The effect of regionalization upon the quality of trauma care assessed by concurrent audit before and after institution of a trauma system. A preliminary report. *Journal of Trauma – Injury Infection and Critical Care* 26, 812–820.

Todder, D., Matar, M. and Kaplan, Z. (2007) Acute-phase trauma intervention using a videoconference link circumvents compromised access to expert trauma care. *Telemedicine Journal E-Health* 13, 65–67.

Waeckerle, J.F. (1991) Disaster planning and response. *New England Journal of Medicine* 324, 815–821.

Chapter 13

Process Management of Multiple Casualty Events

Miklosh Bala, Yuval Weiss and Yoram G. Weiss

Introduction

A decade ago, Jerusalem was the site of recurrent multiple mass casualty incidents (MCIs), most of them related to the Israeli–Palestinian conflict. However, the most significant event was man-made, the collapse of the Versailles Wedding Hall. Within a matter of 2 h more than 250 injured were evacuated to the Jerusalem area hospitals. This work focuses on the Hadassah-Hebrew University Medical Centre at Ein Karem, part of a not-for-profit organization – the Hadassah Medical Organization (HMO) – in Jerusalem, Israel. The Ein Karem Hospital is the only level one trauma centre in the greater Jerusalem area. Hence, these events gave us a rare opportunity to re-examine the effectiveness of our MCI preparedness and MCI process control procedures.

There are no places that are immune to man-made (transportation accidents and acts of terrorism) or natural (tornadoes and earthquakes) disasters, culminating in an MCI scenario. Most disasters occur with little or no warning, hence the importance of preparedness. Much has been written on the importance of preparedness for an MCI response. This review will attempt to emphasize aspects of in-hospital MCI process control and possible pitfalls in management based on the literature dedicated to MCI management and our personal experience. This review will not address non-conventional events (nuclear, chemical or biological).

Definition of Multiple Casualty Incidents

There are several definitions of MCIs and their magnitude (Bonnett *et al.*, 2007). In this review we will use the US Joint Commission on Accreditation of Health Care Organizations (JCAHO) one, which places the term disaster in a spectrum of incrementally worsening emergency events (Joint Commission on Accreditation of Healthcare Organizations, 2006). The first level of emergency is defined as a major incident, such as a school bus rollover. This is a short-lived situation lasting up to 24 h and does not disrupt the operations of a hospital. A disaster is defined as a community-wide event that disrupts the healthcare system and the infrastructure of the community. A recent example of such events is the mayhem created by some gigantic tornados in the USA. Finally, the term catastrophe is used to describe a series of disasters affecting the same community in a short period. The best example for this in modern times is the recent series of natural followed by man-made catastrophes in Japan: a 9.1 earthquake followed by a huge tidal wave tsunami followed by a breakdown of the nuclear centre and leakage to the environment of radioactive material.

Viewed from this perspective it is obvious that all of the terror-associated MCIs presented in this chapter are from the first order of emergency – major incidents (Tables 13.1–13.4). Only the Versailles Wedding Hall disaster may be defined as a disaster as it nearly disrupted the Jerusalem area healthcare system.

Numbers

Patients

A retrospective review of the hospital's response to multiple-casualty terror incidents occurring between 1 October 2000 and 1 April 2011 was performed. Only incidents that resulted in more than 20 admissions to our emergency room were included in this analysis. Information was assembled from our medical centre's trauma registry.

A comparison between three types of attacks is presented: a large building collapse (Versailles Wedding Hall), open space explosions and closed space. The Versailles Wedding Hall collapse will be discussed separately at the end of this section. The information we collected includes: number of victims at the location, number of patients treated and admitted to the ICU, location before ICU admission (operating rooms, imaging department or emergency department), Trauma Injury Severity Score (ISS), time for emergency room admission, time to ICU admission, ICU length of stay and ICU mortality.

Included in the analysis were 13 major terror-related major incidents and one incident meeting the criteria of a disaster. Tables 13.1–13.4 summarize the clinical information. Table 13.1 presents data on the number and type of admissions, ISS and on-site mortality. Of note is the ISS score among all three groups of patients (Table 13.1). As previously published, patients hospitalized after terror events sustained more severe injuries (74% versus 10% in other types of trauma with ISS >16) and had twice the mortality (6.2% versus 3%) compared with motor vehicle accident survivors (Shamir *et al.*, 2004; Aschkenasy-Steuer *et al.*, 2005). This is a surrogate marker for the burden and complexity these patients present later on for the medical teams. Thanks to the scoop and run methodology applied by Israeli paramedics some patients had to be intubated upon arrival to the emergency room. The severity of injuries is demonstrated by the fact that nearly a third of injured patients admitted had to be intubated in the emergency department in addition to those already intubated at the scene. Twelve patients admitted to our centre were intubated at the scene. Of note is also the relatively high rate of dead on-site in both open and closed space bomb attacks. Less severely injured patients were diverted by the emergency medical services to other regional trauma centres in the Jerusalem area, but 16 patients were admitted as secondary transfers after initial resuscitation at other hospitals. This highlights the importance of preparing for secondary transfers following MCIs by level one trauma centres.

Table 13.1. Admissions, Trauma Injury Severity Score (ISS) and on-site mortality.

	Closed (8)	Open (5)	Versailles Wedding Hall
Total number of injured	77.2 ± 30	113.6 ± 50	380
On-site mortality	12.9 ± 6	11.4 ± 8.6	23
ER admissions	26.5 ± 12.27	30.8 ± 19.6	111
Hospital admissions	12.12 ± 3.7	14 ± 9.3	73
ER intubation	5.38 ± 2.77	4.0 ± 2.83	2
ISS 1–8 (%)	31.92 ± 13.38	24.74 ± 13.05	42.5
ISS 9–14 (%)	17.88 ± 16.2	32.04 ± 20.06	41
ISS 16–24 (%)	21.9 ± 13.37	14.02 ± 8.4	15.1
ISS >25 (%)	30.76 ± 15.32	29.18 ± 17.9	1.4

ER, emergency room.

Data on the types of injury are presented in Table 13.2. The hallmark of these injuries was a combination of blunt trauma and penetrating injuries due to bolts. The injuries could be divided into three categories: blunt trauma including blast injuries, burns and penetrating injuries. Commonly victims suffered injuries originating from more than one mechanism of injury. Moreover, victims, both in terror and collapse scenarios, commonly had injuries to several parts of the body (Table 13.2).

Table 13.2. Mechanism of injury (blunt, burn, penetrating) and body area injured.

		Closed (8)	Open (5)	Versailles Wedding Hall
Mechanism of injury	Blunt	5.5 ± 3.7	7.6 ± 9.86	73
	Burn	3.37 ± 3.37	4.2 ± 4.32	–
	Penetrating	10.62 ± 3.11	9.8 ± 6.98	–
Body area injury	Head	4.13 ± 1.64	3.8 ± 2.95	25
	Neck and face	7.5 ± 3.92	5.0 ± 3.08	26
	Chest	5.0 ± 2.78	3.8 ± 2.95	24
	Abdomen	2.75 ± 0.71	4.0 ± 2.9	10
	Spine	0.88 ± 1.36	0.4 ± 0.55	14
	Extremities	11.0 ± 13.44	9.6 ± 7.8	63
	Burn	3.37 ± 3.37	5.2 ± 6.38	–

Table 13.3 presents data on the use of *operating rooms and types of surgeries*. In both closed and open space explosions only a handful of patients needed to be taken directly into the operating room (Table 13.3). As previously published the mean time from the incident to the beginning of the first surgery was 124 ± 81 min (range 37–360 min) after the event (Shamir *et al.*, 2004). Surgeries lasted for 172 ± 110 min (range 40–645 min) (Shamir *et al.*, 2004). The peak number of ORs used simultaneously was 17 in one open space incident. A total of 56% of the patients admitted to our level one trauma centre needed surgery within the first 8 h after the attack.

Table 13.3. Operating room cases and times.

		Closed (8)	Open (5)	Versailles Wedding Hall (73)
OR data	OR cases	8.0 ± 2.72	10.6 ± 6.91	29 (39.7%)
	Time to OR	109.25 ± 57.26	136.6 ± 62.2	197
	Direct to OR	5.25 ± 2.66	7.8 ± 4.97	11 (15%)
Area-specific OR procedures	Head and neck	1.37 ± 1.51	2.2 ± 1.92	3
	Chest	1.13 ± 1.25	1.4 ± 1.52	–
	Abdomen	2.0 ± 1.6	2.2 ± 1.79	–
	Extremities	2.87 ± 1.25	3.8 ± 2.77	20
	Plastic	4.87 ± 2.7	7.6 ± 6.23	5

OR, operating room.

Intensive care

The hospital intensive care facilities include 32 surgical ICU beds (11 general, 8 paediatric, 7 neurosurgical and 6 cardiothoracic). When these ICUs are full, patients are treated in the 16-bed post-anaesthesia care unit (PACU), which is adjacent to the GICU. In addition, nine medical intensive care beds are available. The GICU is part of the Department of Anaesthesiology and Critical Care Medicine. Most ICU attending physicians in the GICU are board-certified anaesthesiologists. All anaesthesiologists had some intensive care training of at least 6 months of an ICU rotation during their residency. Most anaesthesiology senior residents are routinely involved in the daily care of patients in the GICU.

In preparation for admission of critically injured terror victims, patients were transferred out of the GICU either to a regular ward (75%) or to another ICU (25%). Post-operative patients were discharged from the PACU if their condition was deemed stable. This was done to increase the capacity of GICU beds. Table 13.4 presents information related to their ICU stay. The age distribution of terror victims was skewed towards the younger generation (80% aged 15–44 years, compared with 37% for other traumas) (Shamir *et al.*, 2004). A total of 56% of patients were admitted from the operating rooms, 10% from the angiography suite and the rest (34%) were admitted directly from the emergency department (Shamir *et al.*, 2004).

Table 13.4. ICU and hospital length of stay and in-hospital mortality.

	Closed (8)	Open (5)	Versailles Wedding Hall (73)
LOS	11.5 ± 5.29	20.6 ± 6.19	8
ICU (pts)	5.88 ± 2.3	7.4 ± 5.32	13 (17.8%)
ICU (days)	44.75 ± 43.25	96.8 ± 61.4	39
ICU (aver days)	6.25 ± 4.83	13.4 ± 2.7	3
In-hospital mortality	0.88 ± 0.83	1.2 ± 1.1	0

LOS, length of stay.

The average time from the initial trauma to admission to the GICU was 5.5 ± 3.1 h (range 1–13 h). Patients admitted directly from the emergency department or from imaging (including computerized tomography or angiography suite) were admitted earlier than those from the operating rooms (Shamir *et al.*, 2004; Aschkeansy-Steuer *et al.*, 2005). Note that terror victims from open space explosions stayed in the GICU for the longest time (Table 13.4), whereas the median length of stay for our entire GICU population was 3 days. Note the overall low mortality rate among trauma patients admitted to an ICU.

The Versailles Wedding Hall Disaster

The Versailles Wedding Hall in Jerusalem was the site of the worst civil disaster in Israel's history. The Versailles Wedding Hall disaster is the only incident meeting the definition of a disaster as it nearly disrupted the Jerusalem area healthcare system. It resulted in about 380 casualties, of whom 23 died. Injuries were mainly caused by the fall itself, and by the crushing of one person into another. Even though patients were distributed among all four hospitals serving the Jerusalem area, the influx of casualties was particularly heavy to the level one trauma centre lasting from 1–3 h after the event. In total, there were 111 emergency room admissions, exceeding the regular capacity of the emergency room. Of all casualties admitted to the emergency room, 73 (66%) were hospitalized. Most suffered from mild to moderate injuries and 16% had an ISS of 16 or higher. Blunt trauma was a predominant mechanism of injury, no burns were recorded. Most of the hospitalized patients suffered from multiple injuries: almost 70% had head and neck trauma, 41% had torso injury and 86% suffered extremity injuries. Injuries in the lower limbs were the most frequent.

The hospital resources utilization in the Versailles disaster compared with terror-related events (OR, LOS, ICU needs) are shown in Tables 13.1, 13.2 and 13.4. For the first time an auxiliary emergency room area had to be activated. A total of 17.8% of the patients were hospitalized in different ICUs. No in-hospital mortality was recorded.

Impact of Setting on Injury Type and Severity

Patients injured following suicide bombing attacks present with a wide variety of wounds ranging from minor cuts, bruises and foreign bodies, to severe blast lung injuries, intracranial, abdominal and thoracic injuries caused by primarily blast injuries, heat wave or by flying debris. In the Jerusalem terror wave penetrating injuries caused by flying debris and bomb fragments were present in more than 85% of the patients and other external injury such as burns were also very common among survivors (Almogy *et al.*, 2004; 2006).

The physical characteristics of the setting also have implications on the type of primary, secondary, tertiary and quaternary blast injuries. In Israel three types of attack settings were identified: buses, semi-confined spaces (SCS) such as covered open markets, restaurants and indoor cafés, and open spaces (OS) such as outdoor cafés, open markets and bus stops (Shamir *et al.*, 2004). Leibovici and colleagues have shown that explosions inside confined spaces, such as the interior of a bus, have resulted in significantly higher mortality rates compared with similar open space explosions (Leibovici *et al.*, 1996). The mortality following five separate bus explosions was 19% compared with 8.5% in open spaces. These differences were attributed to reflection of the blast wave in a confined space and the relatively shorter distance between the victims and the explosive device. Almogy and colleagues have shown that the incidence of moderate and severe blast lung injuries inside a bus and in a semi-confined space was significantly higher compared with open space explosions (Almogy *et al.*, 2006).

The pattern of penetrating injury also changes in accordance with the attack setting. The head typically sustains a higher percentage of penetrating wounds than its relative body surface area in all settings (Rignault and Deligny, 1989). Penetrating torso injuries are more common in semi-confined spaces (40%). Victims injured in open space blasts are more likely to suffer from penetrating extremity and soft tissue injury and less likely to suffer from the effects of the blast wave (burns, blast lung injury and tympanic membrane rupture) compared with patients injured in semi-confined spaces and bus blasts. A meta-analysis of 29 worldwide terrorist bombing attacks showed that the incidence of burns and tympanic membrane rupture inside a confined space was 22% and 35%, respectively, compared with 1% and 5%, respectively, in open space blasts (Arnold *et al.*, 2004).

The collapse of a building is a dramatic event that can result in large numbers of casualties. Similarly, an earthquake, a technological accident or a large-scale act of international terrorism can all result in a large numbers of casualties. Even though the collapse of a building is not an uncommon phenomenon, the medical literature contains only a few articles on the subject (Rokach *et al.*, 2009). Building collapse associated with a terror-related event (like the Oklahoma city bombing) represents a quaternary blast mechanism of injury. These include injuries from structural collapse or burn secondary to the detonation. Crush, traumatic amputation, compartment syndromes and other blunt and penetrating injuries can be common sequela of structural collapse.

The World Trade Center attack on 11 September 2001 was the worst terror-related disaster. Of the World Trade Center survivors, 43.6% reported sustaining an injury (Brackbill *et al.*, 2006). The most commonly reported injuries were eye injury/eye irritation (31.6%); sprain or strain (13.6%); and cut, abrasion or puncture wound (9.7%). Few survivors reported sustaining more serious injuries (e.g. burns, broken bones or head injuries). Despite the high on-site mortality in this incident, the number of severe casualties on the first day overwhelmed local hospitals. These examples highlight the importance of preparedness and resource control. These issues will be addressed in the following sections.

Preparedness

Much has been written in the literature on the importance of dry (desk/office) and wet (real simulation) drills. Undoubtedly these drills contribute to preparedness. However, two additional issues should be addressed when discussing preparedness: impact management and medical supply stocks.

In our previous publications we have identified critical areas for the management of an MCI (Shamir *et al.*, 2004, 2006; Aschkenasy-Steuer *et al.*, 2005). The emergency room/trauma bay must be evacuated from medical/surgical patients upon notification of an MCI. Hence, a senior experienced physician must apply a triage routine to quickly evaluate those patients who should be hospitalized as compared with those who should be sent home or to other medical facilities. The word ‘triage’ is derived from the French verb ‘trier’, meaning to sort. In practice it is the method used to identify those in greatest need when faced with multiple or mass casualties. It is the process used throughout all management phases and allows the allocation of priorities for initial treatment, transport and in-hospital management, including access to operating rooms and ICU bed space (Shamir *et al.*, 2005).

In short, it is a method that is applied to get 'the right patient to the right care at the right time' (Shamir *et al.*, 2005).

Similar triage criteria should be applied for patients in the ICU (Ryan, 2008). Those in questionable need should be sent to step-down or regular wards. Only life-saving procedures should proceed in patients waiting for angiography or computerized tomography. It is critical in preparation for an MCI to allow fast admission and diagnosis for the injured and not to clog the system with chronic or routine procedures.

Hospital must identify, prepare and staff in advance an area for the management of those patients who require augmented care but do not meet criteria for ICU admission. We believe that preferentially, this area should be controlled or co-directed by ICU specialists and placed if possible in close proximity to the ICU. A possible option is utilizing the PACU, as the nursing staff is trained for the care of unstable critically ill patients.

Nelson has recently suggested that planning for an MCI should include an impact analysis to identify and prioritize critical services that need to be maintained (Nelson, 2008). Impact analysis should be carried out in concert with the entire healthcare system and not by individual departments. Planning should include addressing inadequate staffing, auxiliary locations, disrupted supply chains and loss of information systems. After recording the effect of a drill on inventories, an impact analysis can be used to determine interdependencies between departments and services. It is used to set criteria for returning critical areas to service in order to meet patient care needs. Impact analysis is done at an institutional level and uses departmental and hospital-wide input. From an information technology perspective, it prioritizes the mission critical systems that need to be operational during a catastrophic MCI, along with an expected time frame. It may include analysis of the impact of an MCI on staffing, i.e. increasing staff working hours, altering routine therapy orders or stopping some procedures altogether. The impact analysis will also define an end point for an event, or what is considered the return to a normal operating state (Nelson, 2008). The definition of 'normal' may well be different for each affected department, so that some departments may be able to recover faster than others.

Inadequate staffing must be planned for ahead of time. It is of critical importance to identify personnel, especially nurses and respiratory therapists, who have been trained in critical services, do not practise them at present, but can be routinely updated so that when the time comes they may be used to staff critical areas such as the OR, ICU or emergency rooms. In preparation for the possible H1N1 influenza epidemic we have implemented a re-education plan. Alternative locations that can serve as support ICU or emergency room locations must be identified. Following the Versailles Wedding Hall disaster we had to open, for the first and last time until now, a previously planned auxiliary emergency room. In these areas care may need to be provided without access to the usual resources. The United States Department of Homeland Security provides on their website best practices and exercise support material to address these issues (US Department of Homeland Security. Lessons learned: information sharing. https://www.llis.dhs.gov).

Hospitals have learned to heavily rely on computerized information systems in their day-to-day operations. These systems cover patient identifications, medical care and supply chain. It is of key importance to address the issues of hospital operations if and when these systems become unoperational.

Influenced by the larger business community *Just in Time* is the buzz phrase among many medical community professionals. Just in time is a production strategy that strives to improve a business return on investment by reducing in-process inventory and associated carrying costs (Shingo, 1989). As depicted in the wake of the Hurricane Katrina (2005) and the recent earthquake in Japan (2011) hospitals must be prepared for a disruption in their supply chains following a catastrophe. In Israel hospitals are expected to maintain an in-house inventory allowing 2–4 weeks of uninterrupted operations. Further, in the case of a catastrophe, as in the recent Japan earthquake, local suppliers may not be able to respond, so a list of vendors outside the region, with the assistance of local providers, should be created. This might include the contact information for national and international sales offices of preferred vendors. If an event is widespread, a plan dependent on sharing supplies and resources with other regional hospitals may fail. The collection and exchange of information with different suppliers is critical to provide responses to changing scenarios.

Management of MCIs depends on the availability of *communication and material preparation protocols* to inform in-house and other emergency response personnel and teams and provide material resources for the first wave of injured. Communications must be addressed during the preparatory phase. Specific protocols must be written to provide a step-by-step description of procedures to be carried out for the activation of the surge capacity. These protocols define the *modus operandi* during an MCI and include hospital-wide and department and unit specialized protocols. An integral part is creation of working rules and communication with the police, fire brigade and other rescue forces.

Short messaging service (SMS) or internet-based messaging systems can be used to send messages to mobile phone users who are included in the MCI response group. These services can be configured for hospital or department staff notifications automatically, thereby replacing traditional phone trees that depend on people to perform the task and allowing those in the hospital to participate in other critical preparatory tasks during the latent phase.

Hospital administrators must consider the availability of alternative *communication systems*. Modern hospitals heavily rely on mobile phone technology. However, we have routinely noticed that immediate following an MCI cellular networks collapse due to the heavy traffic. In contrast, as depicted by the recent 9.1 earthquake in Japan, mobile phone networks can be relatively easily restored compared with cable networks. Hence, a balance must be struck between these two systems.

Patient Flow

Surge capacity

Surge capacity is the ability of a healthcare facility or system to expand its operations to safely treat an abnormally large influx of patients in response to an incident (Bonnet *et al.*, 2007). Well-established communication systems are key for an adequate surge response to occur. Furthermore, disasters and MCIs do not follow predictable, linear progressions, so decisions and actions need to be based on 'what is', not on 'what should be' (Nelson, 2008).

To better understand patient flow during MCIs we have adopted two terms in relationship to patient flow (Shamir *et al.*, 2004):

The latent phase – is the time from the occurrence of an MCI to the admission of the first injured at the trauma bay/emergency room. During the latent phase a quick decision, based on official sources (police, fire brigade, etc.) and the media, must be made with regards to the magnitude of the MCI. This will reflect the policy for emergency room and ICU evacuation and activation of surge capacity recruitment mechanisms of medical and support personnel.

The chaotic phase – is the time from first injured admission to the final clearance of the trauma bay/emergency room following an MCI. Patient flow in the hospital during the chaotic phase is of major importance. However, as the chaotic phase starts, patient flow is unidirectional, patient flow is directed from the emergency room/trauma bay to imaging and from there to the OR, ICU or ward (Fig. 13.1). It is important not to overload the emergency room/trauma bay with patients. Hence, injured patients never return to the emergency room/trauma bay after imaging or any other procedure as in many instances, a second wave of injured may arrive from primary and secondary area hospitals.

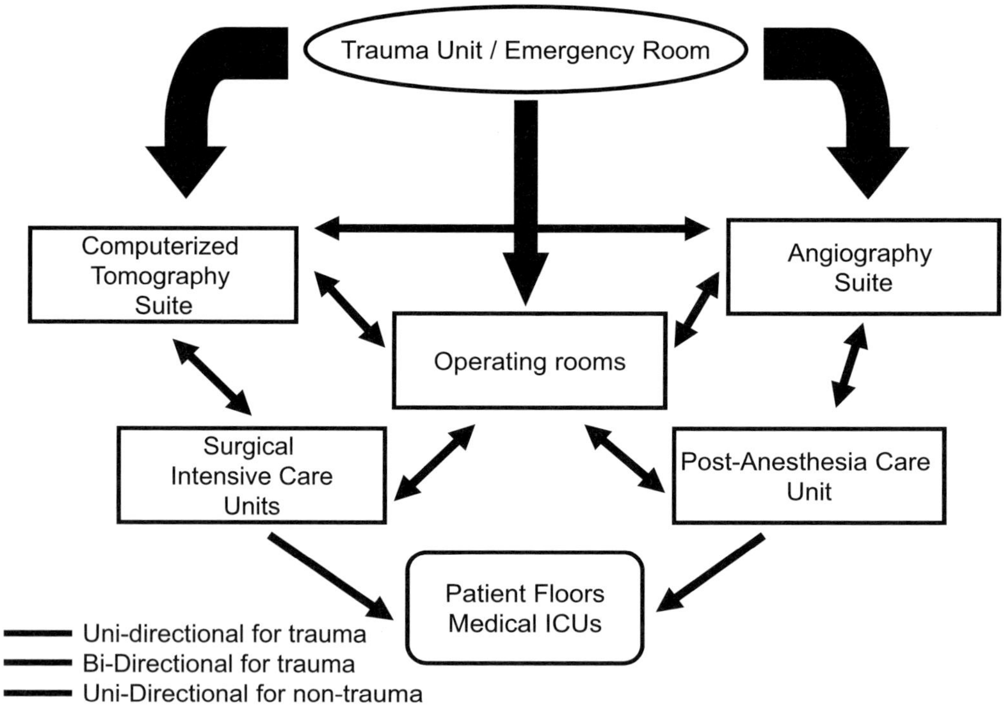

Fig. 13.1. Patient flow during the chaotic phase of an MCI (Published with permission from ICU Management Process Control in Multiple Casualty Events. *ICU Management* Volume 9 - Issue 3 - Autumn 2009).

MCI Macro-process Management

Being repeatedly exposed to MCIs, we came to realize the importance of process control. A key factor for efficiently running an MCI is maintenance of communications between those running the emergency room/trauma bay and those responsible for the functioning of the operating rooms, imaging (specifically computerized tomography and angiography) and ICUs. Clear communication protocols between these important areas are of key importance for the smooth processing of a multitude of severely injured patients and successful management.

To do so we routinely place the most senior anaesthesiologist/ICU physician side by side to the senior triage surgeon evaluating all incoming wounded. Further, a senior anaesthesiologist/ICU physician is also assigned to each area where injured patients are being admitted (trauma bay and regular surgical/internal medicine emergency room).

It is of key importance for the senior triage surgeon and senior anaesthesiologist/ICU physician to perform repeated evaluations of patients in order to prioritize patient care and flow. This assessment provides:

- Decisions on the prioritization of patient flow from the trauma bay/emergency room to imaging, OR and ICUs;
- A direct and *unbiased assessment of patient quantity and severity*;
- Important information on *decisions on the placement of these patients* in the ICU, intermediate unit or regular wards.

It is also important to realize that patients diverted during primary triage to the emergency room may present with severe injuries when undergoing primary and secondary survey. In addition, some patients may present with only minor injuries, but their mechanism of injury and current complaint may signal only the tip of an iceberg of problems to follow within minutes, hours or days. These patients also encompass the inner-hospital second wave of patients requiring imaging evaluation and not uncommonly operations and ICU beds. This is in addition to the second wave of injured admitted on a regular basis from primary and secondary level hospitals.

The information gathered by the senior ICU physician in the trauma bay and emergency room bears directly on the subsequent placement of not only the injured but also on the reorganization the ICU, i.e. other patients' placement in the ICU. Information on the magnitude of the MCI impacts directly the discharge policy of currently admitted patients to other ICUs or regular wards. It is important to realize that some patients being first directed to the operating rooms may arrive at the ICU several hours later, providing an extended time window for patient discharge from the ICU. The information also assists in decision making to direct patient load between different parts of the ICU or other ICUs (cardiothoracic, neurosurgical, medical) based on the type of injury, acuity and the level of required interventions and treatments. Distributing patients based on these criteria is of key importance for nursing to allow adequate care for all patients.

Medical Information Gathering

Much information may get lost during the chaotic phase of an MCI when patients are being admitted and undergoing primary and secondary survey. This is because of the multiple surgical subspecialties that may be involved with evaluation of these severely injured patients. Despite all our attempts, documentation during these initial phases of care is rudimentary as both physicians and nurses are overwhelmed. To remedy this we have adopted a policy of assigning a senior surgery and anaesthesiology resident to each of the severely injured patients immediately upon admission at the trauma bay. They will follow the patient through his entire hospital journey until he is admitted at the OR or ICU. One of their tasks is to summarize all gathered information into the patient's admission letter and present it to the surgery and anaesthesia/ICU attending upon arrival to the OR or ICU.

Informing the Public

Providing information to the public and to concerned families is an aspect that should not be neglected. To prevent collapse of the hospital's switchboard it is recommended to create a dedicated injured identification and missing persons search telephone number for the general public. This telephone line should be published by all electronic media as soon as possible after the MCI. Social workers have a critical role in identification of severely injured patients.

Over- and Under-triage

Several authors advocate a 'minimal work-up approach' following an MCI in order to facilitate the inflow of patients and prevent inundation of the admitting facility (Turégano-Fuentes *et al.*, 2008). The hypothesis is to prevent the improper utilization of limited hospital resources on patients with severe injuries and a lower chance of survival. For example, London EMS teams did few advanced on-scene interventions, but instead focused on identification and extrication of the most severely injured patients. Similarly, access to the computerized tomography scanner was reduced by delaying all non-urgent scans and avoiding abdominal computerized tomography for blast injury in favour of mini-laparotomy (Aylwin *et al.*, 2006). This practice following terrorist attacks has led to a high rate of negative procedures such as was reported following the London attacks (five of five negative laparotomies, 100%) and the Madrid attacks (three of seven negative laparotomies (42.9%) (de Ceballos et al., 2005; Aylwin et al., 2006; Turégano-Fuentes *et al.*, 2008). Patients following negative laparotomies in these circumstances may require ICU admission, and this may shift patients towards over-triage. We have been successful in avoiding high over-triage rates (21% according to our data), compared with over 50% in previous publications (Hirshberg *et al.*, 2010) and minimizing under-triage. This is secondary to several key points. Chiefly, our approach to victims of terrorist explosions is similar to victims of other types of trauma. In practice, this would translate to liberal utilization of advanced imaging modalities and the activation of a multidisciplinary team prior to decision making. Following an MCI we activate all available manpower. As previously mentioned, each moderately to severely injured victim is attended to by a surgical resident and anaesthesiologist/ICU resident. The victim's situation is continuously reassessed by the surgeon and ICU attending-in-charge until a diagnosis is reached and a treatment plan is outlined. This 'restrained' approach lowers the rate of negative surgical explorations while maintaining under-triage at an acceptable level (close to 0% in our experience).

The Day After

As the situation has stabilized it is of key importance to order medical and non-medical staff to leave the hospital. This is to ensure available staff and resources in the coming days.

Post-event Analysis

Recording problems during an MCI is not at the top of any administrative list, since the focus is simply providing medical care to the injured in a situation where the delivery system has become overwhelmed (Nelson, 2008). However, overlooking valuable lessons learned is a mistake. Hence, it is of significant value to perform inter-departmental and hospital-wide reviews on the days immediately following the event with all medical and support functions participants. The United States Department of Homeland Security provides on their website lessons learned, best practices and after-action reports (US Department of Homeland Security. Lessons learned: information sharing. https://www.llis.dhs.gov).

Conclusions

Hospital preparedness for an MCI begins long before the event occurs, and includes: protocols that define the *modus operandi* during an MCI, including hospital-wide and department and unit specialized protocols; creation of in-hospital working rules and communication as well as communication with the police, fire brigade and other rescue forces; preparation and storage of emergency equipment, medical supplies and medications in accessible places. A key component of the preparatory activity is drills that include sand table (management) and 'reality' drill simulations with mock wounded patients.

In the wake of events following recent catastrophes we recommend hospitals maintain an in-house inventory allowing 2–4 weeks of uninterrupted operations. Further, a list of vendors outside the region, with the assistance of local providers, should be created.

When an MCI occurs the first step is to assess its size and severity and accordingly activate a surge capacity plan. Especially during the patient admission phase (the chaotic phase) it is of key importance to get updated real-time information from key points in the hospital: emergency room/trauma bay, ORs, ICUs and the imaging department.

In any MCI, there is an influx of trauma patients commonly followed shortly thereafter by a second wave of patients. This influx of patients is accompanied by a plethora of information (both vital and insignificant), which requires efficient processing and prioritizing. Of core importance is proper process control, which is ideally managed by a senior surgeon together with a senior anaesthesiologist/ICU manager who can assess, prioritize and smooth transfer of patients. Continuous communication is also a crucial element within and between the departments, and facilitates the efficient flow of patients from the emergency room/trauma bay through imaging, the OR and on to the ICU. The preparation and utilization of an auxiliary area for patients who need additional care outside of the ICU also assists in improving the unidirectional patient flow from the trauma bay. While MCIs can test the strengths of any hospital's resources and organizational structure, the adherence to these simple process control guidelines can positively impact the outcome of the patients involved.

Acknowledgements

The authors wish to thank Ms Irina Gertsenshtein for her help in gathering the trauma registry information.

References

Almogy, G., Belzberg, H., Mintz, Y., Pikarsky, A.J., Zamir, G. and Rivkind, A.I. (2004) Suicide bombing attacks: update and modifications to the protocol. *Annals of Surgery* 239, 295–303.

Almogy, G., Mintz, Y., Zamir, G., Bdolah-Abram, T., Elazary, R., Dotan, L., Faruga, M. and Rivkind, A.I. (2006) Suicide bombing attacks: Can external signs predict internal injuries? *Annals of Surgery* 243, 541–546.

Arnold, J.L., Halpern, P., Tsai, M.C. and Smithline, H. (2004) Mass casualty terrorist bombings: a comparison of outcomes by bombing type. *Annals of Emergency Medicine* 43, 263–273.

Aschkenasy-Steuer, G., Shamir, M., Rivkind, A., Mosheiff, R., Shushan, Y., Rosenthal, G., Mintz, Y., Weissman, C., Sprung, C.L. and Weiss, Y.G. (2005) Clinical review: the Israeli experience: conventional terrorism and critical care. *Critical Care* 9, 490–409.

Aylwin, C.J., König, T.C., Brennan, N.W., Shirley, P.J., Davies, G., Walsh, M.S. and Brohi, K. (2006) Reduction in critical mortality in urban mass casualty incidents: analysis of triage, surge, and resource use after the London bombings on July 7, 2005. *Lancet* 368, 2219–2225.

Bonnett, C.J., Peery, B.N., Cantrill, S.V., Pons, P.T., Haukoos, J.S., McVaney, K.E. and Colwell, C.B. (2007) Surge capacity: a proposed conceptual framework. *American Journal of Emergency Medicine* 25, 297–306.

Brackbill, R.M., Thorpe, L.E., DiGrande, L., Perrin, M., Sapp, J.H. 2nd, Wu, D., Campolucci, S., Walker, D.J., Cone, J., Pulliam, P., Thalji, L., Farfel, M.R. and Thomas, P. (2006) Surveillance for World Trade Center disaster health effects among survivors of collapsed and damaged buildings. *Morbidity and Mortality Weekly Report (MMWR) Surveillance Summaries* 55, 1–18.

de Ceballos, J.P., Turégano-Fuentes, F., Perez-Diaz, D., Sanz-Sanchez, M., Martin-Llorente, C. and Guerrero-Sanz, J.E. (2005) 11 March 2004: The terrorist bomb explosions in Madrid, Spain – an analysis of the logistics, injuries sustained and clinical management of casualties treated at the closest hospital. *Critical Care* 9, 104–111.

Hirshberg, A., Frykberg, E.R., Mattox, K.L. and Stein, M. (2010) Triage and trauma workload in mass casualty: a computer model. *Journal of Trauma* 69, 1074–1082.

Joint Commission on Accreditation of Healthcare Organizations (2006) http://www.jointcommission.org/assets/1/18/surge_hospital.pdf (Accessed 29 January 2013).

Leibovici, D., Gofrit, O.N., Stein, M., Shapira, S.C., Noga, Y., Heruti, R.J. and Shemer, J. (1996) Blast injuries: bus versus open-air bombings – a comparative study of injuries in survivors of open-air versus confined-space explosions. *Journal of Trauma* 41, 1030–1035.

Nelson, S.B. (2008) Information management during mass casualty events. *Respiritaory Care* 53, 232–238.

Rignault, D.P. and Deligny, M.C. (1989) The 1986 terrorist bombing experience in Paris. *Annals of Surgery* 209, 368–373.

Rokach, A., Nemet, D., Dudkiewicz, M., Albalansi, A., Pinkert, M., Schwartz, D. and Bar-Dayan, Y. (2009) Advanced rescue techniques: lessons learned from the collapse of a building in Nairobi, Kenya. *Disasters* 33, 171–179.

Ryan, J.M. (2008) Triage: Principles and Pressures. *European Journal of Trauma and Emergency Surgery* 34, 427–432.

Shamir, M.Y., Weiss, Y.G., Willner, D., Mintz, Y., Bloom, A.I., Weiss, Y., Sprung, C.L. and Weissman, C. (2004) Multiple casualty terror events: the anesthesiologist's perspective. *Anesthesia Analgesia* 98, 1746–1752.

Shamir, M.Y., Rivkind, A., Weissman, C., Sprung, C.L. and Weiss, Y.G. (2005) Conventional terrorist bomb incidents and the intensive care unit. *Current Opinion in Critical Care* 11, 580–584.

Shingo, S. (1989) *A Study of the Toyota Production System from an Industrial Engineering Viewpoint*. Productivity Press, Portland, Oregon.

Turégano-Fuentes, F., Caba-Doussoux, P., Jover-Navalón, J.M., Martín-Pérez, E., Fernández-Luengas, D., Díez-Valladares, L., Pérez-Díaz, D., Yuste-García, P., Guadalajara Labajo, H., Ríos-Blanco, R., Hernando-Trancho, F., García-Moreno Nisa, F., Sanz-Sánchez, M., García-Fuentes, C., Martínez-Virto, A., León-Baltasar, J.L. and Vazquez-Estévez, J. (2008) Injury patterns from major urban terrorist bombings in trains: the Madrid experience. *World Journal of Surgery* 32, 1168–1175.

Section 6

Securing the Homeland:

The Medical Way

Chapter 14

Suicide Bombing Response

Aaron Richman, Christopher R. Foerster and Timothy P. Cohen

Introduction

Suicide bombings are a threat that has evolved into a preferred weapon of choice for the adversary at a global level. First responders and receivers in general, and emergency managers and medical responders, specifically, must be prepared to command and respond to this very unique threat. This chapter provides insight for first responder and receiver agencies, particularly those involved in the medical response to suicide attack incidents. It is important in all incidents, and even more so in responses to suicide attacks, that all response agencies are able to launch an effective coordinated response with true interoperability. Thus, having a common framework of important considerations in suicide attack response will help to facilitate a uniform response by all agencies. This is accomplished through outlining a number of important considerations from previous suicide attacks that should be taken into account while developing local response protocols and training plans.

The chapter will begin with an outline of the phases of a suicide bombing attack to provide an important foundation for understanding the response. When examining the important response considerations, we will first examine considerations in the imminent attack phase. These may not be directly applicable to the role of medical responders, but is an important component of the response that should be understood by all responders. This is followed by a discussion of the important considerations for the pre-hospital responders and the on-scene commanders. The specific targeting of these responders by suicide bombers emphasizes the importance of a strong response in both of these areas. The casualties will ultimately be transported to hospitals or other medical facilities, which is the focus of the final section of response considerations.

It is impossible to come to a real understanding of suicide bombing response without examining actual bombing incidents. Throughout the considerations, examples are included from actual suicide attacks. Although the focus of this chapter is suicide *bombings*, much of what is discussed is applicable to other types of suicide attacks where the attacker does not intend on escape, as in various active shooter scenarios. Examples from these other types of attacks have been included when they provide important lessons that are applicable to suicide bombing incidents.

Two case studies of suicide bombing incidents in Israel along with the 7/7 London bombings are included to help to demonstrate how the response considerations presented here can be put into action in the field. This should allow the reader to solidify the knowledge gained from this chapter by considering how these response considerations were implemented in the actual suicide bombing responses.

Phases of Attack

To be an effective part of the response to a suicide bombing incident, it is important to understand the complete continuum of phases in a suicide bombing. Regardless of the motives or structure of the terrorist organization, certain tasks need to be accomplished before the attack can succeed. These tasks are broken up into nine basic phases though it is important to remember that phases may overlap or even be in a slightly different order than is presented below.

Bomber identification

Bomber identification is the phase whereby the cell responsible for recruitment will identify a potential candidate to be used as the suicide bomber. Such candidates may be identified for numerous individual reasons and may be motivated by anything from religious and nationalistic motives to revenge and honour.

Bomber recruitment

Bomber recruitment addresses the need to induct a candidate for the suicide mission. This phase is vulnerable to law enforcement because of the fact that the cell responsible for such recruitment is reaching out to individuals who are not, at this moment, necessarily loyal to the terror cell. Once a potential bomber is located, he or she will be approached by the organizers of the attack, and conditioned to sympathize with the cell's stated cause. The individual will be coached and ultimately convinced that suicide tactics are the only viable approach for the attack. The prospective bomber will be enticed into performing the tactic with promises of rewards in the afterlife, and the legacy that he or she will leave the current life by committing the attack.

Bomber training

Bomber training is mission-specific based on the capability of the bomber and cell, the equipment available and the intended target. Training will address the specific attributes and skills necessary for the suicide bomber to successfully carry out their attack. It will address not only the process that consists of device detonation (pressing the switch), but also the skills necessary to get to device detonation. Training received by the bomber may be minimal, nothing more than a delivery system for the device and a basic understanding of how to detonate it. However, the training process may be made much lengthier, depending on the complexity of the attack, the outward appearance of the bomber, routes of travel and contingencies for modifying the attack.

Target selection

Target selection and reconnaissance is the phase by which teams assigned by the adversary will be dispatched to the field, in order to choose a target and 'learn' the target. The cell responsible for this may not even be aware of why or for whom they are carrying out surveillance. They may be highly skilled surveillance operators. This is a phase in which the adversary is vulnerable to identification and to being thwarted in their plot to attack.

Weapon acquisition

Weapon acquisition is a phase comprising procurement of items that are necessary for the operation. These include the items or components for the explosive device as well as any additional supplies related to the mission. This phase is also vulnerable to early detection in that items to be acquired will be obtained within the community.

Device construction

Device construction by skilled members of the cell, trained in the design and construction of explosive devices, will prepare the device for the last phase. This phase can take place in a home with minimal components from the outside world, preventing suspicion and making detection difficult.

Final preparation

At the final preparation phase, the bomb and bomber are complete and ready for dispatch. The dangers have escalated to proportions that will result in casualties if law enforcement attempts to make any interdiction. Prior to this phase early interdiction would have resulted in the thwarting of the attack with minimal casualties. From this phase on, the danger associated with such intervention is present, because the bomber is trained and ready, and the explosive device is constructed and complete. This may be a time when a martyrdom audio, video or written document is created, to be used for propaganda purposes at a later date. It may also involve a decision for the date and time of the attack and the bringing together of the improvised explosive device (IED) and the bomber. This may be nothing more than having the bomber meet at a location where the IED is located to take custody of it, or it may be a process where the IED is concealed on the person of the bomber.

Movement to target

Depending on the orders of the cell leaders, the bomber will be dispatched either alone, with a handler, or with additional attackers, to the target site. Any attempt to intervene at this phase will result in early detonation of the explosive device. The intended target will be diverted to the officers attempting to make interdiction, resulting in casualties of law enforcement and civilians.

Device detonation

Device detonation is the completion of all the phases and results in adversarial mission success. The detonation of the device will take place once the IED has been delivered to the intended target, or when the bomber is compromised through interdiction. At this final phase the handler who is dispatched may be responsible for triggering the device, thus ensuring that in the event of hesitation on the part of the bomber that the attack is carried to fruition. Post-blast is also pre-blast in such environments and there is always a possibility of multiple devices being used.

Response Considerations

First responders must have a basic knowledge of what to expect during suicide attack incidents along with their specific safety, security and management considerations. Key to this awareness is an understanding of the threat posed by explosive devices specifically targeting first responders. Awareness of the threat of secondary devices is one of the most important aspects of responder awareness and can best be understood through examination of specific incidents. First receivers also need to understand what is occurring pre-hospitally, along with the important in-hospital considerations to allow them to provide the best care for bombing victims while maintaining the safety of the hospital.

In the imminent attack phase

Integrative information collection

Strong intelligence capabilities should integrate into all possible information sources. It is important to recognize and incorporate intelligence that may end up coming from unlikely sources. An example comes from the case of Mike's Place, a bar located in Tel Aviv, which was attacked on 30 April 2003 by one successful suicide bomber along with an unsuccessful second bomber (Israel Ministry of Foreign Affairs, 2003). There were reports that the bombers asked the front desk staff at the hostel where they were staying if they knew a good place to get a drink in order to help them choose their target. There is the potential that further integration of people like the front desk employees could provide important information that may aid in the interdiction of the suicide bomber.

First responders typically know their coverage areas and can detect when something is out of place. They should be given additional training on how to recognize the warning signs of potential terrorism in an integrated multidisciplinary community outreach programme at the service level and increased situational awareness at the personnel level. This will ensure that their observations will be as useful as possible for law enforcement's overall information gathering programmes. While integrating civilian sources into information gathering, the police should also be responsive to the suspicions of other first responders and members of the public.

Trust and support public awareness

Residents know their communities and quickly recognize when someone or something seems out of place. When suspicions arise from residents, they should be taken seriously by the police and should be investigated. In the case of the BeitYisrael bombing in Jerusalem on 2 March 2002 (Israel Ministry of Foreign Affairs, 2002), a resident recognized the suspicious behaviour of the bomber and reported it to the police. Residents had become concerned when they saw someone dressed as an Orthodox Jew in their neighbourhood breaking the Sabbath by smoking, as that behaviour is extremely rare within the Orthodox Jewish community. Unfortunately, in the BeitYisrael incident, the police were waiting for approval to enter the ultra-Orthodox neighbourhood during the Sabbath when the bomber detonated his explosive device.

Encouraging the public to report

Suicide attacks are often well planned and when in the final stages they require swift action to interdict them. Delays in reporting suspicions by members of the public can create missed opportunities for police interdiction prior to an incident. In the case of the Tel Aviv Rosh Ha'ir Shawarma restaurant bombing on 17 April 2006 (Israel Ministry of Foreign Affairs, 2006), many civilians in the area had strong suspicions about the behaviour of the bomber, but failed to report these in advance of the attack. Had the suspicions been reported in this case, the police may have been able to interdict in the final phase of the attack.

The 7/7 bombings in London in 2005 (7 July Review Committee, 2006) prompted renewed efforts to fight terrorism in the UK including encouraging the public to report their suspicions. Many trains on the London Underground now have posters encouraging civilians to report any suspicious activity to the police. A visible police presence may be beneficial in encouraging the public to report, but both overt and covert security measures play an important role in deterring and preventing attackers.

Civilian interdiction

In addition to civilians reporting their suspicions, there have been a number of incidents where civilians who were not part of any official force were critical in actively bringing an end to the attack. One example of this occurred in Jerusalem and although it was not a bombing attack, it was still a suicide attack since the attacker probably had no intention of surviving his attack. In the bulldozer attack of 2 July 2008 (Israel Ministry of Foreign Affairs, 2008), the initial shots at the attacker were fired by a security guard from a nearby bank, with the fatal shots being delivered by an off-duty soldier. This is just one example of the impact of successful civilian interdiction. There is also a more recent example from the USA. The Christmas Day bombing attempt over Detroit in 2009 also showed the important role that civilians can play in the interdiction of suicide bombing attempts (BBC News, 2009). When the attacker attempted to detonate his device in this case, a number of passengers fought with and eventually restrained him. It is not just civilians who have had successes in mitigating the impacts of these suicide attacks, the response from private security guards has also been important.

Private security guards

Private security guards who are able to recognize a threat and are willing to take whatever steps necessary to protect others can be an important mitigating factor in these attacks. The security guard in place at the Rosh Ha'ir Shawarma restaurant in Tel Aviv recognized the bomber as a potential threat due to his behaviour and was successful in preventing him from entering the restaurant. Although the bomber still detonated his device, the success in keeping him outside of the restaurant is credited with saving dozens of lives. Security, however, is only as strong as its weakest point. Attackers can wait for the vulnerable time when the security guard leaves the entrance open for any reason, from a washroom break to a scheduled patrol. This was seen in the bombing of the Park Hotel on 27 March 2002 (Israel Ministry of Foreign Affairs, 2002) in what is commonly referred to as the Passover Massacre. The bomber at this incident did not need to make it past any security guard as he walked through the hotel lobby. There was a security guard at the hotel at the time of the bombing, but he had left his post at the front entrance to perform a routine patrol around the perimeter of the building. This vulnerability was exploited by the attacker who was able to enter the hotel with ease and detonated his explosive device in the dining hall.

Suicide bomber profiles

Although suicide bombers can sometimes be identified by their dress or behaviour, often they are able to reach their target without raising suspicions through blending in or disguising themselves. The Park Hotel bomber is one example of how the outward appearance of the bomber may not meet what we have come to consider the typical suicide bomber profile. The attacker here was disguised as a woman, which also helped him to hide his explosive device and may have helped him to avoid suspicion as he walked past the front desk. In other cases there is nothing substantive that stands out about the bomber. This was also a point that was raised by one of the responders to the Dimona, Israel bombing that occurred on 4 February 2008 (BBC News, 2008). A nurse who responded from a nearby medical centre and began treating the second bomber at this incident later stated that there was nothing different about his appearance that stood out to her until they discovered the suicide belt after lifting up his shirt during treatment. Suicide bombers may be citizens of any country and should not be thought of as coming from one particular area of the world. Both bombers who participated in the attack on Mike's Place in Tel Aviv were UK citizens as were all but one of the 7/7 bombers. As it becomes harder to get terrorists into Western countries from their home countries, terror groups may seek to use Western citizens or permanent residents in their attacks. Though not an attempted suicide attack, a recent example of this was seen in the May 2010 attempted bombing of Times Square by an American citizen who was funded and trained by the Pakistani Taliban (Katz, 2010).

Pre-hospital response

Secondary device threat

First responders must be aware of the threat of secondary devices that are used after the initial explosion in a specific attempt to target first responders. These devices have been used multiple times before with varying degrees of success. In the Dimona and Mike's Place bombings, the second bombers failed to detonate their devices successfully. If the attackers had been able to detonate their devices, the effects on the first responders could have been devastating.

There are multiple examples of the successful detonation of secondary devices. In contrast to the failures of the secondary devices in Dimona and Mike's Place, the bombing of the Ben Yehuda pedestrian mall in Jerusalem on 1 December 2001 (Israel Ministry of Foreign Affairs, 2001a) included multiple devices with greater success. The two concurrent suicide bombings were followed shortly after by a car bomb that appears to have been set to target the location of the incident command post. The 22 January 1995 attack at the Beit Lid junction in Israel used a secondary device on an attacker who approached the scene while the initial casualties were being triaged, killing 21 people in the attack. The adversary can carefully plan secondary devices. In the 13 April 1994 bombing of the Hadera Central Bus Station in Israel a secondary device was left hidden in an ambulance medical bag along the route that the first responders were operating. During the response to the 7/7 bombings, there was largely no consideration given by first responders to the threat of secondary devices after the initial explosions. Had there been any devices targeting first responders, the outcome could have been much worse. As these examples demonstrate, secondary devices pose a real threat that must be considered by all first responders.

First arriving unit beginning the response

Any first arriving unit should be ready and able to begin the response for their specific agency. The first arriving police unit should be capable of staging the initial law enforcement response, just as the first arriving ambulance crew should be able to begin triage and the medical response. Although specialized resources will be available to back up the first arriving vehicles, it is important that these initial first responders be fully capable of handling any incident in its initial stages.

Utilizing diverse resources

Diverse resources should be mobilized to deal with the large number of victims from these types of attacks. As the response is carried out, a reserve capacity must be maintained to ensure that capabilities to respond to day-to-day emergencies and potential subsequent attacks are maintained. Resourceful use of assets that are not typically included in the formal emergency response system can help to meet the needs at the suicide attack response while maintaining reserve capacity. Examples of these might include using family physicians' offices, urgent care centres and specialist hospitals that do not usually accept acutely injured patients to help supplement the hospital's surge capacity plans. An example of these diverse resources being mobilized occurred in the response to the Sbarro Pizzeria bombing that occurred in Jerusalem on 9 August 2001 (Israel Ministry of Foreign Affairs, 2001b). Victims from this bombing were transported to a nearby hospital that did not typically treat trauma patients simply due to the hospital's proximity to the bombing site. It cannot be expected by responders that all hospitals would routinely be able to step up like this, but rather this example should encourage responders to actively investigate what additional resources may be available to them during an incident response. This is no substitute for formal mutual aid agreements but rather is an additional supplement when shortcomings are identified during a response.

Another example of diverse resources being used after a suicide bombing occurred after the 7/7 attacks in the UK. A bus was bombed by a suicide bomber on the upper level as it passed through Tavistock Square, almost directly in front of the British Medical Association building where a meeting of doctors was taking place. The response from the physicians' meeting inside was immediate and they ended up being a valuable resource in the response to this bombing that killed 13 people in addition to the bomber. The leader of this spontaneous response was Dr Peter J.P. Holden who provided his account of the events in the *New England Journal of Medicine* (Holden, 2005). Dr Holden coordinated a group of 14 other doctors, mainly general practitioners, who did their best to treat the casualties initially without any real equipment. Eventually, they helped to set up treatment areas and facilitate transportation to definitive care. It is important to note that Dr Holden did have experience in pre-hospital and emergency care prior to this incident. There may not have been the same benefit from this spontaneous physician assistance had there not been at least one physician with this acute care background who was willing to guide the others.

Incorporating the resources of all hospitals and medical centres to supplement suicide attack responses can be beneficial, but is best done through formal mutual aid agreements. In the Dimona bombing, physicians and nurses from two nearby medical centres rushed to the scene to assist in the initial stages of the response. Although the healthcare professionals who responded did not specialize in emergency medicine, their efforts on the scene provided much-needed assistance during the initial stages of the response. In similar situations, the assistance of allied health professionals and non-emergency physicians may be beneficial when there are large numbers of casualties. If civilians descend on scene, they may also be useful in some circumstances to provide basic assistance to the medical responders. This will depend on the specific circumstances of the attack, resources on scene, and characteristics of the bystanders and will need to be judged by the responders at the time.

Formal mutual aid agreements

Spontaneous mobilization of additional resources cannot be relied on in suicide bombing responses. Not all non-emergency hospitals are ready to be an alternate care site and not all bus bombings occur next to a medical association meeting. Formal mutual aid agreements provide a mechanism for receiving assistance across jurisdictional boundaries from other agencies. These agreements should be decided upon in advance of the incident and put in writing to avoid any potential confusion or disagreement. Efforts should also be made to keep these agreements current and keep both agencies aware of the resources that the other agency has to offer so they can quickly be mobilized by an incident commander when needed.

Confirmation of safety

Ensuring that the threats on scene have been neutralized is one of the most important initial steps in suicide attack responses. There have been numerous cases of wounded suicide attackers attempting to continue their attacks. In Dimona, the second bomber, who was wounded in the initial blast, was attempting to detonate his device while lying injured on the ground. Police were forced to use lethal force to render the threat safe and ensure the safety of the bystanders and first responders. Reports state that the shooter who opened fire with an automatic weapon near the Column Building on Jaffa Road in Jerusalem on 22 January 2002 (Israel Ministry of Foreign Affairs, 2002) continued attempting to fire even after being shot and falling to the ground. Lethal force had to be used to end the attack. Finally, even after being shot at and apparently bleeding from the head, the driver in the bulldozer attack killed one more person before finally being fatally shot by a bystander. As these three examples from three different types of suicide attacks show, these attackers do not intend on coming out of their attacks alive and will often continue to attempt to take lives until their life has been ended.

While considering safety on scene, it is also important to briefly mention the threat of a chemical or radiological attack being integrated into a suicide bombing. Though these have not yet been used with success, it has been attempted in bombings in Iraq using chlorine tankers. Given the labelling requirements for chemical tankers around the world, the adversary can easily identify large quantities of these chemicals. The temptation to rush in without any consideration of scene safety must be avoided and all front line responders must have basic training in chemical, biological, radiological and nuclear (CBRN) recognition.

Unified on-scene commanders

Cooperation and communication on scene

The responses to all large incidents emphasize the importance of strong communication and coordination on scene as should be demonstrated by strong working relationships between all emergency services along with an early establishment of an incident command post. Confusion should be expected in the initial stages. Therefore, one of the immediate objectives should be to simply identify the number and exact locations of the bombs. There was significant confusion over this in the initial response to the 7/7 bombings as casualties surfaced from multiple tube stations. Similar confusion over the number of bombers has been seen in Israeli responses such as during the early stages of the Mahane Yehuda market bombing response on 30 July 1997 when it was not immediately identified as an attack involving two simultaneous bombs (Israel Ministry of Foreign Affairs, 1997). Establishing the number of bombing sites early on is crucial to ensure that appropriate resources will be deployed to each site.

The use of the National Incident Management System (NIMS) that has been mandated in the USA, which includes the use of the Incident Command System (ICS), can help with this coordination on scene. Although the NIMS does not guarantee successful incident management, it offers an important framework for coordination of the response. Personal relationships and familiarity developed between the leadership of the various response organizations during joint training exercises will also contribute to the successful overall coordination and communication between agencies.

In areas where large incidents bring out officials from higher levels of government, these agencies must be capable of integrating into the on-scene command structure and communicating well with all agencies. The effective integration of the command structure with higher levels of government can all be achieved through practice, as is seen in the Israelis' use of frequent exercises and drills and the UK's use of joint training centres, as well as through the use of a system that involves a scaled response to all incidents. The use of frequent joint exercises based on their specific threats in Israel has contributed to their success in being able to respond to these types of incidents. Especially with the expansion of the Fire Service College grounds in England to include training for all first responders rather than just the Fire Service, the UK is moving towards a similar model. All countries should strive to embrace similar models that help to foster cooperation and communication.

Scaled response

The response to a large incident, such as a suicide attack, should be a larger version of a response to a typical incident. A truly scalable response is not something that is often practised. The effectiveness of this strategy may be one of the reasons that the Israelis have been able to stage such strong responses to very large incidents. There will be less confusion on scene in terms of roles and chains of command if these structures are similar to the smaller incidents, only at a larger scale.

Practising a scaled response that all agencies can begin immediately is something that will lead to improvement in all types of mass casualty incident (MCI) responses. The scalability of ICS means that it can be used at small MCIs by the incident commanders simply filling more of the positions themselves rather than delegating them. This would allow pre-hospital medical providers to get into the habit of checking in with the incident commander and understanding the chain of command through practising at the small MCIs.

These same concepts become even more important on the responses to large MCIs, especially suicide bombings.

Promoting a return to normal

The goal of terrorism is very much psychological. Promoting a quick return to normal can contribute to these psychological goals not being met and may increase the resilience of the citizens. During the 7/7 bombing response, authorities made the decision to shut down the entire London Underground system. In this scenario, authorities were forced to balance the desire to maintain as much normality as possible with the potential risks of not shutting down the transit system. As a result, Underground disruptions remained for weeks after the attacks. These disruptions, though they may be warranted at times, contribute to the successes of terrorism.

The goal of the Israeli responders is to return to normal as much as possible with 90 min of the attack. This means within 90 min of an explosion on a bus, the Israeli authorities strive to have the scene cleaned up and the bus route fully operating again. *Returning to normal operations helps to reduce the psychological impacts of terrorism.* This prompt return to normalcy, though, often compromises scene evidence collection. Potentially losing evidence in favour of defeating the goal of the terrorist attack will be a difficult decision to make. In some cases, though, the benefits for the community of returning to normal may outweigh the cost of lost evidence.

Establishing collective knowledge

It is imperative that the lessons learnt from each response be shared with counterparts in other regions. This building up of a collective knowledge within the first responder community can allow for responders who have never responded to suicide attacks to respond with the knowledge of the lessons learnt by other responders in previous incidents. In the Dimona suicide bombing in Israel, this collective knowledge was credited with a strong overall response being staged even though the local commanders had no firsthand response experience with suicide bombing response. The response was not perfect, but it was likely better than any other response would be in an area that had never experienced a suicide attack. The strong networking opportunities within the Israeli security forces though had allowed for the Dimona commanders to already be aware of the lessons learnt from bombings in other areas of the country. Steps should be taken in other areas of the world to establish similar avenues for the development of collective response knowledge.

Since the 7/7 bombings, much more consideration has been given to the development of this type of knowledge in the UK. As previously mentioned, an important component of this can be seen at the Fire Service College in Gloucestershire where firefighters and specialized paramedics train on the same grounds. There are hopes that the training centre will expand in the future to include police training to be a fully integrated services disaster response training centre. Not only would this allow for responders to train alongside each other to be able to work collaboratively in responses, but it would also allow for the personal relationships to be built that will be crucial in the development of a collective knowledge to pass lessons learnt through social networks.

First receivers

Surge capacity

Suicide bombings can cause high numbers of casualties that will tax the resources of any hospital. Facilities must have adequate surge capacity plans in place to deal with this influx.

Types of injuries

Most civilian hospitals are accustomed to dealing primarily with patients suffering from medical problems in their emergency departments with very little time spent dealing with trauma. The injuries from suicide bombing attacks present with a number of unique aspects that first receivers should be aware of, on top of understanding basic blast injuries. First receivers also need to keep in mind that after suicide bombings, like any disaster, patients will probably self-transport to the hospital independent of the organized ambulance system. Blast injuries include the primary injuries from the blast wave, secondary from shrapnel, tertiary from the person being thrown against stationary objects and quaternary from burns (Kluger *et al.*, 2004).

Israeli researchers have described a unique injury pattern in victims of terrorist bombings, particularly with abdominal and thoracic trauma (Bala *et al.*, 2008, 2010). While the focus in treating patients after explosions is often on pulmonary barotrauma, the shrapnel typically added to terrorist bombs creates a unique injury pattern of lung contusion due to the primary blast wave in addition to penetrating injury due to shrapnel. The precise pattern will depend on the specific construction and deployment of the device. The severity of injury depends largely on how close the patient was to the blast, with injuries also depending on the location of the bombing. Patients from bombings in open spaces are more likely to suffer from penetrating injuries and less likely to suffer from the impact of the blast wave than patients from a bombing in an enclosed space (Bala *et al.*, 2008). Overall, the victims of terrorist bombings are more severely injured, arrive with lower Glasgow Coma Scale (GCS) scores, are more likely to be haemodynamically unstable and to need surgical intervention, and generally consume more hospital resources than conventional trauma patients (Kluger *et al.*, 2004).

Case Studies

To help see how these considerations would apply during a real-world suicide bombing response, case studies from three notable suicide bombing incidents are included. While reading these, consider the response considerations discussed previously and how they would apply.

Park Hotel Bombing

Summary

The Park Hotel bombing (also known as the Passover Massacre or the Park Hotel Passover attack) was a suicide bombing carried out by Hamas at the Park Hotel in Netanya, Israel on

27 March 2002, during the Passover Seder. Thirty Israeli civilians were killed in the attack and 140 were injured. It was the deadliest attack against Israelis during the Second Intifada.

Location of the attack

The attack occurred on the night of 27 March, when the Jewish holiday of Passover fell that year. The Park Hotel in Netanya held a large Passover Seder (festive religious meal) for its 250 guests, especially elderly Jews who did not have family or relatives, in the ground-floor dining room.

Method of attack

On 27 March, Passover Eve, around 14:00, suicide bomber Oudeh and his driver Fathi Khatib left Tulkarm and drove to the village of Nazlat 'Isa. In Nazlat 'Isa the two switched into another vehicle prepared in advance and drove towards Herzliya to find an appropriate target.

Upon failing to find an appropriate target in Herzliya, they headed to Tel Aviv, but were unable to find an appropriate target there as well. On their way, Oudeh told Fathi Khatib that he was familiar with Netanya and the two headed off in that direction. Once in Netanya, they headed west and got out of the vehicle next to the Park Hotel. The 'appropriate' place, crowded with people celebrating the Passover Seder, was thus found.

Around 19:30, Oudeh passed a security guard at the hotel's entrance; walked through the lobby passing the reception desk and entered the hotel's dining room where he detonated an explosive device he carried in a suitcase.

Emergency response to the attack

First responders arrived on the scene of the bombing less than 5 min after the explosion. Ten minutes after the bombing, the first patient departed the scene heading to the hospital. Within 20 min, all the seriously wounded (red tags) were removed from the scene and transported to local medical facilities. Approximately 33 min after the explosion all patients were removed from the scene.

Victims of the attack

Twenty-eight people were immediately killed and approximately 140 were injured, of whom 20 were seriously injured. Two of the injured later died from their wounds. Most of the victims were senior citizens (70 and over). The oldest victim was 90 and the youngest was 20 years old. A number of married couples were killed, as well as a father together with his daughter. One of the victims was a Jewish tourist from Sweden who was visiting Israel for Passover.

Responsibility for the attack

Hamas claimed responsibility for the attack. The bomber was identified as Abdel-Basset Odeh, a 25-year-old from the nearby West Bank city of Tulkarm. Hamas claimed that the attack was specifically designed to derail momentum from a recently announced peace initiative of the Saudi Arabian government at the Beirut Summit.

London 7/7 Bombings

Summary

The 7 July 2005 London bombings (commonly referred to as 7/7) were a series of coordinated suicide attacks in London using the public transport system during the morning rush hour. That morning, four suicide bombers detonated four bombs, three on London Underground trains in quick succession with the fourth bomb exploding an hour later in a double-decker bus in Tavistock Square. Fifty-six people, including the four bombers, were killed by the attacks, and about 700 were injured.

Location of the attack

On Thursday, 7 July 2005, a series of four bombs struck London's public transport system during the morning rush hour. At 08:50 (British Summer Time (BST)) three bombs exploded within 50 s of each other on three London Underground trains in the vicinities of the Liverpool Street, Edgeware Road and King's Cross Stations. The final explosion occurred on a double-decker bus in Tavistock Square, not far from King's Cross, around an hour later.

Method of attack

Russell Square

At 08:50 BST suicide bomber Germaine Lindsay entered the Piccadilly Line train number 331 travelling south from King's Cross station to Russell Square. He placed a rucksack containing explosive device made of homemade, organic peroxide-based material next to the rear set of double doors in the front carriage of the train.

Aldgate

At approximately the same time as the Russell Square bombing, bomber Shehzad Tanweer entered on the Circle Line train number 204 travelling east from Liverpool Street station to Aldgate. The bomber used the same type of device as the bomber in Russell Square and placed it on the floor of the rear end of the second carriage.

Edgware Road

Within 50 s of the first two underground explosions, bomber Mohammad Sidique Khan entered the Circle Line train number 216, which had just left Edgware Road station heading west for Paddington. Using the same device as his colleagues, Khan placed the rucksack on the floor of the second carriage, close to the forward set of double doors.

Tavistock Square

At 09:47 BST suicide bomber Hasib Hussain riding the number 30 double-decker bus at the junction of Tavistock Square and Upper Woburn Place detonated another explosive rucksack destroying the roof and rear of the double-decker bus. It was travelling from Marble Arch to Hackney but had been diverted from its normal route because of road closures in the wake of the tube bombings around an hour earlier.

Emergency response to the attack

Paramedics were sent down into the tube system to search for more casualties. St John Ambulance was called out to assist the London Ambulance Service, and hospitals had to call in off-duty staff, plus doctors from as far away as Hampshire and Oxfordshire. The ticket hall and waiting area of King's Cross station was used as a temporary hospital for the victims of the Piccadilly Line explosion. Air ambulances were used extensively to provide rapid transportation of specialist medics to the scenes of the explosions. A number of London buses were also used to transport the 'walking wounded' to hospital.

Royal London Hospital's Helicopter Emergency Medical Service (HEMS) received a call of a 'suspected incident' at 09:07. Forty minutes later, the 'major' incident alarm sounded, and the Accident and Emergency Department (A&E) was closed to all non-major cases related to the incident. The Royal London Hospital was designated as the primary receiving hospital for the victims of the bombings. The HEMS dispatched 18 teams consisting of Medical Incident Officers in fast response cars. Two doctors immediately were mobilized to Aldgate Station, and arrived at Aldgate Station at 09:31. The helicopter transported a team consisting of two doctors and two paramedics to King's Cross Station. Another team was deployed by air to Edgware Road Underground Station. At 10:20, a team of two doctors and one paramedic arrived by a fast response car at the scene of the bus explosion incident at Tavistock Square.

Victims of the attack

Twenty-six people were killed on the Piccadilly Line train, 13 were killed on the No. 30 double-decker bus and 13 were killed on the Circle Line train (Table 14.1).

Table 14.1. The number of people killed in the various transport systems.

Transport system	Travelling from	Travelling to	Time of attack	Number of persons killed
Piccadilly Line Train No. 331	King's Cross Station	Russell Square	08:50 BST	26, plus the bomber
Circle Line train No. 204	Liverpool Street Station	Aldgate	08:50 BST	7, plus the bomber
Circle Line train No. 216	Edgware Road Station	Paddington	08:50 BST	6, plus the bomber
No. 30 double-decker bus	Upper Woburn Place	Tavistock Square	09:47 BST	13, plus the bomber

A total of 700 people were injured in the explosions with 350 being treated on the spot. Two hundred and eight of the injured were treated at Royal London Hospital alone and 100 of them were kept in hospital overnight. Twenty-two were in a serious or critical condition, and one person subsequently died. Many of the injured were foreign nationals, including people from Sierra Leone, Australia, South Africa, Colombia, Poland, New Zealand, Israel and China (Mohammed *et al.*, 2006).

Responsibility for the attack

On 1 September 2005, it was reported that al-Qaeda officially claimed responsibility for the attacks in a videotape broadcasted by the Arab television network Al Jazeera. But an official inquiry by the British government reported that the tape claiming responsibility had been edited after the attacks, and that the bombers did not have direct assistance from al-Qaeda.

Dimona Bombing

Summary

The Dimona bombing was a suicide bombing carried out on 4 February 2008 in the southern Israeli town of Dimona. The attack was carried out by Palestinian militants from the Izzedine al-Qassam Brigades, the military wing of Hamas.

Location of the attack

The attack took place on 4 February 2008, at approximately 10:30 (Israel local time 08:30 GMT), in a shopping mall in the southern Israeli town of Dimona.

Method of the attack

Two suicide bombers, Luay Laghwani and Musa Arafat, entered the shopping mall area in Dimona intending to detonate explosive devices. The first bomber detonated himself on a crowd of innocent bystanders at the open market while inadvertently injuring the second bomber who arrived with him. The planned adversarial operation was designed to be a double suicide attack with the first bomber detonating himself in the open market, and the second bomber targeting first responders operating at the scene. Prior to detonation, the second bomber was identified and, based on their emergency medical training, responders notified the police and lethal force was utilized to neutralize the threat by law enforcement.

Emergency response to the attack

The response was immediately initiated by emergency medical service (EMS) personnel and incident command was established. Even though, for Dimona, it was the first time emergency responders had ever experienced a terror attack, and therefore operating and response procedures could potentially have been slower to coordinate a smooth and safe process, the response was fast by all agencies. EMS was supported by local medical clinics that dispatched 'Good Samaritans' to the scene to assist emergency crews. The Good

Samaritan team comprised a physician and nurse. The pair immediately began to treat the seriously injured, which included the would-be bomber. While treating the injured suicide bomber, the crew identified an imminent threat, evacuated the scene and notified law enforcement. As the team evacuated the scene, and relayed the details of the threat to law enforcement on location, they were able to continue to meet their mission objectives and successfully dragged an additional wounded woman with them to safety.

With the first suicide bomber killed in the primary attack, the second suicide bomber was injured and had been identified by emergency personnel. According to law enforcement personnel on location, the second suicide bomber posed a clear and imminent threat to the rescuers and civilians on location. The intended plan of action of this bomber can only be speculated, but it was believed that he intended to target the first responders entering the scene of the explosion. This is considered a known criterion and a successful tactic perpetrated by adversarial elements globally. The superintendent on the scene used lethal force against the second bomber; but, the threat was not fully neutralized. The danger associated with such an attacker is the potential for the injured bomber to use what strength is left of him to initiate any switch to detonate the explosive device.

Until the threat can be rendered safe, no additional rescue attempts can continue. Identifying the danger to the civilians and rescuers, and adhering to training, a superintendent from the Israeli Police fired several shots, fatally wounding the second suicide bomber before he could detonate his explosive device. As soon as the threat was neutralized, and bomb technicians rendered the explosive device safe, emergency crews were able to re-enter the scene and continue with their overall mission.

Victims of the attack

One female, 73-year-old Lyubov Razdol'skaya, was killed in the suicide bombing. Another 48 civilians were injured including her husband.

Responsibility for the attack

The terror group that planned and executed the attack was the Izzedine al-Qassam Brigades, a terrorist squad from Hebron – the military wing of the Hamas organization.

Conclusion

These case studies along with the considerations presented here emphasize the importance of preparing for suicide bombing incidents. Early planning and training at different levels both together and separately to bring together commanders and first responders and receivers is critical to being able to stage effective suicide bombing responses. All responders must understand their specific role while being aware of the key considerations overall. Continual evaluation of response considerationsis essential to ensure that optimal responses can be staged to evolving terrorist tactics.

Acknowledgements

The foundation of the material in this chapter is the suicide bombing research by Christopher R. Foerster, Johnathon A. Mohr, James E. Patrick and Aaron Richman, presented at the 17th World Congress on Disaster and Emergency Medicine. The authors are grateful for the support of Jennifer Cole, Jason Fenard, Peter House, Rani Tal and Dov Zwerling.

References

7 July Review Committee (2006) *Report of the 7 July Review Committee.* London: Greater London Authority. BBC News What Happened. Available at: http://news.bbc.co.uk/1/shared/spl/hi/uk/05/london_blasts/what_happened/html/default.stm (Accessed 14 April 2011).

Bala, M., Rivkind, A.I., Zamir, G., Hadar, T., Gertsenshtein, I., Mintz, Y., Pikarsky, A.J., Amar, D., Shussman, N., Abu Gazala, M. and Almogy, G. (2008) Abdominal trauma after terrorist bombing attacks exhibits a unique pattern of injury. *Annals of Surgery* 248, 303–309.

Bala, M., Shussman, N., Rivkind, A.I., Izhar, U. and Almogy, G. (2010) The pattern of thoracic trauma after suicide terrorist bombing attacks. *The Journal of Trauma* 69, 1022–1028.

BBC News (2008) Israeli killed in suicide bombing. Available at: http://news.bbc.co.uk/2/hi/7225775.stm (Accessed 26 December 2009).

BBC News (2009) Obama orders air security review after jet bomb attempt. Available at: http://news.bbc.co.uk/2/hi/americas/8431732.stm (Accessed 27 January 2010).

Holden, P.J.P. (2005) The London attacks – a chronicle: improvising in an emergency. *The New England Journal of Medicine* 353, 541–543.

Israel Ministry of Foreign Affairs (1997) *Victims of Mahane Yehuda Bombing.* http://www.mfa.gov.il/MFA/MFAArchive/1990_1999/1998/7/Victims%20of%20Mahane%20Y e huda%20Bombing (Accessed December 28, 2009).

Israel Ministry of Foreign Affairs (2001a) Suicide bombing at the Ben-Yehuda pedestrian mall in Jerusalem. Available at: http://www.mfa.gov.il/MFA/MFAArchive/2000_2009/2001/12/Suicide%20bombing%20at%20t h e%20Ben-Yehuda%20pedestrian%20mall (Accessed 26 December 2009).

Israel Ministry of Foreign Affairs (2001b) Suicide bombing at the Sbarro pizzeria in Jerusalem. Available at: http://www.mfa.gov.il/MFA/MFAArchive/2000_2009/2000/10/Suicide+bombing+at+the+Sbarr o +pizzeria+in+Jerusale.htm (Accessed 26 December 2009).

Israel Ministry of Foreign Affairs (2002) A week of terror: January 22–27, 2002. Available at: http://www.mfa.gov.il/MFA/MFAArchive/2000_2009/2002/1/Palestinian+Terrorism-+Photos+-+January+22-27-+200.htm (Accessed 25 June 2011).

Israel Ministry of Foreign Affairs (2003) Details of April 30, 2003 Tel Aviv suicide bombing. Available at: http://www.mfa.gov.il/MFA/Government/Communiques/2003/Details+of+April+30+2003+Tel+Aviv+suicide+bombing.htm (Accessed 26 December 2009).

Israel Ministry of Foreign Affairs (2006) Suicide bombing at 'Rosh Ha'ir'shawarma restaurant in Tel Aviv. Available at: http://www.mfa.gov.il/MFA/MFAArchive/2000_2009/2006/Suicide+bombing+at+Tel+Aviv+sh a warma+restaurant+17-Apr-2006.htm?WBCMODE=Pr (Accessed 26 December 2009).

Israel Ministry of Foreign Affairs (2008) Terrorist attack on Jaffa Road, Jerusalem. Available at: http://www.mfa.gov.il/MFA/TerrorismObstacle+to+Peace/Palestinian+terror+since+2000/Terror ist+attack+on+Jaffa+Road+Jerusalem +2-Jul-2008.htm (Accessed 26 December 2009).

Katz, B. (2010) Times Square bomber pleads guilty. Reuters. Available at: http://www.reuters.com/article/idUSTRE65K68420100621 (Accessed 20 July 2010).

Kluger, Y., Peleg, K., Daniel-Aharonson, L., Mayo, A. and the Israeli Trauma Group (2004) The special injury pattern in terrorist bombings. *Journal of the American College of Surgeons* 199, 875–879.

Mohammed, A., Mann, H.B., Nawabi, D.H., Goodier, D.W. and Ang, S.C. (2006) Impact of London's terrorist attacks on a major trauma center in London. *Prehospital and Disaster Medicine* 21, 5, 340–344.

Chapter 15

Hospital Triage and Bottlenecks to the Flow of Casualties: A Review

Fernando Turégano and Itamar Ashkenazi

Introduction: Objective of the Hospital Response in Mass Casualty Incidents

The quantitative definition of a mass casualty incident (MCI) is determined by the capability of the receiving institution to care for the victims. Two severely injured patients arriving simultaneously can overwhelm a small community hospital. Even in a large urban trauma centre, if one assumes that each severely injured patient requires a trauma resuscitation bay and a dedicated trauma team, then the routine trauma response envelope extends to no more than three or four severely injured patients arriving together (Hirshberg *et al.*, 2001).

Most of us would agree on the statement that the objective of the hospital response in MCIs would ideally be to provide severely wounded victims with a level of care that approximates the level of care provided under normal circumstances. In favour of this statement is the fact that during terrorist explosions, the most frequent form of man-made MCI, the number of critical patients rarely exceeds 10–15% of the load. Most of the deaths occur on the scene, and only a few occur in hospital. The magnitude of the medical problem is not dictated by the number of those dying on-site.

In most articles written to date on this subject most authors, including Israeli authors, advocate the use of tools of catastrophe management (Frykberg, 2002; Committee on Trauma-American College of Surgeons, 2003; Michaelson *et al.*, 2003; Peleg *et al.*, 2004) but, according to others, this seems inappropriate in MCIs (Ashkenazi *et al.*, 2008). Peleg promotes the provision of 'minimal acceptable care' as long as there is an on-going flow of casualties and the eventual number of victims is unknown. The fact that the majority of casualties always overwhelm the closest hospital adds substance to this statement. Nevertheless, clear guidelines that define what precisely constitutes minimal acceptable trauma care are an obvious necessity that has not been addressed in detail (Hirshberg *et al.*, 2001). Frykberg even advocates avoiding blood transfusions, endotracheal intubations and emergency room thoracotomies during the initial phase of casualty influx. Since no definition is offered as to what transforms a particular terrorist attack into a disaster, these and other similar messages are misinterpreted as recommendations that injuries of moderate severity, rather than greatest severity, should take priority (Ashkenazi *et al.*, 2008). The magnitude of destruction and death tolls seen in the terrorist attacks on the Madrid trains in 2004 (Gutierrez de Ceballos *et al.*, 2005; Turégano *et al.*, 2008a,b), the London Underground in 2005 (Aylwin *et al.*, 2006), India (Deshpande *et al.*, 2007), Pakistan (Umer *et al.*, 2009), Bali (Palmer *et al.*, 2003), the World Trade Center in New York in 2001 (Cushman *et al.*, 2003), the Murrah Federal Building in the Oklahoma City bombing in 1995 (Hogan *et al.*, 1999), the American embassies in Kenya and Tanzania in 1998 (Njenga *et al.*, 2004) and the US Marines barracks in Beirut in 1983 (Frykberg *et al.*, 1989), only add to the catastrophic vision of the medical consequences of terrorist attacks.

The reality in Israel has been different. Based on the experience of managing more than 20 such events during the last decade, Ashkenazi *et al.* understand that an MCI is an event in which there may be many victims, but only a few actually suffer from life-threatening injuries. Relying on this observation, these authors conclude that it is unacceptable to deny these patients timely optimal treatment only because their injuries occur in the context of an MCI. Withholding timely, optimal treatment from those identified with severe injuries, just because other seriously injured victims may eventually be admitted, makes no sense and is not supported by the numbers of seriously injured victims commonly encountered. In fact, Almogy has shown that the average number of casualties per attack was only 38 (Almogy *et al.*, 2004). Based on a retrospective review of 62 MCIs recorded between 2000 and 2003, Kosashvili and colleagues found that the mean number of arriving casualties to a single hospital was 20, and that only 20% of them required immediate medical treatment. They state that hospital preparedness can be better defined by a fixed number of casualties rather than a percentile of its bed capacity, although acknowledging that the actual number of casualties arriving to hospital may vary in each country based on many parameters (Kosashvili *et al.*, 2009).

In summary, in small-scale MCIs the objective of the hospital response should probably be to provide the greatest good to the few severely wounded, devoting all trauma resources to their care. On the contrary, in large-scale MCIs, where local trauma resources are likely to be depleted quickly, the objective should probably be to provide the greatest good to the greatest number, and minimal acceptable care should be given while the situation unfolds.

Metrics to Judge the Efficacy of the Medical Response to an MCI

The two main metrics are the critical mortality rate (CMR) and the surge capacity (SC). The CMR measures the percentage of severely wounded patients (Injury Severity Score (ISS) >15) who die after their medical care has begun (Frykberg and Tepas, 1988). In a classic 2002 article analysing a series of ten terrorist bombings from 1969 to 1995, Frykberg described a positive linear relationship between over-triage and mortality among critically injured victims of MCIs (Frykberg, 2002). Nevertheless, several subsequent reports of mass casualty response have postulated alternative relationships between over-triage and clinical outcomes (Rodoplu *et al.*, 2005; Aylwin *et al.*, 2006).

SC is a hospital's capacity to treat newly arriving severely wounded victims without degradation in the care they receive. It is an arrival rate (Hirshberg *et al.*, 2005, 2010), and requires a method for measuring quality of care. In fact, most reports of MCIs describe injury patterns and casualty profiles, but the quality of trauma care has only rarely been addressed (Hirshberg *et al.*, 2001; Auf der Heide, 2006). This quality of care remains an unpopular discussion topic because of its public implications. No hospital official will ever willingly admit that care of casualties from a high-visibility MCI was anything less than optimal. In reality, the quality of trauma care in MCIs is inversely proportional to the caseload simply because the number of trauma-trained staff and trauma-related resources is limited. The eighth critical patient will be treated in an improvised resuscitation bay by a reinforcement team that may not even include a surgeon with trauma experience. Even the most creative disaster plan in the best trauma centre will not prevent this decline in the quality of trauma care during an MCI (Hirshberg *et al.*, 2001). Also, the notion that the hospital capacity for severely injured patients can be expanded by reinforcement with personnel who do not deal with trauma on a daily basis is a dangerous misconception (Hirshberg *et al.*, 2001).

Tadmor states that SC possesses two distinct but highly connected elements: the technical or 'scientific' element, which refers to physical aspects such as numbers and benchmarks (patients, beds and so forth), and the 'artistic' element, which refers to the art of collaboration, cooperation, joint venture and decision-making processes. Thus, there is both a science and an art to surge (Tadmor *et al.*, 2006).

Israel is unique in that it possesses one national system of first responders and one system of hospitals. Israel has fewer than 30 general acute care hospitals in the entire country, and all are civilian. During a suicide bombing event, an MCI is declared when the hospital receives more than ten casualties if at least four of them are declared 'immediate' (ISS > 15). The Israeli Minister of Health defines adequate surge capacity for a hospital in peacetime to be the ability to augment bed capacity by 20%. A review of suicide bombing events from 2000 to 2003 showed that the 20% threshold was rarely exceeded, and these occurrences were in remote rural hospitals.

When capacity is exhausted, based on experience gleaned from drills, the affected hospital is declared a 'triage hospital' (Rozin and Kleinman, 1987). The concept of transporting the victims to the nearest medical facility, from where, after the primary medical treatment is given, they are secondarily distributed to other medical facilities, was developed in military medicine in the Korean War. American wounded soldiers were removed to a military hospital near the front line, where primary stabilization was achieved and only later were the wounded transported to hospitals in the rear. This system enabled a decrease in mortality from 4% in the Second World War to 2.4% (King and Jatoi, 2005). This system was re-employed by the American Army in Vietnam and in Lebanon, and by the Israeli Army in both the October War in 1973 and the Lebanese War in 1982, with similar results.

Secondary victim distribution, in the civilian urban setting, was first described by Klausner and Rozin (1986). Forty victims were evacuated to a small city hospital after a bomb exploded in a nearby populated market. Only basic procedures were performed, such as securing airway, control of external bleeding, volume replacement, chest drainage and fracture splinting. Four per cent of the casualties needed emergency surgery for progressive respiratory difficulties and uncontrollable bleeding. Seventeen victims were redistributed to other hospitals. The military experience shows that the severely wounded, once stabilized, can be safely transported several hours from the medical facilities in the front, to the hospitals in the rear. Klausner and Rozin advocate the use of the primary medical facility as an 'evacuation hospital' (i.e. 'triage hospital'). Even so, only 17 out of the 40 victims were secondarily distributed to other hospitals. It is unclear from Klausner and Rozin's paper what were the injuries of the victims who were redistributed to other medical facilities.

The Israeli experience following various MCIs in the 1990s and first decade of this century reveals that employing a plan of 'triage hospital' is unnecessary in small-scale MCIs. Nevertheless, long-term improvement of care is facilitated by adopting a policy of simultaneous treatment and selective secondary evacuation for victims who are stable but demand complex care such as those with orthopaedic and penetrating ophthalmologic trauma.

To overcome the methodological obstacles encountered in the conduct of studies on the role of triage performance, several authors have used computer simulation and mathematical programming techniques. The simulation model of single-hospital trauma care created by Hirshberg and colleagues confirms the importance of treatment capability (i.e. radiological capacity, staffing levels) in determining the quality of trauma care, which may determine the rates of preventable morbidity and mortality (Hirshberg *et al.*, 1999). Hupert created a simulation model that includes three essential components of mass casualty care: the number and distribution of patients by casualty type, the triage process and the treatment capability of the trauma care system. In all of the modelled scenarios, the ratio of critical patients to treatment capability has a greater impact on critical mortality than over-triage level or time-dependent mortality assumption. He defined a new metric to describe trauma system response after MCIs, the critical surge to capability ratio (CSCR), or the relative number of critical patients to available and staffed treatment units, which exhibits a consistent and non-linear association with critical mortality in their model (Hupert *et al.*, 2007).

Triage and SC: Computer Modelling and Facts

Effective triage at the emergency department entrance is the key to successfully dealing with an MCI. One of the major reasons for the high over-triage rates is the fact that in the real world (as opposed to during disaster drills), it is difficult to distinguish between casualties requiring immediate and delayed treatments by means of a rapid and cursory examination of a few seconds. It is also often impossible to determine that a casualty is hopeless or dead without a cardiac monitor and a more thorough examination (Kennedy *et al.*, 1996). The definition of a patient as 'hopeless' or 'expected to die' is not absolute but relative to the caseload, something difficult to know from the beginning due to the usual lack of accurate information from the field (Hirshberg *et al.*, 2001).

Disaster planning continues to rely primarily on mock disaster drills, conducted in unrealistic time frames and often treated with complacency by the medical and nursing staff. A more powerful planning tool is discrete-event simulation, a methodology for the study of the flow of objects through a system. It is actually a computer program that moves objects through the system while keeping track of their flow and interactions (Hirshberg *et al.*, 2001).

Hirshberg translated the disaster plan of a US level I trauma centre into a computer model and challenged it with simulated casualties based on 223 patients from 22 bombing incidents treated in one Israeli hospital. The model computes the level of care for each critical casualty from six variables that reflect the composition of the trauma team and access to facilities. The model predicts a sigmoid-shaped relationship between casualty load and the level of care, with the upper flat portion of the curve corresponding to the surge capacity of the trauma assets of the hospital (Fig. 15.1).

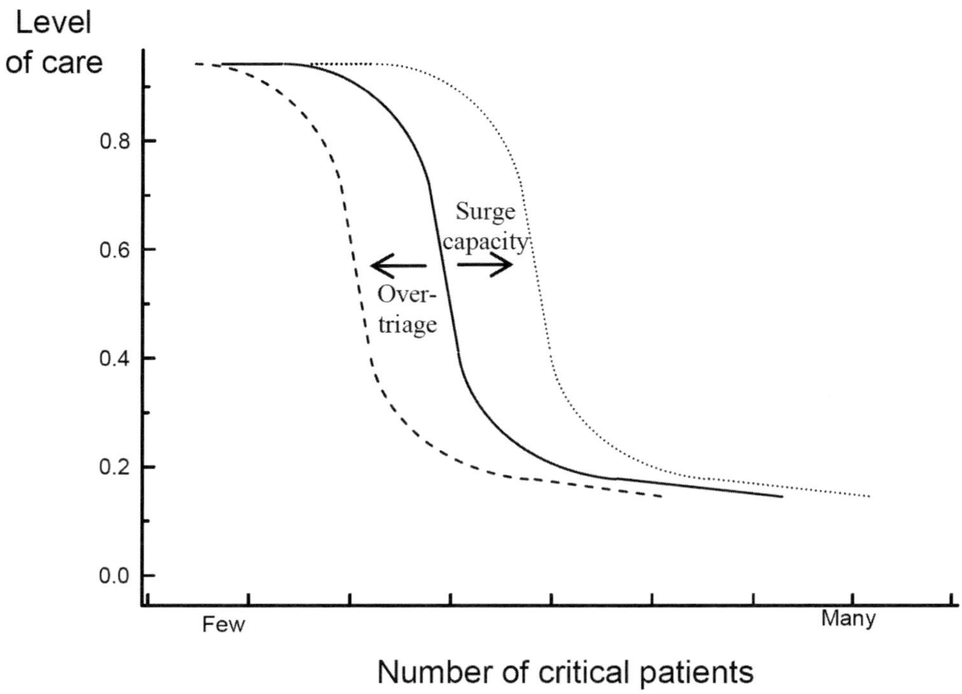

Fig. 15.1. Level of care dependence on number of critical patients, surge capacity and over-triage.

A fully deployed disaster plan shifts the curve to the right while over-triage will shift the curve to the left (Hirshberg *et al*., 2005). This model calculated that an over-triage rate of 50–75% will decrease the capacity to offer optimal care by 15–30%. The model defines the SC of the hospital trauma assets as a rate of casualty arrival rather than a number of beds, and they claim that the study demonstrates the value of dynamic computer modelling as an important tool in disaster planning. The traditional distinction between multiple and MCIs is based on the ability of the hospital to manage the casualty load using local resources. They propose a quantitative definition whereby an MCI is represented by the upper flat portion of the curve, where the inflow of casualties is less than the surge capacity of the trauma assets. In a mass casualty situation, this capacity is exceeded, as represented by the steep portion of the curve. A major medical disaster corresponds to the lower flat portion of the curve (Fig. 15.1). The study also indicates that it is possible to mitigate the effects of over-triage by using means that will shift the curve to the right. One example is reducing processing times or adding parallel servers (like improvised shock rooms) that will increase the throughput of the shock rooms. However, the predicted increase in SC from increased shock room throughput is relatively modest, underscoring the limited ability of a hospital to continue providing competent trauma teams and an optimal initial care environment for a sudden large influx of severe casualties.

This type of computer model can easily be criticized on almost every level (Hirshberg *et al.*, 2005):

- It assumes a continuous flow of casualties when in real incidents casualties typically arrive in several large clusters.
- It does not account for variability in individual performance and disregards important elements of the trauma response envelope such as anaesthesia, surgical subspecialties and blood banking.
- The model is also limited to the initial care phase and disregards later stages.
- Most importantly, the level of trauma care is calculated from a subjective grading system developed by consensus rather than from a universally accepted objective standard (which does not exist).

As said, instead of focusing on subjective measures of over- and under-triage, Hirshberg and colleagues attempt to simplify and quantify the decision-making process by means of a computer model (Hirshberg *et al.*, 2010). In another recent paper they describe either a one-step or a two-step triage process, both of which are reduced to binary decisions, which can be modelled for computer analysis and interpreted for triage accuracy and mode with regard to a centre's ability to cope with the surge. The model predicts that one-step triage works well for limited incidents (up to roughly 30 casualties per hour for a five-team emergency department). Thus, a simplified triage scheme with only two categories (patients requiring care in shock rooms and all others) may be a more practical alternative for triage at the hospital gate than an elaborate multiple-component scheme such as Simple Triage and Rapid Treatment (START). Simplified triage with only the ability to follow commands (the motor response component of the Glasgow Coma Scale (GCS)) has been shown to have excellent predictive power in identifying patients who require urgent trauma care (Meredith *et al.*, 1995). Likely predictors of urgent trauma care are patients being unable to walk, signs of external haemorrhage, coma, tachycardia, tachypnea and also 'clinical intuition'. Following suicide bombing attacks (SBA), Almogy and Rivkind demonstrated that easily recognizable external signs of trauma, such as penetrating head and abdominal wounds and injuries to four or more body regions, are associated with an increased risk of blast lung injury (BLI) and abdominal injuries requiring laparotomy (Almogy and Rivkind, 2006).

In larger events, where the number of severely wounded victims outnumbers the number of available trauma teams, the only feasible option is to switch to a two-step or sequential triage scheme. The first step of the sequence separates the severely wounded victims from all the others, and the second step concentrates on those severely wounded, sorting out those in need of immediate care versus those whose injuries allow delayed care. Cardiorespiratory status, external injuries in four or more body regions, and penetrating injuries to the head and abdomen would help with this distinction (Avidan *et al.*, 2007).

This switch from a one-step to a two-step triage is considered as a major qualitative change in trauma care because two of every three severely injured patients will temporarily receive a lower level of care than they would get on a normal working day. Thus, sequential triage means that trauma care for severe casualties becomes rationed. The decision to use a sequential triage scheme is the most important leadership decision during the early stages of the hospital response, with implications well beyond triage only (Hirshberg *et al.*, 2010). Although the simultaneous urban bombings in London (Aylwin *et al.*, 2006) and Madrid (Turégano *et al.*, 2008a,b) were large-scale incidents, the overwhelming majority of MCIs that any hospital is likely to face will be limited MCIs where effective single-step triage and an ED-based response would suffice.

Sequential triage involves a trade-off between increasing the capacity of the system and decreasing the time that trauma team members spend with each urgent casualty. In other words, the theoretical surge capacity depends on the team-to-casualty ratio. A severely injured patient spends roughly slightly less than an hour in the trauma resuscitation area, on average, and this is based on multiple reports from the literature, most notably the report from the London bombings. If you know the number of available teams in your emergency department, you know your theoretical surge capacity given perfect triage. It is roughly one severe casualty, per team, per hour, an estimate very close to De Boer's empirical estimate of hospital capacity (De Boer, 1999). A calculation consistent across multiple reports is that you roughly have one trauma team per 100 hospital beds (Hirshberg *et al*., 2010).

According to Ashkenazi, all patients entering the emergency department should be assessed by the triage officer. Primary and secondary surveys should be conducted on all patients within minutes, with the aim of identifying those who are severely wounded. The proper evaluation of symptoms and detailed physical examination are the keys to identifying the real magnitude of injury (Ashkenazi *et al*., 2008).

A change in the strategy of patient management may also increase hospital SC, as a paper by Einav *et al*. (2009) demonstrates. This study is the first to point out that the assignment of case managers may improve patient management and flow during MCIs, provided the MCI is of a limited nature. These improvements were achieved with a similar number of staff members and no added equipment. They argue that during an MCI there is a large influx of casualties being transferred from one treatment station to another. From the medical professional's viewpoint, appointment of a case manager turns an MCI into a series of single cases. Once a staff member is given a manageable assignment, the degree of distraction caused by the large number of casualties is significantly reduced. Case management appeared to improve the quality of information transfer but not necessarily through improved documentation during patient workup, it improves the continuity of care and possibly reduces the risk of medical error. Assignment of case managers also decreases the stress associated with uncertainty regarding the hierarchy of care and scope of responsibility. Although case managers need not necessarily be surgeons, they believe that individual patients with critical injuries receive better care from experienced surgeons. Reductions were observed in: the number of X-rays/patient/first 24-h, time to performance of first chest X-ray, time from first chest X-ray to arrival at the next diagnostic/treatment location, time from emergency department arrival to surgery and hospital lengths of stay for critically injured casualties. Most interviewed staff noted improved patient care, communication and documentation (Einav *et al*., 2009).

Bottlenecks to the Flow of Casualties

Traditionally these bottlenecks have been the trauma teams and trauma bays, radiology, operating theatres and intensive care unit (ICU) beds.

Trauma teams and trauma bays

To make an impact on survival, one must identify those who are severely wounded as quickly as possible and offer those patients optimal care. Experienced trauma physicians are the most important trauma resource available to achieve this objective, and they should be allocated to the treatment of seriously injured victims instead of more traditional management roles such as triage and incident manager (Ashkenazi *et al*., 2008).

The prevailing strategy of a 'unidirectional flow plan' (UFP) is advocated by many authors, and aims at facilitating the rapid workup of all of the victims, both seriously and non-seriously injured, with the purpose of keeping to a minimum the missed injuries. This common belief that life-threatening injuries often are missed during the primary evaluation never has been supported by concrete evidence. Out of 78 severely and moderately injured victims in 20 different MCIs, Ashkenazi has experienced only three cases in which primary evaluation did not reveal the real severity of the injury (Ashkenazi *et al*., 2008). Thus, it is a mistake to prioritize repeated assessments if one wants to make an impact on survival. Instead of investing the most capable trauma physicians in a management role, as advocated by those supporting the UFP, the 'customized plan' (CP) takes into consideration that the most important limited resource is experienced trauma leaders, whether these are surgeons, emergency physicians, intensivists or anaesthesiologists. The few experienced in trauma care are placed in direct charge of the treatment of the severely injured victims once they are identified. The main objective emphasized by the CP is that severely injured victims should be identified and all needed resources should be allocated to their treatment. The others can wait. Hospitalizing most of the victims and performing a tertiary survey within several hours can adequately address the shortcomings of the CP (emergency department congestion and missed injuries) (Ashkenazi *et al*., 2008).

Improvised trauma bays can be both a necessity and a means to increase the surge capacity of critical patients, as was experienced at the closest hospital during the Madrid bombings (Turégano *et al*., 2008a).

Radiology

The radiologist has a central role in attempting to reduce the mortality and morbidity in MCIs (Martí *et al*., 2006; Hare *et al*., 2007), and the provision of radiographic services affects forward patient flow in an MCI (Raja *et al*., 2010). Administrators often underestimate the importance of radiology in disaster management plans (Benjaminov *et al*., 2006), possibly because of outdated estimates of the utilization of emergency radiology during MCIs. Hirshberg also suggests that most disaster plans underestimate the need for radiography and computerized tomography, and also emphasizes the importance of not hampering patient flow through the hospital by over-use of radiology (Hirshberg *et al*., 1999).

Previously published reports from the Oklahoma City bombing in 1995 (Hogan *et al*., 1999), the Madrid trains bombings in 2004 (Gutierrez de Ceballos *et al*., 2005; Turégano *et al*., 2008a,b) and the London Underground bombings in 2005 (Aylwin *et al*., 2006) noted that between 45% and 81% of patients required X-ray imaging, 7% to 22% required computerized tomography and 12% to 20% required ultrasound Focused Assessment with Sonography for Trauma (FAST). A recent assessment of civilian victims of improvised explosive devices (IEDs) treated at a modern US military trauma hospital in Iraq found a much higher rate of imaging used. Almost half of the injuries found on computerized tomography were clinically relevant, and the computerized tomography results played a key role in determining the treatment of victims of explosive MCIs (Raja *et al*., 2010).

Fragment injuries commonly involve flying pieces of metal and glass fragments and can be extremely difficult to evaluate on external physical examination. The role of radiology is not only to identify all of the possible flying fragments, but also to help surgeons decide which fragments need to be removed during thorough surgical debridement (all foreign debris removed needs to be preserved for forensic purposes) (Hare *et al.*, 2007). All bony fragments should be removed because of the high risk of infection associated with them but, while all penetrating missile wounds should be thoroughly explored, not all other foreign material needs to be removed. The decision on whether to leave fragments or pursue them depends on accessibility of the fragments, and risk of damage to the surrounding structures during surgery, compared with the risk of infection secondary to skin or clothing, which enters tissue cavities with flying fragments (Spalding *et al.*, 1991).

Experts believe that computerized tomography imaging is the most important radiological tool available for the evaluation of explosive MCI victims, because explosive blasts produce concussive forces that can cause blunt organ injury without any external evidence (Wolf *et al.*, 2009). Hirshberg suggested that the increasing need for diagnostic computerized tomography will make imaging the main bottleneck of patient management during MCIs (Hirshberg *et al.*, 1999). In the Madrid bombings 75 helical computerized tomography scans were done by the end of the day, together with a magnetic resonance imaging (MRI) scan. The abundance of metallic shrapnel precluded a more frequent use of MRI during the first 24 h, and removal of metallic fragments in order to allow MRI to be done to assess a spinal cord injury is a theoretical possibility (Turégano *et al.*, 2008a).

The use of ultrasound FAST for the evaluation of explosive MCI victims is well documented. Although only 12% (63/512) of patients from the Madrid bombings and 12% (102/849) of patients from a series of MCIs treated by Israeli physicians during the second Lebanon War had ultrasound examinations (Gutierrez de Ceballos *et al.*, 2005; Beck-Razi *et al.*, 2007; Turégano *et al.*, 2008a,b), 30% (8/27) of patients from the London Underground bombings were evaluated using bedside ultrasound. A radiologist should be stationed in the major trauma bays to perform FAST to exclude free abdominal fluid or haemodynamically significant abdominal injury (Hare *et al.*, 2007). Extensive and successful ultrasonographic examination was recently reported after the Wenchuan earthquake, without false positive results and a false negative rate of only 5.6% (5 of 89 victims), and it is thought to have played a great role in the management of the victims (Dan *et al.*, 2010). Having said that, FAST is time-consuming and should be prioritized first to workup of unstable patients who could be suffering from significant intra-abdominal haemorrhage. Stable patients suffering from multiple penetrating injuries are best assessed with computerized tomography. In this later group, FAST may aid identify those patients with intra-abdominal injury, information that may lead one to prioritize computerized tomography imaging of these over others.

The role of mandatory chest X-ray is questionable in the setting of MCI, even following an explosion. Patients suffering from BLI manifest early with dyspnoea, haemoptysis or frank hypoxic respiratory failure (Pizov *et al.*, 1999). Patients who are stable and suffer none of these symptoms can be discharged following 4–6 h of observation without imaging (Alfici *et al.*, 2006).

Operating theatres

In a report from the Israeli Trauma Group data were collected from 325 casualties who were either admitted or died in all six level 1 trauma centres following injury in 32 MCIs from suicide bombings (1 October 2000 to 30 June 2003). A total of 34% of casualties had an ISS > 16, operative procedures were performed on 60% of patients and 36% were transferred directly from the emergency department to the OR. A third of the patients were admitted to ICUs, often (31%) directly from the emergency department. Anaesthesiologists, general, thoracic and vascular surgeons were in immediate demand, and most patients operated on within the first 2 h required multidisciplinary teams. Demand for orthopaedic and plastic surgery and anaesthesiology services continued for > 24 h. The authors warn that caution should nevertheless be exercised in extrapolating the findings of that study to different scenarios (Einav *et al.*, 2006b). In the Madrid bombings 124 major surgical interventions were performed on 82 casualties during the first 24 h at the seven hospitals that received most of the victims. In contrast to the Israeli Trauma Group experience with victims of suicide bombings, there was almost no need for thoracic and little need for vascular procedures, whereas orthopaedic, general-abdominal, plastic, maxillofacial and neurosurgery specialists were actively involved in OR procedures from early on. In only about 20% of the patients was the reason for early or immediate intervention a life-threatening problem, mainly intra-abdominal bleeding, intracranial haematoma and extensive extremity trauma with multiple bleeding sites. The large size of the closest hospitals and the early hour of the blasts allowed for a large number of empty ORs waiting for the scheduled cases of the day (Gutierrez de Ceballos *et al.*, 2005; Turégano *et al.*, 2008a,b).

Evaluation of patients admitted to one regional hospital in Israel that responded to over 20 MCIs following terror attacks reveals that 69 (13%) of 532 underwent operations (Ashkenazi, unpublished data). The discrepancy between these data and Einav *et al.*'s data detailed above can be explained by different patterns of transfer between level 1 trauma centres and level 2 trauma centres following MCIs. Need for operation for each patient was classified as follows:

1. Immediate – patient unstable and needs an immediate life-saving operation: for haemodynamic shock, significant external bleeding that cannot be controlled with non-surgical means and neurosurgical patients with anisocuria.
2. Urgent – patient stable but needs to be operated on as soon as possible (in less than 2 h) since if not operated on there is a good probability that he/she will become unstable: patient with signs of active bleeding but responsive to fluids, stable neurosurgical patient with significant pathology in need of surgery.
3. High priority – patient is stable but needs to be operated on within 2–4 h to avoid untoward complications: patients with penetrating injury to the trunk leading to gastrointestinal perforations.
4. Delayed – stable patients who can wait 4–12 h before being operated such as orthopaedic patients in need of debridement of soft tissue and fracture fixation of long bones, suture of eye-globe perforation.
5. Non-urgent – stable patients who can wait > 12 h before being operated on without untoward complications, such as removal of foreign bodies, fracture fixation of small bones.

Escharotomies for circumferential burns were judged as being either immediate, urgent or high priority on a case by case basis. The data for patients known to have undergone surgery are presented in Table 15.1.

Table 15.1. Data pertaining to 69 patients known to have undergone surgery.

Classification of patient	Number of patients
Immediate	14 (20%)
Urgent	10 (14%)
High priority	5 (7%)
Delayed	28 (41%)
Non-urgent	12 (17%)

According to these data, operations need to be prioritized according to urgency. Of 532 patients, there were 11 (2.1%) victims in extremis, 45 (8.5%) were severely injured, 44 (8.3%) were moderately injured and 432 (81.2%) were mildly injured. Twenty four (4.9%) patients needed an operation within 2 h of their arrival. Five (0.9%) other patients could be delayed a little but should have been operated on within 4 h. The rest could wait till the first wave of operations has finished.

In a survey of 60 hospital physicians selected for their experience in terrorist multiple-casualty incidents, Einav states that some ethical dilemmas should be addressed in the future. These dilemmas include the treatment of patients who are already anaesthetized but in whom surgery has not yet commenced at the time of the MCI, the option of shortening operative procedures already underway, guidelines for patient transfer from the PACU and the ICU to evacuate beds for arriving injured patients, and recommendations for continuous monitoring and treatment of these patients. They advise that anaesthetized patients who are not considered high risk for anaesthesia and who are about to undergo elective procedures should emerge from anaesthesia and be extubated until it is possible to proceed with elective surgery without endangering patients who may lose life or limb because of insufficient resources. Surgery for anaesthetized patients who are considered a high anaesthesia risk or who are scheduled for semi-emergent procedures should proceed. Patients already undergoing surgery at the time of the MCI should not undergo a truncated procedure but rather the procedure that is considered optimal for the patient by the operating surgeon regardless of the MCI. ICU facilities should be expanded into the PACU and even into the OR if necessary, rather than transferring critically ill patients from a monitored to an unsafe environment (Einav *et al.*, 2006a).

ICU beds

The victims of terror bombings tend to be young, arriving in the emergency department with a low GCS and hypotension. They are injured in multiple body regions and have a high ISS. As a result, the rate of surgical interventions is high, as is the need for ICU admission. The mortality is higher, and the ICU length of stay and hospital length of stay are longer than with other trauma victims. The large retrospective study by Kluger and colleagues was the first to show the different patterns of injury inflicted by terror bombings (Kluger *et al.*, 2004). St Vincent's hospital in New York reported that it needed nine beds (11.5% of hospitalized patients) over the first 24 h, eight of them ventilated (Kirschenbaum *et al.*, 2005). This number is low because the World Trade Center disaster was of a different category: a building collapse. In Jerusalem, 49% of hospitalized victims needed ICU care (Aschkenasy-Steuer *et al.*, 2005). In the Madrid bombings there were 78 patients admitted to ICUs (15%) and their ISSs varied from 11 to 75, with an average score of 29 (Turégano *et al.*, 2008a).

Intensivists have been provided with a rough preliminary tool to predict patients in need of ICU admission. It was found that following suicide bombings, specific external signs of trauma (penetrating head injury, skull fractures and burns) were associated with a high rate of BLI, although this is not the only reason for ICU admission (Almogy *et al.*, 2005). The PACU was found to be an excellent location for the care of patients in an unstable condition or receiving ventilation while awaiting surgery or an ICU bed (Shamir *et al.*, 2005).

Liberal use of ICU beds is probably unavoidable in MCIs because of diagnostic uncertainty in the initial phase of treatment. In the series of Avidan *et al.* the most common reason for ICU care was BLI. Of their patients presenting to the emergency department after an MCI, only 4.7% required ICU care. Seventy-three per cent of the ICU patients required mechanical ventilation (Avidan *et al.*, 2007). Early knowledge of the bomb location and number of survivors may help the ICU director estimate the need for ICU care, since it is known that closed space explosions are associated with a higher mortality rate and increased incidence of BLI (Leibovici *et al.*, 1996). In a recent report of a US trauma hospital in Iraq (Propper *et al.*, 2009) where they assess their MCIs following explosions in civilian settings, half of the transfused blood went to 8% of casualties, a finding consistent with that of an Israeli group in civilian casualties from MCIs (Soffer *et al.*, 2008). Their 50% ICU admission rate is significantly higher than the 4.3% of the Shaare Zedak Medical Center in Israel (Avidan *et al.*, 2007), although in the later study they include all walking wounded patients seen at the hospital.

Are we ready for MCIs?

In 2008, the House of Representatives in the USA conducted a survey of seven cities, five considered at highest risk for a terrorist strike, and compared it with the 2004 Madrid bombing. The survey occurred at a set time on 25 March 2008. The results of the survey demonstrated that none of the hospitals surveyed in the seven cities had enough emergency care capacity to respond to an attack like Madrid. In addition, more than half of the emergency departments in the level 1 trauma centres were operating above capacity; in Los Angeles three of five hospitals were on diversion; in Washington, DC there were no available emergency department spaces at two level 1 trauma centres, none of the trauma centres had enough critical care capacity or regular in-patient beds, and combined emergency department spaces from all seven cities was less than the number treated at a single Madrid hospital (Nager and Khanna, 2009). Nevertheless, we should not forget that in Madrid the bombings occurred shortly before the start of a midweek workday, when most clinicians and medical personnel were on their way to work or already in the hospital, and night shifts were still on duty. This, together with empty ORs and personnel waiting for the first scheduled cases, proved decisive for the adequacy of the medical and surgical response at the closest hospital. Had the blasts occurred just 1 h later, the whole situation would have been much worse and very difficult to handle (Gutierrez de Ceballos *et al.*, 2005).

In 2007, the United States Department of Health and Human Services and the Centers for Disease Control and Prevention outlined the concerns imposed regarding SC from a terrorist bombing. The healthcare system, emergency departments and ICUs of acute care hospitals are chronically overcrowded and resource-strained. Emergency departments divert ambulances, at times up to 50%, and personnel shortages for nurses and physicians in certain regions, do not fulfil usual daily demands. In addition, three-quarters of hospitals had disaster plans that addressed explosives, but simulated explosives were only found in one in five of disaster drills or practice sessions (Sasser *et al.*, 2007).

A survey of the National Foundation for Trauma Care (NFTC) on the US trauma centres' preparation for a terrorist attack in the community was recently reported (Trunkey, 2009). The survey was answered by 33% (175) of all level I and level II trauma centres. A high level of preparation for an MCI was already in place in many leading trauma hospitals, but further attention to specific areas is needed, like in sustainability of the response (operating at maximum capacity for over 72 h), family care plan for children of injured patients or staff, or special populations (children, pregnant women, psuchiatric patients, disabled, obese patients), and several suggestions have been made to improve preparedness.

From a trauma care perspective, the ultimate success or failure of hospital deployment for an MCI hinges on the coordinated action of a small core of key individuals (Hirshberg *et al.*, 2001). A core group consisting of a command physician, a triage officer and the charge nurse is the true engine behind the medical effort. Perhaps the most effective method to train this core group in the decision-making skills required is the simulated war game, a method akin to a military tabletop exercise. This war game, pioneered by Professor Sten Lennquist of the University of Linköping in Sweden, is aimed at pivotal decision makers (Ergo-Train system, 2001).

Conclusion

An effective triage at the entrance to the emergency department is the key in the management of the MCI, and should be flexible and variable according to the caseload and available resources. In small-scale MCIs a one-step binary triage system is all that is needed, but in a large-scale MCI a two-step binary triage should be adopted. Attention should be directed to the potential bottlenecks to the flow of casualties, and appropriate measures should be taken to increase the SC of the receiving institution.

The best way to be prepared for a large-scale MCI is to have an integrated trauma system, practical and detailed hospital disaster plans and professionals who are knowledgeable in the specifics of disaster medicine.

References

Alfici, R., Ashkenazi, I. and Kessel, B. (2006) Management of victims in a mass casualty incident caused by terrorist bombing: treatment algorithms for stable, unstable and in-extremis victims. *Military Medicine* 171, 1155–1162.

Almogy, G. and Rivkind, A.I. (2006) Surgical lessons learned from suicide bombing attacks. *Journal of the American College of Surgeons* 202(2), 313–319.

Almogy, G., Belzberg, H., Minz, Y., Pikarsky, A.K., Zamir, G. and Rivkind, A.I. (2004) Suicide bombing attacks: update and modification of the protocol. *Annals of Surgery* 239, 295–303.

Almogy, G., Luria, T., Richter, E., Pizov, R., Bdolah-Abram, T., Mintz, Y., Zamir, G. and Rivkind, A.I. (2005) Can external signs of trauma guide management? Lessons learned from suicide bombing attacks in Israel. *Archives of Surgery* 140, 390–393.

Aschkenasy-Steuer, G., Shamir, M., Rivkind, A., Mosheiff, R., Shushan, Y., Rosenthal, G., Mintz, Y., Weissman, C., Sprung, C.L. and Weiss, Y.G. (2005) The Israeli experience: conventional terrorism and critical care. *Critical Care* 9, 490–499.

Ashkenazi, I., Kessel, B., Khashan, B., Haspel, J., Oren, M., Olsha, O. and Alfici, R. (2006) Precision of in-hospital triage in mass-casualty incidents after terror attacks. *Prehospital Disaster Medicine* 21, 20–23.

Ashkenazi, I., Kessel, B., Olsha, O., Khashan, B., Oren, M., Haspel, J. and Alfici, R. (2008) Defining the problem, main objective, and strategies of medical management in mass casualty incidents caused by terrorist events. *Prehospital Disaster Medicine* 23, 82–89.

Auf der Heide, E. (2006) The importance of evidence-based disaster planning. *Annals of Emergency Medicine* 47, 34–49.

Avidan, V., Hersch, M., Spira, R.M., Einav, S.H., Goldberg, S. and Schechter, W. (2007) Civilian hospital response to a mass casualty event: the role of the intensive care unit. *Journal of Trauma* 62, 1234–1239.

Aylwin, C.J., Konig, T.C., Brennan, N.W., Shirley, P.J., Davies, G., Walsh, M.S. and Brohi, K. (2006) Reduction in critical mortality in urban mass casualty incidents: analysis of triage, surge, and resource use after the London bombings on July 7, 2005. *Lancet* 368, 2219–2225.

Beck-Razi, N., Fischer, D., Mickaelson, M., Engel, A. and Gaitini, D. (2007) The utility of focused assessment with sonography for trauma as a triage tool in multiple-casualty incidents during the second Lebanon war. *Journal of Ultrasound Medicine* 26, 1149–1156.

Benjaminov, O., Sklair-Levy, M., Rivkind, A., Cohen, M., Bar-Tal, G. and Stein, M. (2006) Role of radiology in evaluation of terror attack victims. *American Journal of Roentgenology* 187, 609–616.

Committee on Trauma (2003) American College of Surgeons Statement on disaster and mass casualty management. *Journal of the American College of Surgeons* 197, 855–856.

Cushman, J.G., Pachter, H.L. and Beaton, H.L. (2003) Two New York city hospital's surgical response to the September 11, 2001, terrorist attack in New York City. *The Journal of Trauma* 54, 147–155.

Dan, D., Mingsong, L., Jie, T., Xiaobo, W., Zhong, C., Yan, L., Xiaojin, L. and Ming, C. (2010) Ultrasonographic applications after mass casualty incident caused by Wenchuan earthquake. *Journal of Trauma* 68, 1417–1420.

De Boer, J. (1999) Order in chaos: modelling medical management in disasters. *European Journal of Emergency Medicine* 6, 141–148.

Deshpande, A.A., Mehta, S. and Kshirsagar, N.A. (2007) Hospital management of Mumbay train blast victims. *The Lancet* 369, 639–640.

Einav, S., Spira, R.M., Hersh, M., Reissman, P. and Schechter, W. (2006a) Surgeon and hospital leadership during terrorist-related multiple-casualty event. *Archives of Surgery* 141, 815–822.

Einav, S., Aharonson-Daniel, L., Weissman, C., Freund, H.R., Peleg, K. and the Israeli Trauma Group (2006b) In-hospital resource utilization during multiple casualty incidents. *Annals of Surgery* 243, 533–540.

Einav, S., Schechter, W.P., Matot, I., Horn, J.K., Hersch, M., Reissman, P., Spira, R.M. (2009) Case managers in mass casualty incidents. *Annals of Surgery* 249, 496–501.

Ergo-Train system (2001) Available at: http://emergotrain.com.

Frykberg, E.R. (2002) Medical management of disasters and mass casualties from terrorist bombings: how can we cope? *Journal of Trauma* 53, 201–212.

Frykberg, E.R. and Tepas, J.J. (1988) Terrorist bombings: lessons learned from Belfast to Beirut. *Annals of Surgery* 208, 569–576.

Frykberg, E.R., Tepas, J.J. and Alexander, R.H. (1989) The 1983 Beirut airport terrorist bombing. Injury patterns and implications for disaster management. *The American Surgeon* 55, 134–141.

Gutierrez de Ceballos, J.P., Turégano, F., Pérez-Díaz, D., Sanz Sanchez, M., Martin Llorente, C. and Guerrero Sanz, J.E. (2005) Casualties treated at the closest hospital in the Madrid, March 11, terrorist bombings. *Critical Care Medicine* 33, S107–S112.

Hare, S.S., Goddard, I., Ward, P., Naraghi, A. and Dick, E.A. (2007) The radiological management of bomb blast injury. *Clinical Radiology* 62, 1–9.

Hirshberg, A., Stein, M. and Walden, R. (1999) Surgical resource utilization in urban terrorist bombings: a computer simulation. *Journal of Trauma* 47, 545–550.

Hirshberg, A., Holcomb, J.B. and Mattox, K.L. (2001) Hospital trauma care in multiple-casualty incidents: a critical review. *Annals of Emergency Medicine* 37, 647–652.

Hirshberg, A., Scott, B.G., Granchi, T., Wall, M.J., Mattox, K.L. and Stein, M. (2005) How does casualty load affect trauma care in urban bombing incidents? A quantitative analysis. *Journal of Trauma* 58, 686–695.

Hirshberg, A., Frykberg, E.R., Mattox, K.L. and Stein, M. (2010) Triage and trauma workload in mass casualty: a computer model. *Journal of Trauma* 69, 1074–1082.

Hogan, D.E., Waeckerle, J.F., Dire, D.J. and Lillibridge, S.R. (1999) Emergency department impact of the Oklahoma City terrorist bombing. *Annals of Emergency Medicine* 34, 160–167.

Hupert, N., Hollingsworth, E. and Xiong, W. (2007) Is overtriage associated with increased mortality? Insights from a simulation model of mass casualty trauma care. *Disaster Medicine Public Health Preparedness* 1(Suppl. 1), S14–S24.

Kennedy, K., Aghababian, R.V., Gans, L. and Lewis, C.P. (1996) Triage: techniques and applications in decision making. *Annals of Emergency Medicine* 28, 136–144.

King, B. and Jatoi, I. (2005) The mobile army surgical hospital (MASH): a military and surgical legacy. *Journal of the National Medical Association* 97, 648–656.

Kirschenbaum, L., Keene, A., O'Neill, P., Westfal, R. and Astiz, M.E. (2005) The experience at St. Vincent's Hospital, Manhattan, on September 11, 2001: preparedness, response, and lessons learned. *Critical Care Medicine* 33(Suppl.), S48–S52.

Klausner, J.M. and Rozin, R.R. (1986) The evacuation hospital in civilian disasters. *Israeli Journal of Medical Sciences* 22, 365–369.

Kluger, Y., Peleg, K., Daniel-Aharonson, L., Mayo, A. and Israeli Trauma Group (2004) The especial injury pattern in terrorist bombings. *Journal of the American College of Surgeons* 199, 875–879.

Kosashvili, Y., Daniel, L.A., Peleg, K., Horowitz, A., Laor, D. and Blumenfeld, A. (2009) Israel hospital preparedness for terrorism-related multiple casualty incidents: can the surge capacity and injury severity distribution be better predicted? *Injury* 40, 727–731.

Leibovici, D., Gofrit, O.N., Stein, M., Shapira, S.C., Noga, Y., Heruti, R.J. and Shemer, J. (1996) Blast injuries: bus versus open-air bombing – a comparative study of injuries in survivors of open-air versus confined-space explosions. *Journal of Trauma* 41, 1030–1035.

Martí, M., Parrón, M., Baudraxler, F., Royo, A., Gómez-León, N. and Alvarez-Sala, R. (2006) Blast injuries from Madrid terrorist bombing attacks. *Emergency Radiology* 13, 113–122.

Meredith, W., Rutledge, R. and Hansen, A.R. (1995) Field triage of trauma patients based upon the ability to follow commands: a study in 29,573 injured patients. *Journal of Trauma* 38, 129–135.

Michaelson, M., Olin, N. and Hyams, G. (2003) Preparedness for mass casualty situations – the key to success. In: Shemer, J. and Shoenfeld, Y. (eds) *Terror and Medicine*. PABST Science Publisher, Lengerich, pp. 359–360.

Nager, A.L. and Khanna, K. (2009) Emergency department surge: models and practical implications. *Journal of Trauma* 67, S96–S99.

Njenga, F.G., Nicholls, P.J., Nyamai, C., Kigamwa, P. and Davidson, J.R. (2004) Post-traumatic stress after terrorist attack: psychological reactions following the US embassy bombing in Nairobi: naturalistic study. *British Journal of Psychiatry* 185, 328–333.

Palmer, D.J., Stephens, D., Fisher, D.A., Spain, B., Read, D.J. and Notaras, L. (2003) The Bali bombing: the Royal Darwin Hospital response. *The Medical Journal of Australia* 179, 358–361.

Peleg, K., Aharonson-Daniel, L., Stein, M., Michaelson, M., Kluger, Y., Simon, D., Noji, E.K. and Israeli Trauma group (ITG) (2004) Gunshot and explosion injuries: characteristics, outcomes, and implications for care of terror-related injuries in Israel. *Annals of Surgery* 239, 311–318.

Pizov, R., Oppenheim-Eden, A., Matot, I., Weiss, Y.G., Eidelman, L.A., Rivkind, A.I. and Sprung, C.L. (1999) Blast lung injury from an explosion on a civilian bus. *Chest* 115, 165–172.

Propper, B.W., Rasmussen, T.E., Davidson, S.B., Vandenberg, S.L., Clouse, W.D., Burkhardt, G.E., Gifford, S.M. and Johannigman, J.A. (2009) Surgical response to multiple casualty incidents following single explosive events. *Annals of Surgery* 250, 311–315.

Raja, A.S., Propper, B.W., Vandenberg, S.L., Matchette, M.W., Rasmussen, T.E., Johannigman, J.A. and Davidson, S.B. (2010) Imaging utilization during explosive multiple casualty incidents. *Journal of Trauma* 68, 1421–1424.

Rodoplu, U., Arnold, J.L., Yucel, T., Tokyay, R., Ersoy, G. and Cetiner, S. (2005) Impact of the terrorist bombings of the Hong Kong Shanghai Bank Corporation headquarters and the British Consulate on two hospitals in Istanbul, Turkey, in November 2003. *Journal of Trauma* 59, 195–201.

Rozin, R.R. and Kleinman, Y. (1987) Surgical priorities of abdominal wounded in a combat situation. *Journal of Trauma* 27, 656–660.

Sasser, S., Hunt, R., Bailey, B. *et al.* (2007) *In a Moment's Notice: Surge Capacity for Terrorist Bombings, Challenges and Proposed solutions.* US Department of Health and Human Services and the Centers for Disease Control and Prevention, Atlanta, Georgia, pp. 1–37.

Shamir, M.Y., Rivkind, A., Weissman, C., Sprung, C.L. and Weiss, Y.G. (2005) Conventional terrorist bomb incidents and the intensive care unit. *Current Opinion in Critical Care* 11, 580–584.

Soffer, D., Klausner, J., Bar-Zohar, D., Szold, O., Schulman, C.I., Halpern, P., Shimonov, A., Hareuveni, M. and Ben-Tal, O. (2008) Usage of blood products in multiple-casualty incidents. The experience of a level I trauma center in Israel. *Archives of Surgery* 143, 983–989.

Spalding, T.J., Stewart, M.P., Tulloch, D.N. and Stephens, K.M. (1991) Penetrating missile injuries in the Gulf war 1991. *British Journal of Surgery* 78, 1102–1104.

Tadmor, B., McManus, J. and Koenig, K.L. (2006) The art and science of surge: experience from Israel and the U.S. Military. *Academic Emergency Medicine* 13, 1130–1134.

Trunkey, D.D. (2009) US Trauma Center preparation for a terrorist attack in the community. *European Journal of Trauma and Emergency Surgery* 35, 244–264.

Turégano, F., Caba-Doussoux, P., Jover-Navalon, J.M., Martín-Perez, E., Fernandez-Luengas, D., Diez-Valladares, L., Perez-Diaz, D., Yuste-Garcia, P., Guadalajara-Labajo, H., Rios-Blanco, R., Hernando-Trancho, F., Garcia-Moreno Nisa, F., Sanz-Sanchez, M., Garcia-Fuentes, C., Martinez-Virto, A., Leon-Baltasar, J.L. and Vazquea-Estevez, J. (2008a) Injury patterns from major urban terrorist bombings in trains: the Madrid experience. *World Journal of Surgery* 32, 1168–1175.

Turégano, F., Pérez-Diaz, D., Sanz-Sánchez, M. and Ortiz-Alonso, J. (2008b) Overall assessment of the response to terrorist bombings in trains, Madrid, 11 March 2004. *European Journal of Trauma and Emergency Surgery* 34, 433–441.

Umer, M., Sepah, Y.J., Shahpurwala, M.M. and Zafar, H. (2009) Suicide bombings: process of care of mass casualties in the developing world. *Disasters* 33, 809–821.

Wolf, S.J., Bebarta, V.S., Bonnett, C.J., Pons, P.T. and Cantrill, S.V. (2009) Blast injuries. *Lancet* 374, 405–415.

Chapter 16

Role of Military Hospitals in Handling Chemical and Biological Disasters

Mesut Ortatatli and Levent Kenar

General Characteristics of Chemical Weapons

The deliberate use of chemical toxic agents – so-called chemical weapons – and microbiological agents including bacteria, viruses, rickettsia and toxins has emerged as a significant threat especially in the past decades, mainly after the terrorist attack on 11 September 2011, and the use of these agents in future wars and terror attacks remains a realistic concern. Despite the fact that there are lots of conventions and agreements against the use of chem-bio weapons, they have been used in a number of wars and conflicts (Hu *et al.*, 1989; Kenar and Karayilanoglu, 2005b). Although death and disability with emotional stress are known immediate effects of these agents, there may also be long-term adverse effects as a result of exposure. In this chapter, we aim to give a summary of the effects of very well-known chem-bio agents and give guidance on medical management after exposure to these agents.

Chemical warfare agents are toxic chemical substances that can produce incapacitation, serious injury and death. They may be used in a battlefield, in a terrorist attack or in individual assassinations.

These chemical warfare agents can be classified based on their mechanism of action (Karayilanoglu *et al.*, 2003a; Kenar *et al.*, 2004):

- Nerve agents (tabun, sarin, soman, VX);
- Vesicants (sulphur mustard, lewisite);
- Choking agents (chlorine, phosgene);
- Cyanides (hydrogen and cyanogen chloride);
- Incapacitants (3-quinoclinidinyl benzoate-BZ, lysergic acid diethylamide (LSD));
- Riot control agents (lachrymators and vomiting agents);
- Herbicides (cacodylic acid, picloram).

Nerve agents

Organophosphorus nerve agents are chemically related to organophosphates used as pesticides. Nerve agents are classified as G agents (tabun GA, sarin GB, soman GD, GE and GF), which are relatively volatile, and V agents (VE, VG, VM, VX), which are more persistent. In battlefield conditions, nerve agents can be dispersed from missiles, rockets, bombs, spray tanks, land mines and any other munitions. Route of exposure has a major effect on the persistency of agents in the body. The greatest effect from volatile nerve gases like sarin is caused by inhalation of agent vapours or aerosols where absorption through the lungs occurs in few minutes. Low-volatility V-type agents are probably more effective but cutaneous exposure and several hours are required for absorption (Karayilanoglu *et al.*, 2003a; Cosar and Kenar, 2006).

Nerve agents phosphorylate and hence inactivate acetylcholinesterase (AChE) enzyme, which is responsible for the breakdown of neurotransmitters. Then, these neurotransmitters, mainly acetylcholine (ACh) accumulate at neural synapses in muscle and glandular tissues and in organs including the heart and skeletal muscles. The clinical effects following a nerve agent intoxication may occur in three defined stages (Karalliedde *et al.*, 2000; Sidell *et al.*, 2008).

1. Acute cholinergic phase occurs immediately after exposure and usually lasts 12–24 h. Main symptoms are due to muscarinic effects (tightness in chest, wheezing, cough, nausea, vomiting, diarrhoea, sweating, salivation, miosis, blurring of vision, urinary incontinence), nicotinic effects (muscle twitching, fasciculation, muscle weakness) and central nervous system effects including emotional lability, insomnia, confusion, drowsiness, slurred speech, convulsions, coma and death.
2. Intermediate syndrome may occur 1–4 days after the acute cholinergic phase. Difficulty in breathing may lead to respiratory failure following paralysis of the diaphragm. Following organophosphorus insecticide poisoning in humans, it has been reported that 10–30% of patients may develop intermediate syndrome.
3. Delayed polyneuropathy may be seen 7–14 days after exposure possibly due to the phosphorylation of neuropathy target esterase enzyme found in nerve tissue.

Other than the central nervous system effect, genotoxic and carcinogenic effects are reported. In addition, VX and sarin especially have the potential to produce fatal dysrhythmia (ventricular premature beats) in humans (Saadeh *et al.*, 1997).

Detection of nerve agent exposure

Signs and symptoms

Many individuals showing a group of signs and symptoms involving a feeling of tightness of constriction in the chest, unexplained runny nose, difficulty in breathing, small pinpoint size pupils, a slight sensation of pain in the eyes and frontal area should lead military doctors to suspect a nerve agent poisoning.

Determination of plasma and erythrocyte cholinesterase (ChE) activity is a guide of some value in detecting systemic absorption of a nerve agent and the persistency of its effects. Erythrocyte ChE and, to a lesser extent, plasma cholinesterase remain at a low level of activity long after symptoms disappear. As well as detecting nerve gas exposure, ChE determination is also valuable in patients undergoing surgery with succinylcholine, a muscle relaxant, in order to prevent prolonged neuromuscular blockade and apnoea, and to confirm neural tube defects with increased amniotic α-fetoprotein. A decrease of 50–75% in ChE activity should be taken as a life-threatening threshold in clinical practice. So, a military hospital should have an analytical laboratory capable of studying ChE measurements for variable clinical and chemical incidents. The spectrophotometrical Ellman method is commonly used, in which propionylthiocholine or acetylthiocholine as a substrate is measured at 410 nm. It should be mentioned here, however, that determination of ACh in red blood cells is a more analytically and clinically sensitive indicator when comparing the value of enzymes in plasma after acute exposure to nerve agents (Jortani *et al.*, 2000; Kenar and Karayilanoglu, 2005a).

Detectors and analytical measures

Since one of the main tasks of a military hospital is to provide medical management of patients or casualties exposed to chem-bio weapons, it should possess all detection and identification methods for diagnosing nerve agent exposure. Detectors including paper detectors and handheld chemical agent monitors (CAM) can be used in the field and pre-hospital area by any health staff for detecting agents in vapour and in liquid forms, respectively. Assaying of biomedical samples cannot identify the nerve agent itself and instead measure the concentrations of its metabolites since nerve agents decompose and hydrolyse spontaneously in the body with alkylmethylphosphonic acids as primary metabolic products. This serves as a kind of biomarker of nerve agent exposure. Chromatographic methods such as high-performance liquid chromatography (HPLC), gas chromatography–mass spectrometry (GC-MS) and liquid chromatography–mass spectrometry (LC-MS) may be used to monitor the presence and levels of metabolites in large hospital laboratories in the lab network. Meanwhile, a laminair flow head should be set up in a laboratory analysing chem-bio exposure to provide a safe place to study any suspected material that gives off dangerous vapours (Driskell *et al.*, 2002; Karayilanoglu *et al.*, 2003b).

Medical management and treatment of nerve agent casualties

Self-protection

Military health personnel must not forget that the first and most important concept in the medical management of nerve agent casualties is to protect themselves. Although liquid contaminated casualties are unlikely to present directly to the hospital emergency department prior to decontamination by emergency responders, medical personnel should always protect themselves. Whenever possible, areas of liquid contamination should be decontaminated prior to patient handling to minimize spread of contamination and cross-contamination of other providers.

Decontamination

In the immediate aftermath of the sarin nerve agent attack in Tokyo, over 650 patients presented to St Luke's Hospital within several hours after the release of sarin. With high numbers of vapour-exposed patients presenting to a medical facility under these conditions, minimum decontamination should include removal of patients' clothing. This will hopefully prevent secondary chemical exposure of hospital personnel due to vapour offgassing. If the patient has been exposed to liquid nerve agent (such as spraying or an explosion), survivors will require complete decontamination of skin and hair with water, soap and water, and a water rinse at the incident site prior to evacuation. Patients arriving at the emergency department with an unclear exposure history who are symptomatic from nerve agent exposure should be fully decontaminated as above before entering treatment areas (Okumura *et al.*, 1998; Baysallar and Kenar, 2006).

Airway and ventilation

Establishment of an airway is essential for the survival of the severely exposed patient. Severely intoxicated patients will die if aggressive airway management is not rapidly available. With large numbers of victims, rapid scene and resource assessment will influence triage decisions regarding interventional therapy. Because of the intense bronchoconstriction and secretions associated with nerve agent exposure, effective ventilation may not be initially possible due to high airway resistance. Adequate atropinization will reverse muscarinic effects; therefore, atropine should be administered before any other measures are attempted. Endotracheal intubation, followed by positive pressure ventilation with a bag valve mask, should be performed as quickly as possible. Periodic suctioning of secretions will help to improve ventilation and air exchange. Patients with seizures and respiratory failure can be rescued with immediate and adequate intervention (Karayilanoglu *et al.*, 2003b; Cosar and Kenar, 2006).

Antidote administration

Standard therapy consists of the administration of anticholinergics, reactivators of AChE, anticonvulsants and pretreatment with reversible enzyme blockers. Type of these treatment vehicles may be different according to country structures and conditions. For example, in the Turkish army, only atropine as an anticholinergic, obidoxime as a reactivator, diazepam as an anticonvulsive drug and pyridostigmine bromide as a pre-treatment medicine are still in use. The general indications for use of these antidotes will be presented first, followed by a discussion of their use in the treatment of nerve agent intoxication (Bajgar, 2004).

Atropine

Atropine works by blocking the effect of the accumulated neurotransmitter, ACh, at muscarinic sites. The more ACh at the sites, the more atropine is required to counteract its effects. Atropine can be administered intravenously (IV), intramuscularly (IM) or endotracheally (ET). Parenteral atropine will reverse muscarinic effects such as rhinorrhoea, salivation, sweating, bronchoconstriction, bronchorrhoea, nausea, vomiting and diarrhoea. The IV route of atropine administration is preferred but it can also be given IM or intrathecally, but only until IV access is established. The initial parenteral dose of atropine is 2–6 mg in adults, with subsequent doses titrated to the severity of the nerve agent signs and symptoms. Treatment for chemical nerve agent exposure might require up to 40 mg of atropine. Patients poisoned with insecticides may require large doses; over 1000 mg of atropine has been used to treat insecticide poisoning. When atropine therapy exceeds the amount necessary to reverse the effect of the cholinergic hyperstimulation, it may cause toxicity manifested by dry mouth, flushing and diminished sweating, but this would be extremely unlikely in a patient poisoned by an organophosphate (OP) compound including nerve agents. Side-effects in unexposed people include mydriasis, blurred vision, tachycardia and diminished secretions. Atropine dosing is guided by the patient's clinical presentation and should be given until secretions are dry or drying and ventilation becomes less laboured. When shortness of breath, increased airway resistance and secretions are reduced and the patient is breathing more easily, it should be considered that he or she has received enough atropine. It should be noted here that heart rate and pupillary size, which are ordinarily accurate reflections of atropine dosing, are not useful for clinical monitoring after nerve agent exposure. Atropine cannot reverse nicotinic effects such as fasciculations, twitching or muscle weakness (Karayilanoglu *et al.*, 2003a; Cannard, 2006).

AChE reactivators

Also known as oximes, these antidotes work as nucleophilic agents that specifically break the chemical bond between the nerve agent and the enzyme AChE and thus restore the activity of the inhibited enzyme and re-establish its physiological activity by removing the agent. In practice, this will therapeutically decrease muscle twitching, improve muscle strength and allow the patient to breathe more easily. The bond between the phosphorylated enzyme and the nerve agent can 'age', that is, monophosphoric acid residue bound to enzyme protein is generated and the enzyme and agent complex become irreversibly bound. This means that if the antidote is not administered within 5 h of sarin exposure (meaning the ageing time for the sarin–enzyme complex is between 4 and 6 h) or within about 40 h after VX or tabun exposure, the bond becomes permanent. Usually, there is a comfortable time for medical staff to treat patients with oximes after exposure, with the exception of soman (GD) where the soman–enzyme complex can age in about 2 min. Since pralidoxime takes time to become effective, atropine administration should be the first priority (Kenar and Karayilanoglu 2005a; Marrs *et al.*, 2006).

Atropine-obidoxim autoinjector kit

In the Turkish army, an autoinjector for nerve agent treatment is provided by Military Drug Factory, which includes 2 mg of atropine sulphate and 200 mg obidoxime chloride. The atropine autoinjector content is administered IM by pressing the end of the device on to the thigh. A spring pushes the needle into the muscle and causes the atropine to be injected. This device causes atropine to be absorbed more rapidly than when administered by a conventional needle and syringe (Karayilanoglu *et al.*, 2003a).

Diazepam

Seizures are treated with benzodiazepines such as diazepam. These medications can be used IV or via an autoinjector that contains 10 mg of diazepam. Some authorities recommend treating all severely exposed patients with diazepam whether they are convulsing or not. If three atropine autoinjectors kits are required initially, because of the victim's clinical presentation, diazepam should be administered immediately thereafter (Kenar and Karayilanoglu, 2005a).

Pre-treatment

Pyridostigmine bromide, a carbamate derivative, occupies the active site of AChE and reversibly carbamylates the enzyme protein, thus preventing binding of the agent and enzyme if there is any exposure to nerve agents in the near future. Treatment of soman intoxicated victims is facilitated and the outcome is improved in pre-treated victims of this type of nerve agent. Pyridostigmine bromide tablets of 30 mg are recommended for prophylaxis every 8 h for a week. Side-effects including nausea, vomiting, coordination disorder, intestinal spasm, bradycardia and myosis should be noted here for operational purposes (Kenar and Karayilanoglu, 2005a).

Vesicants

These are so-called because of the vesicles (blisters) they cause on the skin. Vesicants include sulphur mustard, HD, nitrogen mustard and lewisite. Sulphur mustard (2,2-di(chloroethyl) sulphide) is chemically and toxicologically similar to nitrogen mustard, which is a cytotoxic and anti-tumoral agent (Karayilanoglu *et al.*, 2003a; Kenar *et al.*, 2005).

Sulphur mustard (SM)

SM has a long-lasting effect and incapacitates rather than kills living organisms. Since it is an oily volatile liquid with low solubility in water, it can easily penetrate through the skin within 30 min of exposure. In vapour form, it is also absorbed through the skin; nearly 20% of the total agent penetrates inside the skin and the rest goes through the systemic absorption. It is a strong alkylating agent and reacts with –SH, amino, carboxy, hydroxyl and primary phosphate groups found in DNA and other macromolecules by binding irreversibly. This mechanism may lead to the development of cytostatic, mutagenic and cytotoxic effects of chronic duration. Other than DNA alkylation, various glycolytic enzymes may be inhibited and cause impairment in glucose uptake. This cellular damage negatively affects basal cell proliferation causing separation of the epidermis from the dermis leading to blister generation. Energy metabolism is also deteriorated and anaerobic glycolysis predominates in severe intoxication with a mustard agent. Most studies in this area have focused on SM as opposed to other chemical agents (Dacre and Goldman, 1996; Kenar *et al.*, 2006).

Depending on the magnitude of exposure to mustard gas there can be a latent period of more than 2 h. SM has acute effects mainly on the respiratory system, skin and eyes. Any local contact with SM vapours or liquids may initiate erythema formation and give rise to oedema, ulceration and finally necrosis of the skin tissue. Typical vesicles appear about 18 h after contamination and large painless blisters are formed, which are pendulous and full of clear yellow fluid. As the exposure proceeds or remains untreated, the casualties begin coughing, expectorating and undergoing changes in skin pigmentation followed by the collapse of vesicles and necrosis, and eschar formation within 72 h. Profound burns due to mustard gas may cause full thickness skin loss on the penis, scrotum, axilla and areas where tight dressings are worn. Respiratory symptoms including severe coughing, a prulent sputum, rhinorrhoea, epistaxis, dyspnoea and mechanical airway obstruction due to pseudomembranes of inflammatory necrosis may be observed. Death can occur owing to respiratory failure or secondary bacterial pneumonia, which stimulates bone marrow depression (Karayilanoglu *et al.*, 2003a; Hurst *et al.*, 2008).

Eyes, the most sensitive organ to SM vapours, show symptoms varying in severity from reddening, conjunctival irritation, eye pain, photophobia and blepharospasm to corneal perforation, panophtalmitis and permanent blindness. Systemic absorption may cause bone marrow depression giving rise to agranulocytosis, neutropenia, thrombocytopenia and lymphopenia and suppression of the immune system (Safarinejad *et al.*, 2001; Kenar and Karayilanoglu, 2005a).

For diagnosis of SM casualties, other than the signs and symptoms mentioned, on-site detection with handheld detectors or paper detectors is available. Laboratory identification consists specifically of the analysis of SM and its degradation products, mainly thiodyglycol in urine samples by using chromatographic techniques (GC-MS or capillary GC-MS) with very low detection limits. SM adducts formed by alkylation of haemoglobin, serum albumin and DNA have also recently been identified as potential biomarkers for chronic exposure to vesicants (Black *et al.*, 1997; Kenar and Alp, 2011).

Medical management and treatment for a mustard gas casualty requires prompt and extensive decontamination, and supportive and symptomatic care including burn treatment, use of systemic analgesics and antipruritics, maintenance of fluid and electrolyte balance and oxygen support. For decontamination, removal of clothing and the use of copious amounts of water with liquid soap and drying should be carried out within the first 5 min. If possible it should be confirmed with detectors that the patient is thoroughly decontaminated before he or she is accepted to emergency room and hospital services. Dakin solution, chloramine-T solution, 1% silver sulphadiazine and aluminium silicate powders can be used as topical cleaners. Mucous membranes and eyes should be rinsed with saline or isotonic sodium bicarbonate along with water. For skin decontamination, Fuller's earth and hypochloride solutions followed by washing with abundant amounts of water is strongly recommended (Kenar and Karayilanoglu, 2004a; Kenar *et al.*, 2004).

For the treatment of pulmonary symptoms, a wide spectrum of management methods involving steam inhalation, cough suppressants, bronchodilators and steroids should be considered. Intubation is to be performed before laryngeal spasm or oedema occurs. Sometimes early use of positive end-expiratory pressure (PEEP) or continuous positive airway pressure (CPAP) may be beneficial (Kenar and Karayilanoglu, 2005a).

What is important for military hospitals is that traumatic wounds contaminated with mustard gas or any chemical warfare agent (CWA) following the release of vapour or liquid droplets from a chemical storage cylinders or their dispersal via aerial sprays, chemical bombs or mortar shells should be treated with isotonic sodium bicarbonate or 0.5% hypochlorite solution irrigation and lavage. This will prevent or minimize surgical team exposure while treatment is conducted. The main goals from a surgical perspective are to control haemorrhage and contamination and to correct the lethal triad of hypothermia, acidosis and coagulopathy (Graham *et al.*, 2008).

Lewisite

Lewisite, a vesicant damaging the eyes, skin and airways by direct contact, is an oily colourless liquid with a geranium-like odour. It is more volatile than mustard gas and decomposes in liquid solutions. It is readily absorbed from the skin, eyes and respiratory tract, as well as by ingestion and via wounds (Kenar and Karayilanoglu, 2005a; Hurst *et al.*, 2008).

It has been alleged that lewisite inhibits enzymes carrying –SH (thiol) groups such as pyruvic oxidase, alcohol dehydrogenase, succinic oxidase and hexokinase. In fact, the exact mechanism of cellular damage by lewisite has not been fully determined. Another main factor is the inactivation of carbohydrate metabolism due to the inhibition of the pyruvate dehydrogenase complex, thus causing pyruvate to be shunted to lactic acidosis, which inhibits the tricarboxylic acid cycle (TCA) cycle from generating energy leading to acidosis (Karayilanoglu *et al.*, 2003a).

Unlike mustard gas effects, lewisite causes more immediate pain or irritation. Erythaema and blister formation follow more rapidly than in similar lesions, which leads to more tissue necrosis and tissue sloughing. On eyes, it causes pain and blepharospasm followed by oedema of conjunctiva and eyelids and corneal damage when the dose is high. The airway mucosa are the primary target and lewisite causes the same pulmonary signs and symptoms as seen in mustard gas exposure. Other findings are haemolysis, hypotension and anuria due to arsenic intoxication. No specific laboratory finding is available (Karalliedde *et al.*, 2000).

Medical management of lewisite casualties can be summarized as early decontamination, correction of pulmonary functions and dehydration, antidote – British Anti Lewisite – administration. Dimercaprol (BAL), a chelator for heavy metals like arsenic is applied IM while monitoring renal functions and arterial pressure. However, BAL injection is painful and has some toxic effects so novel antidotes such as meso-dimercaptosuccinic acid (DMSA), N-(2,3-dimercaptopropyl)-phthalamidic acid (DMPA) and 2,3-dimercapto-1-propanesulfonic acid (DMPS), which are more potent than BAL, have been developed for systemic use (Aposhian *et al.*, 1984).

Choking agents

Phosgene and chlorine agents are common CWAs that military hospitals may encounter. These agents also generate some of the toxic industrial chemicals, which are a wide variety of lung damaging agents or choking agents used in manufacturing petroleum, textiles, paper, plastics, fertilizers, pesticides and so on.

Phosgene was the main CWA used in the First World War. This agent accounted for about 85% of all deaths and injuries due to chemical weapons during the war. Phosgene applies its effects by damaging the lungs and causing pulmonary oedema. Chronic exposure to phosgene may result in broncholitis, alveolar bronchiolarization, ciliated cysts and emphysaema. At normal temperatures and pressures, phosgene is a colourless gas giving off a suffocating odour, similar to that of mouldy hay. Exposure can produce some local effects on the eyes including lacrimation and chemical conjunctivitis. This transient burning feeling in the eyes may coexist with mild, early onset cough and a sternal pressure sensation. Exposure to very large concentrations may cause sudden laryngeal spasm and eventually death. Dyspnoea – shortness of breath – with or without chest lightness is the most prominent symptom. Death may result from respiratory failure, hypoxaemia, hypovolaemia or from a combination of all of these. Progression of these pulmonary signs and symptoms within 4 h of exposure suggests an indication of poor prognosis. The initiation of symptoms may be triggered by exercise and supermotility (Kenar and Karayilanoglu, 2005a).

However, the majority of phosgene intoxications show a good prognosis. Occasional impairment of pulmonary function depends on smoking habits more than on severity of the main phosgene exposure. There is no specific laboratory test for indicating phosgene exposure; however, non-specific laboratory tests including increased haematocrit, low PaO_2 or $PaCO_2$ and decreased peak respiratory flow rate can alert military health staff to the possibility of phosgene inhalation. Chest X-ray shows hyperinflation followed by pulmonary oedema without any cardiac signs (Karayilanoglu *et al.*, 2003b).

Medical first aid includes termination of exposure, removal of the casualty from the contaminated field, decontamination of the agent on clothing or skin and the application of the ABCs (airways, breathing and circulation) of resuscitation with the aim of establishing a clear airway (Table 16.1). In addition to these steps, the casualty should be made to rest and hypotension should be treated by using intravenous administration of either crystalloids or colloids. Steroid therapy is also indicated especially to prevent bronchospasm depending on the severity of pulmonary oedema. Aerosol beclametasone in 50 μg doses can be applied via inhalation apparatus for up to 5 days. In heavy exposures, systemic prednisolone may be given IV followed by gradually decreased doses throughout the duration of clinical illness. For decontamination, since phosgene cannot physicochemically remain in liquid form for a long time, no decontamination is required. But, in some extreme conditions, contaminated eyes and skin should be washed with copious amounts of water for 5–15 min (Karayilanoglu *et al.*, 2003b; Sciuto and Hurt, 2004).

Table 16.1. Important points in the medical management of lung irritant exposures.

1.	No expectorant is given.
2.	Local anaesthesia is administered when surgical intervention is required.
3.	Cardiac and respiratory stimulating agents are contraindicated.
4.	Protective masks can provide perfect protection.
5.	Patients should be transported in a reclined position.

Chlorine gas

Chlorine (Cl) is a greenish-yellow gas that is heavier than air and has a characteristic odour. Cl has a corrosive effect mainly on the airways and mucous membranes. It is also reported that Cl gas impairs capillary permeability and generates oxygen radicals as a pathophysiological mechanism. Chlorine was used as a CWA during the First World War especially in lower-lying battlefield parries. However, many incidents involving mild to toxic chlorine exposure have occurred worldwide since the First World War (Karayilanoglu *et al.*, 2003b).

Symptoms due to chlorine exposure are mostly dependent on the intake or inhaled concentration. Burning sensation in airways and coughing can be seen with deep hypoxia. Tachycardia and collapse may be followed by syncope and immediate death in heavy exposures without any medical intervention. Dermal erythaema, pain and irritation and neurological symptoms like agitation and anxiety are the other major complaints accompanied by metabolic acidosis findings (Evans, 2005; Kenar and Karayilanoglu, 2005a).

For medical management, protective equipment and decontamination should be provided, with other treatment methods involving administration of 10% nebulized oxygen and a prophylactic bronchitis and pneumonia treatment regimen against progression of pulmonary oedema. It should be noted that copious soapy water should be applied to skin, and water or saline solution to eyes for a complete intervention (Karayilanoglu *et al.*, 2003a; Russell *et al.*, 2006).

Blood agents (cyanides)

Three chemical warfare compounds are of importance as blood intoxicating agents: hydrogen cyanide (HCN), cyanogen chloride and cyanogen bromide.

HCN is a rapidly acting lethal agent and is classed as a non-persistent substance. It is a colourless or yellow-brown liquid and smells like bitter almond, marzipan, ratafia or peach kernels. Cyanides are found as liquids in weapons and rapidly vaporize upon detonation of the munitions, which can cause a real threat. Cyanide has a high affinity for compounds carrying –SH atoms and certain metallic complexes containing Fe^{3+}. Thus, it strongly combines with iron in cytochrome a3 or in cytochrome oxidase complex in mitochondria and prevents cellular oxygen utilization. This process then increases the formation of lactic acid leading to metabolic acidosis (Champe *et al.*, 2005; Baskin *et al.*, 2008).

The central nervous system (CNS) is very vulnerable to this anoxic status, which leads to death through respiratory failure. Since the CNS and the heart are thc organs most susceptable to cyanide, most of the clinical effects are of CNS origin. Signs of cyanide intoxication include headache, vertigo, agitation, confusion, coma and convulsions. Initially, hyperventilation and unconsciousness are described and a metallic taste in the mouth is sensed with a concentration of 10 mg/l in air. With a concentration of 5 g/m^3, death is expected within a minute. Cardiac symptoms are hypertension and tachycardia progressively followed by bradycardia and hypotension, resulting in cardiac arrhythmia and ST wave depression in electrocardiogram monitoring (Karayilanoglu *et al.*, 2003a).

Medical management for cyanide casualties includes complete ventilation support, antidotal therapy, correction of acidosis, management of methaemoglobinaemia and hypotension, decontamination and lavage in any oral ingestion case. After administration of 100% oxygen, antidotes containing amyl nitrite, sodium nitrite and sodium thiosulphate should be administered. Here, nitrites are used to increase methaemoglobine formation since the cyanide ion has more affinity to MetHb than that of cytochrome oxidase. Thiosulphate then generates non-toxic compounds thus forming thiocyanate followed by excretion in the urine (Kenar and Karayilanoglu, 2005a).

Inhalation of amyl nitrite is provided by crushing the ampoules in the hollow of the hand and inhaling nasally for a period of 30 s. This can be repeated until a total of 8 ampoules have been inhaled. Sodium nitrite is administered IV for 3–5 min at a volume of 10 ml for adults and 0.33 ml/kg for children assuming a Hb concentration of 12 g/dl. The second step is IV injection of sodium thiosulphate solution (25%) at a dose of 1.65 ml/kg, which is utilized as a substrate by rhodanese for its conversion of cyanide to thiocyanide. Some other alternative therapeutic antidotes used are dimethylaminophenol (DMAP) and dicobalt edetate, which are a rapid MetHb former and a cobalt chelater, respectively. A water and soap decontamination should also be applied for removal of skin and eye contamination. IV $NaHCO_3$ (1 mEq/kg) and diazepam (10 mg for adults and 0.1–0.3 mg/kg for children) for convulsions should be considered as part of clinical practice (Karayilanoglu *et al.*, 2003a).

Incapacitating agents

Incapacitating agents are those causing psychological stimulation or depression by affecting the central nervous system (CNS). 3-Quinuclidinyl benzilate (BZ) and lysergic acid diethylamide (LSD) are the well-known agents used for this aim; however, since LSD is no longer in use for warfare purposes, medical management for BZ is summarized below (Karayilanoglu *et al.*, 2003a).

BZ is a glycolic ester anticholinergic compound that is odourless and stable in most solvents. It has a maximum persistency in soil and water and on most surfaces. It is an aerosolized solid dispersed for inhalation or absorbed by ingestion or skin. The mechanism of action of BZ is via prevention of cholinergic transmission in muscarinic sites in both the autonomic nervous system and the brain and spinal cord. So, it acts as a competitive inhibitor of acetylcholine at the postsynaptic and postjunctional muscarinic receptors in smooth muscle, exocrine glands, autonomic ganglia and the brain. Peripheral nervous system effects of BZ are the opposite of those seen in nerve agent exposure. Patients exposed to BZ may show initially peripheral effects including mydriasis, blurred vision, dry mouth and skin, and an atropine flush – 'red as a beet' – due to decreased sweating and partly to compensatory cutaneous vasodilatation. Patients with BZ exposure are sometimes described as being as 'blind as a bat' due to the paralysis of eye accommodation. Effects progress to CNS signs that include a dose-dependent decrease in consciousness starting from drowsiness and leading through sedation to stupor and coma. Patient may have short-term memory loss. Other CNS effects are slurred speech, disorientation, ataxia and poor judgement and insight. Medical management of BZ-exposed patients includes decontamination of skin and clothing, confiscation of weapons, physical rest, management of heat stress and antidote administration. Physostigmine is very effective as an antidote after 4 h of exposure and should be applied at a dosage of 45 μg/kg IM for adults (20 μg/kg for children). Pysostigmine, a carbamate anticholinesterase, temporarily raises acetylcholine concentration by binding reversibly to AchE on the post-synaptic or post-junctional membrane (Kenar and Karayilanoglu, 2005a; Ketchum and Salem, 2008).

Riot control agents

Riot control agents, also known as irritants or tear gas, cause pain, a burning sensation or discomfort in exposed mucous membranes and skin. These substances are in solid form with low vapour pressures and are dispersed in fine particles or in solution. The most commonly used types of crowd control agents are o-chloro-benzylidine malononitrile (CS gas), 1-chloroacetophenone (CN gas), dibenzoxazepine (CR gas) and bromoacetonone. Of these agents, CN is reported as more toxic than CS. CS and CN are alkylating agents reacting readily at nucleophilic sites. It has been suggested that tissue injury may be related to inactivation of certain enzyme systems. But pain occurs without any tissue injury and it is perhaps bardykinin-mediated. The main effects are pain, burning and irritation of mucous membranes and skin. Eyes are most sensitive to riot control agents. A sensation of conjunctival and corneal burning leads to tearing, blepharospasm and transient blindness. Rhinorrhoea, nasal discomfort, sore throat, chest tightness and coughing can be seen with bronchospasm and laryngospasm. CS gas may cause erythematous dermatitis and allergic contact dermatitis when exposed to high concentrations. Medical management includes rapid evacuation from the incident zone, removal of clothing, decontamination of skin, eyes and mouth with copious amounts of water and soapy water, administration of steroid ointments and symptomatic treatment (Karayilanoglu *et al.*, 2003b).

Military Hospitals: How to Get Ready for Chemical Terrorism

The threat from unconventional warfare agents including radiological, chemical and biological agents has traditionally been considered as a military issue (Sidell *et al.*, 1997). However, several recent events have shown that civilians may also be exposed to these agents. Potential sources of exposure for civilian populations include acts of terrorism, direct military attacks and industrial accidents. The intentional release of chemical and biological weapons might lead to thousands of casualties, thereby overwhelming local health and medical resources, particularly military medical facilities. Accordingly, setting up medical defence and first aid systems, especially in military hospitals, should be a priority to prepare for a possible chem-bio attack. Although medical defence approaches against the various biological and chemical weapons have some common countermeasures that need to be taken, these measures including medical care, triage, treatment and decontamination are all different from each other. From this point of view, military hospitals must be prepared against these chem-bio disasters with a detailed preparedness plan. The aim of this chapter is to illustrate the relative importance of the role of military hospitals following a chem-bio attack compared with that of civilian medical facilities, as well as discussing the effects, methods of detection and medical management of the agents, and outlining the elementary issues concerning planning, preparedness and response to such disasters (Brennan *et al.*, 1999; Macintyre *et al.*, 2000; Jernigan *et al.*, 2001).

Hospitals were considered as sacred areas both in peace and war times, and in the urban environment or in the operational field. But in a war scenario, military hospitals represent one of the attractive soft targets for both modern terrorists and enemies. By attacking hospitals one can kill the hope for the people involved in a CBRN incident so it is like killing them twice. So, military hospitals should take protective measures with respect to both protecting themselves and increasing their preparedness levels to give the required medical assistance (US Army Medical Research Institute of Chemical Defense, Chemical Casualty Care Division, 2007).

A military hospital might be very close or adjacent to the incident site or very far away. If the location is very close, then reaction and response time could be minimal to none. This means that the rapid response team of the hospital must be able to go to 'red alert' within minutes. This takes a lot of training, specialized equipment, modern planning and open-minded individuals who understand the magnitude and nature of the event. Hospitals that are in more distant areas might have enough time to prepare although in many instances nobody will go there no matter how prepared they are. It is obvious that all hospitals, both public and military, should be equally prepared to accept massive CBRN casualties in case of a terrorist event (The Battlebook Project Team, 2000).

The chemical and biological agents with potential for use in a deliberate release have been discussed earlier in the chapter. The impact of the attack depends on a number of factors such as the type of agent used, method of dispersal and the responsiveness of the health system. In cases involving the intentional release of chem-bio agents, effective management has to include a rapid and coordinated response amongst state, local and military foundations. From the perspective of disaster planning and preparedness, these should cover training of medical care providers, establishment of a chem-bio Medical Response Team, emergency department preparedness, the provision of a pharmaceutical stockpile containing antibiotics, antidotes, vaccines and personal protective equipment (PPE), the setting up of a medical care and decontamination unit including shower system, analytical and detection laboratories and linkage with other military healthcare facilities in addition to surveillance systems of long-term medical sequelae (Grabenstein, 1998; Evans *et al.*, 2002).

What is most important in an emergency response is to organize and coordinate these elements. If this is done well, effective emergency management in the chem-bio defence is possible, particularly in military hospitals.

Certain statistics have estimated that after a CBRN incident approximately 20% of the casualties will remain in place (dead, severely wounded and/or contaminated) and the remaining 80% will move in all possible directions seeking medical assistance or will go home if they are not wounded or contaminated. Another important estimate is that the ratio of the truly contaminated versus the 'worried well' would be 1:5. These people will soon overwhelm hospitals and collapse even the most organized and advanced medical systems worldwide. The lessons learned from the Tokyo sarin release event showed that 84.5% of those involved went to 169 hospitals and clinics all over the city by their own means. A number beyond this would emphasize the need to invest in hospitals' CBRN defence instead of in classic 'golden hour' first responders. The latter will certainly go to the incident site but they will arrive late (due to very heavy traffic and the large dimensions of decontamination vehicles) and most probably those who are severely contaminated/wounded would be dead (Kenar, 2002; Fry, 2006).

Chemical and biological warfare agents (CBWAs) are weapons that can be used not only for military purposes, but also for civilian populations owing to their toxicities/infectivities and destructive effects. Terrorist interest in the use of chem-bio weapons has grown substantially since the Tokyo Subway attack in 1995 and the attack on the twin towers on 11 September 2001 in New York City. The recent war between the USA and Iraq and the current threat of further US military involvement with Iraq has reportedly raised the prospect of the use of chem-bio weapons both on the battlefield and in terrorist attacks on civilian populations anywhere in the world. In addition to the death and physical injury they cause, the use of CBWAs may also give rise to fear, panic and psychological trauma throughout the entire population. It also causes the state and public to take several measures against any possible attack including purchasing protective equipment, giving lectures and any other items that might be related to the economical implications caused due to the use of CBWAs. Beyond this, medical preparedness is a very essential countermeasure, which needs to be carried out in advance. Successful management of casualties in a chem-bio attack depends on planning, preparation and training. Medical care of casualties depends on knowledge of the agent and timely intervention. The next section of the chapter aims to present an overview of the highlights of the emergency medical and first aid issues that should be noted related to preparedness and response against CBWAs (Kawana *et al.*, 2001; Kenar and Karayilanoglu, 2005b, 2006).

Potential sources of exposure to chem-bio agents include accidental release from military factories and stockpiles, direct military attacks, industrial accidents and intentional release as an act of terrorism (Table 16.2).

Table 16.2. Potential sources for an incident where a chem-bio weapon can be released.

• Crowded places	• Embassies/diplomats' residencies
• Subways	• Governmental facilities
• Airports	• Ceremonies
• Shopping malls	• Universities/schools
• Research/medical facilities	• Amusement parks
• Theatres, movie theatres	• Sport stadiums/arenas

It has been widely accepted that most pre-hospital and emergency medical personnel should be well-prepared, trained or equipped to respond to such incidents. These personnel should be mainly emergency medical technicians, emergency physicians and emergency nurses and they have to be aware of the following medical issues regarding to pre-hospital management of attack:

- Event recognition;
- Incident medical command and control;
- Safety and protection;
- Decontamination;
- Isolation of the incident area;
- Sampling and detection;
- Psychological management;
- Communication and coordination;
- Triage;
- Treatment;
- Transportation;
- Recovery activities;
- Fatality management.

First of all, the attack must be well recognized as a chem-bio attack and medical responders should be familiar with the indicators of possible agent use (Table 16.3). If the incident is related to use of a CBWA, the medical personnel should perform the required first aid and treatment interventions (Kenar, 2002; Kenar and Karayilanoglu, 2004a).

Table 16. 3. General indicators of possible chem-bio agent use.

• Unusual occurrence of dead or dying animals (like dead birds)
• Unexplained casualties (multiple victims with similar signs and symptoms)
• Unusual liquid or vapour (droplets, unexplained odour)
• Suspicious dispersal devices or packages (spray devices and munitions)
• Data suggesting a massive point-source outbreak
• High morbidity and mortality relative to the number of personnel at risk
• Multiple disease entities in the same patients
• Sudden appearance of a disease that is unusual or that does not occur naturally in a certain geographic area

To enable an effective medical approach after a weapon of mass destruction (WMD) incident, the affected zone must also be established. For example, in a chemical incident, a ‘hot line’ concept is used. People on one side of this clearly demarcated line are considered ‘dirty’ (contaminated), and people on the other side are considered ‘clean’. The line should be upwind of the accident (Fig. 16.1).

The most important parameter in hospital defence is to avoid contamination of the hospital site, working medical personnel and existing patients. In that respect the CBRN response unit of the hospital should be deployed outside the hospital. The response unit is composed of several stations that facilitate the arriving casualties. At this point, it would be appropriate to give some information regarding the Medical CBRN Response Team

(MedCBRN RT) established in our military medical facility, which has been very active for about 10 years (Kenar and Karayilanoglu, 2004b).

Since CBRN warfare agents are still accepted as a threat that all healthcare units should be prepared for, our military medical facility established a medical CBRN response team in order to provide medical first aid and perform medical procedures in the event of a CBRN incident. The team is composed of military physicians and military nurses to perform medical aid and paramedics specifically to conduct decontamination. The team serves all military assets and civilian populations (with the permission of the Commandership of Gülhane Military Medical Academy (GATA)) in any CBRN incident.

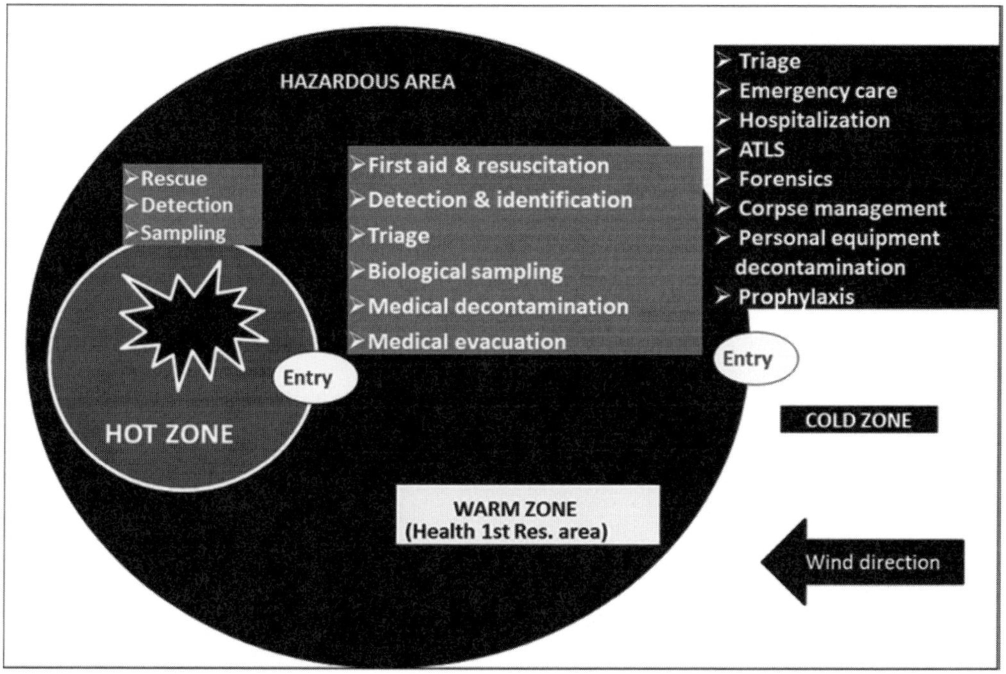

Fig. 16.1. After a WMD incident, the zones where medical intervention differs must be established.

Anyone including medical people entering the dirty area must wear protective clothing and must be very well decontaminated before coming back to the clean area. In the hot zone (fully contaminated zone), demarcated by the detection team with special detectors such as chemical agent monitors (CAMs) and sensors, the main objective is to remove the victims to the clean area immediately. Specific first aid and antidotal treatment can be applied simultaneously.

Decontamination, which is a special aspect in the response to a WMD incident, is a neutralization process performed by application of a decontaminating compound or thorough flushing with water depending on the type of agent. Transferring the patients from the incident site directly to a hospital might be a mistake. Taking into consideration that patients are generally poorly decontaminated at the site, military hospitals have to be ready with a decontamination facility and personnel trained and assigned to do this task and have to conduct these functions based on a specified decontamination protocol (Table 16.4). A

0.5% solution of hypochlorite (one part household bleach to nine parts water) should be gently applied and rinsed off with water at the last station. That rubbing and scrubbing the skin may sometimes enhance the agent absorption must be kept in mind (Raber *et al.*, 2001).

Table 16.4. A hospital decontamination protocol specified for each hospital should be organized and practised as a countermeasure against CBWA terrorism.

- Hospital staff must be familiar with the protocol
- A decontamination area and a route that will be used to take the patient to that area should be determined
- A sufficient warning system should be established
- Adequate information about the agents involved, mechanism of contamination, degree of contamination, patient status and any suspected coexisting injuries or illnesses should be given to concerned staff
- The members of the decontamination or medical response team should be set up along with the necessary clean-up procedures
- All clothes and disposable suits should be placed in specially marked containers
- The routes of removal for waste items should be arranged

In the event of an attack with CBWA, medical rescuers and healthcare providers must also consider first aid and treatment approaches in the overall evaluation of contaminated casualties.

Elementary vital functions should be aggressively supported and ABC should be corrected. Antidotal therapy is not concerned for either chemical warfare agent. The antidotal regimen recommended for a chemical casualty is given in Table 16.5 (Karayilanoglu *et al.*, 2003a; Kenar and Karayilanoglu, 2004a; Kenar *et al.*, 2004).

Table 16.5. Antidotal treatment available for the chemical warfare agents.

Agents	**Antidote**	**Dosage**
Nerve agents	Atropine	2–8 mg IM/IV. Full atropinization maintained at 2 mg doses every 3–8 min for several hours
	Pralidoxime	1–2 g IV (0.5 g/min) in saline
	Diazepam (valium)	5–10 mg IV/IM/p.o.
	Pyridostigmine bromide	30 mg every 8 h
Lewisite	BAL (dimercaprol)	Commercial preparation of 10% BAL in peanut oil up to 4.0 ml IM. Repeat in 4, 8, 12 h
	BAL analogues (DMPS, DMSA, DMPA)	DMSA 300 mg orally every 6 h for 3 days
Hydrogen cyanide	Amyl nitrite	Inhaled for 30 s/min and maintained until the initiation of Na nitrite
	Sodium nitrite	IV infusion of 10 ml over 3–5 min
	Sodium thiosulphate (25 %)	IV infusion of 50 ml
	4-DMAP	3 mg/kg IV injection
BZ (incapacitant)	Physostigmine	2 mg in 10 ml saline IV (over 5 min)

The most important rule for any responder to a WMD event is self-protection. There are two basic methods of self-protection:

1. Wearing an adequate protective suit;
2. Ensuring that the casualty is thoroughly decontaminated.

The protective suit has an interior layer of activated carbon that adsorbs CWAs. Staff should wear protective clothing of at least level C (Table 16.6). One piece of protective equipment especially effective against volatile agents is a gas mask; improper fitting of the mask may cause psychological stress and possible exposure. Continuous exercises and training with this equipment are essential to overcome discomfort and reduction in performance related to its incorrect use (Kenar and Karayilanoglu, 2004a, 2005b).

Table 16.6. The levels of protection in a chemical incident.

Level A	Maximum level of protection and used with very high concentrations of toxic agents	Fully chemical protective suit, positive pressure self-contained breathing apparatus, double layers of chemical resistant gloves and boots. Airtight seals between the suit and inner layer of face, hand and foot protection
Level B	Used when the dangers to the skin are less	Full respiratory protection similar to level A excluding airtight seals
Level C	Used when air concentration of the agent is much lower	Face cartridge mask, chemical resistant suit with gloves and boots
Level D	Used only when there is no danger of chemical exposure	Latex gloves, eye splash protection and no respiratory protection

After a CWA release, a triage station should be established in the warm zone to determine the priorities for resuscitation, decontamination, pharmacological therapy and transport to hospital (Table 16.7). Triage is a dynamic process and should be performed in both hot and warm zones, and be conducted by specially trained medical personnel who know the effects and treatment of CWAs.

Table 16.7. Some items that have to be considered in minimal patient care at the incident site if available.

- Enough decontamination (15–30 min if available)
- Basic life support measures and life-saving procedures must be performed in the decontamination area
- If medically indicated, cardiac monitorization, IV access route and oxygen support should be administered
- Conditions such as tension pneumothorax or respiratory distress should be treated immediately
- In the case of trauma, blood for haemoglobin determination and cross-match should be sent
- Anything in the decontamination area should be considered potentially contaminated
- Patient decontamination should be performed by first removing all the patient's clothes, this will take care of 70–85% of the contaminant. After being sufficiently washed off, the patient may be transferred to the emergency department

Triage is to classify the mass casualties in accordance with medical care priorities by taking into consideration the neurological, respiratory and circulatory status of the injured people and the available medical supplies that the government can provide. The main aim is to provide life-saving medical intervention to those who need treatment immediately.

The triage system commonly used by medical units includes four categories that are based on the need for medical care: immediate, delayed, minimal and expectant (Karayilanoglu *et al.*, 2003a; Ramesh and Kumar, 2010):

- T1 (immediate): casualties who require medical care and advanced life support within a short time on the incident site and further in the hospital.
- T2 (delayed): casualties with injuries who are in need of prolonged care and require hospitalization. Delay of this care does not affect the prognosis of the injury negatively.
- T3 (minimal): casualties who have minor injuries who will not be evacuated and will be able to return to duty in a short time.
- T4 (expectant): casualties with fatal injuries who will possibly not survive with standard medical care.

Detection and diagnosis of illness and injury caused by chemical terrorism constitute a complex process that involves activities of many local and community resources to assist in resolving the situation (Kenar, 2002). These include:

- Public health organizations;
- Poison control centres;
- Medical research centres;
- Professional societies;
- Emergency response units;
- First responder organizations;
- Safety and medical equipment manufacturers;
- Military organizations;
- Intelligence services;
- Law facilities.

Some critical information should also be provided, which may be useful for hospitals or other local centres. If available, the following data should be obtained and transmitted:

- Number and types of casualties;
- Chemical substance involved;
- Estimated time of arrival of the casualty at the hospital;
- Time of incident and location of incident site;
- Method of contamination (vapour or liquid);
- Hazards to healthcare providers.

However, most hospitals or medical facilities even in developed countries are unfortunately insufficient and poorly prepared to set up effective medical defence including decontamination, treatment and laboratory services. Thus, military hospitals, in particular, should have a plan that includes medical treatment and service units with specialized staff experienced in the medical care of chem-bio casualties, as well as analytical laboratories and a decontamination unit. Taking different medical management requirements for intervention in such casualties into consideration, different facilities may be required for each group showing different signs and symptoms. Military hospitals should have capability at various levels in terms of medical care, treatment, laboratory support and mobilized response teams. They should be better organized and have much more capability compared with civilian hospitals in the event of a mass casualty incident (Cancio, 1993; Macintyre *et al.*, 2000).

Triage, emergency medical care and decontamination elements are also be needed in order to save the lives of people exposed to chemical agents. Prior to transport of patients (evacuation) to the appropriate hospital, victims must be subjected to, first of all, triage to determine the medical care priorities by taking into consideration available medical sources. On the incident site, an emergency medical responder may provide medical care for stabilization of injuries and the casualty should be decontaminated and then evacuated to appropriate medical facilities (Kenar and Karayilanoglu, 2004a; Ramesh and Kumar, 2010). First aid and rescue teams assigned in military hospitals should be ready permanently, if necessary, to mobilize to an incident site.

The emergency department of a military medical unit must be prepared against chem-bio disasters with a detailed incident plan, decontamination facilities and protective equipment for all staff involved. These agents can cause life-threatening disease and necessitate intensive hospital care, local availability of intensive care unit (ICU) beds, ventilators and drugs in order to treat potentially hundreds or thousands of ill people. This preparedness has to include methods to protect the hospital from contamination and how to prevent its personnel from becoming secondary casualties. Since hospitals could be overwhelmed with casualties, hospital contamination might occur due to delay in recognizing CBWA exposure (Karayilanoglu *et al.*, 2003b).

In the hospital response plan, some specific sites related to potential disasters should be separated, such as an initial triage site located just outside the hospital building, a decontamination site, secondary triage site and treatment site.

Decontamination unit

A military hospital must have the ability to immediately decontaminate and treat those exposed to an agent. Decontamination is the procedure for removal of nuclear, biological and chemical (NBC) agents to mediate further medical care. Decontamination methods that are applied in the hospital environment have some specific requirements different from those used at the incident site – there should be a shower system with specialized water and chemical containers in which the chemical content must be removed following a neutralization process. A specific decontamination site must be established close to a appropriate place where the victims could be taken under care before medical maintenance is provided prior to acceptance to the hospital interior. In this decontamination centre, the required equipment and drugs must be provided as soon as possible. A similar decon system is under service in our military medical academy, which is strongly connected with the emergency department. A total of 420 conscious and 60 patients on stretchers (littered) can be thoroughly decontaminated in an hour before acceptance to the hospital interior (Baysallar and Kenar, 2006).

The decontamination facility should be operational within 2–3 min. Decontamination solutions used for chemical decontamination will usually also be suitable for biological decontamination. Chlorine is the recommended disinfectant and decontaminant for use in outbreak response. An all-purpose disinfectant should have a concentration of 0.05% (i.e. 1 g/l) of available chlorine, a stronger solution with a concentration of 0.5% (i.e. 10 g/l) available chlorine being used, for example, in suspected outbreaks of Lassa and Ebola virus diseases. Use of the solution with 0.5% available chlorine is recommended for disinfecting excreta, cadavers and spills of blood and body fluids (Macintyre *et al.*, 2000; Raber *et al.*, 2001; Baysallar and Kenar, 2006).

Mass casualties requiring specific chemical antidotes, vaccinations or antibiotics will quickly use up available supplies. So, hospital pharmacies will be required to provide antidotes, antibiotics, antitoxins and other pharmaceuticals in large amounts and have the capability for accurate procurement. Staff should also become aware of medical treatment methods against such threats with respect to nerve agents, cyanide, pulmonary irritants, anthrax, botulism and possible other WMD (Macintyre *et al.*, 2000).

Together with those mentioned above, the most effective CBRN defence is, above all, the training and education of first aid and rescue teams including triage officers, emergency medical responders and other paramedical personnel responsible for decontamination.

General Characteristics of Biological Weapons

Biological warfare agents (BWAs) are microorganisms or their toxic products that cause death, disability or damage in man, animals or plants. Biological weapons are characterized by low visibility, high potency, substantial accessibility and relatively easy delivery. A definitive and complete prevention to make these agents ineffective is not practically currently available. Agents are generally used via the aerosol route, and intake of the agent via inhalation may cause clinical patterns with high mortality rates and severe courses. Disasters due to bioweapons are generally supposed to be contagious and may give rise to chaos and panic amongst the population. In case of a major outbreak of infectious diseases, causing massive loss of lives, such cases should be suspected as a man-made deliberate disaster (Kortepeter *et al.*, 2001; Ashford *et al.*, 2003; Thavaselvam and Vijayaraghavan, 2010).

The impact on the healthcare system, whether it is a man-made or naturally occurring disaster, will be tremendous. In any biological attack, it is clear that hospitals may be overwhelmed with casualties. As considered in any disaster, the response to a bioterrorist event needs to be an integrated response by local public health teams, emergency management, community resources and hospitals (Shoaf and Rottman, 2000; Perry and Lindell, 2007).

It is essential that hospitals are prepared to respond to a large-scale contagious disease outbreak. When preparing for a response to bioterrorism, hospitals should prepare similarly to how emergency management prepares for any kind of disaster. The principles of the İncident Command System should be incorporated into the emergency preparedness plan. An emergency management plan should possess the four phases of emergency management to effectively prepare and respond to emergencies: mitigation, preparedness, response and recovery (Table 16.8) (Shoaf and Rottman, 2000).

Table 16.8. The four phases of emergency management.

Mitigation	Preventing future emergencies or minimizing their effects
	Includes any activities that prevent an emergency, reduce the chance of an emergency happening or reduce the damaging effects of unavoidable emergencies
	Mitigation activities take place before and after emergencies
Preparedness	Preparing to handle an emergency
	Includes plans or preparations made to save lives and to help response and rescue operations
	Preparedness activities take place before an emergency occurs
Response	Responding safely to an emergency
	Includes actions taken to save lives and prevent further property damage in an emergency situation. Response is putting your preparedness plans into action
	Response activities take place during an emergency
Recovery	Recovering from an emergency
	Includes actions taken to return to a normal or an even safer situation following an emergency
	Recovery activities take place after an emergency

Preparedness consists of a continuous cycle of planning, organizing, training, equipping, exercising, evaluating and taking corrective action in an effort to ensure effective coordination during incident response (Shoaf and Rottman, 2000; Perry and Lindell, 2007).

Although preventive measures taken by military hospitals are similar to the readiness measures used by civilian health centres, the most important difference is that military hospitals need to be prepared against not only any disaster in their province, but also any war or conflict that may emerge in any region of the world they may deploy. In that area of incident, any kind of WMD agent may be used. Thus, the main roles of a hospital in the event of use of a chem-bio agent would be to protect the casualties and staff from the hazardous effects of these agents and to apply medical procedures including triaging the casualties, first aid, decontamination of victims and detection of the type of substance for a proper further diagnosis and treatment (Higgins *et al*., 2004).

The effects of BWA attacks on humans may not immediately be recognized or differentiated from naturally occurring epidemics (Selvamurthy *et al*., 2013). Biological warfare agents differ from chemical weapons with respect to time duration of the appearance of symptoms. Due to the specific incubation period of each agent, delayed effects are a great concern in biowarfare, while the effects of chemical weapons are initiated more acutely. Bioterrorism victims may admit or be hospitalized following a reasonable time lag after the attack, which is characteristic for each agent. Clinical presentation will be like an outbreak that could occur owing to a similar agent. For this reason, the medical response in a bioterror incident should be similar to the chain of procedures that should be performed in the event of any epidemic. So, being aware of and well-trained on the main characteristics of bioagents and their differentiation from natural outbreaks is of great importance (Ortatatli, 2005).

Biological warfare agents are relatively inexpensive and do not require sophisticated production and delivery systems. They have an insidious onset and mimic natural epidemics. Based on the ease of transmission, severity of morbidity, mortality, likelihood of use and capability for causing public pain, biological agents can be classified into three categories according to the Centers for Disease Control and Prevention (CDC) (Table 16.9; Khan *et al.*, 2000; Rotz, 2002).

Table 16.9. Classification of biological warfare agents.

Biothreat level A (agents that pose the greatest threat due to their infectiousness, relative ease of transmission or a high rate of mortality)	**Biothreat level B** (agents having a moderate ease of transmission and morbidity with a low rate of mortality)	**Biothreat level C** (emerging pathogens and potential risks for the future)
Anthrax (*Bacillus anthracis*)	Brucellosis (*Brucella* species)	Hantavirus
Botulism (*Clostridium botulinum* toxin)	Epsilon toxin of *Clostridium perfringens*	Yellow fever virus
Plague (*Yersinia pestis*)	Glanders (*Burkholderia mallei*)	Encephalomyelitis (Nipah virus)
Smallpox (*Variola major*)	Q fever (*Coxiella burnetii*)	Tick-borne viruses
Tularaemia (*Francisella tularensis*)	Ricin toxin from *Ricinus communis* (castor bean)	Cryptosporidiosis (*Cryptosporidium parvum*)
Viral haemorrhagic fevers (filoviruses (e.g. Ebola, Marburg) and arenaviruses (e.g. Lassa, machupo))	Enterotoxin B (*Staphylococcus aureus*)	Multidrug-resistant tuberculosis (*Mycobacterium tuberculosis*)

Biological warfare agents enter the body via: the respiratory tract following inhalation of an aerosolized BWA; the exposed mucosal surfaces (mouth, noise, and eyes); the digestive tract following ingestion of contaminated food or water; or inadvertent swallowing of an agent delivered as an aerosol (Table 16.10). Exposure of intact skin to the primary aerosol presents insignificant risk, except for mycotoxins. However, traumatic wounds, superficial abrasions and cuts can provide portals of entry (Keim and Kaufmann, 1999). To be maximally effective, an agent must have some of the following properties (Kortepeter and Parker, 1999; Kortepeter *et al.*, 2001; Dembek *et al.*, 2006):

- Biological agents are those that can be easily produced, stored and applied, but need very expensive measures against them.
- Biological warfare agents may be hidden behind some humanitarian purposes such as biotechnology, vaccine and drug production, agriculture and animal livestock.
- Despite being non-pathogenic in nature, microorganisms and their toxins can be used after becoming disease-causative as a result of genetic manipulations.
- They may possess highly lethal characteristics (e.g. Botulinum A toxin is 100,000 times more toxic than sarin nerve agent).
- They may show a wide distribution, but often do not penetrate through the intact skin unless skin sores and cracks occur.
- Their effects do not necessarily appear immediately. Depending on the type of disease and microorganism virulence the incubation time varies from several days to several months. This feature of biological weapons is one of the important ones separating them from chemical weapons.
- It is difficult and time-consuming to identify the agents in open spaces. They are not recognized by the human senses.

- They may be spread to other regions through the water and nutrients or by sick people and vector animals (like porters, reservoir, vector insects) from the region in which they are used. Tourism and international trade and fast transportation vehicles make this spread more effective.
- They may be fast-acting and disappear from the ambient environment like Staphylococcus toxin or they can cause serious environmental pollution like anthrax spores for many years.
- They can lead to much panic in the population.
- It is not easy to determine the exact use of these weapons since there is always a possibility of a natural outbreak.

Table 16.10. Mode of transmission and infection control precautions for diseases caused by potential biological threat agents (from Garner, 1996; Keim and Kaufmann, 1999).

Microorganism	Entrance		Precaution type[a]
	Aerosol	Other routes	
Bacillus anthracis	Inhalation	Mouth, skin	S
Brucella spp.	Inhalation	Mouth, skin, eyes	S
Yersinia pestis	Inhalation	Bite of vector	S, D
Coxiella burnetii	Inhalation	Ingestion	S
Francisella tularensis	Inhalation	Mouth, animal, vector	S
Vibrio cholerae	None	Mouth	S
Marburg – Ebola viruses	Unknown	Unknown	S, A, C
Lassa virus	Inhalation	Fomites	S, A, C
Smallpox	Inhalation	Contact/ mucous membranes	S, A, C
Botulinum toxin	Inhalation	Mouth, wound	S
Venezuelan equine encephalitis		Vector	S
Chickenpox[b]			S, A, C
Mycoplasma pneumoniae[b]			S, D
Streptococcus pneumoniae[b]			S

[a] A, Airborne; C, contact; D, droplet; S, standard.
[b] This is a rather common illness that is provided here for comparison.

BWAs are thousands of microorganisms typically found in nature, which can be modified to increase their virulence and resistance to current antibiotics or vaccines, and enhance their ability to be disseminated into the environment so they can be used for the purpose of a biological attack.

Bacillus anthracis

Bacillus anthracis is a Gram-positive, non-motile, aerobic, spore-forming, rod-shaped bacterium that causes an infectious disease of herbivores that can be transmitted to humans. The bacterium often penetrates the body via wounds in the skin and may also infect humans as aerosol or ingestion (Lucey, 2005). After spores enter into the body germination occurs within hours, and vegetative cells produce the anthrax toxin. Depending on the route of transmission, anthrax cases have very different clinical manifestations.

Cutaneous anthrax is the most common manifestation of infection. Cutaneous infection usually presents as a small, painless, pruritic papule that develops into a vesicle, which then develops into a blackened necrotic eschar surrounded by significant oedema with regional lymphadenopathy. Mortality occures in 25% of untreated cases; treated, this decreases to 1%. When bacteraemia develops, it leads to high fever and death (Klietmann and Ruoff, 2001; Cahill, 2006).

Respiratory anthrax occurs with inhalation of spores from contaminated animal products or as a potential biological weapon. The incubation period is often only several days. Early symptoms of inhalational disease (fever, malaise, myalgias and an unproductive cough) are hard to distinguish from influenza-like illness and community-acquired pneumonia. Clinically, this rapidly leads to dyspnoea and hypoxia, which may lead to respiratory failure. Haemorrhagic mediastinitis, thoracic haemorrhagic lymphadenitis and pleural effusions may develop (Ortatatli, 2005). Symmetrical mediastinal widening is very characteristic of this manifestation on chest radiographs. Antibiotic treatment with penicillin, ciprofloxacin, doxycycline or tetracycline is highly effective in the early stages of the disease and becomes largely ineffective in later stages with severe complications. There is no person-to-person spread of inhalation anthrax (Cahill, 2006; Pien *et al.*, 2006).

Gastrointestinal anthrax occurs via the ingestion of contaminated undercooked meat. The symptoms are variable and include fever, pharyngitis, severe neck swelling, vomiting, abdominal pain, bloody diarrhoea and ascites. Mortality rates can be quite significant and approach 50–75% (Thavaselvam and Vijayaraghavan, 2010).

Anthrax in all forms can lead to septicaemia, and meningitis may also occur as a complication.

Depending on the type of infection, anthrax is diagnosed by culturing cutaneous lesions, sputum, pleural fluid, stool or other gastrointestinal specimens, cerebrospinal fluid and blood.

Attenuated spore-based vaccine is available for use in animals. Recently, recombinant proteins, mainly the recombinant protective antigen, have been used effectively to protect from human anthrax. The drawbacks with the recombinant protein-based vaccines are short protective efficacy, need of yearly booster doses, side-effects and poor tolerance in individuals (Klietmann and Ruoff, 2001; Lucey, 2005; Thavaselvam and Vijayaraghavan 2010).

Differentiation of epidemics due to the use of biowarfare agents and natural outbreaks

In the case of the use of biological weapons, it is difficult to differentiate whether the event is the result of a natural outbreak or the use of a BWA since they become invisible, odourless and tasteless, they do not give any immediate signs and symptoms, and thus the incident region is not very well identified and there exists a possibility of a natural outbreak in the mentioned area. Epidemiological studies should be initiated immediately when faced with a pandemic. It can be evaluated with a developed surveillance system whether the outbreak is unique to the region. When it is considered that a biological agent attack occurs in the form of aerosol spraying, the observance of rarely seen clinical patterns might be good indicators that a biological agent attack has taken place (Ortatatli, 2005). Emergency medicine physicians and other primary healthcare providers, including clinical microbiology laboratory staff, are the sentinels or medical first responders and will most likely identify the initial cases (Snyder, 2003). Detection and recognition of a suspicious event is also dependent on a vigilant laboratory staff comprising well-trained personnel who are capable of recognizing unusual circumstances and possess a high index of suspicion. Occasions that may cause health staff to suspect a possible biological attack are listed below (Kortepeter and Parker, 1999; Snyder, 2003; Treadwell *et al.*, 2003; Dembek *et al.*, 2006):

- A disease entity that is unusual or that does not occur naturally in a given geographical area, or combinations of unusual disease entities in the same population;
- Higher morbidity and mortality in association with a common disease or syndrome or failure of such patients to respond to usual therapy;
- Disease with an unusual geographical or seasonal distribution;
- Absence of a competent natural vector in the area of the outbreak for those biological agents;
- Unusual, atypical, genetically engineered, increased antibiotic resistance pattern, or antiquated strain of an agent;
- Unusual disease presentation (e.g. pulmonary instead of cutaneous anthrax);
- Similar genetic type among agents isolated from the distinct sources at different times or locations;
- Atypical disease transmission through aerosols, food or water, which suggests deliberate sabotage;
- Illness that is unusual (or atypical) for a given population or age group;
- Illness in persons suggesting a common exposure (e.g. same office building, meal, sporting event or social event);
- Simultaneous clusters of similar illness in non-contiguous areas, domestic or foreign.

Military hospitals: how to get ready for bioterrorism

The presentation of the casualties of bioterror agents will be similar to those seen due to any epidemics. The bioterror incident will either disseminate or limit itself depending on the transmission characteristics of the causal agent (person-to-person, infected by a vector). The resulting response should the same as for any disaster. In this context, the response plan should include pre-incident, on-site (on-event) and post-response steps. Thus, civilian hospitals need to be involved in only the 'In the hospital' step listed in Table 16.11, however, military hospitals are required to become prepared for all steps indicated below by taking into consideration that they may be assigned in any military operation.

Table 16.11. Medical CBRN response planning steps for military hospitals.

BEFORE THE EVENT	MOMENT OF THE EVENT	AFTER THE INCIDENT	
Risk management		Pre-hospital	In the hospital
		Search and rescue	Medical assistance

Hospital disaster plan

Establishing a hospital disaster planning committee or group is a critical step in achieving preparedness. It should include broad representation from the institution, including the medical staff, administration, nursing staff, infection control, emergency department, security, communications, public relations, laboratory/radiology, engineering and maintenance, and medical records and admissions (Perry and Lindell, 2007).

Military healthcare facilities (MHCFs) are essential components of the emergency response system to give healthcare for BWA casualties in the field. Key elements of an effective MHCF response plan include prompt recognition of the incident, laboratory preparedness, surge capacity, coordination with external emergency response and civilian public health agencies, patient decontamination and triage, staff and facility protection, medical therapy and training (Macintyre *et al.*, 2000).

Recognition

In a biological attack, an infectious agent may be released surreptitiously and discovered after the incubation period, when patients start presenting with illness. Diagnosis of the first illness in an outbreak may occur before the epidemic is recognized and is often determined retrospectively. BWAs are relatively easy to produce, inexpensive and can be deployed covertly. Most significantly, the widespread release of these weapons could be time-consuming and expensive, and their dispersal can be complicated with efficient response systems in place in several advanced nations. Decontamination tents, trailers and isolation rooms are expensive, require prolonged set-up time and can be inadequate for large numbers of patients (Kenar *et al.*, 2004).

The most critical components for bioterrorism outbreak detection and reporting are the frontline healthcare professionals and the local health departments. Emergency physicians confronted with the situation of an alleged community-based biological agent should immediately notify an infectious disease consultant, the hospital laboratory officer and the administration. Bioterrorism preparedness should emphasize education and support of the frontline healthcare professionals as well as methods to shorten the time between outbreak and reporting (Ashford *et al.*, 2003).

Laboratory preparedness

The hospital-based clinical microbiology laboratory should have a bioterrorism response plan and a standing operating procedure. This plan includes event recognition, access to and interaction with the other laboratories, communication protocols, safety guidelines, training of personnel to ensure competence and awareness, packaging and shipment of infectious substances and laboratory security (Snyder, 2003).

A major concern for testing environmental samples in a hospital-based microbiology laboratory is the unknown nature of the sample. The sample could be explosive or a volatile, toxic chemical or contain a radioactive substance.

The hospital-based clinical microbiology laboratory must be familiar with the general morphological, cultural and Gram stain characteristics of these agents and perform common conventional diagnostic test protocols for the bacterial agents of anthrax, brucellosis, plague and tularaemia.

Patient specimens or isolates should be forwarded to higher-level laboratories for further analysis and for confirmatory testing in an advisory capacity. Specimens and agents must be packaged and shipped in accordance with guidelines specified by the International Air Transport Association and United Nations 6.2 packaging regulations. All specimens, including pure cultures, are classified as infectious substances and must be packaged and transported in the same manner, whether their destination is intra- or international (Snyder, 2003).

In the event that a suspicious agent is detected, the first priority of the laboratory, as always, should be to notify the treating clinician of test results so that they can initiate appropriate management of patients. Additional security measures should be taken including the detention of unauthorized personnel. Other security measures include locking all storage cabinets, refrigerators, incubators and doors to sensitive areas (Henchal *et al.*, 2001; Snyder, 2003).

Surge capacity

Biological and chemical agents often require patient isolation and observation, which demands still more capacity. Military hospitals should have surge capacity plans to care for an influx of any number of patients at a non-healthcare facility, such as a community centre, sports arena or hotel. Space can sometimes be created through early discharge of inpatients (Perry and Lindell, 2007; Rebmann *et al.*, 2007).

A sudden biological event may require administration of prophylactic medications and vaccines and could place extraordinary demands on medical and public health staff and facilities (Macintyre *et al.*, 2000; Perry and Lindell, 2007). Mass casualties requiring antibiotics and vaccinations will quickly deplete available supplies. In most cases, current hospital stocks of medications would be inadequate to meet the needs of even a few of these patients. Vaccination for prophylaxis against potential biological agents and antibiotic stockpile/supplies for medical responders and workers under risk in hospital environment are also important for effective biological defence (Macintyre *et al.*, 2000).

A bioterrorism attack or outbreak of an emerging infection involving an agent that is transmitted by way of the airborne route would require the use of negative pressure rooms and would be expected to exceed hospitals' current capacity to house potentially contagious patients (Rebmann *et al.*, 2007).

Expansion of capacity demands personnel, and the disaster plan should examine measures such as expansion of staff work shift hours, call-back of off-duty employees, and adapting non-clinical staff to clinical roles. The hospital's disaster plan should include incentives for encouraging healthcare workers to continue working during an infectious disease emergency. It is critical that hospitals continue to develop plans for obtaining extra staff to respond during an infectious disease emergency, because this will affect a hospital's ability to care for patients (Perry and Lindell, 2007; Rebmann *et al.*, 2007).

Military hospitals need to plan for surge capacity for ventilators, respiratory protection equipment as a precaution against airborne agents, and surgical masks as precautions against droplet infection. Many potential bioterrorism agents cause diseases that result in severe respiratory distress or failure that would require prolonged intensive care for patients, including the use of mechanical ventilation. Without ventilator surge capacity, patient care could be compromised severely and result in increased morbidity and mortality (Rebmann *et al.*, 2007).

Ventilators and other critical care supplies may be needed in large quantities. This problem could be resolved in part through mutual aid agreements between healthcare facilities.

Coordination

Connecting hospitals to the larger community through the mutual planning process is also an important priority in WMD preparedness. Mutual aid agreements and pre-planning allow for systematic redistribution of patients, pharmaceuticals, equipment, medical staff or support staff to relieve overtaxed hospitals (Perry and Lindell, 2007).

Communication capabilities are an important component of hospital disaster plans and the majority of attention is given to establishing communication links with intrafacility departments, local emergency operations centres, other hospitals, and medical institutions, emergency medical service providers (including ambulance services) and government authorities. Because mobility and low cost are key features of hospital disaster planning, radios are most often adopted as a means of communicating within the facility (Perry and Lindell, 2007).

Decontamination and triage

A brief sign-in process before decontamination should capture name and date of birth (full registration can occur after decontamination). The purpose of decontamination after exposure to an aerosolized biological weapon is to remove or reduce any potential contaminant on the patient's body or clothing and thus prevent re-aerosolization and further respiratory exposure (Keim and Kaufmann, 1999).

Decontamination of personnel and equipment after a biological warfare attack is a lesser concern than after a chemical warfare attack because most BWAs (except trichothecene mycotoxins) are not dermally active or volatile. Still, decontamination remains an effective way to reduce the spread of infection from potential secondary aerosolization. The procedure could be as simple as taking a shower and changing clothes (Keim and Kaufmann, 1999; Macintyre *et al.*, 2000; Ramesh and Kumar, 2010).

Some authors suggest that as much as 75–90% of the hazardous agent may be removed by disrobing (Macintyre *et al.*, 2000; Levitin *et al.*, 2003). In the case of visible contamination of the victim, skin should be thoroughly washed and sterilized by swabbing with a sporicidal/bactericidal solution (e.g. 5% sodium hypochlorite or other approved products), and then rinsed with water to minimize cutaneous irritation by the solution. Eye and inhalational exposures to the solution should be avoided. Eyes may be rinsed with water or saline solution. Clothing should be removed and disinfected or discarded. Decisions about whether people exposed in such incidents require chemoprophylaxis depend on additional considerations, particularly the suspected identity of the agent (Keim and Kaufmann, 1999; Kenar *et al.*, 2004).

A biological attack might involve an area encompassing many square metres. A massive aerosol exposure of many people would be beyond the capacity of any healthcare facilities. Under these circumstances some recommendations include instructing people who may have been exposed to contaminated materials to: (i) wash their hands; (ii) change their clothing and place potentially contaminated clothing in a sealed plastic bag; and (iii) conduct pre-hospital decontamination by showering with soap and water. Although the risk of re-aerosolization of an infective level of *B. anthracis* spores from clothing or human body is negligible, these simple methods will reduce the potential for secondary transmission of biological threat agents (Keim and Kaufmann, 1999).

All exposed and potentially exposed individuals should receive an initial brief triage, performed by medical personnel in PPE, before decontamination (Fig. 16.2). The uninjured, those with minor injuries requiring no medical intervention during decontamination, and the majority of ambulatory patients will be assigned to non-medical decontamination. Those with injuries or illness potentially requiring medical intervention will be assigned to medical decontamination by staff. Throughout the decontamination process, attention must be given to symptoms of exposure to biological agents that may indicate early life-threatening deterioration (e.g. a sore throat or mild shortness of breath after exposure to pulmonary or laryngeal irritants) (Macintyre *et al.*, 2000).

In the decontamination zone there should be a computer system, tables, chairs, stationery and medical equipment and supplies to function as an isolation and triage area. After triage, at-risk patients should be directed to the decontamination unit (Tham, 2004).

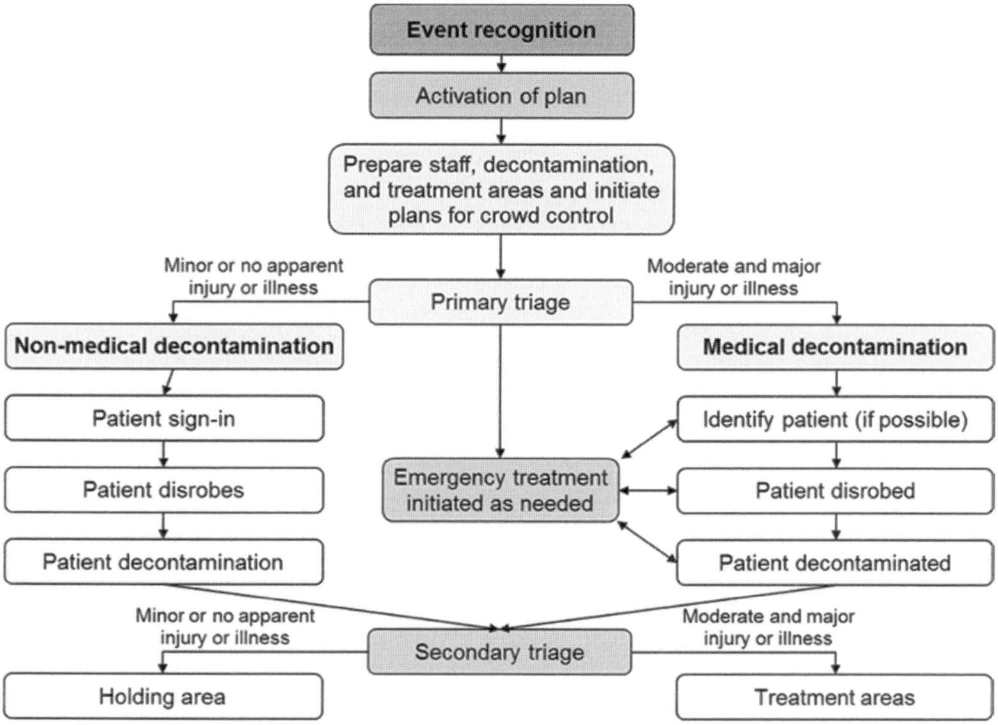

Fig. 16.2. Healthcare facility response plan for chemical or biological weapons release.

Staff and facility protection

For HCF workers conducting treatment of decontaminated patients, level D PPE (standard work clothes) plus latex gloves, eye splash protection and N-95 respiratory masks should be adequate. If the agent class for a sudden release cannot be identified, level C PPE with an organic vapour/high-efficiency particulate air (HEPA) filter cartridge mask is recommended. Since PPE face masks muffle the voice, loudspeakers should be provided to personnel directing contaminated patients (Macintyre *et al.*, 2000).

Work times and conditions must be monitored while personnel are using PPE to prevent fatigue or heat stress. Providing food and hydration in a hygienic manner will enhance staff performance. Psychological support for staff should be available. Personnel should be rotated if decontamination operations are prolonged (Macintyre *et al.*, 2000).

Two types of precautionary methods can be suggested as standard or transmission-based precautions (Table 16.12). Standard precautions are the first and most important tier and are designed for use during the care of pre-hospital and hospital patients regardless of their diagnosis or presumed infection status. Transmission-based precautions are disease-specific and are designed only for the care of those patients known or suspected to be infected with epidemiologically important pathogens that can be transmitted by airborne or droplet transmission or by contact with dry skin or contaminated surfaces (Garner, 1996; Keim and Kaufmann, 1999).

Table 16.12. Isolation precautions for infection control (from Garner, 1996).

Standard precautions for infection control
1. Hand washing after touching potentially contaminated materials, regardless of whether gloves were worn 2. Wearing gloves when touching potentially contaminated materials 3. Wearing a mask and eye protection or a face shield to protect mucous membranes of the eyes, nose and mouth during procedures and patient care activities that are likely to produce potentially infectious splashes or sprays 4. Wearing a gown to prevent soiling of clothing during procedures and patient care activities that are likely to produce potentially infectious splashes or sprays 5. Handling patient care equipment soiled with potentially infectious material in a manner that prevents secondary transmission 6. Routinely using environmental surface cleaning and disinfecting 7. Handling, processing and transporting used linen that has been soiled with potentially infectious materials in a manner that prevents secondary transmission 8. Following occupational health and bloodborne pathogens requirements to reduce the risk for infection from contaminated equipment and inherently risky patient care procedures 9. Placing patients who present risk of environmental contamination in a private or cohort room
Transmission-based precautions for infection control
Airborne precautions include (in addition to standard precautions): 1. Patient placement in a negative-pressure room 2. Respiratory protection including N95 high-efficiency particulate air filter respirators 3. Limit patient transport. When transport is necessary, place a surgical mask on the patient 4. Additional guidlines for specific prevention of tuberculosis

Droplet precautions include (in addition to standard precautions):

1. Patient placement in a private or cohort room
2. Wearing masks, eye protection and face shield when within 1 m of patient
3. Limit patient transport. When transport is necessary, place a surgical mask on the patient

Contact precautions include (in addition to standard precautions):

1. Patient placement in a private or cohort room
2. Gloves and hand washing
3. Gown
4. Limit patient transport. When transport is necessary, place a surgical mask on the patient
5. Dedicate use of patient care equipment to one patient whenever possible. If common use of equipment among patients is unavoidable, clean and disinfect equipment before use on another patient
6. Additional requirements specifically for preventing the spread of vancomycin resistance

Medical therapy

Medical biological defence requires isolation rooms in infectious diseases departments, a specifically designed morgue, a microbiological laboratory with Biosafety Level III, a surveillance system to recognize unexplained epidemic outbreaks and a vaccination programme. Specific therapies for biological agent casualties vary according to the aetiological agent (Table 16.13). The use of a screening questionnaire and admission criteria enables the emergency room to screen, treat and safely discharge the majority of patients (Tham, 2004).

Table 16.13. Clinical and microbiological characteristics of possible biological warfare agents (adapted from Pien *et al.*, 2006).

Agent	Infective dose	Incubation period	Clinical presentation	Treatment
B. anthracis	8,000–50,000 spores	Cutaneous: 1–14 days inhalational: 1–60 days	Haemorrhagic mediastinitis; septicaemia; meningitis; necrotic eschar; dysentery	Ciprofloxacin or doxycycline
Y. pestis	< 100 organisms	1–7 days	Buboes; pneumonia; septicaemia; meningitis	Ciprofloxacin or doxycycline
F. tularemia	10–50 organisms	1–14 days	Ulceroglandular; oculoglandular; pneumonia; septicaemia; meningitis	Streptomycin or ciprofloxacin or doxycycline
Brucella spp.	10–100 organisms	5–60 days	Isolated fever; orchitis; pancytopenia; endocarditis; osteomyelitis	Doxycycline + rifampin or streptomycin

Q fever	1–10 organisms	1–14 days	Q fever, atypical pneumonia	Doxycycline or tetracycline
Smallpox	10–100 viruses	7–17 days	Smallpox	Supportive care, cidofovir (not FDA approved)
Viral haemorrhagic fever	1–10 viruses	2–21 days	Haemorrhagic fever; multisystem organ failure	Supportive care, ribavirin
C. botulinum	0.001 mcg/kg of Type A toxin	1–5 days	Cranial nerve palsy; descending flaccid paralysis; autonomic dysfunction	Supportive care and trivalent or heptavalent equine botulinum
Staphylococcal enterotoxin B	30 ng incapacitates; 1.7 mcg kills	3–12 h	ARDS; toxic shock; gastroenteritis	Supportive care

ARDS, acute respiratory distress syndrome.

Training

Training of the emergency services personel such as emergency physicians, first responders and hazardous materials response teams is required to best ensure and manage patient and worker safety in the case of suspected exposure to biological threat agents.

Drills constitute a simultaneous and comprehensive test of emergency plans, staffing levels, personnel training, procedures, facilities, equipment and materials (Perry and Lindell, 2007).

Laboratory personnel should receive specialized training in the recognition of targeted agents, and the application of the test protocols for ruling out and referring suspicious isolates (Snyder, 2003).

Limitations to the use of PPE are restriction of physical activity, dehydration, heat-related illness and psychological effect. To avoid this, emergency personnel should be trained to use PPE appropriately (Ramesh and Kumar, 2010).

References

Aposhian, Carter, D.E., Hoover, T.D., Hsu, C.A., Maiorino, R.M. and Stine, E. (1984) DMSA, DMPS, and DMPA – as arsenic antidotes. *Fundamental and Applied Toxicology: Official Journal of the Society of Toxicology*, 4(2 Pt 2), S58–S70.

Ashford, D.A., Kaiser, R.M., Bales, M.E., Shutt, K., Patrawalla, A., McShan, A., Tappero, J.W., Perkins, B.A. and Dannenberg, A.L. (2003) Planning against biological terrorism: lessons from outbreak investigations. *Emerging Infectious Diseases* 9(5), 515–519.

Bajgar, J. (2004) Organophosphates/nerve agent poisoning: mechanism of action, diagnosis, prophylaxis, and treatment. *Advances in Clinical Chemistry* 38, 151–216.

Baskin, S.I., Kelly, J.B., Maliner, B.I., Rockwood, G.A. and Zoltani, C.K. (2008) Cyanide poisoning. In: Tuorinsky, S.D. (ed.) *Medical Aspects of Chemical Warfare*. Office of the Surgeon General, Virginia, pp. 371–411.

Baysallar, M. and Kenar, L. (2006) Bioterrorism and management of decontamination. *Turkish Bulletin of Hygiene and Experimental Biology* 63(1,2,3), 115–128.

Black, R.M., Clarke, R.J., Harrison, J.M. and Read, R.W. (1997) Biological fate of sulphur mustard: identification of valine and histidine adducts in haemoglobin from casualties of sulphur mustard poisoning. *Xenobiotica; the Fate of Foreign Compounds in Biological Systems* 27(5), 499–512.

Brennan, R.J., Waeckerle, J.F., Sharp, T.W. and Lillibridge, S.R. (1999) Chemical warfare agents: emergency medical and emergency public health issues. *Annals of Emergency Medicine* 34(2), 191–204.

Cahill, J.D. (2006) Bioevents and manmade disasters. In: Antosia, R. and Cahill, J.D. (eds) *Handbook of Bioterrorism and Disaster Medicine*. Springer Science and Business Media, LLC, New York, pp. 89–202.

Cancio, L.C. (1993) Chemical casualty decontamination by medical platoons in the 82nd Airborne Division. *Military Medicine* 158(1), 1–5.

Cannard, K. (2006) The acute treatment of nerve agent exposure. *Journal of the Neurological Sciences* 249(1), 86–94.

Champe, P.C., Harvey, R.A. and Ferrier, D.R. (2005) Tricarboxylic acid cycle. In: Harvey, R.A. and Champe, P.C. (eds) *Biochemistry*. Lippincott Williams & Wilkins, Philadelphia, Pennsylvania, USA.

Cosar, A. and Kenar, L. (2006) An anesthesiological approach to nerve agent victims. *Military Medicine* 171(1), 7–11.

Dacre, J.C. and Goldman, M. (1996) Toxicology and pharmacology of the chemical warfare agent sulfur mustard. *Pharmacological Reviews* 48(2), 289–326.

Dembek, Z.F., Kortepeter, M.G. and Pavlin, J.A. (2006) Discernment between deliberate and natural infectious disease outbreaks. *Epidemiology and Infection* 135(03), 353–357.

Driskell, W.J. *et al.* (2002) Quantitation of organophosphorus nerve agent metabolites in human urine using isotope dilution gas chromatography-tandem mass spectrometry. *Journal of Analytical Toxicology* 26(1), 6–10.

Evans, R.B. (2005) Chlorine: state of the art. *Lung* 183(3), 151–167.

Evans, R.G., Crutcher, J.M., Shadel, B., Clements, B. and Bronze, M.S. (2002) Terrorism from a public health perspective. *The American Journal of the Medical Sciences* 323(6), 291–298.

Fry, D.E. (2006) Chemical threats. *The Surgical Clinics of North America* 86(3), 637–647.

Garner, J.S. (1996) Guideline for isolation precautions in hospitals. The Hospital Infection Control Practices Advisory Committee. *Infection Control and Hospital Epidemiology: The Official Journal of the Society of Hospital Epidemiologists of America* 17(1), 53–80.

Grabenstein, J. (1998) The pharmacist's response to biological or chemical terrorism: developing a preparedness plan. *Hospital Pharmacy* 33(11), 1423–1431.

Graham, J.S., Gerlach, T.W., Logan, T.P., Bonar, J.P., Fugo, R.J., Lee, R.B. and Coatsworth, M.A. (2008) Methods of advanced wound management for care of combined traumatic and chemical warfare injuries. *Eplasty* 8, e34.

Henchal, E.A., Teska, J.D., Ludwig, G.V., Shoemaker, D.R. and Ezzell, J.W. (2001) Current laboratory methods for biological threat agent identification. *Clinics in Laboratory Medicine* 21(3), 661–678.

Higgins, W., Wainright, C., Lu, N. and Carrico, R. (2004) Assessing hospital preparedness using an instrument based on the Mass Casualty Disaster Plan Checklist: results of a statewide survey. *American Journal of Infection Control* 32(6), 327–332.

Hu, H., Cook-Deegan, R. and Shukri, A. (1989) The use of chemical weapons. Conducting an investigation using survey epidemiology. *JAMA: The Journal of the American Medical Association* 262(5), 640–643.

Hurst, C.G., Petrali, J.B., Levine, E.S., Barillo, D.J., Graham, J.S., Smith, W.J., Urbanetti, J.S. and Sidell, F.R. (2008) Vesicants. In: Tuorinsky, S.D. (ed.) *Medical Aspects of Chemical Warfare*. Office of the Surgeon General, Virginia, pp. 259–311.

Jernigan, J.A., Stephens, D.S., Ashford, D.A., Omenaca, C., Topiel, M.S., Galbraith, M., Tapper, M., Fisk, T.L., Zaki, S., Popovic, T., Meyer, R.F., Quinn, C.P., Harper, S.A., Fridkin, S.K., Sejvar, J.J., Shepard, C.W., McConnell, M., Guarner, J., Shieh, W.J., Malecki, J.M., Gerberding, J.L., Hughes, J.M. and Perkins, B.A. (2001) Bioterrorism-related inhalational anthrax: the first 10 cases reported in the United States. *Emerging Infectious Diseases* 7(6), 933–944.

Jortani, S.A., Snyder, J.W. and Valdes, R., Jr (2000) The role of the clinical laboratory in managing chemical or biological terrorism. *Clinical Chemistry* 46(12), 1883–1893.

Karalliedde, L., Wheeler, H., Maclehose, R. and Murray, V. (2000) Possible immediate and long-term health effects following exposure to chemical warfare agents. *Public Health* 114(4), 238–248.

Karayilanoglu, T., Saygı, S., Kenar, L. and Baykal, B. (2003a) Chemical warfare agents. In: Karayilanoglu, T. (ed.) *Medical Defence in Chemical Attack and Pesticides*. Gulhane Military Medical Academy Publishing Center, Ankara, Turkey.

Karayilanoglu, T., Kenar, L. and Gulec, M. (2003b) Evaluations over the medical emergency responding to chemical terrorist attack. *Military Medicine* 168(8), 591–594.

Kawana, N., Ishimatsu, S. and Kanda, K. (2001) Psycho-physiological effects of the terrorist sarin attack on the Tokyo subway system. *Military Medicine* 166(12 Suppl), 23–26.

Keim, M. and Kaufmann, A.F. (1999) Principles for emergency response to bioterrorism. *Annals of Emergency Medicine* 34(2), 177–182.

Kenar, L. (2002) Establishment of a national NBC defense and first-aid system against an NBC attack for Turkey. PhD Thesis. Gulhane Military Medical Academy, Ankara, Turkey.

Kenar, L. and Alp, O. (2011) Determination of nitrogen mustard hydrolysis products in rat urine samples using GC-MS. *Journal of Chromatographic Science* 49(5), 361–364.

Kenar, L. and Karayilanoglu, T. (2004a) Prehospital management and medical intervention after a chemical attack. *Emergency Medicine Journal* 21(1), 84–88.

Kenar, L. and Karayilanoglu, T. (2004b) A Turkish medical rescue team against nuclear, biological, and chemical weapons. *Military Medicine* 169(2), 94–96.

Kenar, L. and Karayilanoglu, T. (2005a) Chemical weapons. In: Eryilmaz, M. and Dizer, U. (eds) *Disaster Medicine*. Unsal Publishing, Ankara, Turkey, pp. 1255–1286.

Kenar, L. and Karayilanoglu, T. (2005b) Medical defence against chemical threat. In: Eryilmaz, M. and Dizer, U. (eds) *Disaster Medicine*. Unsal Publishing, Ankara, Turkey, pp. 1287–1374.

Kenar, L. and Karayilanoglu, T. (2006) Medical preparedness against chemical and biological incidents for the NATO Summit in Istanbul and lessons learned. *Prehospital and Disaster Medicine* 21(4), 268–271.

Kenar, L., Karayilanoglu, T. and Gulec, M. (2004) How would military hospitals cope with a nuclear, biological, or chemical disaster? *Military Medicine* 169(10), 757–760.

Kenar, L., Karayilanoğlu, T., Yuksel, A., Gunhan, O., Kose, S. and Kurt, B. (2005) Evaluation of protective ointments used against dermal effects of nitrogen mustard, a vesicant warfare agent. *Military Medicine* 170(1), 1–6.

Kenar, L., Boyunaga, H., Serdar, M., Karayilanoglu, T. and Erbil, M.K. (2006) Effect of nitrogen mustard, a vesicant agent, on lymphocyte energy metabolism. *Clinical Chemistry and Laboratory Medicine: CCLM / FESCC* 44(10), 1253–1257.

Ketchum, J.S. and Salem, H. (2008) Incapacitating agents. In: Tuorinsky, S.D. (ed.) *Medical Aspects of Chemical Warfare*. Office of the Surgeon General, Virginia, pp. 411–441.

Khan, A.S., Morse, S. and Lillibridge, S. (2000) Public-health preparedness for biological terrorism in the USA. *The Lancet* 356(9236), 1179–1182.

Klietmann, W.F. and Ruoff, K.L. (2001) Bioterrorism: implications for the Clinical Microbiologist. *Clinical Microbiology Reviews* 14(2), 364–381.

Kortepeter, M.G. and Parker, G.W. (1999) Potential biological weapons threats. *Emerging Infectious Diseases* 5(4), 523–527.

Kortepeter, M.G., Cieslak, T.J. and Eitzen, E.M. (2001) Bioterrorism. *Journal of Environmental Health* 63(6), 21–24.

Levitin, H.W., Siegelson, H.J., Dickinson, S., Halpern, P., Haraguchi, Y., Nocera, A. and Turineck, D. (2003) Decontamination of mass casualties – re-evaluating existing dogma. *Prehospital and Disaster Medicine* 18(3), 200–207.

Lucey, D. (2005) *Bacillus anthracis*. In: Mandell, G.L., Bennett, J.E. and Dolin, R. (eds) *Principles and Practice of Infectious Disease*. Churchill Livingstone, New York, pp. 2485–2491.

Macintyre, A.G., Christopher, G.W., Eitzen, E., Jr, Gum, R., Weir, S., DeAtley, C., Tonat, K. and Barbera, J.A. (2000) Weapons of mass destruction events with contaminated casualties: effective planning for health care facilities. *The Journal of the American Medical Association* 283(2), 242–249.

Marrs, T.C., Rice, P. and Vale, J.A. (2006) The role of oximes in the treatment of nerve agent poisoning in civilian casualties. *Toxicological Reviews* 25(4), 297–323.

Okumura, T., Suzuki, K., Fukuda, A., Kohama, A., Takasu, N., Ishimatsu, S. and Hinohara, S. (1998) The Tokyo subway sarin attack: disaster management, Part 1: Community emergency response. *Academic Emergency Medicine: Official Journal of the Society for Academic Emergency Medicine* 5(6), 613–617.

Ortatatli, M. (2005) Biological warfare agents. In: Eryilmaz, M. and Dizer, U. (eds) *Disaster Medicine*. Unsal Publishing, Ankara, Turkey, pp. 1207–1255.

Perry, R.W. and Lindell, M.K. (2007) Hospital planning for weapons of mass destruction incidents. *Journal of Healthcare Protection Management: Publication of the International Association for Hospital Security* 23(1), 27–39.

Pien, B.C., Saah, J.R., Miller, S.E. and Woods, C.W. (2006) Use of sentinel laboratories by clinicians to evaluate potential bioterrorism and emerging infections. *Clinical Infectious Diseases: An Official Publication of the Infectious Diseases Society of America* 42(9), 1311–1324.

Raber, E., Jin, A., Noonan, K., McGuire, R. and Kirvel, R.D. (2001) Decontamination issues for chemical and biological warfare agents: how clean is clean enough? *International Journal of Environmental Health Research* 11(2), 128–148.

Ramesh, A. and Kumar, S. (2010) Triage, monitoring, and treatment of mass casualty events involving chemical, biological, radiological, or nuclear agents. *Journal of Pharmacy and Bioallied Sciences* 2(3), 239.

Rebmann, T., Carrico, R. and English, J.F. (2007) Hospital infectious disease emergency preparedness: a survey of infection control professionals. *American Journal of Infection Control* 35(1), 25–32.

Rotz, L.D. (2002) Public health assessment of potential biological terrorism agents. *Emerging Infectious Diseases* 8(2), 225–230.

Russell, D., Blain, P.G. and Rice, P. (2006) Clinical management of casualties exposed to lung damaging agents: a critical review. *Emergency Medicine Journal* 23(6), 421–424.

Saadeh, A.M., Farsakh, N.A. and al-Ali, M.K. (1997) Cardiac manifestations of acute carbamate and organophosphate poisoning. *Heart (British Cardiac Society)* 77(5), 461–464.

Safarinejad, M.R., Moosavi, S.A. and Montazeri, B. (2001) Ocular injuries caused by mustard gas: diagnosis, treatment, and medical defense. *Military Medicine* 166(1), 67–70.

Sciuto, A.M. and Hurt, H.H. (2004) Therapeutic treatments of phosgene-induced lung injury. *Inhalation Toxicology* 16(8), 565–580.

Selvamurthy, W., Arora, R. and Rao, P.V.L. (2013) Dual-use of Technology in Bioterrorism: Issues in Biosecurity and Biosafety. In: Talwar, G.P., Sarin, S.K. and Hasnain, S.E. (eds) *Text Book of Biochemistry, Biotechnology, Allied and Molecular Medicine*. Prentice Hall of India, New Delhi, India (in press).

Shoaf, K.I. and Rottman, S.J. (2000) The role of public health in disaster preparedness, mitigation, response, and recovery. *Prehospital and Disaster Medicine* 15(4), 144–146.

Sidell, F.R., Takafuji, E.T. and Franz, D.R. (1997) *Medical Aspects of Chemical and Biological Warfare*. Borden Institute, Walter Reed Army Medical Center, Washington, DC.

Sidell, F.R., Newmark, J., Levine, E.S. and Filbert, M.G. (2008) Nerve agents. In: Tuorinsky, S.D. (ed.) *Medical Aspects of Chemical Warfare*. Office of the Surgeon General, Falls Church, Virginia, pp. 155–221.

Snyder, J.W. (2003) Role of the hospital-based microbiology laboratory in preparation for and response to a bioterrorism event. *Journal of Clinical Microbiology* 41(1), 1–4.

Tham, K.-Y. (2004) An emergency department response to severe acute respiratory syndrome: a prototype response to bioterrorism. *Annals of Emergency Medicine* 43(1), 6–14.

Thavaselvam, D. and Vijayaraghavan, R. (2010) Biological warfare agents. *Journal of Pharmacy and Bioallied Sciences* 2(3), 179.

The Battlebook Project Team (2000) *The Medical NBC Battlebook*. US Army Center for Health Promotion and Preventive Medicine, Aberdeen Proving Ground, Maryland.

Treadwell, T.A., Koo, D., Kuker, K. and Khan, A.S. (2003) Epidemiologic clues to bioterrorism. *Public Health Reports (Washington, DC: 1974)* 118(2), 92–98.

US Army Medical Research Institute of Chemical Defense. Chemical Casualty Care Division (2007) *Medical Management of Chemical Casualties Handbook,* 4th edn. Chemical Chemical Casualty Care Division, USAMRICD, Aberdeen Proving Ground, Maryland.

Chapter 17

Initial Management of Mass Casualty Incidents

Robert P. Chilcott

Introduction

The threat from global terrorism has increased over the last decade. In particular, it has become apparent that certain organizations may wish to seek injury or death to unprotected civilians through the deliberate release of hazardous substances such as chemical warfare (CW) agents or toxic industrial chemicals (TICs). Indeed, such deplorable events have already occurred, most notably during the Tokyo subway attack using sarin, a volatile nerve agent (Okumura *et al.*, 1998a,b,c) Less well publicized were several previous attacks (by the same organization) using the persistent nerve agent VX (Tsuchihashi *et al.*, 1998).

Whilst still relatively uncommon, mass poisonings have highlighted the need to ensure that first responders have both the training to recognize incidents and the available resources to mitigate the health effects of exposure to toxic materials (Burgess *et al.*, 1999; Simon, 1999; Totenhofer and Kierce, 1999; Tur-Kaspa *et al.*, 1999; Bradley, 2000). The potential impact of such events has led many governments to review existing response arrangements and to develop, where necessary, new and improved means of dealing with major incidents. The purpose of this chapter will be to review some of the more common features and problems inherent to mounting an effective response against the deliberate release of hazardous substances.

Threat Materials and Associated Challenges

There are three main categories of hazardous materials that could potentially be used in a deliberate release incident: chemical, biological or radiological (Thornton *et al.*, 2004). Reviews of such materials have been presented elsewhere (Marrs *et al.*, 2008; Gupta, 2009; Maynard and Chilcott, 2009; Chilcott, 2010). Whilst radiological and biological contaminants are clearly of concern, exposure to chemicals will, in general, require more rapid clinical intervention to mitigate potential health effects. For example, inhalation of hydrogen cyanide or certain organophosphorus compounds may be lethal within minutes (Maynard and Chilcott, 2009). In contrast, there may be a potential therapeutic window of several days or more for the effective administration of medical countermeasures against biological or radiological contaminants. Therefore, this chapter will focus on chemical incidents rather than those involving radiological or biological materials.

Chemicals likely to be of interest to terrorist groups can be generally categorized as CW agents or TICs. The former generally have little or no application other than to cause incapacitation or death, tend to be more toxic than TICs and have been comprehensively banned under international legislation (Anonymous, 2005). In contrast, TICs may be subject to extensive and perfectly legitimate use within the chemical industry and so may be ubiquitous within many countries (Russell and Simpson, 2010). Sadly, there is a long history of incidents involving the accidental release of TICs and so many countries have well-developed and practised response protocols for such 'hazmat' incidents (Annelli, 2006).

As already mentioned, the rapidity with which some chemicals exert pathological effects poses a considerable challenge when planning for (and responding to) a deliberate release incident. In this respect there should, at least in theory, be much to learn from military doctrine gained from many decades of research, development and operational experience. However, there are many considerable and necessary dichotomies between military and civilian preparedness: military personnel tend to be young, healthy, highly trained individuals who, under certain conditions, may carry detection equipment, personal protective equipment (PPE), decontamination kits and antidotes specific to many threat agents. Thus overall, a military response to a chemical exposure should be swift and effective. In contrast, whilst a civilian response may draw upon such military experience in terms of effective medical countermeasures and decontamination systems, there will necessarily be a delay between initial exposure and arrival on-scene of appropriate equipment, countermeasures and trained personnel. Furthermore, it cannot be assumed that all members of the general public will have the cognitive or physical ability to comply with procedures. In addition, there may be potential complications as a result of religious/spiritual beliefs, language barriers and other confounding factors such as heightened susceptibility to certain chemicals (due to pre-existing diseases).

Incident Recognition

Although it is obvious to state that an appropriate response is critical to mitigating the public health effects of a chemical, biological, radiological or nuclear (CBRN) incident, such a response can only be of value if implemented in a timely manner. Therefore, the most critical event following the deliberate release of a toxic material would be the recognition that an incident has actually occurred. Whilst many chemicals may provoke immediate signs or symptoms of intoxication (and may thus raise suspicion of an exposure), there are a number of chemicals that have a latent period during which pathological changes may develop in the absence of overt clinical features or other warning signs such as unusual or pungent odours. Classic examples of chemicals that have such a characteristic delay include phosgene and sulphur mustard (Marrs *et al.*, 2008; Maynard and Chilcott, 2009). Moreover, the onset of clinical effects following exposure to chemicals that act predominantly via dermal absorption (such as the nerve agent VX) may also be subject to a latent period, which will be dependent on the anatomical location of the exposure and the environmental conditions (Craig *et al.*, 1977; Duncan *et al.*, 2002; Hamilton *et al.*, 2004). Fortunately, the effects of many chemicals can be effectively mitigated through the process of disrobing and decontamination, even after a delay of several hours.[1]

Clearly, adequate training of first responders is vital in facilitating the process of incident recognition and many countries have developed appropriate procedures. For example, the UK emergency services have adopted an initial response based on the Safety Triggers for Emergency Personnel or 'STEP 1-2-3' procedure (Table 17.1).

Table 17.1. Outline of UK initial emergency response procedure (STEP; safety triggers for emergency personnel). The basic response applies to casualties exhibiting the same signs/symptoms at the same location at the same time.

Casualty status	Basic response
One casualty	Treat as normal
Two casualties	Approach with caution
Three casualties	Do not approach and request specialist support

A small number of chemicals have relatively specific signs and symptoms of exposure (toxidromes), which may aid detection of an incident and be of possible diagnostic utility. For example, nerve agents (and other chemicals that act via inhibition of cholinesterase) may produce overt signs of poisoning consistent with nicotinic or muscarinic stimulation such as miosis and hypersalivation, respectively. Indeed, several countries have developed algorithms to assist in the recognition of exposure to key threat agents (Cieslak *et al.*, 2000; Krivoy *et al.*, 2005; Heptonstall and Gent, 2006) but it must be noted that only a relatively small group of chemicals have such characteristic toxidromes; there are literally thousands of chemicals that could potentially be used in a deliberate release incident and their effects may be non-specific such as coughing, headache, nausea and dizziness. Therefore, recognizing that an incident has occurred requires a combination of vigilance, experience, training and common sense.

---

[1] The unpublished data referred to in this and subsequent sections relate to research performed in support of the ORCHIDS 1; project, conducted between 2008 and 2011, which was co-funded by the European Union (Executive Agency for Health and Consumer) and the Department of Health (England, UK). The overall aim of the project was to establish the optimum means of performing mass casualty decontamination. The primary project partners were the Health Protection Agency (UK), Faculty of Military Health Sciences, University of Defence (Czech Republic), Institut de Recherche Biologique des Armées (France) and the Swedish Defence Research Agency. For supplementary information, refer to www.orchidsproject.eu.

Initial Response

Many countries have developed national or regional plans for responding to a CBRN incident (Annelli, 2006; Baker, 2007; Anonymous, 2010). Whilst such plans vary in detail, all have generic features, which will now be presented in 'ideal' chronological order. It should be noted that in a real event, the actual sequence of activities may be dictated by on-going risk assessments and availability of resources: incident commanders must be prepared for *ad hoc* changes to long-standing plans and have the presence of mind not to delay individual elements of a response by doggedly adhering to written procedures.

The following outline of events makes the assumption that an incident has been recognized and that appropriately equipped responders are available on scene. This represents an idealized scenario. In a real situation, life-saving actions may be performed by first responders equipped with minimal levels of PPE operating to country-specific guidelines such as the '3/30' rule (Anonymous, 1999) under which short-duration 'snatch' rescues may be performed prior to the arrival of incident-trained responders with access to high level PPE.

Evacuation of ambulant casualties

The primary response to any CBRN incident should be to immediately facilitate the self-extraction of casualties from the point of contamination (commonly referred to as the 'hot zone' or 'red zone') to the relative safety of a 'warm zone' (or 'white zone'). In practice, such an apparently simple step can present a number of problems. For example, is the source/location of the contaminant known? How far upwind from the point of release is deemed safe? Such questions are likely to be site-specific and can only be addressed at the time of an incident. Moreover, it is conceivable that pre-planned or *ad hoc* evacuation points may need to be relocated during the course of an incident due to changes in wind direction (which can be an inherent challenge in built-up areas) or as a result of the subsequent identification of additional, 'secondary devices'.

Evacuation of non-ambulant casualties

The evacuation of non-ambulant casualties may pose two problems. The first would be the clinical impact of moving casualties with immediately life-threatening injuries (such as catastrophic haemorrhage) or other circumstances (such as spinal trauma) that would normally necessitate stabilization prior to movement of the patient. Such considerations may be particularly relevant to incidents involving the energetic (explosive) dissemination of contaminants. However, if the immediate environment were overtly life-threatening then evacuation should become a priority over stabilization of the non-ambulant patient. The second problem relates to the availability of appropriate protective equipment to first responders during the initial stages of an incident. If a toxic gas, aerosol or vapour were known to be present (for example, as confirmed by overt physiological effects on casualties), then it would be inappropriate for a responder to attempt a snatch rescue of a non-ambulant casualty in the absence of *at least* an 'escape hood', full-face respirator or self-contained breathing apparatus without running the risk of becoming a casualty. This may pose a considerable personal dilemma, as the *raison d'être* of the emergency medical services is to save lives.

Zoning

In parallel to evacuation, the outer area peripheral to the incident should be immediately cordoned off to prevent further, accidental exposure of unaffected individuals to the contaminant. The distance from the contaminant source to the outer cordon varies according to country-specific guidelines. For example, Canada, Mexico and the USA employ cordon distances that are specific to individual chemicals (Anonymous, 2008), whereas UK emergency services use an initial, generic cordon distance of 400 m. Historically, the latter was probably derived in the 19th century as the minimum distance that an individual could stand from a barrel of gunpowder without risk of shrapnel injury.

When the extent and nature of a contaminant source has been ascertained, an inner cordon should be imposed, which is generally a 25–50 m radius around the contaminant. This inner area is then referred to as the ‘hot zone’ or ‘red zone’, with the area between the hot zone and the outer cordon being termed the ‘warm zone’ or ‘white zone’. The area outside the warm zone is referred to as the ‘cold zone’ or ‘blue zone’ (Fig. 17.1).

In addition to preventing ingress of individuals, cordons provide the opportunity to prevent the egress of potentially contaminated individuals, although the ability to effectively enforce this measure varies considerably between countries as it has potential implications for the personal rights of the affected individuals. However, there are many advantages to secure zoning. These include:

- Preventing further, unintentional spread of contamination (by people or vehicles) to unaffected areas. Limiting contamination to a relatively small area may enhance effectiveness and reduce costs associated with post-incident (environmental) decontamination.
- Reducing or eliminating arrival of ‘worried well’ and/or potentially contaminated casualties at multiple medical facilities. The uncontrolled migration of potentially contaminated individuals to multiple medical facilities could result in a number of problems such as crowd control (security of staff and buildings), overwhelming of capacity and contamination of hospital infrastructure.
- Providing an area within which the emergency services can operate effectively under appropriate safety guidelines (such as wearing of hazard-specific PPE in accordance with extant procedures).

Whilst the enforcement of zones can undoubtedly improve the overall effectiveness of an incident response, there are some attendant disadvantages. These include the physiological burden on responders (carrying non-ambulant casualties over relatively long distances imposed by the cordons whilst wearing full PPE) and the resource-intensive effort required to enforce what could potentially be a large warm-zone perimeter.

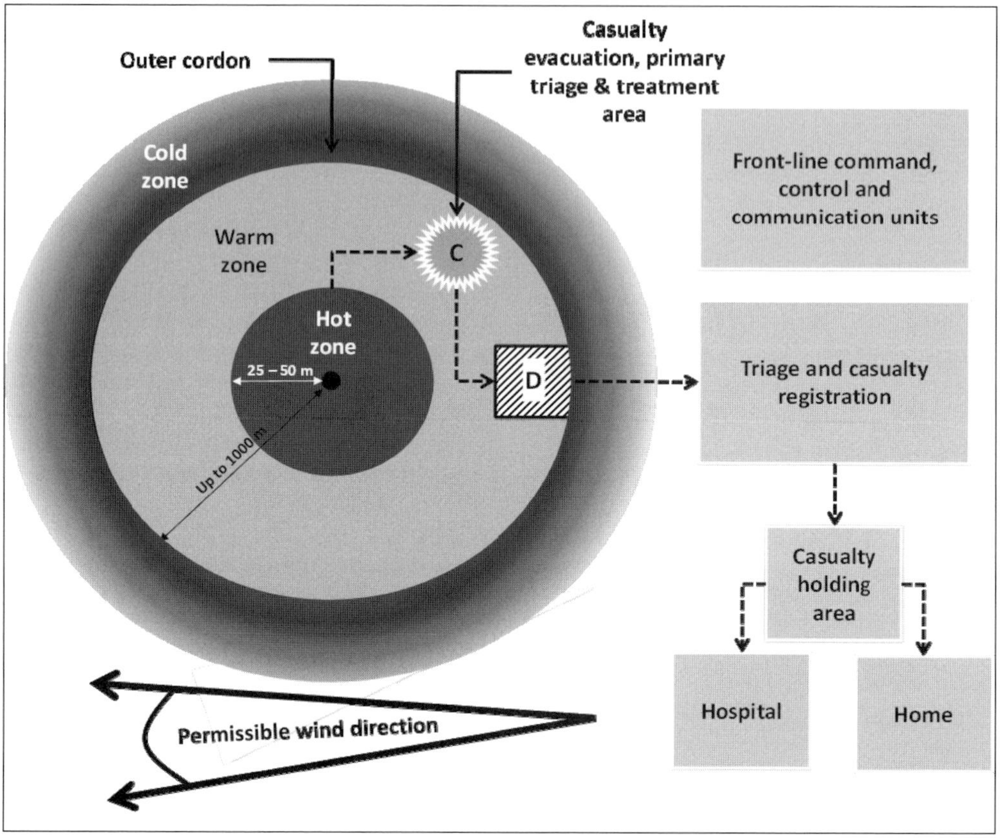

Fig. 17.1. Schematic representation of cold, warm and hot incident zones. 'C' approximates to the evacuation and initial triage area. Dotted lines represent flow of casualties through the incident zones, via decontamination units ('D'). The casualty registration point allows collection of personal data, which may be used as part of criminal investigation and to facilitate future health surveillance. The casualty holding area should provide a comfortable environment within which casualties await onward transport to hospital, home or alternative residence.

Administration of medical countermeasures

Advanced medical care has traditionally been limited to the cold zone following evacuation and decontamination of casualties. However, there has been a growing recognition that advanced clinical support needs to occur in the hot or warm zone, especially with non-ambulant, high-priority patients. In the UK, hot zone medical treatment is performed by specialist units of the Ambulance Service known as 'special operations response teams' or 'hazardous area response teams' (Fig. 17.2) who are trained to perform procedures including intubation, intra-osseous drug administration and haemostatic interventions, as well as administer medical countermeasures such as antidotes.

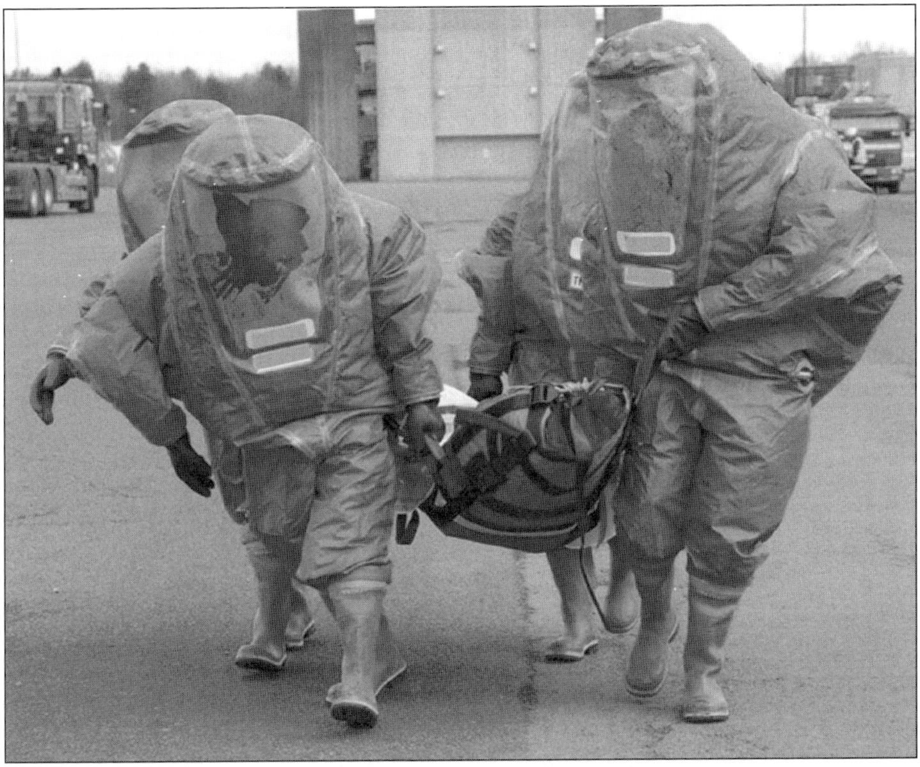

Fig. 17.2. Hazardous area response team (HART) members extracting a non-ambulant casualty from the hot zone of a chemical incident exercise. In the UK, HART and special operation response teams (SORT) provide advanced medical care capability within the hot zone and so may substantially improve survival rates for high priority casualties. In this photograph, each team member is wearing a chemically inert, gas-tight suit with an internal source of air (self-contained breathing apparatus; SCBA). (Picture reproduced with permission of the Department of Health, England, UK)

Disrobing

Disrobing (removal of clothing) is arguably the most effective means of mitigating the health effects of exposure to toxic aerosols, liquids or solid materials and, as such, should be given the highest priority if a CBRN incident is suspected or known to be in progress (Clarke *et al.*, 2008). It is commonly claimed that disrobing removes 75–90% of contaminants from an individual (Wolbarst *et al.*, 2010). This figure is likely to be derived from the 'rule of nines' (Knaysi *et al.*, 1968) on the assumption that all areas of the body except the hands and face are covered in relatively impermeable clothing. However, there does not appear to be a definitive study to support this degree of effectiveness. Indeed, recent (unpublished) studies[1] (Chilcott, 2009) have indicated that the proportion of a contaminant that can be removed by disrobing is in the region of 45–70%, depending on the conditions of the exposure. However, removal of such a proportion of contaminant may still be of clinical relevance if performed with minimal delay.

For exposure to liquid contaminants in particular, the delay between initial exposure and subsequent disrobing should be as short as practically possible. This is because liquids can diffuse through normal fabric layers and so the effectiveness of disrobing decreases with time (Matar *et al.*, 2010). As a rough rule of thumb, the effectiveness of disrobing has a half-life of approximately 30 min. In other words, the amount of liquid contaminant that can be effectively removed by disrobing will decrease by half for every 30-min delay.[2] Therefore, it is essential that disrobing be considered a primary action in response to an incident involving the release of a hazardous substance in order to maximize effectiveness. In addition to the clear clinical benefits, disrobing will substantially reduce the risk of secondary contamination to medical staff and associated infrastructure. Disrobing should also be considered following putative exposure to gases and vapours. The Tokyo subway incident clearly demonstrated that when multiple casualties (exposed to nerve agent vapour) congregated at hospital emergency departments, there was sufficient off-gassing of contaminant to cause incapacitation of medical staff (Nozaki *et al.*, 1995).

Clearly, there are many practical challenges associated with disrobing, least of all privacy issues and the availability of clean replacement garments. In the UK, specialist emergency response vehicles carry 'disrobe packs', the contents of which include a cutting tool (to facilitate removal of contaminated garments) and a high-visibility poncho for re-robing (Fig. 17.3).

Where such a specialist response is not available, consideration should be given to requesting or commandeering articles of clothing from local retail outlets. Given the urgency with which disrobing should be performed, any form of replacement clothing should be considered. For example, blankets or foil sheets (often carried as standard equipment by emergency response services) or even opaque 'bin liners' (refuse sacks) would provide an adequate, if temporary, re-robing capacity.

Decontamination

Decontamination is generally performed in the warm zone following evacuation from the hot zone (Fig. 17.1). Passage through a decontamination facility represents transfer from the warm zone to the cold zone.

Decontamination can be defined as the process of removing hazardous material(s) both on or available to the external surfaces of the body in order to reduce local or systemic exposure to a contaminant and thus minimize the risk of subsequent adverse health effects. It is perhaps worth differentiating between mass decontamination (performed on groups of individuals sometime after exposure) and 'interim' (or 'immediate') decontamination. The latter generally refers to *ad hoc* methods such as a bucket and sponge, municipal shower or fire hose ('ladder-pipe method'; Lake *et al.*, 2000). This section will focus on the treatment of large numbers of casualties at the scene of an incident ('mass decontamination').

---

[2] It is important to note that this half-life refers specifically to the *amount* of contaminant removed, *not clinical efficacy*. The latter will be dependent on the extent of contamination and the percutaneous toxicity and volatility of the contaminant.

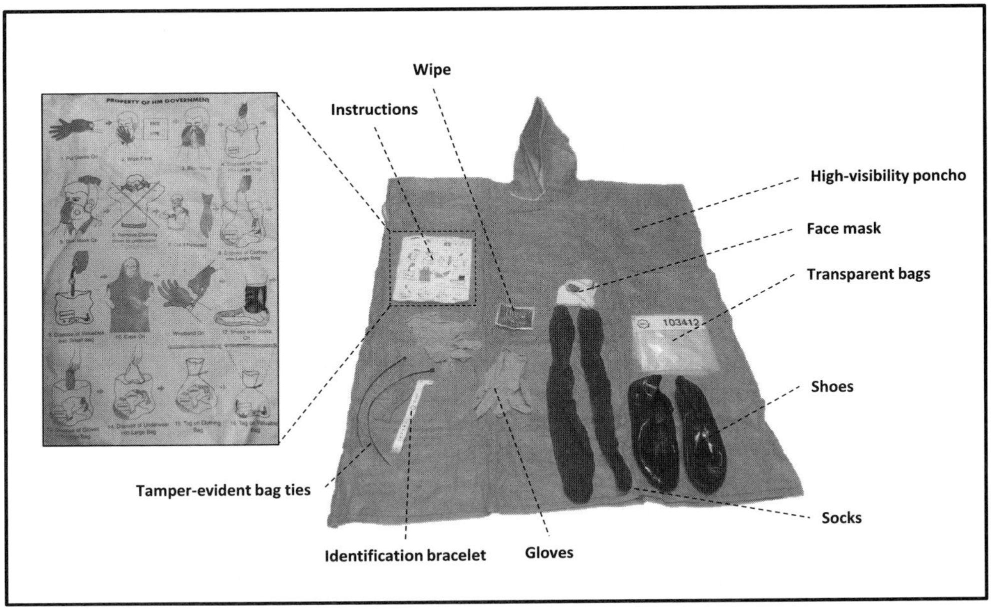

Fig.17.3. Articles contained in the UK's mass casualty decontamination 'disrobe pack'. The packs are individually vacuum-sealed to reduce storage requirements. Instructions (inset left) are printed on waterproof paper. Two transparent bags are included; one large (for contaminated clothing) and one small (for personal effects). The bracelet and bag ties have the same unique identification number.

It should be noted that a small number of countries (for example, Israel) have a doctrine of extracting casualties, via pre-planned transport systems, to large-scale decontamination facilities at nominated medical institutes rather than performing decontamination at the scene of an incident. Both on-scene and hospital decontamination have theoretical merits and disadvantages, although there is little practical experience upon which to base a rational comparison.

Hospital emergency departments should have standard procedures for performing decontamination on small numbers of individuals ('clinical decontamination') and so local guidelines should be consulted where available. However, this limited approach should not be considered part of an integral response to a major incident, as it would be rapidly overwhelmed.

Decontamination is commonly thought of as a stand-alone process. However, decontamination should be considered to be one aspect of a combined 'disrobe and decontaminate' procedure. It is important to disrobe casualties prior to decontamination for the following practical reasons:

- Contaminated clothing represents a potential contact and/or off-gassing hazard to both casualties and emergency response personnel.

- Decontamination may be rendered ineffective in the presence of clothing. Moreover, water-based decontamination may facilitate transfer of contaminants from the outer layers of clothing to the skin surface and so negate the transient protective effects offered by civilian attire.

As with disrobing, decontamination must be performed as soon as reasonably possible in order to maximize efficacy.

Wet and dry decontamination processes

Decontamination can be broadly categorized as 'wet' or 'dry'. Wet, or aqueous-based decontamination, relies on the use of water (optionally containing detergents or other excipients such as bleach) to wash and rinse potentially contaminated areas of hair and skin. The over-riding advantage of wet decontamination is that thc raw matcrial (water) is ubiquitous in developed countries and so access to municipal or domestic supplies can generally be assured during an incident. However, wet decontamination has several challenges:

- There may be uncontrolled run-off of waste water, which could increase the mobility of the contaminant.
- There may be some difficulty in removing lipophilic (oily) substances from the skin due to limited dissolution. In extreme cases, this could potentially lead to increased areas of skin contamination.
- In the absence of a heated water supply and/or adequate shelter, showering of individuals may lead to hypothermia, especially when deployed in colder climates on vulnerable populations such as the elderly and very young. The optimal water temperature[1] for performing skin decontamination is 35°C.
- In order to effectively remove lipophilic (oily) substances, an adequate supply of soap or detergent should be available to improve dissolution of contaminants. As a general rule, detergent solutions remove approximately 40% more skin contamination compared to water alone.[1]
- Some studies have indicated that water may enhance the dermal absorption of certain contaminants (Moody and Maibach, 2006). This effect can be markedly reduced by limiting the duration of wet decontamination to under 90 s.[1]

The use of bleach (hypochlorite) has been suggested as a means of neutralizing chemical contaminants, and animal studies have confirmed some degree of effectiveness (Bjarnason *et al.*, 2008). However, the tolerable concentration of hypochlorite[3] (0.5%) in shower water (for mass decontamination purposes) is of questionable relevance for the rapid and complete neutralization of chemicals on the skin surface.

A recent, comprehensive study[1] has produced evidence-based recommendations on the optimal conditions for shower-based, mass casualty decontamination. In summary, these are:

---

[3] Tolerable concentration in this context refers to the threshold concentration for ocular toxicity.

- Shower water temperature of 35°C;
- Shower duration of 60 (minimum) to 90 (maximum) s;
- Addition of a detergent to the shower water at the manufacturer's recommended concentration;
- Provision of a washing aid, such as a flannel (wash cloth).

The latter point is important, as use of a washing aid can improve the effectiveness of decontamination by ~20% (Amlot *et al.*, 2010). Thus, the act of providing a washing aid is a simple yet cost effective means of substantially improving the efficacy of mass casualty decontamination. Finally, it is worth considering the impact of drying the skin after wet decontamination. In the absence of a washing aid, absorbent materials such as a towel can remove up to 30% of a skin contaminant after showering[1] and so active drying is a major factor controlling the outcome of wet decontamination.

There are many commercial suppliers of portable, wet-decontamination equipment offering a range of products such as single stands, rapid-deployment tents and hard-walled units. Commercial mass decontamination systems often comprise separate disrobing, showering and re-robing areas, acquire pressurized water from fire appliances or municipal hydrants and can adjust the flow rate, duration, temperature and composition (detergent concentration) of the shower water. Thus overall, bespoke systems provide an ideal environment within which to perform mass casualty decontamination. However, a disadvantage of such systems may be the time taken to deploy and become operational at an incident. For this reason, immediate (or 'interim') decontamination may be required to supplement an incident response.

Dry decontamination generally utilizes the absorbent properties of powders or fabrics to passively draw contaminants from the skin surface (Chilcott, 2007). In the case of liquid skin contaminants, this can be an effective means of mitigating dermal exposure.[4] Indeed, a number of military organizations use commercial (powder-based) decontamination systems such as Fuller's earth. In theory, any absorbent material may demonstrate some degree of effectiveness and should be considered if other, more conventional means of decontamination are unavailable. Practical examples of absorbent materials include cotton wool, sponges, flour, paper towels, tissue paper, blotting paper and dry earth. However, the use of such interim products has not been subject to extensive evaluation and extreme caution would need to be exercised when handling or disposing of used material, as passive absorbents do not deactivate, degrade or otherwise neutralize chemical contaminants and, therefore, may represent a significant contact or respiratory hazard.

Subsequent Actions

Following decontamination and re-robing, ambulant casualties should be transferred to a comfortable environment where personal details, witness statements (if required for criminal investigations), clinical observation, further triage and medical treatment may be

---

[4] In certain regions of France, the emergency services employ a combination of dry decontamination with Fuller's earth ('*Gant Poudre*') followed by wet (shower-based) decontamination (Dr Denis Josse, personal communication, 2010).

performed prior to onward transport. Whilst seemingly of trivial relevance during a major incident, the acquisition of personal information is essential to facilitate future health surveillance – this is an important aspect, as toxic materials may have chronic, as well as acute health effects.

Conclusion

Recognizing the onset of a mass casualty incident is key to implementing an effective response. In the first instance, evacuation and cordoning of the affected area(s) should be undertaken. When the safety of casualties and responders has been established, disrobing of contaminated individuals should be undertaken as soon as practically possible followed rapidly by decontamination. Following transfer to a safe area, personal details should be acquired to ensure future contact for health surveillance to counter any potential chronic health effects.

Acknowledgements

The author wishes to acknowledge the European Union's Executive Agency for Health and Consumers, the Department of Health (England) and the UK's Home Office for funding the (unpublished) experimental work cited in this chapter.

References

Amlot, R., Larner, J., Matar, H., Jones, D.R., Carter, H., Turner, E.A., Price, S.C. and Chilcott, R.P. (2010) Comparative analysis of showering protocols for mass-casualty decontamination. *Prehospital Disaster Medicine* 25(5), 435–439.

Annelli, J.F. (2006) The national incident management system: a multi-agency approach to emergency response in the United States of America. *Review of Science and Technology* 25(1), 223–231.

Anonymous (1999) U.S. ARMY SBCCOM Domestic Preparedness Chemical Team. Guidelines for Incident Commander's use of firefighter protective ensemble (FFPE) with self-contained breathing apparatus (SCBA) for rescue operations during a terrorist chemical agent incident. Available at: http://www.chem-bio.com/resource/1999/cw_irp_final_incident_cmd.pdf (Accessed 31 January 2013).

Anonymous (2005) Convention on the prohibition of the development, production, stockpiling and use of chemical weapons and their destruction. Organisation for the Prohibition of Chemical Weapons (OPCW). Available at: http://www.opcw.org/index.php?eID=dam_frontend_push&docID=6357 (Accessed 31 January 2013).

Anonymous (2008) The 2008 Emergency Response Guidebook (ERG2008). Transport Canada, the US Department of Transportation, and the Secretariat of Communications and Transport of Mexico. Available at: http://www.ehso.com/ehsodot.php?URL=http%3A%2F%2Fphmsa.dot.gov/staticfiles/PHMSA/DownloadableFiles/Files/erg2008_eng.pdf (Accessed 31 January 2013).

Anonymous (2010) The United Kingdom's strategy for countering chemical, biological, radiological and nuclear (CBRN) terrorism. HM Government. Available at:

http://webarchive.nationalarchives.gov.uk/20100418065544/http:/security.homeoffice.gov.uk/news-publications/publication-search/cbrn-guidance/strat-countering-use-of-CBRN?view=Binary (Accessed 31 January 2013).

Baker, D.J. (2007) The management of casualties following toxic agent release: the approach adopted in France. In: Marrs, T.C., Maynard, R.L. and Sidell, F.R. (eds) *Chemical Warfare Agents: Toxicology and Treatment*, 2nd edn. John Wiley & Sons, , Chichester, UK, pp. 261–276.

Bjarnason, S., Mikler, J., Hill, I., Tenn, C., Garrett, M., Caddy, N. and Sawyer, T.W. (2008) Comparison of selected skin decontaminant products and regimens against VX in domestic swine. *Human and Experimental Toxicology* 27(3), 253–261.

Bradley, R.N. (2000) Health care facility preparation for weapons of mass destruction. *Prehospital and Emergency Care* 4(3), 261–269.

Burgess, J.L., Kirk, M., Borron, S.W. and Cisek, J. (1999) Emergency department hazardous materials protocol for contaminated patients. *Annals of Emergency Medicine* 34(2), 205–212.

Chilcott, R.P. (2007) Dermal aspects of chemical warfare agents. In: Marrs, T.C., Maynard, R.L. and Sidell, F.R. (eds) *Chemical Warfare Agents: Toxicology and Treatment*, 2nd edn. John Wiley & Sons, Chichester, UK, pp. 409–422.

Chilcott, R.P. (2009) An overview of the Health Protection Agency's research and development programme on decontamination. *Chemical Hazards and Poisons Report* 15, 26–28.

Chilcott, R.P. (2010) CBRN contamination. In: Ayres, J., Harrison, R., Nichols, G. and Maynard, R.L. (eds) *Textbook of Environmental Medicine*. Hodder Arnold, London.

Cieslak, T.J., Rowe, J.R., Kortepeter, M.G., Madsen, J.M., Newmark, J., Christopher, G.W., Culpepper, R.C. and Eitzen, E.M. Jr (2000) A field-expedient algorithmic approach to the clinical management of chemical and biological casualties. *Military Medicine* 165(9), 659–662.

Clarke, S.F., Chilcott, R.P., Wilson, J.C., Kamanyire, R., Baker, D.J. and Hallett, A. (2008) Decontamination of multiple casualties who are chemically contaminated: a challenge for acute hospitals. *Prehospital and Disaster Medicine* 23(2), 175–181.

Craig, F.N., Cummings, E.G. and Sim, V.M. (1977) Environmental temperature and the percutaneous absorption of a cholinesterase inhibitor, VX. *Journal of Investigative Dermatology* 68(6), 357–361.

Duncan, E.J., Brown, A., Lundy, P., Sawyer, T.W., Hamilton, M., Hill, I. and Conley, J.D. (2002) Site-specific percutaneous absorption of methyl salicylate and VX in domestic swine. *Journal of Applied Toxicology* 22(3), 141–148.

Gupta, R.C. (2009) *Handbook of Toxicology of Chemical Warfare Agents*. Academic Press, London..

Hamilton, M.G., Hill, I., Conley, J., Sawyer, T.W., Caneva, D.C. and Lundy, P.M. (2004) Clinical aspects of percutaneous poisoning by the chemical warfare agent VX: effects of application site and decontamination. *Military Medicine* 169(11), 856–862.

Heptonstall, J. and Gent, N. (2006) CRBN incidents: clinical management and health protection. Health Protection Agency, London.

Knaysi, G.A., Crikelair, G.F. and Cosman, B. (1968) The rule of nines: its history and accuracy. *Plastic and Reconstructive Surgery* 41, 560–563.

Krivoy, A., Layish, I., Rotman, E., Goldberg, A. and Yehezkelli, Y. (2005) OP or not OP: the medical challenge at the chemical terrorism scene. *Prehospital and Disaster Medicine* 20(3), 155–158.

Lake, W.A., Fedele, P.D. and Marshall, S.M. (2000) Guidelines for mass casualty decontamination during a terrorist chemical agent incident. ECBC-TR-125. Available at: http://www.dtic.mil/cgi-bin/GetTRDoc?AD=ADA387193. From http://www.ecbc.army.mil/downloads/cwirp/ECBC_cwirp_gls_mass_casualty_decon.pdf (Accessed 31 January 2013).

Marrs, T.C., Maynard, R.L. and Sidell, F.R. (2008) *Chemical Warfare Agents: Toxicology and Treatment*, 2nd edn. John Wiley & Sons, Ltd, Chichester, UK.

Matar, H., Price, S.C. and Chilcott, R.P. (2010) Temporal effects of disrobing on the skin absorption of chemical warfare agents and CW agent simulants [abstract]. *Toxicology* 278, 344–345.

Maynard, R.L. and Chilcott, R.P. (2009) Toxicology of chemical warfare agents. In: Ballantyne, B., Marrs, T.C. and Syversen, T. (eds) *General and Applied Toxicology*, 3rd edn. John Wiley & Sons, Chichester, UK, pp. 2875–2911.

Moody, R.P. and Maibach, H.I. (2006) Skin decontamination: importance of the wash-in effect. *Food and Chemical Toxicology* 44(11), 1783–1788.

Nozaki, H., Hori, S., Shinozawa, Y., Fujishima, S., Takuma, K., Sagoh, M., Kimura, H., Ohki, T., Suzuki, M. and Aikawa, N. (1995) Secondary exposure of medical staff to sarin vapor in the emergency room. *Intensive Care Medicine* 21(12), 1032–1035.

Okumura, T., Suzuki, K., Fukuda, A., Kohama, A., Takasu, N., Ishimatsu, S. and Hinohara, S. (1998a) The Tokyo subway sarin attack: disaster management, Part 1: Community emergency response. *Academic Emergency Medicine* 5(6), 613–617.

Okumura, T., Suzuki, K., Fukuda, A., Kohama, A., Takasu, N., Ishimatsu, S. and Hinohara, S. (1998b) The Tokyo subway sarin attack: disaster management, Part 2: Hospital response. *Academic Emergency Medicine* 5(6), 618–624.

Okumura, T., Suzuki, K., Fukuda, A., Kohama, A., Takasu, N., Ishimatsu, S. and Hinohara, S. (1998c) The Tokyo subway sarin attack: disaster management, Part 3: National and international responses. *Academic Emergency Medicine* 5(6), 625–628.

Russell, D. and Simpson, J. (2010) Emergency planning and preparedness for the deliberate release of toxic industrial chemicals. *Clinical Toxicology (Phila)* 48(3), 171–176.

Simon, J.D. (1999) Nuclear, biological, and chemical terrorism: understanding the threat and designing responses. *International Journal of Emergency Mental Health* 1(2), 81–89.

Thornton, R., Court, B., Meara, J., Murray, V., Palmer, I., Scott, R., Wlae, M. and Wright, D. (2004) Chemical, biological, radiological and nuclear terrorism: an introduction for occupational physicians. *Occupational Medicine (London)* 54(2), 101–109.

Totenhofer, R.I. and Kierce, M. (1999) It's a disaster: emergency departments' preparation for a chemical incident or disaster. *Accident and Emergency Nursing* 7(3), 141–147.

Tsuchihashi, H., Katagi, M., Nishikawa, M. and Tatsuno, M. (1998) Identification of metabolites of nerve agent VX in serum collected from a victim. *Journal of Analalytical Toxicology* 22(5), 383–388.

Tur-Kaspa, I., Lev, E.I., Hendler, I., Siebner, R., Shapira, Y. and Shemer, J. (1999) Preparing hospitals for toxicological mass casualties events. *Critical Care Medicine* 27(5), 1004–1008.

Wolbarst, A.B., Wiley, A.L., Jr, Nemhauser, J.B., Christensen, D.M. and Hendee, W.R. (2010) Medical response to a major radiologic emergency: a primer for medical and public health practitioners. *Radiology* 254(3), 660–677.

Chapter 18

Emergency Decontamination in Low-resource Settings

Denis Josse and Gilles Barrier

Introduction

Human exposure to toxic chemical (C), radiological (R) or highly infectious biological (B) agents used to mainly concern the military on battlefields (Szinicz, 2005). When a threat is established, the military can be individually equipped with emergency decontamination (ED) and treatment kits (Hurst, 1997). They are trained to use them in order to adequately and quickly respond to CBR attacks.

Recent history has shown that civilian populations can also be exposed to CBR agents. Exposures can occur in specific workplaces (Harper, 2004), or following small- or large-scale accidents (Varma and Guest, 1993; Pesatori *et al.*, 2003; Moysich *et al.*, 2011), or terrorist acts (Okumura *et al.*, 1998; Inglesby *et al.*, 2002; Tokuda *et al.*, 2006). In industrial environments or laboratories, where workers can be potentially exposed to CBR agents, personal protective equipment and prepositioned ED systems, such as showers or eyewash stations or specific decontaminants (Hall and Maibach, 2006; Nehles *et al.*, 2006; Spagnul *et al.*, 2010), are immediately available close to the working area (Fig 18.1). Safety procedures are taught to workers and can be found in pathogen (biological) or material (chemical) safety data sheets for an immediate response to exposure by the victims themselves and rescuers (Elliott, 2001; Hayes, 2011). In non-professional settings, following unexpected exposure to initially non-identified agents, ED might not always be performed, particularly if the symptoms of exposure do not quickly appear or if the victims are not sufficiently educated in first-aid measures. In the presence of a limited or large number of symptomatic victims on the incident site, the first emergency measures that it is recommended to take in order to limit the severity of any potential intoxication, irradiation or infection are the extraction of victims from the 'hot zone', i.e. an exclusion area where they could be directly exposed to the vapour, liquid or dust forms of the agents, into a 'warm zone' where the victims are decontaminated and eventually treated before entering a 'cold zone', i.e. a contamination-free area.

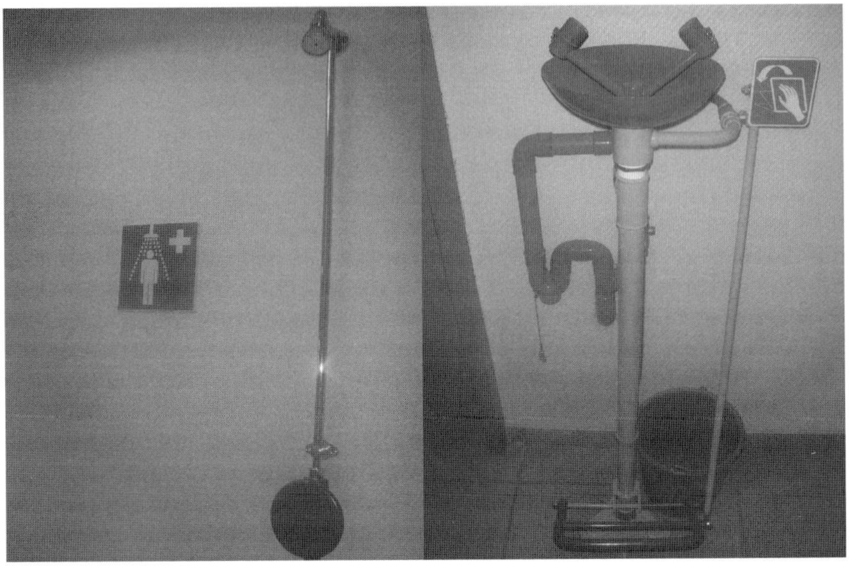

(a) (b)

Fig. 18.1. Emergency decontamination shower (a) and eye wash station (b) for emergency decontamination at work (Source: Laboratory of Dr Denis Josse).

Emergency Decontamination: A Life-saving Decontamination Procedure

Decontamination is a critical part of victim care management. It is defined as a procedure aimed at removing or neutralizing any C, R or B agents present on the body surface (Braue *et al.*, 2009). It can be viewed as a two-step process: first, ED, which is a life-saving decontamination procedure, and second, thorough decontamination or full body decontamination performed to avoid the transfer of contamination in the cold zone, particularly in medical units, and the secondary contamination of responders, unexposed population, equipment and environment (Lukey *et al.*, 2008). The objectives of ED are to remove as much contamination as possible from the body surface, including clothes, but not necessarily all of it. Following ED, the level of contamination should be low enough to allow the victims' survival and to limit irreversible damage of victims' skin, eyes and mucosal membranes.

In a military or professional context, ED can usually be performed in the first minute following contamination: it is immediate decontamination. In contrast, in a civilian or homeland defence scenario, the first decontamination may not occur until emergency responders arrive on the incident site, which might take more than 30 min after the exposure. Furthermore, for most ambulatory victims who might have escaped the incident site and reached the closest medical units, the first decontamination, which might be put in place in a dedicated space near the hospital entrance, might only start more than 1 h after the exposure. Whether performed immediately or delayed following contamination, the first decontamination could be considered as ED as long as its main outcome is the victims' survival.

In low-resource settings, i.e. in the absence of specifically dedicated equipment such as decontamination shelters, or fast transportation vehicles to hospitals, or large water supplies (pool, river, car-wash site, etc.) in the vicinity, the victims themselves and emergency responders, possibly not equipped with decontamination kits or informed of the agent's identity, might therefore have to find or design and use as quickly and effectively as possible any potential decontamination systems present on-site to perform ED.

The objective of this chapter is to review ED principles, procedures and systems and to provide ED guidelines to victims and responders in a low-resource setting.

ED Principles

When performing ED, a few principles are consistently recommended to be followed. These principles are mostly common sense-based, more rarely evidence-based.

First principle: ED should be performed with the shortest possible delay following contamination (Hurst, 1997)

Due to the intrinsic properties of contaminants such as skin reactivity, absorption and volatility, the amount of contaminants present on the body surface, i.e. potentially available to the decontaminant, could quickly become low 15 to 30 min post-exposure. Consequently, the victims' survival rate and possibility of irreversible injuries will strictly depend on how quickly ED is performed following an exposure to contaminants. This has clearly been demonstrated in animals exposed to nerve agents (soman, VX) (Bjarnason *et al.*, 2008; Braue *et al.*, 2011a,b) or the vesicant sulphur mustard (SM) (Taysse *et al.*, 2011). The main operational consequences of this rule are that ED systems should be easily and quickly available to victims. In addition, ED systems and procedures should be sufficiently polyvalent to be implemented before any agent's identification. In a mass casualty incident (MCI), the symptomatic victims, i.e. the most likely contaminated victims, should be treated and decontaminated first. Consequently, decontamination triage should be viewed as a critical part of victim care management since, if correctly and quickly performed, it should shorten the time between exposure and decontamination for the most contaminated.

Second principle: Removal of contamination is the main rule of ED (Lukey *et al.*, 2008)

Physical removal is imperative since none of the biocompatible decontaminants destroy the agents instantaneously (Hurst, 1997). It includes disrobing, scraping or blotting off visible agent from the skin, using adsorbents to soak up the agent, and flushing or showering with large quantities of water (Schulze and Lake, 2009).

Third principle: ED should be easy to perform in order to facilitate personal self-decontamination, even for non-educated people, possibly with low autonomy

In certain situations, decontamination could be best achieved using a 'buddy system', i.e. one individual will decontaminate the other and then switch place to allow access to skin sites frequently missed, e.g. the back (Pulley and Jones, 2008). In addition, ED procedure could be demonstrated (mimicked) by emergency responders to groups of victims.

Fourth principle: ED mostly applies for C agents

Decontamination following an exposure to R or B agents does not require the same degree of emergency as it does for C agents since the acute toxicity of R or B agents is much lower than that of highly toxic and reactive C agents. However, after an exposure to radioactive contaminants, it is crucial to first prevent the inhalation of dust (Arora *et al.*, 2010; Kumar *et al.*, 2010). In addition, it has been shown that some radioactive compounds have a high affinity for biological components, which make them difficult to remove if the decontamination is not quickly performed (Bolzinger *et al.*, 2010), others can significantly penetrate through the skin (Petitot *et al.*, 2010). Among the C agents, the nerve agents, such as soman and VX, the vesicants, such as SM and lewisite, but also strong irritants, such as riot control agents (Pesonen *et al.*, 2010), corrosives, strong acids and bases specifically require ED.

ED Systems and Procedures

The objective of this section is not to provide an exhaustive list of currently available ED kits and to introduce their components. Instead, we will focus on two groups of ED systems, which are potentially available in most environments, i.e. dry decontaminants and water.

Before introducing the ED systems and as outlined in the current US guidelines for mass casualty decontamination (Schulze and Lake, 2008), it should be remembered that the most critical step of decontamination is the removal of the outer clothing since clothes trap most contaminants (Hao *et al.*, 2007; Feldman, 2010). It is generally assumed that removal of outer clothing removes at least 80% of contamination.

Clothing removal

Victims should be encouraged to immediately remove as much clothing as possible, at least the outer garments, including hat, shoes, gloves, as well as potentially contaminated jewellery (watches, necklaces, etc.) and place them in closed bags. Ideally, disrobing should be performed from head to toe. Contact between the external part of clothing, which is potentially contaminated, and the skin, i.e. contamination transfer, should be limited as much as possible. Lifting the clothes over the head should be avoided to reduce the transfer of contamination to the face, eyes and scalp. In a mass casualty situation, self-disrobing should be promoted. However, partial disrobing of people with low autonomy (children, the elderly, the disabled) will require assistance by another victim or, if present in sufficient number, by a rescuer (Rotenberg *et al.*, 2003).

After exposure to radioactive contaminants, it is recommended that the protection of the respiratory route be followed with water spraying of clothes before their removal, since this will limit the dispersion of dust.

Emergency decontamination of the exposed body surface (i.e. not covered with clothes)

Wound ED

Since wounds represent a direct route of entry into the systemic circulation, wound decontamination should be performed first, before that of intact skin. Wound ED should at least consist of the removal of any potentially contaminated foreign bodies. Ideally, this should be followed by saline or water flushing, gentle scrubbing with a surgical sponge and disinfection (Bushberg *et al.*, 2007). Alternatively, wounds potentially contaminated with radioactive agents should first be covered with a clean dressing since radioactive material will often exude from wounds into dressings. Frequent changing of dressings may aid wound decontamination. Selective decontaminants such as diethylene triamine pentaacetic acid (DTPA) or calixarene-based formulations have been demonstrated to be effective on wounds (Tymen *et al.*, 2000; Schadilov *et al.*, 2010; Spagnul *et al.*, 2011). Thermal burns should be decontaminated by gently rinsing with clean water.

Eye ED

Eye contamination with irritants will require water flushing with a large volume of clean water as an emergency measure (Chau *et al.*, 2012). Commercial eye decontaminants such as Diphoterine® (Fig. 18.2) or Hexafluorine® have been found to be effective against caustic chemicals (Hall *et al.*, 2002; Horton *et al.*, 2002; Soderberg *et al.*, 2004; Carron and Yersin, 2009).

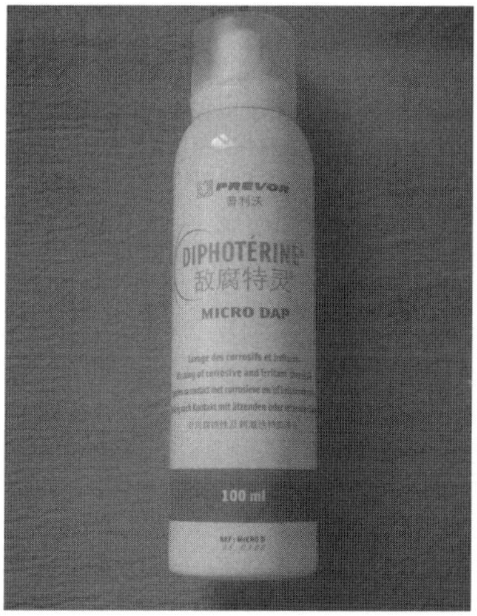

Fig.18.2. Example of eye emergency decontaminant against caustic chemicals (Diphoterine®) (picture by Dr Denis Josse).

Hair ED

Hair potentially adsorbs C agents (DeLauder and Kidwell, 2000). This can lead to the permeation of chemicals through the scalp, desorption of chemical vapours and secondary contamination. Pouring adsorbent powder on the hair might limit chemical absorption and desorption. Powdered hair could then be covered until a shower could be performed (i.e. thorough decontamination). Powders should not be used on hair potentially contaminated with R or B particles. In this case, hair should only be covered to limit the agent's dispersion until a shower can be performed.

Intact skin ED

As demonstrated by van Hooidonk *et al.* (1983), the removal of any visible potential contamination present on the skin by using any adsorbent or absorbent system available, i.e. handkerchief, paper, towel, clean fabric, is quite an effective ED measure. The ad- or absorbent should only be blotted on the skin to avoid the spreading of contamination on the skin surface and any enhancement of skin permeation. The decontamination procedure should preserve the skin integrity as much as possible. It could be repeated several times, each time with a clean system. This especially applies following skin contamination with lipophilic compounds such as VX and SM. The waste should be collected in a closed bag in order to avoid secondary exposure. Alternatively, adsorbent powders such as flour, talcum powder, clean sand, cat litter could be used. These powders usually have selective affinity for hydrophilic or lipophilic chemicals. In a few countries, adsorbent powders are used by the military as skin emergency decontaminant (Fig. 18.3).

For instance, Fuller's earth has a relatively high affinity for lipophilic chemical and has been shown to be highly effective as a skin decontaminant against SM and VX (Taysse *et al.*, 2007, 2011). However, if the decontamination is delayed, it is slightly less effective than the RSDL® kit (Fig. 18.4), which consists of a polylethylene glycol (PEG)- and oximate-based lotion and a sponge (Bjarnason *et al.*, 2008; Braue *et al.*, 2011a; Taysse *et al.*, 2011). Adsorbent powders are poured on the contaminated area, then either left until a shower can be performed or, after a short contact time, removed with a towel or more effectively with water.

Water as an effective emergency skin decontaminant?

Thanks to its diluting and mechanical effects when applied on the body surface as a jet, water is often viewed as one of the most convenient and effective emergency decontaminants. Standard first aid guidelines following skin and eye exposure to toxic chemicals is to flush the affected areas with copious amounts of water for 15 min (Hall and Maibach, 2006). However, it is recommended that chemicals that create significant exothermy when combined with water, e.g. white phosphorus, or that have a very low solubility in water, e.g. phenol or SM, should be blotted off prior to lavage with water (Segal, 2007; Palao *et al.*, 2010). This is supported by recent work from Lademann *et al.* (2011) who showed that after a short exposure to an oily chemical, absorbing materials are better suited than the water washing process for skin decontamination.

(a)

(b)

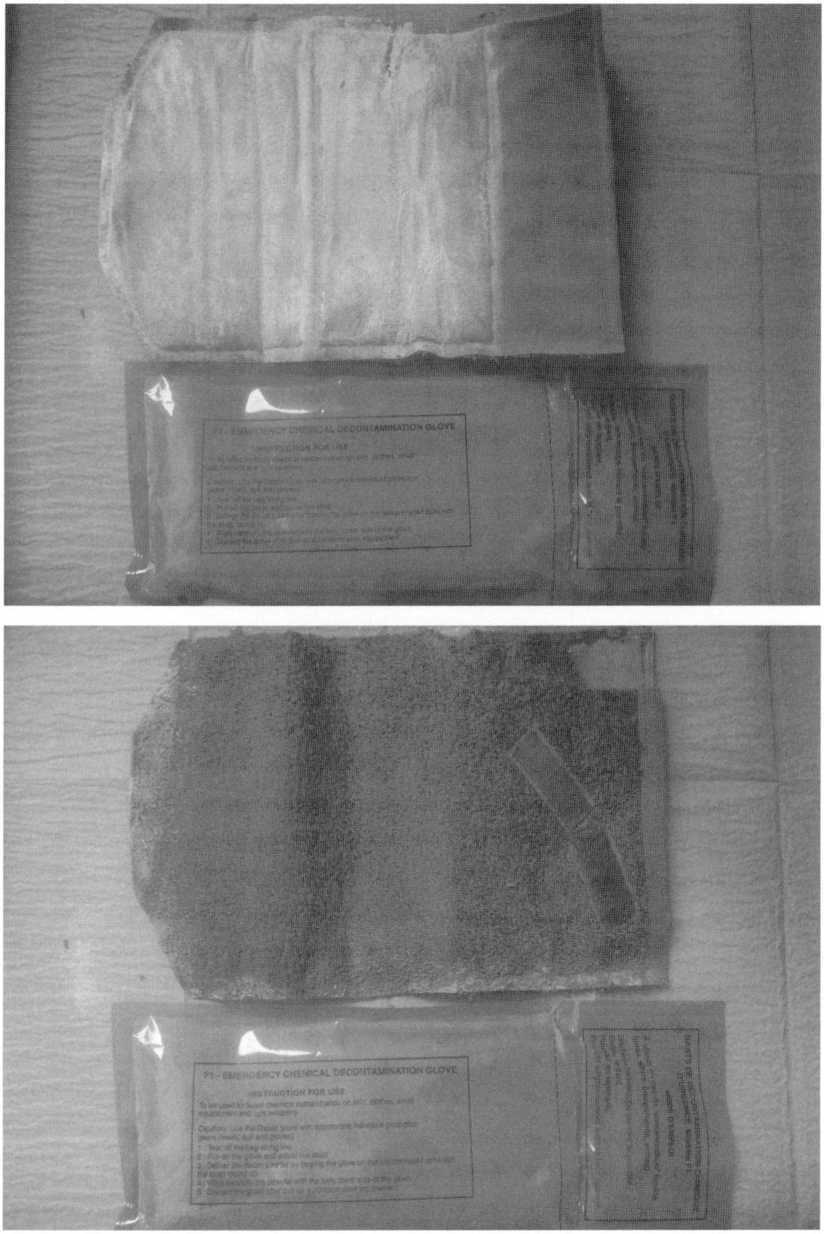

Fig. 18.3. French Army emergency decontamination kit: (a) sponge (glove external side); (b) Fuller's earth-containing porous fabric (glove internal side) (pictures by Dr Denis Josse).

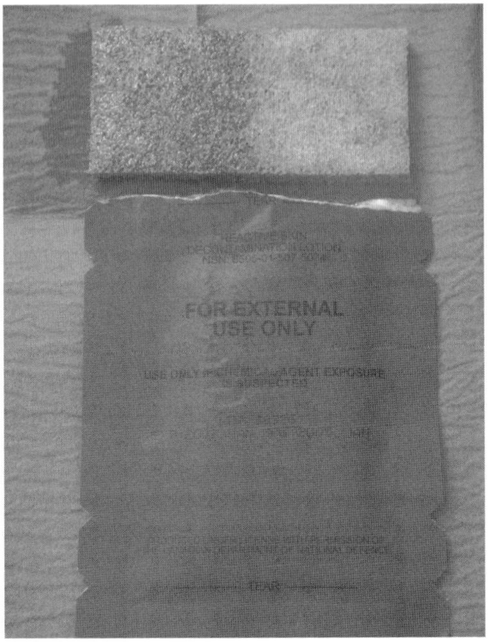

Fig. 18.4. US Army emergency decontamination kit. Reactive Skin Decontamination Lotion (RSDL®) kit. (Picture by Dr Denis Josse.)

With contaminants of low water solubility, addition of soap or any other detergent to water, at a concentration of about 0.5%, and use of a soft sponge to aid friction with the contaminated skin are strongly recommended since water only can spread the contamination on the skin and enhance the skin absorption of contaminants (Houston and Hendrickson, 2005; Amlot *et al.*, 2010). Ideally, water decontamination should not be delayed since any delay between contamination and decontamination could enhance the wash-in effect, i.e. an increase of the skin permeation rate of chemicals stored in the lipophilic stratum corneum (Moody and Maibach, 2006).

ED Guidelines for Rescuers and Victims in a Low-resource Setting

First, it should be remembered that following exposure to highly toxic chemicals such as the nerve agents sarin and soman, the implementation of ED should not prevent or delay that of emergency treatments if available.

In a low-resource setting, the systems and procedures must be adapted as a function of what is readily available in a close environment. If we assume that specific decontaminants or equipments are not available to the victims and rescuers and that the contaminant's identity is unknown, which might actually be the most frequent situation, then knowledge of the agent's physical state, water solubility, corrosivity/irritability and reactivity with water will be important in determining first aid measures (Segal, 2007).

In the case of liquid or vapour exposure to chemicals, the simplest ED measures to be performed either by the victim her or himself or by a rescuer could consist of the following sequence of tasks:

- Remove the foreign bodies from contaminated wounds;
- Cover the wounds with a clean, i.e. non-contaminated, sponge-cloth;
- Remove the outer clothing;
- Blot any visible contamination present on the exposed skin with a sponge-cloth;
- Pour absorbing powder (e.g. sand, flour) on the hair, then cover with a clean fabric.

Casualties could then be directed to a water source, since clean water could be quickly required for eye washing. Water accessibility will be urgently required after exposure to strong irritants.

If neither clean fabric, nor water are available close to the incident site, but transportation means are, it could be envisaged, as planned in Israel (Markel *et al.*, 2008), to quickly transport the partially disrobed symptomatic victims to the closest hospital, where they could be fully decontaminated.

After exposure to particles, the implementation of ED procedure should include the prevention of internal contamination and that of contamination spreading. It could consist of:

- Quick face washing with a clean cloth;
- Protection of the respiratory routes (mouth and nose), hair and ears with a clean cloth.

Then, with the exception of hair decontamination, which should not be performed with a powder, the ED measures described for liquids or vapours could be applied.

Conclusion

After exposure to any life-threatening RBC contaminant, ED should be performed without delay. Removing clothes is the golden rule of ED. In most cases, it will be sufficient to save lives and very effective to limit the agent's dispersion and potential inhalation by unexposed people. Ideally, it should be followed by gentle rubbing or blotting of the contaminated skin with a clean cloth, then showering with soap and shampooing of hair.

In a low-resource setting, the outcome of ED will depend on the rapidity of implementing self-decontamination, which will rely on the victims' education, i.e. awareness of potential exposures and hazards, and training. It will also depend on the arrival and aid of educated and trained emergency responders on the incident scene. In a MCI, decontamination triage, i.e. 'the symptomatics first', in the warm zone will be a crucial part of victim care management. The availability or on-site improvisation of ED tools such as polyvalent absorbents and water availability could also be critical for the outcome of ED.

In most large cities, more and more attention has been paid to the preparation by emergency response services and evaluation during drills of mass decontamination plans specific to incident locations. However, to our knowledge, ED plans, including casualties' self-decontamination, are not often part of the evaluation process as opposed to delayed decontamination by showering in specifically designed shelters. Obviously, most ED systems and procedures currently planned to be used in different contexts, including occupational ones, are common sense-based. Therefore, research, performed on relevant *in vitro* or *in vivo* models with real agents and on human volunteers with agent surrogates, is required to evaluate and improve existing or proposed systems and procedures. As an illustration of current research on the topics of decontamination, it should be mentioned that, thanks to the support of the European Commission, the effectiveness of showering for delayed decontamination has recently been evaluated both at the laboratory scale with real agents and in the field in order to validate and improve current guidelines (for more details, see the website www.orchidsproject.eu). Finally, as a crucial part of ED preparedness, we should not forget education on ED principles, which could probably start with that of children at school and at home. From a long-term perspective, this would ensure significant ED effectiveness in any context, even in the lowest resource setting.

References

Amlot, R., Larner, J., Matar, H., Jones, D.R., Carter, H., Turner, E.A., Price, S.C. and Chilcott, R.P. (2010) Comparative analysis of showering protocols for mass-casualty decontamination. *Prehospital Disaster Medicine* 25(5), 435–439.

Arora, R., Chawla, R., Marwah, R., Kumar, V., Goel, R., Arora, P., Jaiswal, S. and Sharma, R.K. (2010) Medical radiation countermeasures for nuclear and radiological emergencies: Current status and future perspectives. *Journal of Pharmacy and Bioallied Sciences* 2(3), 202–212.

Bjarnason, S., Mikler, J., Hill, I., Tenn, C., Garrett, M., Caddy, N. and Sawyer, T.W. (2008) Comparison of selected skin decontamination products and regimens against VX in domestic swine. *Human and Experimental Toxicology* 27, 253–261.

Bolzinger, M.A., Bolot, C., Galy, G., Chabanel, A., Pelletier, J. and Briançon, S. (2010) Skin contamination by radiopharmaceuticals and decontamination strategies. *International Journal of Pharmaceutics* 402(1–2), 44–49.

Braue, E.H., Boardman, C.H. and Hurst, C.G. (2009) Decontamination of chemical casualties. In: Tuorinsky, S.D. (ed.) *Medical Aspects of Chemical Warfare*. Borden Institute, Washington, DC, pp. 527–558.

Braue, E.H., Smith, K.H., Doxzon, B.F., Lumpkin, H.L. and Clarkson, E.D. (2011a) Efficacy studies of reactive skin decontamination lotion, M291 skin decontamination kit, 0.5% bleach, 1% soapy water, and skin exposure reduction paste against chemical warfare agents, part 2: guinea pigs challenged with soman. *Cutaneous and Ocular Toxicology* 30(1), 29–37.

Braue, E.H., Smith, K.H., Doxzon, B.F., Lumpkin, H.L. and Clarkson, E.D. (2011b) Efficacy studies of reactive skin decontamination lotion, M291 skin decontamination kit, 0.5% bleach, 1% soapy water, and skin exposure reduction paste against chemical warfare agents, part 1: guinea pigs challenged with VX. *Cutaneous and Ocular Toxicology* 30(1), 15–28.

Bushberg, J.T., Kroger, L.A., Hartman, M.B., Leidholdt, E.M., Miller, K.L., Derlet, R. and Wraa, C. (2007) Nuclear/radiological terrorism: emergency department management of radiation casualties. *Journal of Emergency Medicine* 32(1), 71–85.

Carron, P.N. and Yersin, B. (2009) Management of the effects of exposure to tear gas. *British Medical Journal* 338, b2283.

Chau, J.P., Lee, D.T. and Lo, S.H. (2012) A systematic review of methods of eye irrigation for adults and children with ocular chemical burns. *Worldviews on Evidence-Based Nursing* 9(3), 129–138.

DeLauder, S.F. and Kidwell, D.A. (2000) The incorporation of dyes into hair as a model for drug binding. *Forensic Science International* 107, 93–104.

Elliott, F. (2001) The eyewash imperative. *Occupational Health and Safety* 70(10), 60–63.

Feldman, R.J. (2010) Chemical agent simulant release from clothing following vapor exposure. *Academic Emergency Medicine* 17(2), 221–224.

Hall, A.H. and Maibach, H.I. (2006) Water decontamination of chemical skin/eye splashes: a critical review. *Cutaneous and Ocular Toxicology* 25(2), 67–83.

Hall, A.H., Blomet, J. and Mathieu, L. (2002) Diphoterine for emergent eye/skin chemical splash decontamination: a review. *Veterinary and Human Toxicology* 44(4), 228–231.

Hao, R.Z., Cheng, Z.X., Zhu, H.Y., Zuo, G.M. and Zhang, C.M. (2007) Transportation of sulfur mustard (HD) in alkyd coating. *Journal of Physical Chemistry A* 111(22), 4786–4791.

Harper, M. (2004) Assessing workplace chemical exposures: the role of exposure monitoring. *Journal of Environmental Monitoring* 5, 404–12.

Hayes, C. (2011) The ultimate emergency shower. *Occupational Health and Safety* 80(5), 20–22.

Horton, D.K., Berkowitz, Z. and Kaye, W.E. (2002) The public health consequences from acute chlorine releases, 1993–2000. *The Journal of Occupational and Environmental Medicine* 44(10), 906–913.

Houston, M. and Hendrickson, R.G. (2005) Decontamination. *Critical Care Clinics* 21(4), 653–672.

Hurst, C.G. (1997) Decontamination. In: Zajtchuk, R. and Bellamy, R.F. (eds) *Medical Aspects of Chemical and Biological Warfare*. Borden Institute, Washington, DC, pp. 351–359.

Inglesby, T.V., O'Toole, T., Henderson, D.A., Bartlett, J.G., Ascher, M.S., Eitzen, E., Friedlander, A.M., Gerberding, J., Hauer, J., Hughes, J., McDade, J., Osterholm, M.T., Parker, G., Perl, T.M., Russell, P.K. and Tonat, K. (2002) Anthrax as a biological weapon, 2002: updated recommendations for management. *JAMA* 287(17), 2236–2252.

Kumar, V., Goel, R., Chawla, R., Silambarasan, M. and Sharma, R.K. (2010) Chemical, biological, radiological, and nuclear decontamination: Recent trends and future perspective. *Journal of Pharmacy and Bioallied Science* 2(3), 220–238.

Lademann, J., Patzelt, A., Schanzer, S., Richter, H., Gross, I., Menting, K.H., Frazier, L., Sterry, W. and Antoniou, C. (2011) Decontamination of the skin with absorbing materials. *Skin Pharmacology and Physiology* 24(2), 87–92.

Lukey, B.J., Slife, H.F., Clarkson, E.D., Hurst, C.G. and Braue, E.H. (2008) Chemical warfare agent decontamination from skin. In: Romano, J.A. and Lukey, B.J. (eds) *Chemical Warfare Agents: Chemistry, Pharmacology, Toxicology, and Therapeutics*. CRC Press, Taylor/Francis Group, Boca Raton, Florida, pp. 611–625.

Markel, G., Krivoy, A., Rotman, E., Schein, O., Shrot, S., Brosh-Nissimov, T., Dushnitsky, T. and Eisenkraft, A. (2008) Medical management of toxicological mass casualty events. *Israelian Medical Association Journal* 10(11), 761–766.

Moody, R.P. and Maibach, H.I. (2006) Skin decontamination: importance of the wash-in effect. *Food and Chemical Toxicology* 44(11), 1783–1788.

Moysich, K.B., McCarthy, P. and Hall, P. (2011) 25 years after Chernobyl: lessons for Japan? *The Lancet Oncology* 12(5), 416–418.

Nehles, J., Hall, A.H., Blomet, J. and Mathieu, L. (2006) Diphoterine for emergent decontamination of skin/eye chemical splashes: 24 cases. *Cutaneous and Ocular Toxicology* 25(4), 249–258.

Okumura, T., Suzuki, K., Fukuda, A., Kohama, A., Takasu, N., Ishimatsu, S. and Hinohara, S. (1998) The Tokyo subway sarin attack: disaster management, Part 1: Community emergency response. *Academic Emergency Medicine* 5(6), 613–617.

Palao, R., Monge, I., Ruiz, M. and Barret, J.P. (2010) Chemical burns: pathophysiology and treatment. *Burns* 36(3), 295–304.

Pesatori, A.C., Consonni, D., Bachetti, S., Zocchetti, C., Bonzini, M., Baccarelli, A. and Bertazzi, P.A. (2003) Short- and long-term morbidity and mortality in the population exposed to dioxin after the 'Seveso accident'. *Indian Health* 41(3), 127–138.

Pesonen, M., Vähäkangas, K., Halme, M., Vanninen, P., Seulanto, H., Hemmilä, M., Pasanen, M. and Kuitunen, T. (2010) Capsaicinoids, chloropicrin and sulfur mustard: possibilities for exposure Biomarkers. *Frontiers in Pharmacology* 1, 140.

Petitot, F., Moreels, A.M. and Paquet, F. (2010) Evolution of the percutaneous penetration and distribution of uranyl nitrate as a function of skin-barrier integrity: an *in vitro* assessment. *Drug and Chemical Toxicology* 33(3), 316–324.

Pulley, S.A. and Jones, M.R. (2008) Emergency medical response to a chemical terrorist attack. In: Romano, J.A. and Lukey, B.J. (eds) *Chemical Warfare Agents: Chemistry, Pharmacology, Toxicology, and Therapeutics*. CRC Press, Taylor/Francis Group, Boca Raton, Florida, pp. 675–711.

Rotenberg, J.S., Burklow, T.R. and Selanikio, J.S. (2003) Weapons of mass destruction: the decontamination of children. *Pediatric Annals* 32(4), 260–267.

Schadilov, A.E., Belosokhov, M.V. and Levina, E.S. (2010) A case of wound intake of plutonium isotopes and ^{241}Am in a human: application and improvement of the NCRP wound model. *Health Physics* 99(4), 560–567.

Schulze, P. and Lake, W. (2009) Guidelines for mass casualty decontamination during a hazmat/weapon of mass destruction incident, ECBC SP-024, volume I.

Segal, E.B. (2007) First aid for skin/eye decontamination: are the present practices effective? *Journal of Chemical Health and Safety* 14(4), 16–22.

Soderberg, K., Kuusinen, P., Mathieu, L. and Hall, A.H. (2004) An improved method for emergent decontamination of ocular and dermal hydrofluoric acid splashes. *Veterinary and Human Toxicology* 46(4), 216–218.

Spagnul, A., Bouvier-Capely, C., Phan, G., Rebière, F. and Fattal, E. (2010) A new formulation containing calixarene molecules as an emergency treatment of uranium skin contamination. *Health Physics* 99(3), 430–434.

Spagnul, A., Bouvier-Capely, C., Phan, G., Landon, G., Tessier, C., Suhard, D., Rebière, F., Agarande, M. and Fattal, E. (2011) Ex vivo decrease in uranium diffusion through intact and excoriated pig ear skin by a calixarene nanoemulsion. *European Journal of Pharmaceutics and Biopharmaceutics* 79(2), 258–267.

Szinicz, L. (2005) History of chemical and biological warfare agents. *Toxicology* 214(3), 167–181.

Taysse, L., Daulon, S., Delamanche, S., Bellier, B. and Breton, P. (2007) Skin decontamination of mustards and organophosphates: comparative efficiency of RSDL and Fuller's earth in domestic swine. *Human and Experimental Toxicology* 26, 135–141.

Taysse, L., Dorandeu, F., Daulon, S., Foquin, A., Perrier, N., Lallement, G. and Breton, P. (2011) Cutaneous challenge with chemical warfare agent in the SKH-I hairless mouse (II): Effects of some currently used skin decontaminants (RSDL and Fuller's earth) against liquid sulphur mustard and VX exposure. *Human and Experimental Toxicology* 30(6), 470–490.

Tokuda, Y., Kikuchi, M., Takahashi, O. and Stein, G.H. (2006) Prehospital management of sarin nerve gas terrorism in urban settings: 10 years of progress after the Tokyo subway sarin attack. *Resuscitation* 68(2), 193–202.

Tymen, H., Gerasimo, P. and Hoffschir, D. (2000) Contamination and decontamination of rat and human skin with plutonium and uranium, studied with a Franz's chamber. *International Journal of Radiation Biology* 76(10), 1417–1424.

Van Hooidonk, C., Ceulen, B.I., Bock, J. and van Genderen, J. (1983) Agents and the skin. In: *Proceedings of an International Symposium on Protection against chemical warfare agents* – Stockholm (Sweden), 6–9 June, 153–160.

Varma, D.R. and Guest, I. (1993) The Bhopal accident and methyl isocyanate toxicity. *Journal of Toxicology and Environmental Health* 40(4), 513–529.

Chapter 19

Radiological Contaminants: Triage, Treatment and Medical Management of Exposed Persons

Edward Joseph Waller

Introduction

A disaster may be defined as a sudden event causing a great amount of damage, hardship and/or loss of life, and, as such, may have either natural or anthropogenic origins. A radiological disaster may, therefore, be defined as a disaster involving radiological material. Radiological material is any material that is, or has components that are, radioactive.

A radiological disaster may expose persons directly to ionizing radiation without contaminating them, or can generate contamination fields from aerosol dispersion. The radioactive materials in these aerosols can be deposited on the ground, surround a person in a cloud, be inhaled or be ingested. Although response to a disaster involves triage and initial treatment of the wounded, this response can be confounded by the presence of radioactive materials in the location of the disaster and on the victims. Therefore, careful medical management plans are required to appropriately address all of the issues surrounding the response.

Trauma injuries may be prevalent in a radiological disaster, and it is imperative that first responders and medical personnel be educated to treat the patients' traditional or conventional injuries before addressing radiological injury, as radiation injury and most scenarios involving a contaminated patient do not pose a health hazard to medical staff who employ standard pathogen precautions (surgical mask, gloves, gown). Education, training and policy must be examined over all aspects of medical care, including transport. There is evidence that medical transport, such as ambulances, will not accept contaminated patients until decontaminated, which can be a major factor in providing early treatment to the injured (Wells *et al.*, 2007).

Studies have indicated that stress can also be a major factor related to the medical well-being of persons following a disaster (Schuster *et al.*, 2001) and care must be provided early to mitigate symptoms both of the exposed population and the 'worried well'. As such radiological disaster management is a synergy of classical trauma triage/treatment, radiological assessment, psychosocial counselling and long-term management of radiation exposure.

Injury from exposure to radiation can vary from no detectable injury (with the possibility of latent stochastic effects, such as cancer induction), to acute radiation syndrome (ARS) for the most severely exposed. For those with no observable effects of exposure, triage and treatment plans may be generated through patient interview, dose interview, or bioassay results. For those with large acute exposures, the presentation may be divided into two phases:

- Prodromal (initial) phase;
- Manifest (illness) phase.

The approximate dose ranges and estimated symptoms for prodromal and manifest effects are given in Table19.1.

Table 19.1. Dose ranges for acute effects.

Dose range (Gy)	Symptoms	
	Prodromal	Manifest
0.5–1.0	Mild	Slight decrease in blood cell count
1.0–2.0	Mild to Moderate	Beginning to severe bone marrow damage
2.0–3.5	Moderate	Moderate to severe bone marrow damage
3.5–5.5	Severe	Severe bone marrow damage
5.5–7.5	Severe	Bone marrow pancytopenia and moderate intestinal damage
7.5–10.0	Severe	Combined gastrointestinal damage and bone marrow damage; hypotension
10.0–20.0	Severe gastrointestinal damage; early transient damage; gastrointestinal death	
20.0–30.0	Gastrointestinal and cardiovascular damage	

Expression of severity (mild, moderate, severe) is a qualitative marker of severity. For example, mild vomiting or diarrhoea can suggest a few episodes, moderate several episodes and severe many profuse episodes. Some effects can be semi-qualitative. For example, mild hypotension may be an approximate 10% drop in blood pressure, whereas severe hypotension can refer to a drop of 30% or more.

Medical personnel must be able to interpret the symptoms of acute radiation injury in light of an unfolding radiological disaster response and determine appropriate treatment plans. In addition, issues related to personnel protective equipment and facility decontamination need to be addressed to ensure continuity of the disaster management plan within a hospital and emergency department environment. The following sections consider the various phases of a response to a radiological disaster from a medical management perspective.

Radiological Disaster Management

There are numerous facets to disaster management involving radioactive material that extend beyond traditional disaster management. For example, a radiological disaster can yield conventional injuries and trauma, which are complicated by the presence of radiological contaminants. In addition, since radiological agents can be spread by mechanical disturbances or wind-driven mixing, proper decontamination and monitoring must be employed for the reduction of hazard to victims, first responders and medical personnel. The International Atomic Energy Agency (IAEA) provides generic guidance for response to radiological emergencies (for example IAEA, 2000, 2002a,b), first response guidance (for example IAEA, 2006b) and guidance for medical response (for example IAEA, 2005).

There are three phases to medical management in radiological disasters: (i) pre-event; (ii) event; and (iii) post-event. The three phases have specific considerations with respect to planning, actions and follow-up, which will be considered in the following sections. In this section, background foundations related to radiological disaster management are presented.

Disaster categories involving radioactive materials

There are three types of events involving radioactive material that may be considered as disasters: (i) nuclear reactor accidents; (ii) nuclear weapon detonation; and (iii) radiological dispersal device (RDD) use. Other events involving radiation or radioactive material, such as inadvertent exposure from lost or orphan sources, are generally of medical concern for a small number of persons involved in a specific incident and therefore would not satisfy the requirement of definition of a disaster.

Nuclear reactor accidents

There have been relatively few nuclear reactor accidents worldwide, especially compared with other industrial accidents (WNO, 2011). Using fatality statistics from 1969 to 2000, it is found that hydroelectric power has a factor of over 200 times more fatal accidents per unit electrical production compared with nuclear power generation, and coal has a factor of 16 times more fatal accidents compared with nuclear power generation (OECD/NEA, 2010).However, accidents such as have happened at Chernobyl NPP Unit 4 (UNSCEAR, 2000) and at Fukushima Daiichi Units 1–6 (NN, 2011) demonstrate that the potential for widespread radiological contamination, health detriment, environmental impact and social disruption require comprehensive disaster management plans. Nuclear reactor accidents and incidents are categorized by the International Nuclear Event Scale (INES), which is a scale ranging from ‘Level 0 – Deviation’, indicating no safety relevance, to ‘Level 7 – Major Accident’, indicating widespread health and environmental effects (IAEA, 2009).Both Chernobyl and Fukushima were categorized as INES Level 7 events (WNO, 2011).

Nuclear weapon detonation

The only time nuclear weapons have been used in a time of war was in the Second World War when the USA detonated two nuclear weapons against Japan, on 6 August 1945 (weapon code name: Little Boy, 13 kt yield) and on 9 August 1945 (weapon code name: Fat Man, 22 kt yield) (Glasstone and Dolan, 1977).The weapons generated approximately

106,000 deaths and 110,000 injured from the initial detonation (Loper, 1951). In general, the detonation of a nuclear weapon generates four unique effects that are responsible for human casualties: (i) air blast (55% fatalities); (ii) thermal radiation (30% fatalities); residual radioactivity; (iii) fallout (10% fatalities); (iv) and instantaneous radiation (5% fatalities) (Loper, 1951). Owing to both the instantaneous and long-term detrimental health effects, and the massive amount of persons that can be affected by nuclear weapon detonation, most countries have developed planning guidance documents for nuclear weapon detonations (FEMA, 2010), which include the potential use of improvised nuclear devices, which are crude nuclear bombs based upon illicitly acquired highly enriched fissile material (Ferguson and Potter, 2004).

Radiological dispersal devices

A radiological dispersal device (RDD), radiological dispersal weapon (RDW) or 'dirty bomb' may be defined as 'Any device, including any weapon or equipment, other than a nuclear explosive device, specifically designed to employ radioactive material by disseminating it to cause destruction, damage, or injury by means of the radiation produced by the decay of such material' (Ford, 1998). Any anthropogenic radioactive material can be used for an RDD. Weapons grade materials such as highly enriched uranium or plutonium are less advantageous for this type of weapon since they are not very radioactive and have higher value for use with improvised nuclear devices. A typical RDD design would be to fabricate an explosive package using radioactive material as a dispersant; however, it is also possible to disperse radioactive material as a powder or liquid aerosol. It is assumed that in order for an RDD to be effective in doing harm to human health, it must have a relatively large activity within an exposed population. As such, consequence management for disasters involving RDDs is an extremely active area (Musolino and Harper, 2006) as is medical resource management for response to radiological terrorism (Mettler, 2005).

Radiological exposure scenarios

Radiation may be defined as kinetic particles and quanta of energy that are emitted through the radioactive decay of unstable nuclei, through particle interactions with the atomic nucleus or orbital electrons, or through nuclear fission processes. Radioactive material can be in solid, liquid or gas form, can exist elementally or as a compound, and can be naturally occurring or human made. An isotope (same number of protons; different number of neutrons) of an element is radioactive if it has an unstable nucleus and decays with a characteristic half-life (the amount of time it takes for half of a number of atoms to transmute, or, decay). Therefore, radioisotopes are radioactive isotopes. Energetic radiations can interact with water molecules in the body, producing hydroxyl radicals which can damage DNA, or alternatively the radiation can interact directly with the DNA. Radiation interacts in tissue differently depending upon the type of radiation. Most isotopes decay by emitting charged particles in the form of alpha particles (helium nucleus) or beta particles (electron) from the nucleus, and usually photons (gamma rays from the nucleus) are emitted in the decay process. Charged particles interact continuously as they slow down in material, and therefore have a short range. Photons (gamma rays) on the other hand are uncharged quanta of energy and interact probabilistically. As a result of the type of interactions, charged alpha particles cannot penetrate the dead layer of skin covering the body and are therefore only a hazard when taken into the body. Charged beta particles can penetrate the skin depending upon their energy, but are more hazardous when internalized.

The (uncharged) photons can interact equally with tissue well whether inside or outside the body, although the most probably outcome of a photon entering tissue is for it to pass through the tissue without interacting at all. The characteristics of nuclear radiation interactions are summarized in Table 19.2.

Table 19.2. Nuclear radiation characteristics.

Type	Tissue penetration	Radiation stopped by
Alpha	First layer of dead skin	Clothing or paper
Beta	Several layers of skin	Clothing; plastic; rubber
Gamma	Total body	Several inches of iron; several feet of concrete or earth
Neutron	Total body	Several feet of water, concrete or earth

Radiation interactions with tissue can cause a multitude of effects, ranging from no effect at all, deterministic effects (erythaema, oedema, nausea, etc.) for large acute exposures, to stochastic effects (typically cancer) for chronic and/or low dose/dose rate exposures. Radiation can interact with the human body as an external source (either partial or whole-body), as an external contamination field (partial or whole-body) or as an internal contamination source (through inhalation, ingestion, wound or skin absorption). The three primary scenarios for radiation interaction in human tissue are described below.

External exposure

External exposure can be caused by a point source of radiation, by proximity to a contaminated plane (i.e. ground contamination) or by being under an overhead plume of radiation (cloudshine). The scenarios may be seen in Fig. 19.1 (left). In this case the source of radiation is at some stand-off distance from the receptor. Although energetic beta particles may be an external hazard, the primary hazard from this scenario is from photon-emitting sources. Generally speaking, from a medical management perspective, the treatment for external exposure involves treating the symptoms related to the exposure, including haematological changes (Gusev *et al.*, 2001). There is no danger from radiation to first responders or medical personnel from a person who has been externally irradiated. Secondary external contamination hazard may exist if radioactive material has been externally deposited from a ground plane (e.g. via resuspension) or from an overhead plume (for example, through gravitational settling).

External contamination

When radioactive material deposits on the skin or clothing from airborne contamination (accidental reactor release; nuclear weapon fallout; RDD aerosol) energetic beta radiation and photon radiation can interact with the receptor. This close proximity to the receptor, as depicted in Fig. 19.1 (centre), suggests that high dose rates may be delivered to tissue (Cember and Johnson, 2009). As opposed to the external exposure scenario where the hazard exists only as long as the receptor is near the source of radiation, the hazard from an external contamination scenario exists as long as the person is contaminated. The hazard can be removed through proper decontamination (removal of contaminated clothing, washing of contaminated skin surfaces). Secondary internal contamination hazard may exist if radioactive material is ingested or inhaled through mechanical resuspension from the clothing of the victim, or through the decontamination process.

Internal contamination

Internal contamination can result from breathing radiologically contaminated air, ingesting radiologically contaminated food, water or other ingestibles such as swimming water, and wound or skin absorption. In this case, the radioactive material enters the body and either gets deposited long term in the lungs (for highly insoluble inhaled materials) or transports into the blood after crossing the lung–blood barrier or directly from the gastrointestinal tract, wound or skin. Although some of the internalized material will be excreted (typically through the urine or faeces), a portion will circulate through the extracellular fluids until finally depositing at target locations in the body. The biological half-life is the time it takes for half the quantity of internalized radioisotopes to exit the human body via excretory pathways (Cember and Johnson, 2009). There are numerous methods for reducing the body burden of radioactive contaminants in the body (thereby reducing dose) which will be discussed in the section entitled 'Event response considerations'.

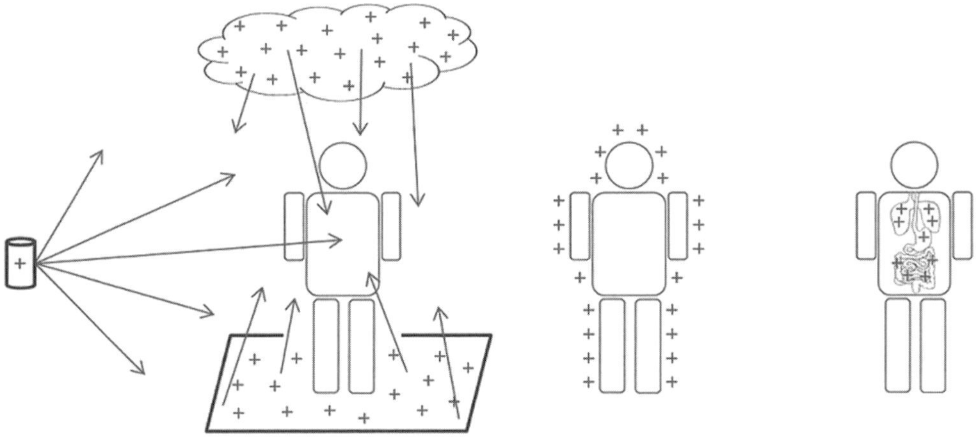

Fig. 19.1. External exposure (left), external contamination (centre) and internal contamination (right) scenarios.

Personnel resources for radiological disaster response

There are a number of assets, agencies and departments that will take part in a comprehensive response to a radiological disaster. The varied groups and their interactions will vary from country to country and jurisdiction to jurisdiction. Starting with the radiological contamination event, the critical response groups are depicted in Fig. 19.2 along with their relative locations, which may be interpreted both spatially and temporally with respect to the event location and time of initiation. For example, the first-on-the-scene responders will be involved in the disaster management both from a time perspective and geographical perspective, whereas the radiation biodosimetry resources will not be invoked until later in the response and not necessarily geo-located with the event. The forensic investigation will begin as soon as law enforcement is involved in the response and will be present in varying degrees throughout the entirety of the response to the disaster. The response categories are briefly discussed below (Waller *et al.*, 2009).

First-on-the-scene radiological incident responders are generally from the cohort of 'traditional' first responders, such as emergency medical service (EMS), fire and police personnel. It is not uncommon for first-on-the-scene responders of this category to have little-to-no training in radiological response or not to have access to radiation detection equipment or personal dosimetry. First-on-the-scene responders will provide initial critical first care for trauma, but generally provide no medical management for radiological injury. Suitably equipped and trained first-on-the-scene responders may be able to provide triage assessment. Chemical, biological, radiological, nuclear (CBRN) responders are well trained to provide rudimentary medical management for radiologically contaminated victims. CBRN personnel will be able to mitigate cross-contamination, reduce hazard to the primary and secondary sources of radiation, establish personal protective equipment measures, and make preliminary measurements of hazard and dose. CBRN personnel, however, will not be first on the scene and will generally arrive at some time after the initial event. Health physics support and the incident CBRN incident command should arrive at approximately the same time as the CBRN responders. Health physics support can be from the CBRN cohort, or may be from the command infrastructure. The health physicists will be responsible for predicting plumes and contamination migration, establishing extent of condition of the radiological disaster, assisting the management of assets required by the CBRN teams and ensuring personal protective equipment and decontamination protocols are being met. Health physicists can also assist with the triage and/or treatment recommendations for exposed victims. Incident Commanders will be required to coordinate the response actions of the groups involved, including victim management and transport to reach-back medical teams. There will probably need to be coordination of various Incident Commanders, and turnover of responsibilities as new agencies take the lead on the response (e.g. the initial Incident Commander may be local officials such as fire, the second Incident Commander may be military, the third Incident Commander may be lead government agency for disasters, etc. as per an established disaster management plan). Hospital emergency services may include (military) field hospitals, local civilian hospitals, or even ad hoc medical facilities established by local physicians and nurses. Of special value to the management of radiological disaster victims will be facilities that have nuclear medicine departments that are well trained in handling loose radioisotopes, oncology departments that are familiar with high dose/dose rate applications of radiation and most importantly facilities in which training and exercising for radiological emergencies have taken place. Of principal importance is to have a well-developed hospital emergency department plan for handling radiological disasters (Tan and Fitzgerald, 2002). Medical personnel will also include medical examiners/pathologists who may have special responsibilities to handle the contaminated deceased, and will require the assistance of health physics support (Horan and Gammill, 1963). Radiation biodosimetry encompasses observation of prodromal clinical signs/symptoms, following lymphocyte counts, performing cytogenetic investigations, and/or chromosome aberration analysis studies (IAEA, 2001). Since most radiological disasters will not have any physical dosimetry at the time of the event, retrospective dosimetry will be the only way to determine a dose for long-term medical management of exposed victims. Finally, although not involved in the medical management, the forensic teams will require access throughout all stages of the disaster response, which may include interaction with the medical personnel and/or the exposed victims (IAEA, 2006a).

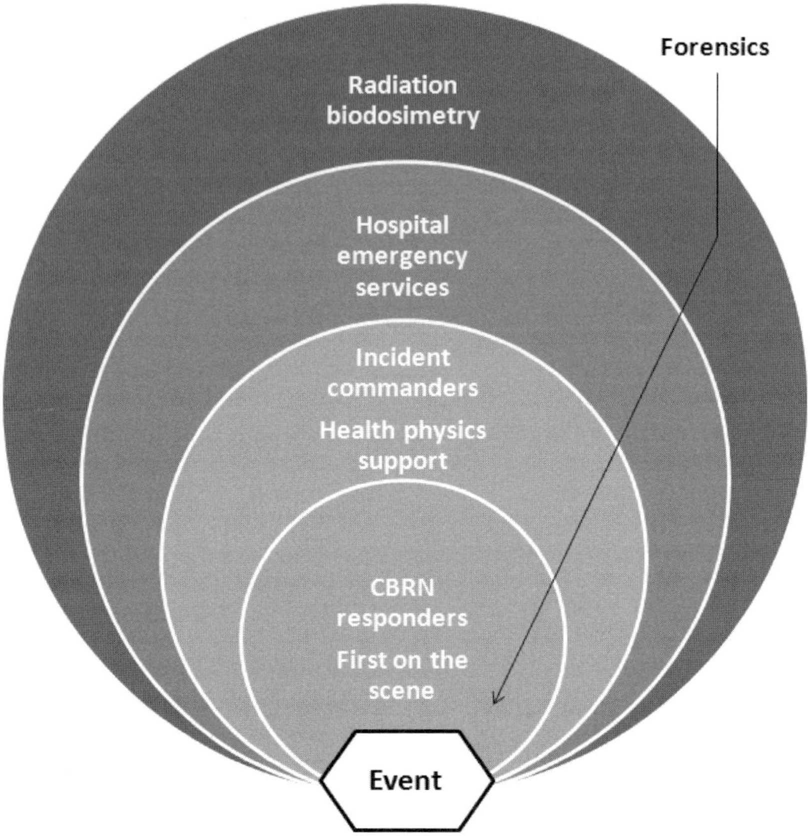

Fig.19.2. Critical response groups for a radiological contamination disaster.

Phases of a radiological disaster

The progression of medical response to a radiological disaster encompasses early, intermediate and late phases (NCRP, 2001) and is graphically represented in Fig. 19.3. The focus of the early phase is on life saving. The first responders must first consider that trauma and other traditional injury takes precedence over any radiological injury or exposure for the simple reason that even extremely large radiation exposures have a latency period (even for fatal exposures), whereas a traumatic injury can produce a fatality in a very short period of time post-event. This phase can last from immediate post-event extending for several hours. Ideally all (traditional and radiological) triage will occur during the first 24 h, although this depends upon the number of persons exposed. In addition, it is important to clear the non-injured from the response scene as quickly as possible. This includes the so-called 'worried well' – persons who have not been exposed to a radiological contaminant but believe they may have been, and often present with symptoms similar to persons who have had acute, large exposures. In addition, medically stabilized persons who will be transferred to reach-back medical facilities will either require decontamination or be wrapped to prevent the spread of contamination. In the intermediate phase, which extends from hours to days post-event, focus is on the treatment of radiologically contaminated persons and improving the quality of life of those exposed. In this phase it will be required to treat the symptoms of exposure and consider using pharmaceuticals (decorporation therapies) for reduction of internal dose. In this phase it will be realistically possible to initiate bioassay sampling (for example, 24 h urine or 72 h faecal) in order to obtain magnitude of internal dose. Psychological counselling may be required for exposure persons at this time, with special emphasis on vulnerable populations such as children (Becker, 2005). In the late phase of medical management, which can extend years post-event, the focus is initially on the preservation of life (for acute exposures) and for long-term dosimetry to properly assess the dose. This may include long-term epidemiology studies of the exposed cohort to verify risk.

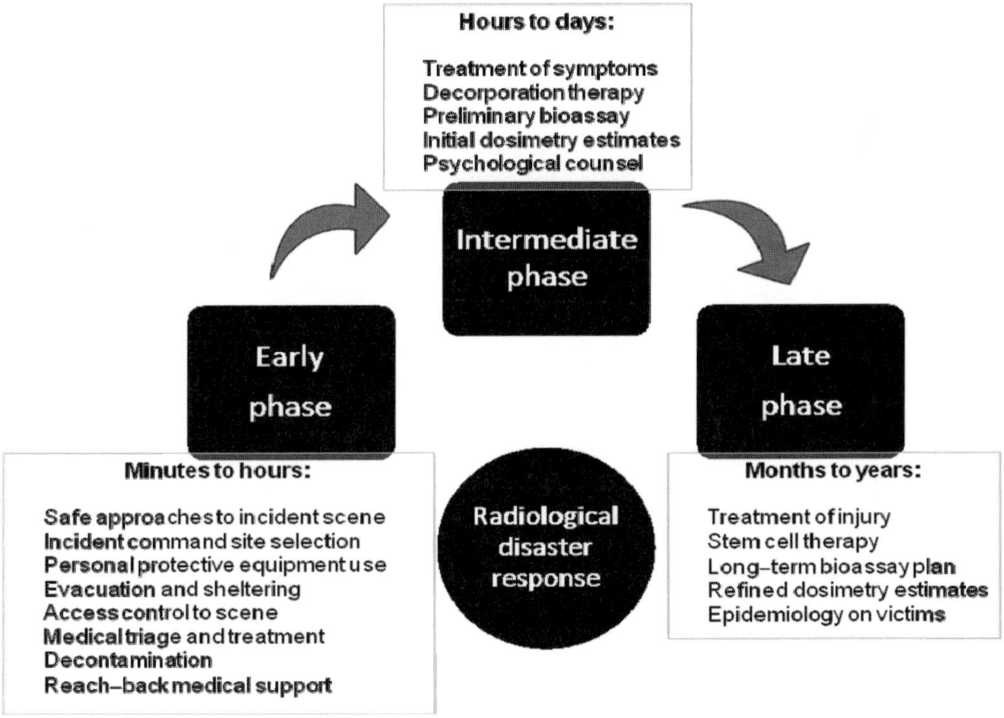

Fig. 19.3. Phases of medical response to a radiological disaster.

Tools for managing radiological disasters

Planning response to a radiological disaster involves detailed management plans that consider inter-agency operational issues. In addition, planning and preparation must take place regarding the variety of toolsets needed to adequately manage the first response, including the medical response. Waller *et al.* (2009) have discussed software tools available for various radiological responder end-user groups, ranging from first-on-the-scene responder tools, hazard planning tools, medical management tools to biodosimetry tools. There are a number of hardware resources for detection and quantification of radiation fields for the purpose of hazard assessment, medical triage, determination of contamination and decontamination efficacy and dosimetry (Weiss, 1997). Some paraphernalia especially useful for medical management include portal monitors for preliminary identification of contaminated persons, hand-held contamination instruments (for performing body frisks on contaminated persons and identifying hot spots), gamma survey meters for assessing the ambient radiation field and hand-held isotope identifiers (useful for identifying isotopes which will aid in treatment decision making). Advances in hardware technology are driven by testing standards and there are very few readily available consumer-oriented documents to assist disaster planners in appropriate equipment selection (Unterweger and Pibida, 2005). There are, unfortunately, very few instruments that are available from manufacturers specifically for the medical triage and treatment mission of a radiological disaster (Waller, 2010a).

A sample model for radiological disaster response assets is presented by Remick *et al.* (2005). This model describes a variety of government assets, the radiation monitoring equipment, medical management assets and software utilized for comprehensive response to a radiological disaster. In addition, Remick *et al.* (2005) outline a prediction of the approximate response times for the various assets. It is worthy to note that the organization of assets will vary from country to country and will be dependent upon structure of the disaster response organization within each country. Generalized comprehensive guidance for planning radiological disaster response, principally from a medical perspective, is provided in the Triage, Monitoring and Treatment (TMT) Handbook (Liland *et al.*, 2009).

Pre-disaster Event Considerations

Planning for radiological disasters is the first step to improving the quality of life for those that may be exposed to radiological insults. After the 11 September 2001 terrorist attacks on the USA, much emphasis has been given to disaster management plans and incident management systems (IMS), which are tools for identifying and marshalling resources and assets to the emergency or disaster (Perry, 2003). Specific to radiological disasters, the following section will discuss the development of disaster response management plans, personnel training, stockpiling of treatment pharmaceuticals, plan exercising and considerations for vulnerable populations.

Management plan

A generalized incident management structure, adapted from Perry (2003), is depicted in Fig. 19.4. It may be seen that between incident command and the primary management layer are a number of agency liaisons that will vary from country to country depending upon resources. Under operations, there is a medical management structure that involves first response and extrication of individuals from the scene (this may be a joint task with rescue), followed by triage assessment and then medical treatment management (first trauma management and then radiological considerations). The exposed victims and the non-exposed ‘worried well’ may require psychological counselling and/or education on the effects of exposure prior to transport from the scene. Finally, the medical management will be concerned with refined dosimetry estimates that will assist in continuing care of the exposure victims. Decontamination may be the responsibility of a Hazmat team, with specific guidance from CBRN responders, or other response personnel knowledgeable in radiological exposure and contamination. Decontamination may be required initially to attempt to avert doses from the exposure victims, the first responders and medical personnel. After triage, contaminated victims may require additional decontamination.

There will be a variety of management plans that will be invoked by various agencies in radiological disaster management, such as government disaster management plans, local response plans and hospital management plans. It is essential that the plans be developed with consideration to other agencies and jurisdictions, and validated through exercises.

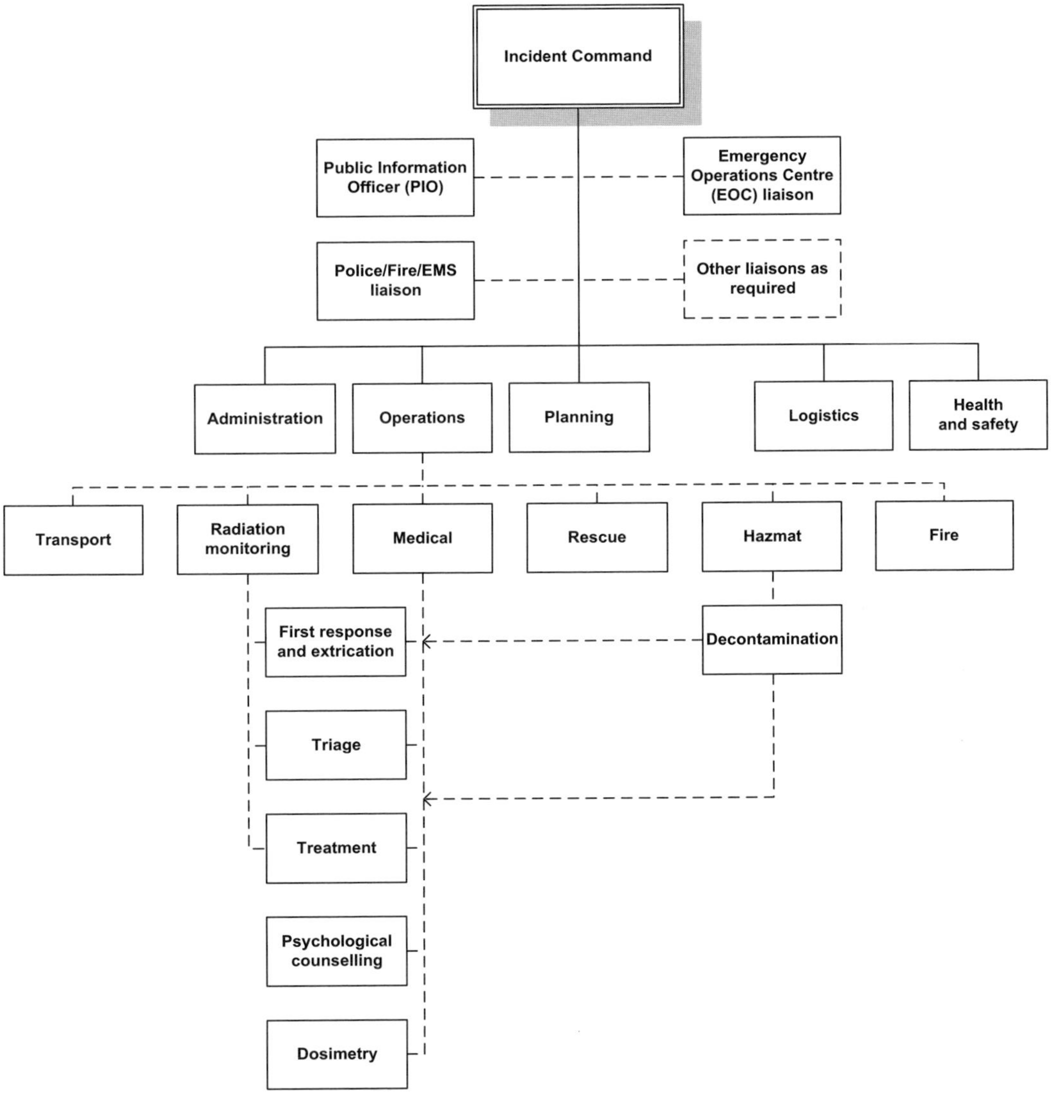

Fig. 19.4. General incident management organization chart (adapted from Perry, 2003).

Alternative models for disaster management plans, especially as related to mass fatality incidents, are discussed by Jensen (1999).

Personnel training

Training is an essential ingredient to ensure the success of a radiological disaster response plan. In a study exploring CBRN education of medical staff it was found that US Emergency Medical Technicians (EMT) were 9–13% less willing to respond to terrorist-related radiological, biological or chemical incidents, whereas EMTs who had received related continuing medical education within the previous 2 years were twice as likely to respond (DiMaggio *et al.*, 2005), which underscores the need for adequate and continuing education of the medical personnel that may be involved in the response. In addition to the hands-on training conducted for medical personnel, a number of simulation tools (Lake *et al.*, 2008), including virtual training (Berry and Hilgers, 2004) and mixed reality (Chroust *et al.*, 2009) environments, are available and/or under development. Unfortunately, training in the medical field for response to radiological disasters, although improving, has been historically lacking (Turai *et al.*, 2004). Current emphasis has been on training first responders, CBRN specialists and emergency department medical personnel (Bushberg *et al.*, 2007), and recurrent testing through periodic drills. To improve radiological disaster preparedness and increase confidence in the staff responding to this type of disaster, medical personnel must be provided with current training in readiness, contamination control, self-protection and medical management of the exposed (Becker and Middleton, 2008).

Exercises

To exercise is to 'use or apply'. In terms of radiological disaster response, an exercise is to test the operation of the disaster plan, the interaction of agencies, the deployment of personnel and the training of responders. Exercises can be useful to develop inter-agency cooperation, to increase the confidence of planners and responders to the plan, and to identify weaknesses in the plan. The three principal categories of exercises are discussed below (EPA, 2011).

Table Top Exercise (TTX)

The purpose of a TTX is to test the disaster response plan and standard operating procedures (SOPs) by informally 'walking through' a hypothetical disaster. The TTX allows disaster managers, policy makers and key staff with disaster management responsibilities to identify and resolve problems with the disaster plan. A TTX can be conducted in any location that is large enough to host the participants.

Command Post Exercise (CPX)

A CPX is more extensive than a TTX and is often located in a disaster response operations centre or other response asset. It typically focuses on a single response or activity, for example, command and control. A CPX may also be used to exercise limited deployment of equipment for a specific mission.

Full Field Exercise (FFX)

An FFX is more extensive and realistic than either a TTX or CPX. Activities extend beyond a conference room or operations centre, and take place in a field environment over several days, utilizing actual response assets and often simulated victims (using moulage techniques and appropriate coaching of the simulated victims). An FFX tests many functions of a disaster plan under realistic conditions. This is the 'gold standard' of exercising.

In field exercising radiological disaster response plans, care must be taken to ensure that the exercise is realistic and the assessment objective. It is vital to ensure that the participants are not informed in advance of the exercise, as this will improve the ability to respond through *a priori* preparation, both psychologically and administratively. The purpose of a field exercise is to identify both strengths and weaknesses in the medical response. A large-scale hospital exercise in Philadelphia, USA demonstrated that the hospitals involved were not adequately prepared to manage mass casualties from a radiological disaster (Jasper *et al.*, 2005), and exercises have identified weak areas such as inadequate communications, lapses in logistical support, lack of coordination of patient movements, insufficient staff both in terms of quantity and training (Schleipman *et al.*, 2004).

Pharmaceutical stockpiles

It may be assumed that in any radiological disaster, a number of persons will become internally contaminated, primarily from inhalation of aerosols containing radioactive contaminants, and possibly by ingesting contaminated food or water. Treatment of internally contaminated victims included utilizing decorporation agents (Fisher, 2000), which are pharmaceuticals that accelerate the removal of radioactive atoms from the body. Rapid application of a decorporating agent post-exposure can significantly reduce the total radiation dose victims receive, hence reducing the total risk to the individual for both deleterious deterministic and stochastic effects. The advantage of early decorporation is depicted in Fig. 19.5. The exposure from internalized radionuclides will decrease in time both by radioactive decay and excretion from the body. The amount of radioactive material remaining in the body, integrated over time, is directly proportional to the total radiation dose received and hence is proportional to the risk from the exposure. Early application of

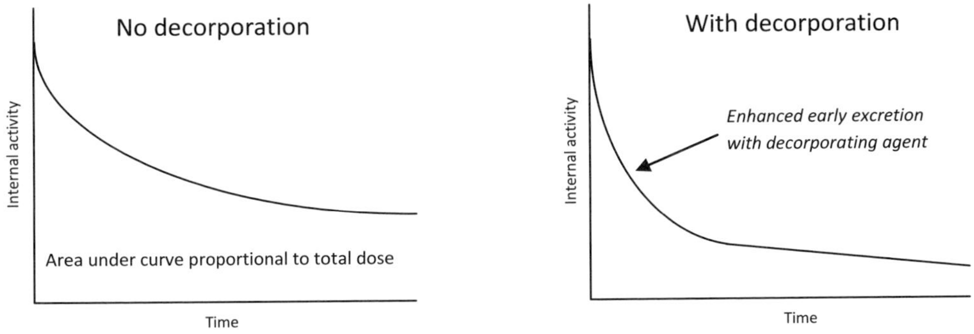

Fig. 19.5. Advantage of early decorporation to dose savings.

decorporating agents can accelerate removal of radionuclides from the body by various mechanisms (discussed in 'Event response considerations'), hence reducing the dose and risk from exposure (Cassatt *et al.*, 2008).

An essential component to a comprehensive radiological disaster response plan is, therefore, the stockpiling of radiological decorporation pharmaceuticals and planning for their rapid deployment.

Specific details of a nation's strategic stockpile are normally not generally widely disseminated so as to prevent a terrorist or other aggressor from using this information in developing malevolent plans. However, access to stockpile information between local, state, territorial, tribal and federal agencies can be obtained generally through official channels. By way of example, the USA initiated the National Pharmaceutical Stockpile Program (NPS) in 1999 (subsequently renamed the Strategic National Stockpile Program (SNS) under the Department of Homeland Security) as a way to oversee the stockpile of pharmaceutical agents, vaccines, medical supplies and equipment that may be made available to states in time of disaster once local supplies have been depleted (Esbitt, 2003). It has, however, been acknowledged that national stockpiles of certain decorporating agents that are not normally maintained locally do not meet the mission of rapid administration, and some emphasis is being placed upon local stockpiling of decorporating agents (Koenig *et al.*, 2008). To address medical management issues, the SNS convened a Radiation Working Group in 2002 to specifically address radiological insult, and generated clinical guidelines for the medical management of acute radiation syndrome (Waselenko *et al.*, 2004). It may be readily seen that there is a lifecycle of needs assessment, decorporation research, approval for mission, stockpiling, training and replenishing stocks at end of shelf-life (Fig. 19.6).

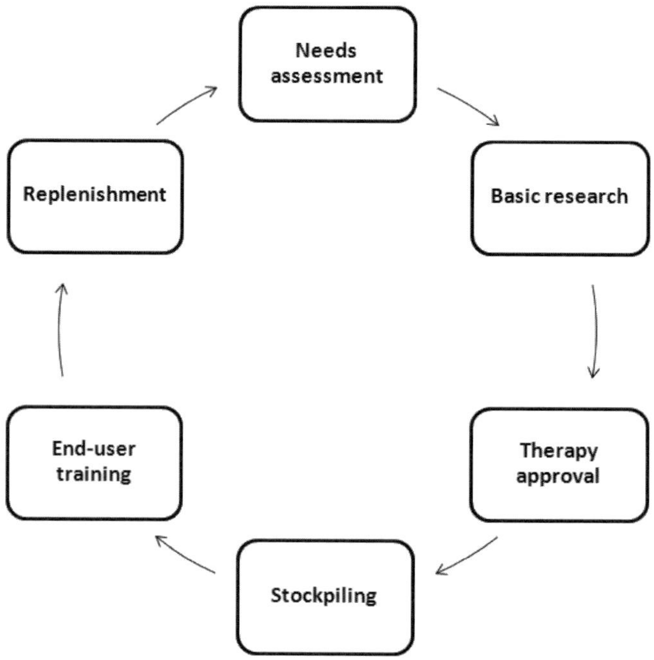

Fig. 19.6. Decorporation pharmaceutical life cycle.

The use of a specific drug for treating internalized radioactive contaminants relies on the fact that the drugs are available, tested, approved for use and stockpiled. The limiting step in the critical path to decorporation therapy stockpiling is the approval process. The acceptances of drugs into a pharmacopeia vary from nation to nation, however a generalized process, adapted from Hafer *et al.* (2010), is depicted in Fig. 19.7. Basic research and non-clinical drug development is normally undertaken by universities and pharmaceutical companies. The new drug application for an investigational new drug (IND) would be submitted to the regulatory agency overseeing the licensure. If approval to proceed is granted, the process continues to clinical development and trials, and afterwards if the drug is found to be safe and effective, it may be licensed for manufacture and subsequent procurement for stockpiling.

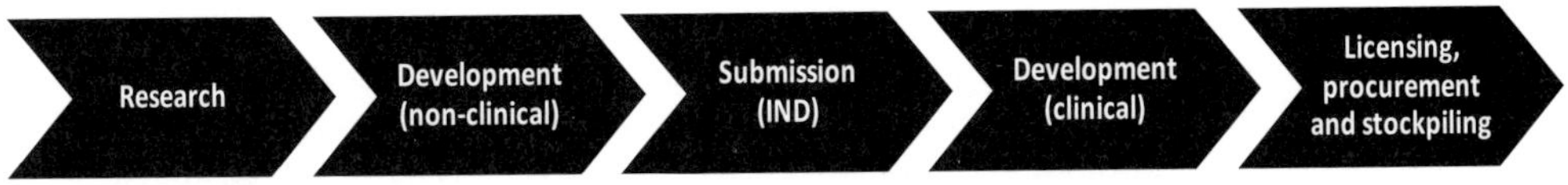

Fig. 19.7. Decorporation therapy development (adapted from Hafer *et al.*, 2010).

It may be seen that the path to stockpiling adequate supply of decorporating agents as medical countermeasures for radiological disasters can be long and potentially very expensive, especially for short shelf-life drugs that are not constantly consumed. As such, consideration for pharmaceutical stockpiling pre-event is critical to radiological disaster management.

Vulnerable population considerations pre-event

There are numerous vulnerable cohorts in the population as related to emergency preparedness for response to radiological and nuclear disasters. In fact, any group of people possessing characteristics, situations or conditions that deviate from the group average may be at increased risk in a disaster situation (Chen *et al.*, 2009). A convenient definition of a vulnerable group is a population cohort that is likely to have a worse outcome from an event compared with the cohort aggregate outcome. Unfortunately, most disaster response plans are designed and tailored to standard or reference persons, thereby excluding consideration of these vulnerable groups. A number of important studies have been conducted that consider vulnerable populations in a qualitative manner (Sullivan and Häkkinen, 2006; Kollek and Karawowska, 2009; Lemyre *et al.*, 2009; Powell *et al.*, 2009; Wilkinson, 2009), however there are very few studies that examine quantitatively the relationships between vulnerable cohorts, exposure, health risk and mitigation strategies (Richardson, 2009).

For radiological disaster hazards, one might consider first responders as a category of vulnerable population as they put themselves in harm's way. Examples include first responders (fire, police, EMS), first receivers (nurses, physicians) and military personnel. These groups are generally excluded as a vulnerable cohort as they are well-studied and protected groups within emergency and disaster management organizations. In addition, volunteers are excluded due to the fact that they have accepted the risk of insertion into the event, and will probably be included within the emergency disaster management structure. The principal cohorts are, therefore, from the general population. The most common classifications are provided below.

Children

Children are more susceptible to the effects of toxins, biological agents and radiological insults primarily due to the fact that they have more active cell division (mitosis) compared with the adult population and therefore detrimental effects promulgate very quickly. Additionally, physical and social characteristics of children make them more prone to internalize a toxin (e.g. children are closer to the ground where heavy aerosols can collect; children also have more relaxed sanitary habits compared with the adult population, which aids in hand-to-mouth transfer of contaminants). To confound matters, many emergency protocols are based upon a 'reference' adult (ICRP, 2003) as opposed to a child.

Conceptus

The conceptus (zygote, embryo and fetus) is at risk at three distinct phases: (i) interaction of chemical, biological or radiological insult on the fetus (direct possible from external radiation – all possible through contaminants crossing the maternal–placental barrier); (ii) toxins affecting the mother's health, impacting the conceptus' health; and (iii) risk perceptions leading to abortion. It has been shown (Bentur *et al.*, 1991) that before counselling, pregnant women exposed to radiation assigned themselves a higher risk than the non-exposed population, with a concomitant risk of abortion. This demonstrates that early stage communication and risk perception during a radiological disaster event can be critical to vulnerable population outcomes.

Women

The BEIR VII report (BEIR, 2006) presented that women were at higher risk in terms of both cancer morbidity and mortality (especially younger women) as a function of radiation exposure. Women have also been shown to have higher cancer rates when exposed to certain industrial chemicals. Therefore, this group may be considered a vulnerable population for a number of factors (pregnant, young adult, genetic susceptibility).

Elderly

It is said that it is not age that makes this group vulnerable, but a combination of factors associated with age such as deteriorated health, psychological state, physical environments and mobility, and social support circle (Powell *et al.*, 2009). The elderly are an often poorly triaged group in emergency response, especially if they are infirm and immobile, as was observed during the Katrina hurricane (Okie, 2008). The same possibilities hold for radiological disaster events. In addition, the elderly are often immunocompromised, as discussed below.

Immunocompromised

It is well known that immunocompromised persons are less capable of combating systemic insults compared with persons with healthy immune systems. Radiological insults are capable of causing cytopenia, limiting the ability to fight infection. Immunosuppression combined with any other insult can be devastating to the patient condition and therefore persons in this condition require additional considerations with respect to both triage and treatment.

Injured/sick

The injured and sick are a *de facto* vulnerable population. Persons in hospital environments should be processed via hospital protocols. Persons arriving injured or sick at a response station may be misclassified or triaged inappropriately. For example, a person with a mild trauma may enter a low priority triage even though they may have an exposure to a radiological insult that would warrant a higher priority. Synergistic effects of trauma with radiological insults require detailed examination.

Physically disabled

The physically disabled have a disadvantage in so far as in an emergency, when resources are exercised, it may be difficult to impossible for disabled people to achieve the level of care they deserve. For example, normal body frisking procedures for radiological contaminants generally do not have alternate protocols for wheelchair-bound personnel. Additionally, protocols generally do not exist to handle contaminated mobility devices (wheelchairs, walkers, etc.) that cannot pass the 'clean/dirty' boundary in a decontamination procedure.

Mentally disabled

The mentally disabled will require varying levels of assistance concomitant with their degree of disability. Mildly disabled persons that do not normally require assistance for everyday tasks may require additional support in an emergency. Moderate to severely disabled persons will require a support structure, especially if institutionalized.

Isolated populations

An example of an isolated cohort is Aboriginal persons. Often, members of this cohort live on reserves, many located in isolated areas. This population is at risk due to isolation, poor communications and limited understanding of responders to psychological needs.

Other categories

The above lists the most commonly discussed vulnerable populations that may be encountered during a radiological disaster. There are a number of other cohorts that may require additional consideration during an emergency involving radiological insults that will be identified in the first stages of the research (e.g. institutionalized cohorts, the homeless, persons with genetic variability or sensitivity to radiological insults, or domesticated pets; Wilkinson, 2009) as they relate to the human population.

It is not sufficient to assume that an *ad hoc* response to medical management of these vulnerable populations will be appropriate in the time of a radiological disaster. Therefore, it is critical that these groups are incorporated at all planning stages into the radiological disaster management plan. Exercising disaster response plans with vulnerable populations is the most instructive way to train the commanders and responders on dealing with the special needs of these groups (Waller, 2010b).

Event Response Considerations

As a radiological disaster unfolds, whether it is a nuclear reactor accidental release, nuclear weapon detonation, or radiological dispersal device detonation, there will be a number of response functions set into place. One of the initial first responder actions will be to assess and triage casualties for medical care. In the following sections concepts related to external and internal contamination, triage, treatment and morgue as related to radiological disasters will be discussed.

External contamination

External contamination in a radiological disaster can occur from plume deposition, fallout and resuspension processes. Primary decontamination involves removing the outer clothing of the exposed. Decontamination of intact skin is a relatively simple procedure. Complete decontamination, which returns the area to a background survey reading, is not always possible because some radioactive material can remain fixed on the skin surface. Decontamination should be only as thorough as practical, and should begin with the least aggressive method and progress to more aggressive ones. Care must be taken to limit mechanical or chemical irritation of the skin. The standard procedure is to wash the contaminated area gently under a stream of water (avoiding splash) and scrubbing at the same time using a soft brush or surgical sponge. Warm tap water is used, as cold water tends to close the pores, trapping radioactive material within them, whereas hot water causes vasodilatation with increased area blood flow, opening pores, and thereby enhancing the possibility of absorption of the radioactive material through the skin. Aggressive rubbing should be avoided as it tends to cause abrasion and erythaema. If washing with plain water is ineffective, a mild soap (neutral pH) or surgical scrub soap can be used. The area should be scrubbed for 3–4 min, then rinsed for 2–3 min and dried, repeating if necessary. Between each scrub and rinse, the contaminated area should be monitored for decreasing radiation levels. For rough skin, such as found on the hands and feet, very fine sandpaper can be used. The decontamination procedure stops when the radioactivity level does not change between cleanings. Hair, and body areas with abundant hair, can be shampooed several times and then rinsed in a 3% citric acid solution. Contaminated hair can be clipped if shampooing is ineffective. Shaving should be avoided since small nicks or abrasions can lead to internal contamination. When shampooing the head, avoid getting any fluids into the ears, eyes, nose or mouth as this will lead to internal contamination.

Wounds

In a radiological disaster, any wound must be considered contaminated until proven otherwise and should be decontaminated prior to decontaminating intact skin. When wounds are contaminated, it must be assumed that uptake (internal contamination) has occurred. Contaminated wounds are first draped, preferably with a waterproof material, to limit the spread of contamination. Primary wound decontamination is accomplished by gently irrigating with saline, water or a 3% hydrogen peroxide solution. Irrigation fluid should be collected and checked with a radiation detector to assess the effectiveness of decontamination. It is likely that multiple irrigations will be necessary, with the wound monitored after each irrigation procedure. If irrigation decontamination procedures are not successful, debridement of the wound must be considered. Embedded radioactive particles, if visible, can be removed with forceps or tweezers.

Body orifices

Contaminated body orifices, such as the mouth, nose, eyes and ears, require special attention because absorption of radioactive material is likely to be much more rapid in these areas than through the skin. If radioactive material has entered the oral cavity, repetitive brushing of the teeth with toothpaste and frequent rinsing of the mouth with a 3% citric acid solution may reduce radioactivity levels. Gastric lavage can be used if contamination is swallowed. Rinsing the nose, eyes and ears with water or saline can be done with care.

Internal contamination

Internal contamination can occur from: (i) inhalation of contaminants from an aerosol in the breathing space; (ii) ingestion through eating or drinking contaminated consumables or mechanical clearance from the respiratory system after inhalation; (iii) absorption through open wounds; and (iv) through direct absorption through exposed skin. Upon entering the body, the contaminants can either remain deposited in the lungs (for inhaled insoluble particles) or are transported in the extracellular body fluids. Once radioactive contaminants cross cell membranes, they are said to be incorporated. Incorporation is a time-dependent, physiological phenomenon related to both the physical and chemical nature of the contaminant. The rate of incorporation can be rapid (occurring in minutes) or extended (occurring over days to months).

Internal contamination monitoring

There are a variety of ways to determine the presence of internal contamination (Voelz, 1969). Nasal swabs may be used in the field to give an indication of potential intake via inhalation, and health physics personnel may be able to assess potential for intake using hand-held radiation contamination instruments. There are relatively few field *in situ* radiation instruments that are capable of giving an indication of internal contamination; most rely on expert operators such as health physicists, although there is some research and development being conducted in this area (Waller, 2010a). Definitive assessment of internal contamination is performed using various bioassay techniques, outlined below.

Urine

Provided that the sample is collected free from contamination, this is a common method of bioassay. If a radionuclide is found in urine, there is no doubt that the radionuclide was present in extracellular body fluids. The absence of a positive test for radionuclides by urinalysis does not, however, preclude a body burden of any given radionuclide. Although spot urine samples can be collected and analysed, it is more common, and accurate, to request 24-h urine samples.

Faeces

Faecal analysis is most useful in detecting intake of non-transportable material and in providing evidence of the clearance of material from the lungs. It is common to request collection of 72-h faecal samples for analysis.

Whole body counts

This technique can determine intake of transportable material in the body, and is only useful after complete external decontamination.

Lung counts

This technique, similar to whole-body counting, can determine the quantity of inhaled contaminants, and especially if they are insoluble.

Thyroid counts

This technique is useful to determine if inhalation of radioactive iodine has occurred.

Nasal discharge

This technique may be used for detecting significant exposures and identifying the radionuclide involved in an accident, but is very difficult to use to obtain information for a body burden. Nasal, blows, swabs or smears can be useful to triage persons potentially exposed to airborne contamination.

Sputum

May contain insoluble material initially deposited and later eliminated by ciliary action.

Sweat

Sweat may be analysed to detect tritium (^{3}H) contamination.

Breath

Breath may be used to determine ^{14}C (exhaled CO_2) and tritium (exhaled vapour).

Blood and hair

These samples are not commonly analysed. In general, blood and hair is analysed in criticality accidents for neutron activation products. There is little benefit for analysing these samples with an internal contamination scenario.

A comprehensive overview of bioassay techniques is available in NCRP Report 161 (NCRP, 2008).

Triage

Triage is a French origin word meaning to 'separate' or 'to sort'. The concept of medical triage is to sort patients or victims in order of medical priority, with the ultimate goal to minimize preventable morbidity and mortality (Bostick *et al.*, 2008). Most emergency departments utilize the concept of medical triage for routine operations. The principal factor that distinguishes a typical emergency department triage from an MCI triage is the number of patients simultaneously presenting for assessment (Frykberg, 2005).

Two competing factors in triage systems are: (i) rapid evaluation of victims; and (ii) accurate identification of triage priority.

Although different nations utilize different processes and scoring systems (Lanoix *et al.*, 2002), there are five general categories of triage priorities, listed as:

1. Immediate (priority 1, or P1): persons with life-threatening injuries that may be readily stabilized until they can reach comprehensive care. Survival prognosis is possible – good with rapid treatment.
2. Delayed (priority 2, or P2): persons with injuries that are stable enough such that their treatment can be delayed without affecting their medical outcome. Survival prognosis is good to very good.
3. Minimal (priority 3, or P3): persons who may be considered walking wounded, and will be medically attended to after higher priority patients have been treated. Survival prognosis is very good to excellent.
4. Expectant (priority 4, or P4): although not a common category in routine triage for all nations, this category is useful in mass casualty or military events, and includes persons who are considered to be injured to the extent that they will not survive given the absolute resources or treatment time frames available. Survival prognosis is very poor.
5. Deceased (Priority 0, or P0): an obvious triage category that it is important to recognize so that resources are not deviated from triage categories with non-zero survival outcome prognosis.

As evident above, triage decisions are based upon likelihood of survival given available resources. The first responders arriving on the scene of a radiological disaster should conduct the initial assessment in a similar fashion to any other MCI. In fact, the response to a radiological disaster starts with the trauma assessment, which splits to ambulatory and radiation exposure decision trees (Hick *et al.*, 2011). The injury from most, if not all, incidents involving a radiological contamination incident is not immediately life threatening. Even in a nuclear weapon or radiological dispersal device detonation, the primary injuries in terms of triage are from the blast and thermal components of the detonation. Radiation exposure does, however, require triage, but it must take place after trauma injuries have been assessed and treated.

Assessment

Radiological triage should include assessment of: (i) radiation exposure; (ii) external contamination; and (iii) internal contamination. Persons exposed to radiation but not radiological contaminants (such as aerosols) are of no risk to medical personnel, and can generally be assigned as priority 3. However, the symptoms presented will depend upon the level of exposure and, although there is individual variability to radiation exposure, the greater the exposure, the more severe the symptoms and the sooner the onset of symptoms that will require treatment as normal. Persons who are externally contaminated (such as from fallout of radiological material, rainout from suspended aerosols, etc.) will require decontamination to reduce risk from exposure to the patient, the responders and the medical personnel. Although decontamination may remove a great proportion of external contamination, these persons may have residual contamination on their bodies and may also have internalized contamination. A system for radiological disaster medical triage is presented in Fig. 19.8. The initial medical decision is whether the person is injured (in a classical sense) or not. If injured, the person must undergo classical triage for trauma injuries and made stable before a radiological assessment can be made. A stable patient requires two basic assessments, in order of priority: (i) is that person contaminated (first assessing for external contamination and then internal); and (ii) has that person been exposed to radiation (i.e. from an external source). It is presumed *de facto* that a person who has been externally or internally contaminated has been exposed to radiation. After or concomitant with the radiation exposure assessment is examination of latent symptoms (such as nausea or vomiting) that can be indicative of large radiation exposure, or can be indicative of the 'worried well' phenomenon (Wagner and Curran, 1984). The so-called 'worried well' are persons characterized by presenting symptoms that are not related to any exposure, but can be mistaken for a symptom related to exposure. This cohort can also present with evidence of psychological distress and/or depression. In an MCI, the worried well can represent a large fraction of persons presenting for medical assessment, and can rapidly overwhelm triage facilities, emergency departments and other medical services. Unfortunately, it is very difficult to differentiate the worried well from the population of potentially exposed persons, which makes expert assessment and radiation measurements critical in the early radiological triage assessment. In addition, medical resources still must be expended on treating the symptoms of the worried well, and therefore accurate identification is critical to adequate triage priority assignment.

The symptoms that may be exhibited by both the exposed and worried well include those related to the neurovascular systems (nausea, vomiting, anorexia, fatigue, headache, hypotension) and gastrointestinal (diarrhoea, cramps), whereas those exposed to significant ionization radiation also have symptoms related to the cutaneous system (erythaema, oedaema, blistering, desquamation, hair loss, onycholysis). The onset of symptoms varies with the degree of exposure and is specific to individuals. For example, at a total body exposure equivalent to approximately 1–3 Gy, nausea and vomiting may be expected within 48 h of exposure, whereas epilation and erythaema may take hours to days to develop post-exposure. Therefore, initial radiological triage based upon symptoms will only be useful in very high (~ several Gy) levels of exposure, although the usefulness of the symptoms as triage indicators may be improved synergistically when using data collected from patient interview and with a careful examination of all physical data (primarily radiation measurements).

Process

The flow of potentially radiologically contaminated persons into a triage assessment is presented in Fig. 19.9.

At some point in the radiological disaster response, injured persons and those potentially exposed to radiological insults will require triage and treatment. At the triage 1 position, victims are separated into P1 and P2 (often ambulatory) and P3 (walking) lines. It

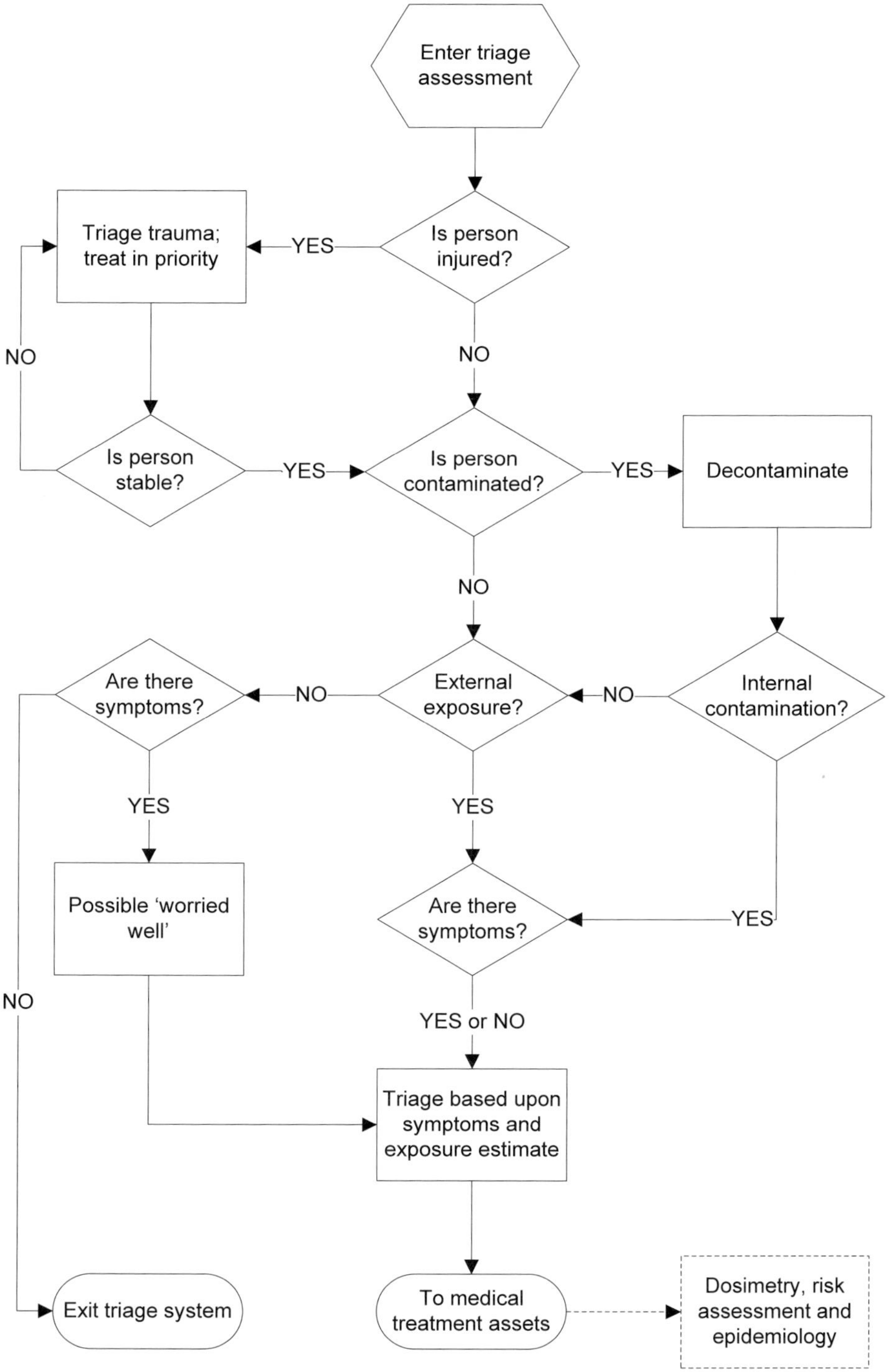

Fig.19.8. System of radiological disaster triage (adapted from NCRP, 2008).

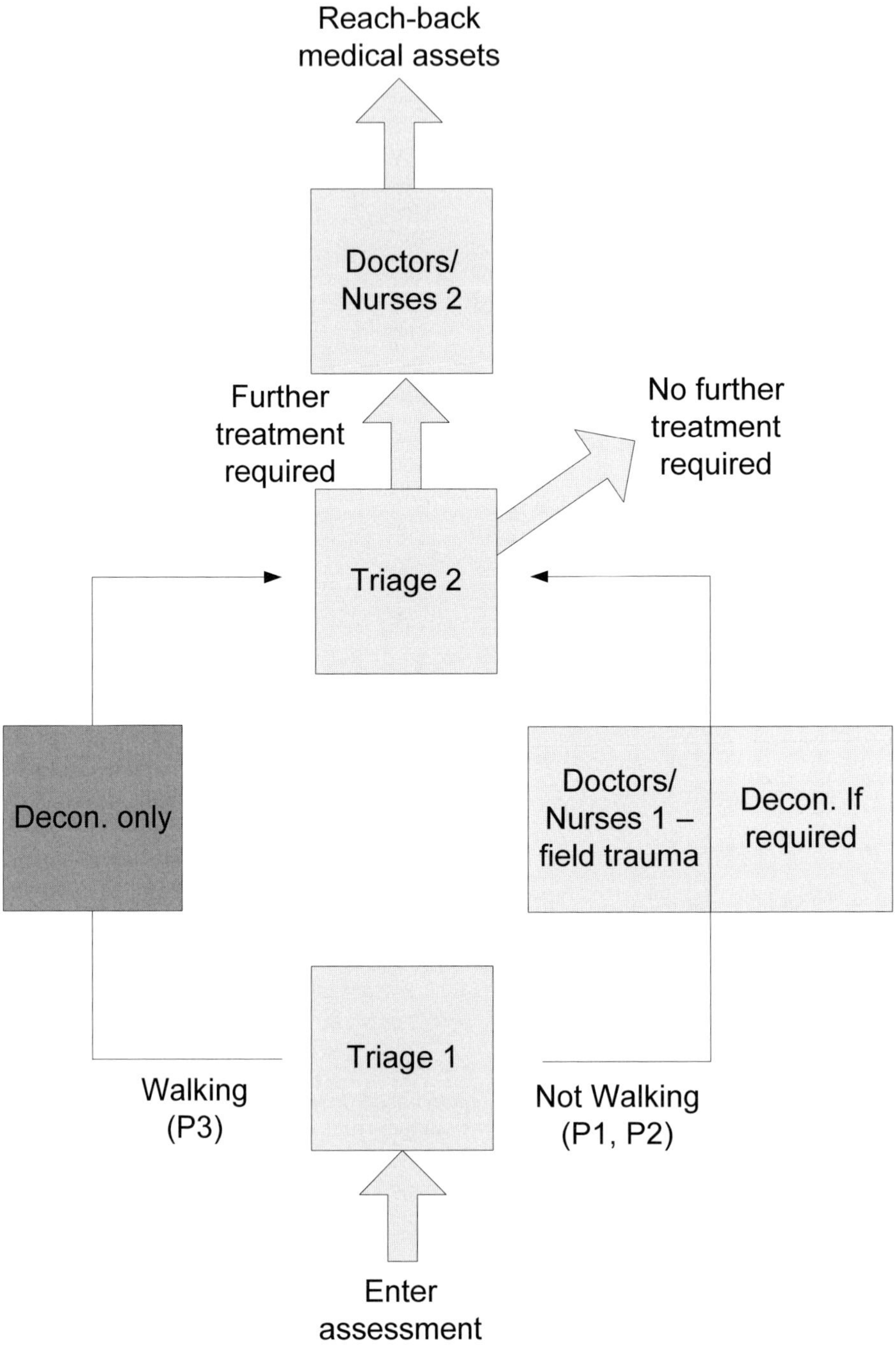

Fig. 19.9. Triage flow in a mass casualty radiological event.

is desirable to have the triage 1 position capability of radiation monitoring with portable portal monitors and contamination meters. The P3 victims proceed to a decontamination station where they will be monitored, decontaminated and then sent to a secondary triage assessment (triage 2) where it is determined if they need reach-back medical care (e.g. if it is believed they have incorporated radionuclides) or if they can be diverted out of the triage system. The P1/P2 victims are taken to field physicians, nurses and/or paramedics where they are stabilized and undergo radiation monitoring and decontamination to the extent possible given the nature of their injuries. These stabilized patients then are processed at the triage 2 position for any further field medical care, and are generally sent in triage priority to reach-back medical assets.

This two-tier triage system should provide a rapid triage and improve triage accuracy by reducing both under-triage and over-triage of patients. If resources are limited then the triage 2 position can be eliminated.

Decontamination

Decontamination of persons exposed to radiological contaminants may be required at the triage phase (often in the field) and at the medical treatment phase (often at or near the hospital). Most of the patient radioactive contamination is removed if the outer layer of clothing is removed. This clothing should be placed into plastic bags in steel or fibreboard drums. Personal items, such as watches, rings and wallets, can be surveyed and returned to patients when convenient. In general, personal objects do not become radioactive, but may become contaminated hence requiring decontamination. Activation may occur in the presence of an intense neutron radiation field, but this would only be possible in a nuclear weapon environment, in which injury will be dominated by blast and thermal effects.

Thorough decontamination typically involves showering with soap, water and perhaps a specially formulated decontamination agent. Best practice when decontaminating a person is to avoid splashing water (or saline), which may be used for a quick rinse on the scene of hands, face, hair. The remainder of the decontamination procedure will involve the shampooing of the hair to remove any further contamination. This can be done at the scene with the ambulatory patients or persons thought to be exposed (depending upon the resources available and the number of patients presenting at triage). Shower lanes with soap/decontamination agent can be used with radiation surveyors at the beginning and end of the decontamination line comparing radiation counts before and after washing. In addition, containment of the effluent water must be considered and this water surveyed.

Estimation of the level of internal contamination is difficult in the initial first response stages. Therefore, all patients at risk of contamination should be monitored by field portable instruments (direct reading or nasal swabs) and all excreta should be preserved (to the greatest extent possible) for biodosimetry. If internal contamination is found, the amount and quantity can be used for both triage of victims and for determining appropriate treatment protocols (Waller and Wilkinson, 2010c).

Although it is desirable for most contamination on personnel to be removed prior to presentation at a medical facility, it is important for hospitals and emergency departments to have decontamination management plans (Koenig *et al.*, 2008) that include location of entry points, radiation monitoring assets, personal protective equipment, security, collection of contaminated personal belongings, collection of contaminated medical supplies, protection of medical equipment from contamination and environmental consideration of contaminated water. There is an abundance of guidance available for assisting in establishing proper decontamination procedures (Severa and Bár, 1991; Gusev *et al.*, 2001; Liland *et al.*, 2009; AFRRI, 2010).

Treatment

Medical management of acute radiation injury that may occur in a radiological disaster involves monitoring depletion of absolute lymphocyte counts (Goans *et al.*, 2001), chromosome aberration analysis (IAEA, 2001), and responding by rapid administration of cytokine therapy (Goans and Waselenko, 2005). Dose action levels have been suggested by the Treatment Initiatives after Radiological Accidents (TIARA) project in the European Union (Ménétrieret *et al.*, 2007) to assist medical personnel in making treatment decisions. The suggested levels, in terms of committed effective dose (CED), are presented as follows (Hodgson *et al.*, 2007):

$$\text{CED} < 1 \text{ mSv}$$

Appropriate for public reassurance that doses pose a minimum risk to health.

$$1 \text{ mSv} < \text{CED} < 20 \text{ mSv}$$

More accurate dose assessment is required. Treatment should not be considered.

$$20 \text{ mSv} < \text{CED} < 200 \text{ mSv}$$

More accurate dose assessment is required. Treatment is subject to medical judgement. Although clinical effects are unlikely to occur, the potential efficacy of initial short-term treatment should be considered.

$$\text{CED} > 200 \text{ mSv}$$

Treatment should be considered. However, psychological factors and the potential efficacy of extended or protracted treatment should also be considered.

External exposures are treated for symptoms and clinical indications. For internal contamination, there are a number of techniques available to reduce the dose by removal of radionuclides from the body.

Internal contamination

There are standard procedures and drugs used to reduce doses from internal contamination by radionuclides (Voelz and Bushberg, 1994), discussed in great detail including specific dose recommendations, in NCRP Report 161 (NCRP, 2008).The principal current standard therapies in decorporation of radionuclides from the human body are presented below.

Chelating agents

Several chemical compounds are known to enhance the elimination of metals from the body by chelation. Chelation is a process by which organic compounds (ligands) exchange less firmly bonded ions for other inorganic ions to form a relatively stable non-ionized ring complex. This soluble complex is excreted readily by the kidney. Chelation therapy is most effective when it is begun immediately after exposure while the metallic ions are still in extracellular fluids before incorporation into cells. The principal chelate used for the removal of radionuclides is diethylenetriaminepentaacetic acid (DTPA). It is effective for transuranic metals (plutonium, americium, curium, californium and neptunium), the rare earths (such as cerium, yttrium, lanthanum, promethium and scandium) and others (such as zirconium and niobium). The effectiveness of DTPA in enhancing excretion of plutonium is affected principally by the chemical form of the plutonium. For exposures to insoluble forms of plutonium, such as plutonium oxide, DTPA is not effective because only tiny amounts of plutonium are present in the blood and extracellular fluids soon after exposure. Soluble compounds of plutonium, such as the nitrate, are taken up much more rapidly in blood, where it is available for chelation. Data from persons treated with Ca-DTPA within about 3 h of exposure indicate that about 60% or more of soluble forms of plutonium are removed. Two forms of DTPA are available for clinical use, calcium salt (Ca-DTPA) and zinc salt (Zn-DTPA). Zn-DTPA, which is less toxic than Ca-DTPA, is recommended for longer-term treatment and pregnant women.Ca-DTPA has been found to be more effective than Zn-DTPA (in animal studies) when given promptly after exposure to transuranium metals. Thus, Ca-DTPA is generally the preferred form of the drug used during the first day or two after exposure.

Mobilizing agents

Mobilizing agents are compounds that increase a natural turnover process, thereby releasing some forms of radionuclides from body tissues and enhancing elimination from the body. An example is ammonium chloride, which acts as a mobilizing agent for radiostrontium in the body. Other examples of mobilizing agents are diuretics for sodium, chlorides, potassium and tritium (radioactive hydrogen), and parathyroid extract for calcium, phosphorus and strontium.

Blocking and diluting agents

A blocking agent saturates the metabolic processes of a specific tissue with the stable element and thereby reduces the uptake of the radioisotopes. Stable potassium iodide (KI) given to prevent the uptake of radioiodine in the thyroid is an example of a blocking agent. To be effective, stable iodide must be administered in a rapidly absorbed form soon after exposure to the radionuclide. Only about 50% of the uptake is blocked if treatment is delayed by 6 h, which may be compared with about 90% reduction if started in less than 1 h. Little reduction is achieved if the delay is 12 h or more. Once started, continuation of stable iodide administration for 7–14 days will prevent recycling of the radioiodine into the thyroid. Isotopic dilution is achieved by the administration of large quantities of the stable element or compound similar to the radionuclides being treated. The presence of a large quantity of the stable element dilutes the smaller quantity of the radioisotope. For example, forcing fluids to tolerance (minimum of 3–4 l daily) reduces the biological half-time of tritium (radioactive hydrogen) in the body due to dilution and enhanced turnover time of water. Displacement therapy is a special form of dilution therapy in which a stable element of a different atomic number successfully competes with a radionuclide for uptake sites. An example is the use of calcium to reduce the deposition of radiostrontium in the bone.

Reduction of uptake

The procedures that may prevent or reduce uptake of radionuclides into the body include skin decontamination, proper management of contaminated wounds and reduction of gastrointestinal absorption. Immediately following an intake, simple procedures such as irrigation of the nose, mouth and pharynx, removal of gastric contents and the use of purgatives can help reduce uptake. Any reduction in the residence time of the radioactivity in the gastrointestinal tract will reduce the resultant absorption, hence the dose. The administration of a laxative (such as magnesium sulphate) may reduce the residence time of radioactive material in the lower segment of the large intestine. Magnesium sulphate may also produce relatively insoluble sulphate with some radionuclides, such as radium or strontium. Several compounds can be used to reduce the gastrointestinal uptake of specificradionuclides. Most notable examples are Prussian Blue (Ferric(III) hexacyanoferrate(II)) for caesium, thallium or rubidium; aluminium-containing antacids for strontium; and barium or magnesium sulphate for strontium or radium.

The availability of various decorporating agents will vary between nations. Some of the more commonly identified (both Food and Drug Administration-approved and off-label) decorporation strategies are provided in Table 19.3 (NCRP, 2008). Some of the therapies have alternative names, and they may be available in different countries' pharmacopeia under different labels.

A great deal of research has been conducted in decorporation therapy and techniques (Durbin *et al.*, 1998; Stradling *et al.*, 1998, 2000; Taylor *et al.*, 2000). A list of select radionuclides that may be internalized by exposed persons, along with the suggested therapy, is provided in Table 19.4. A medical decision to treat using a given therapy will depend upon the availability of the pharmaceutical (if appropriate) and any patient contraindications to the therapy. Guidance regarding appropriate pharmaceutical dose will be available on the package inserts, or may be found in NCRP Report 161 (NCRP, 2008).

Table 19.3. Potential therapy identifiers for radionuclide decorporation.

Therapy long name	Therapy short name	Therapy long name	Therapy short name
Acetycysteine (N-acetyl-L-cysteine)	NAC	Sevelamer HCL	
Aluminium hydroxide		Potassium iodide	KI
Aluminium carbonate		Potassium perchlorate	
Calcium carbonate		Potassium iodate	KIO_3
Calcitonin		Propylthiouracil	
Deferasirox	Exjade	Methimazole	Tapazole
Deferoxamine mesylate	DFOA	Ferric(III) hexacyanoferrate(II)	Prussian blue
Dialysis		Radium and strontium therapy	Aluminium hydroxide
Diethylene triamine pentaacetic acid	DTPA	Saturated solution potassium iodide	SSKI
Dimercaprol	British Anti-Lewisite (BAL)	Sodium bicarbonate	
Diuretic and isotopic dilution with 0.9% NaCl		Sodium thiosulphate	Thiosulphate
Ethylenediaminetetraacet ic acid	EDTA	Succimer	DMSA
Forced diuresis		Barium and calcium therapy	Magnesium or sodium sulphates
Haemodialysis		Trientine	Syprine
Hydration and non-labelled carbons		Water dieresis	
Penicillamine		Zinc sulphate	
Phosphorus therapy			

Table 19.4. Primary therapies for select radionuclides.

Radionuclide	Treatment	Radionuclide	Treatment
Americium-241	DTPA	Mercury-203	British Anti-Lewisite (BAL)
Antimony-124	British Anti-Lewisite (BAL)	Molybdenum-99	n/a
Arsenic-72	British Anti-Lewisite (BAL)	Neptunium-237	DFOA
Barium-133	Magnesium or sodium sulphates	Nickel-63	British Anti-Lewisite (BAL)
Bismuth-210	DMSA	Phosphorus-32	Sevelamer HCL
Cadmium-109	DMSA	Plutonium-239	DTPA
Caesium-137	Prussian blue	Polonium-210	British Anti-Lewisite (BAL)
Calcium-45	Magnesium or sodium sulphates	Potassium-42	n/a
Californium-252	DTPA	Promethium-147	DTPA
Carbon-14	Hydration and non-labelled carbons	Radium-226	Aluminium hydroxide
Cerium-144	DTPA	Rubidium-86	Prussian blue
Chromium-51	DTPA	Ruthenium-106	DTPA
Cobalt-60	DTPA	Scandium-46	DTPA
Copper-64	Penicillamine	Silver-110m	n/a
Curium-244	DTPA	Sodium-24	Diuretic and isotopic dilution with 0.9% NaCl
Europium-152	DTPA	Strontium-90	Aluminium hydroxide
Fluorine-18	n/a	Sulphur-35	Sodium thiosulphate
Gold-198	British Anti-Lewisite (BAL)	Technetium-99m	Potassium perchlorate
Indium-115m	DTPA	Thallium-204	Prussian blue
Iodine-129,131	KI	Thorium-228	DTPA
Iridium-192	DTPA	Tritium (H-3)	Water diuresis
Iron-59	DFOA	Uranium-233,235,238	Sodium bicarbonate
Lanthanum-140	DTPA	Yttrium-88	DTPA
Lead-210	DMSA	Zinc-65	DTPA
Manganese-54	DTPA	Zirconium-95	DTPA

The deceased

In a mass radiological disaster scenario, numerous people may be exposed to radiation and/or contaminated with radionuclides. Deceased victims who have been only externally exposed to ionizing radiation are of no hazard to medical personnel, and there are no special morgue requirements. However, for those victims who have been contaminated with radionuclides, special precautions must be taken regarding exposures and contamination control, especially during autopsy (see also Chapter 32, this volume). In previous incidents of trauma causing death concomitant with radiological contamination, both clothing removal and water decontamination were only partially successful (decontamination factor of 2–3), whereas melting ice used to preserve the bodies proved surprisingly successful (decontamination factors of 20–40) (Horan and Gammill, 1969). Specialized lead autopsy beds were fabricated *ad hoc*, and have been reproduced in function for facilities that may be required to perform post-mortem activities on highly contaminated bodies. An example of a leaded autopsy table may be found in Fig. 19.10 (photographed at the Radiation Emergency Assistance Center/Training Site, REAC/TS in Oak Ridge, Tennessee).The bed itself (which could also serve as a treatment bed for non-deceased, contaminated victims) has lead-lined walls and movable screens with leaded viewing glass. Arm access ports allow medical personnel to examine the deceased while limiting the dose to the major blood-forming organs in the examiner.

If the deceased are identified in the field, it is presumed that they will be transported directly to morgue facilities (Shapira and Shemer, 2002). Standard contamination control procedures should be practised, and external contamination can be addressed with standard decontamination protocols (Jacocks *et al.*, 2008). Remains will need to be identified as contaminated if residual radioactivity persists and, although internal organs will generally not be contaminated, it is possible that the lungs and body fluids could have detectable contamination, so care should be taken with these during autopsy, including consideration of closed-cycle embalming (NCRP, 2008). A comprehensive overview of morgue operations for MCIs is provided by Jensen (1999), and detailed guidance for handling decedents contaminated in a radiological disaster is provided by Wood *et al.* (2007).

Post-disaster Event Considerations

It is known that disasters involving radiological materials can cause population-based widespread confusion, fear and psychological stress, which may generate long-term effects in the population (Hyams *et al.*, 2002). In a radiological disaster, there are three primary areas of medical management to consider post-event: (i) long-term care; (ii) dose reconstruction; and (iii) epidemiology as related to long-term health effects.

Long-term care

For radiation exposure of the order of greater than about 1 Gy, bone marrow damage is possible and may require aggressive treatment using cytokine therapy, stem cell replacement and bone marrow transplant (Moulder, 2004). Local radiation injuries can be treated symptomatically, and internal radionuclides can be treated using decorporation therapy.

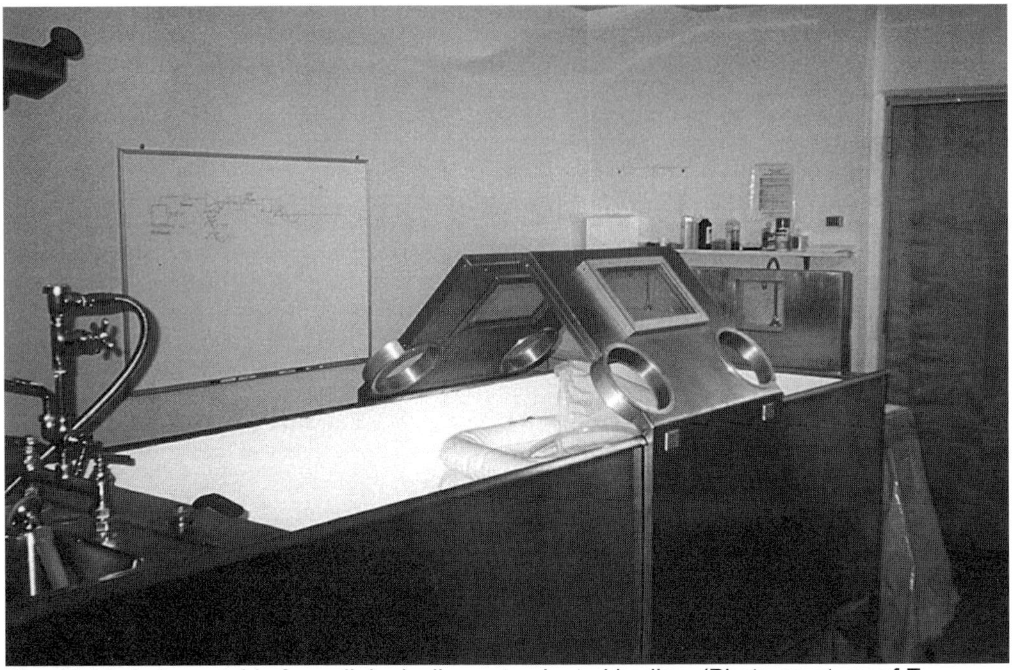

Fig. 19.10. Autopsy table for radiologically contaminated bodies. (Photo courtesy of E. Waller, UOIT.)

Considerations related to the use of decorporation agents

There has not been an abundance of adverse health effects associated with decorporation therapy in humans, and knowledge in this area is limited. The principal consideration with decorporation agents is that they can deplete the body of non-radioactive elements essential to physiological function, and therefore the medical personnel caring for patients utilizing decorporating agents must carefully monitor appropriate haematopoietic components. In addition, risk analysis must be performed to balance therapy risk against radiation risk. Some considerations for specific pharmaceuticals are discussed below.

Ca-DTPA

Ca-DTPA can deplete the body of zinc and, to a lesser extent, manganese with repeated dosing. The amount of zinc lost is determined by the amount of DTPA and the frequency of dosage. By depleting these essential trace metals, Ca-DTPA can then interfere with necessary mitotic cellular processes, over long time periods. No serious toxicity in human subjects has been reported. When given repeatedly, with short intervals for recovery, Ca-DTPA treatment may cause nausea, vomiting, diarrhoea, chills, fever, pruritus and muscle cramps in the first 24 h. Urinary zinc excretion studies suggest that the zinc supply is quickly replenished during this treatment regimen and that any partial depletion of zinc stores, if it occurs at all, would be transient. Ca-DTPA is approximately ten times more effective than Zn-DTPA for initial chelation of transuranics; therefore, Ca-DTPA should be used whenever larger body burdens of transuranics are involved. Ca-DTPA is the form of choice for initial patient management unless contraindicated. Approximately 24 h after exposure, Zn-DTPA is, for all practical purposes, as effective as Ca-DTPA. This comparable efficacy, coupled with its lesser toxicity, makes Zn-DTPA the preferred agent for protracted therapy. Ca-DTPA should not to be used as a chelator for uranium or neptunium. Internal contamination with uranium is currently treated by alkalizing the urine with bicarbonate in order to promote excretion. DTPA has also been postulated to form an unstable complex with neptunium, which may increase bone deposition of this actinide.

Zn-DTPA

No serious toxicity in humans has been reported. When given repeatedly, with short intervals for recovery, Zn-DTPA treatment may cause nausea, vomiting, diarrhoea, chills, fever, pruritus and muscle cramps in the first 24 h. Zn-DTPA should not to be used as a chelator for uranium or neptunium, as above.

Dimercaprol (BAL)

Although BAL is a very powerful chelating agent, especially for arsenic and mercury poisoning, it can have some serious side-effects. BAL treatment may cause nausea, vomiting, burning of lips and throat, salivation, abdominal pain, anxiety, weakness and unrest. Potential effects to the nervous system include headache, conjunctivitis, lacrimation and tingling of the hands. Cardiovascular effects may include a rise in blood pressure and tachycardia. Other miscellaneous effects may include a burning sensation in the penis, sweating of the forehead and hands, feeling of constriction in the chest and throat, pain at the site of injection and renal damage. The risk of toxicity of this drug increases when taken with iron.

Ferric(III) hexacyanoferrate(II)

The medical consideration to using high doses of Prussian blue during treatment over a prolonged period is obstipation. In addition, the patient will observe blue stools, which may be a psychological consideration.

Penicillamine

This drug is a standard therapy for Wilson's disease and severe rheumatoid arthritis. Penicillamine treatment may cause nausea, vomiting, gastric pain, diarrhoea, altered taste perception and oral ulcerations. Nervous system effects include muscle weakening and tinnitus. Various haematological effects include bone marrow depression, leucopenia, thrombocytopenia, red cell aplasia, agranulocytosis and aplastic anaemia. In addition, persons allergic to penicillin are likely also allergic to penicillamine.

Potassium iodide

The side-effects among adults are generally mild and not clinically significant. Side-effects may include gastrointestinal distress and rash. Allergic reactions are possible in persons with known iodine sensitivity.

Psychological effects

There are a number of factors that can contribute to the appearance of psychological health problems, including the duration of the traumatic event, amount of devastation, loss or injury to family, friends and co-workers, and the overall impact on normal life (Leon, 2004). The long-term effects can manifest as feelings of shock/numbness, depression, anxiety, anger, acute stress disorder and/or post-traumatic stress disorder, and ultimately result in health detriment indicators such as alcoholism, suicide, cardiovascular disease and family/vocational problems (Leon, 2004). Psychological and social detriment has been observed in the fatal radiological accident in Goiânia, Brazil in 1987 (Bandeira de Carvalho, 1988) and to a greater extent after the Chernobyl accident in 1986 (Ginzburg, 1993). In both cases it was found that both persons exposed and those unexposed experienced high levels of stress. It is essential that psychological counselling be provided as early as possible in the event of a radiological disaster, and that the counselling continues long after the event has ended, as many of the end-points are only realized months to years post-event.

Dose reconstruction

Estimation of radiation dose is an activity that will take place as soon as is practical after a radiation exposure event, and may continue for many years, potentially extending the lifetime of the individual exposed. The goal of dose estimation in the early stages of an event is for triage and for determining potential treatment strategies (especially if a large dose is expected). At times long after exposure, the dose estimates will be used for long-term care medical management and epidemiology studies. Dose estimation in the early stages post-exposure can be achieved by:

1. Interview of the exposed, situational assessment and calculational reconstruction of dose;
2. Use of radiation dosimeters (if available) or expert radiation metrology;
3. Symptomological assessment (type and onset of symptoms);
4. Haematological indicators (primarily lymphocyte depletion kinetics);
5. Bioassay, principally urinalysis, faecal analysis and whole-body counting for internal contamination.

At times long after exposure, other techniques are available for non-computational retrospective dose assessment (Simon *et al.*, 2007). Viable techniques include: (i) electron paramagnetic (or spin) resonance (EPR; ESR); (ii) cytogenetic dosimetry; (iii) somatic cell assay; (iv) luminescence ions in the form of thermoluminescence (TL) and optically stimulated luminescence (OSL); and (v) long-term bioassay.

Long-term radiation monitoring must be based upon a number of considerations such as ability to accurately monitor, ability to relate monitoring to disease(s)-of-interest end-point(s), the potential that the monitoring may cause harm (either physical or psychological), the ability to act upon monitoring results, the potential for improved clinical outcome and the cost–benefit analysis of the monitoring programme (Gusev *et al.*, 2001).

Follow-up epidemiology

Epidemiology studies the incidence, distribution and subsequent control of diseases in a population. Following an exposed cohort post-radiological disaster is important to: (i) estimate the potential health risk to the population; (ii) add data to the relative dearth of dose-risk model datasets; (iii) provide data that may be used in compensation cases; and (iv) provide data to the scientific community to better understand long-term risk from exposure to radiation. There are two principal and widespread studies related to radiation disasters: (i) the atomic bombs on Hiroshima and Nagasaki in 1945; and (ii) the Chernobyl Unit 4 accident in 1986. These events have provided the epidemiological basis for both the US National Research Council Biological Effects of Ionizing Radiation studies (BEIR, 2006) and the United Nations Scientific Committee on the Effects of Atomic Radiation reports (UNSCEAR, 2006, 2008). Epidemiological studies require careful planning as there are many difficulties, such as: (i) obtaining a population size large enough to detect a statistically significant difference compared with the non-exposed cohort; (ii) ensuring the disease end-point attributable to radiation exposure uniquely; (iii) time between onset of disease (e.g. malignant cancer) and exposure; and (iv) confounding factors that may mask the radiation effect (e.g. smoking) (Gusev *et al.*, 2001). Integral to epidemiological studies is the dosimetry basis, which drives the results. A summary of epidemiology dosimetry issues is provided by Simon *et al.* (2006).

Conclusion

Although there is global threat of radiological dispersal either through accidental, military or terrorist actions, there are gaps in the ability of emergency medical services to appropriately respond (Phelps, 2006). After the 11 September 2001 attacks in the USA, much attention has been focused on CBRN threats, and many nations have prepared emergency response plans for these disaster scenarios. However, areas requiring on-going improvements in this field include:

1. *Education of medical personnel*: although great improvements have been made to dispel fear of radiation in the medical community, this is an on-going effort worldwide. Education on radiation, radioactive materials and medical management of those exposed likely has the most potential for positive outcome to patient health.
2. *Disaster planning*: as discussed, many nations have disaster response plans that deal with radiological emergencies. These plans require periodic review, integration inter-agency and interfacing with international agencies (such as the International Atomic Energy Agency) that may help in time of crisis.
3. *Exercising*: a plan is only a plan until it has been enacted. As such, periodic exercises of radiological disaster plans must be conducted. The most comprehensive exercises include large numbers of actors, inter-agency cooperation and, in some cases, live radiological agents. Exercises must be reviewed with a critical eye to identify what went right and what went wrong, and although tempting, should not be used necessarily as a positive public relations exercise.

4. *Radiation metrology*: although there are a great number of radiation detection instruments available on the market, very few are designed for the specific mission of radiological disasters, especially for triage of potentially exposed persons. This is an area that requires research and development.
5. *Stockpiling*: there are clear challenges to stockpiling decorporation therapies. For example, high cost (especially for so-called orphan drugs), shelf-life and stockpile management all need to be addressed within the disaster response framework.
6. *Decorporation agents*: despite the fact that chelators and decorporating agents have been studied for decades, there are relatively few approved-for-use pharmaceuticals. More research, development, clinical trials and manufacture is required in this area.
7. *Acute exposure care*: those exposed to high radiation doses may need cytokine therapy and/or stem/bone marrow transplant, which are resource-intensive treatments, especially in the aftermath of a mass casualty radiological disaster (Blakely *et al*., 2005).
8. *Retrospective dosimetry*: there are a number of areas in retospective dosimetry that require more research and development for use in a radiological disaster. For example, *in situ* electron paramegnetic resonance, *in situ* optically stimulated luminescence, fluorescent *in situ* hybridization (FISH) assay and glycophorin-A (GPA) somatic mutation assay (Simon *et al*., 2007) have all been evaluated for long-term dosimetry.

In summary, a comprehensive disaster plan requires a unique addressing of radiological insults from a medical management perspective. Thorough preparation and integration of the radiological response plan with the overall plan will ensure the best possible medical outcome for the greatest number of patients.

References

AFRRI (2010) *Medical Management of Radiological Casualties*, 3rd edn.. Armed Forces Radiobiology Research Institute, AFRRI Special Report 10-1. Available at: http://www.afrri.usuhs.mil/outreach/infoprod.htm#guide (Accessed 5 February 2013).

Bandeira de Carvalho, A. (1988) The psychological impact of the radiological accident in Goiânia. National Nuclear Energy Commission. INIS BR 1354. Rio de Janeiro, Brazil.

Becker, S. (2005) Addressing the psychosocial and communication challenges posed by radiological/nuclear terrorism: key developments since NCRP Report No. 138. *Health Physics* 89(5), 521–530.

Becker, S. and Middleton, S. (2008) Improving hospital preparedness for radiological terrorism: perspectives from emergency department physicians and nurses. *Disaster Medicine and Public Health Preparedness* 2(3), 174–184.

BEIR (2006) Health risks from exposure to low levels of ionizing radiation. BEIR VII Phase 2. National Research Council, Washington, DC.

Bentur, Y., Horlatsch, N. and Koren, G. (1991) Exposure to ionizing radiation during pregnancy: perception of teratogenic risk and outcome. *Teratology* 43, 109–112.

Berry, A. and Hilgers, M. (2004) Modeling first responder emergency sensors for virtual training. *Proceedings of the 15th IASTED Modeling and Simulation Conference*, 1–3 March 2004.Marina del Rey, California, pp.234–239.

Blakely, W., Salter, C. and Prasanna, P. (2005) Early-response biological dosimetry – recommended countermeasure enhancements for mass-casualty radiological incidents and terrorism. *Health Physics*89(5), 494–504.

Bostick, N., Subbarao, I., Burkle, F., Hsu, E., Armstrong, J. and James, J. (2008) Disaster triage systems for large-scale catastrophic events. *Disaster Medicine and Public Health Preparedness* 2(suppl. 1), S35–S39.

Bushberg, J., Kroger, L., Hartman, M., Leidholdt, E., Miller, K., Derlet, R. and Wraa, C. (2007) Nuclear/radiological terrorism: emergency department management of radiation casualties. *Journal of Emergency Medicine* 32(1), 71–85.

Cassatt, D., Kaminski, J., Hatchett, R., DiCarlo, A., Benjamin, J. and Maidment, B. (2008) Medical countermeasures against nuclear threats: radionuclide decorporation agents. *Radiation Research* 170(4), 540–548.

Cember, H. and Johnson, T. (2009) *Introduction to Health Physics,* 4th edn. McGraw-Hill, London,.

Chen, J., Wilkinson, D., Richardson, R. and Waruszynski, B. (2009) Issues, considerations, and recommendations on emergency preparedness for vulnerable population groups. *Radiation Protection Dosimetry* 134(3–4), 132–135.

Chroust, G., Schönhacker, S., Rainer, K., Roth, M. and Ziehesberger, P. (2009) Training and supporting first responders by mixed reality environments. *Proceedings of the 53rd Annual Meeting of the International Society for the Systems Sciences (ISSS)*,12–17 July 2009. Brisbane, Australia.

DiMaggio, C., Markenson, D., Loo, G. and Redlener, I. (2005) The willingness of U.S. emergency medical technicians to respond to terrorist incidents. *Biosecurity and Bioterrorism: Biodefense Strategy, Practice, and Science* 3(4), 331–337.

Durbin, P., Kullgren, B., Xu, J. and Raymond, K. (1998) Development of decorporation agents for the actinides. *Radiation Protection Dosimetry* 79(1–4), 433–443.

EPA (2011) Radiation Emergencies – Response Exercises. US Environmental Protection Agency. Available at:http://www.epa.gov/radiation/rert/exercises.html(Accessed15 July 2011).

Esbitt, D. (2003) The strategic national stockpile: roles and responsibilities of health care professionals for receiving the stockpile assets. *Disaster Management and Response* 1(3), 68–70.

FEMA (2010) *Planning Guidance for Response to a Nuclear Detonation,* 2nd edn.. Federal Emergency Management Agency, Hyattsville, Maryland.

Ferguson, C. and Potter,W. (2004) Improvised Nuclear Devices and Nuclear Terrorism. The Weapons of Mass Destruction Commission. Report No. 2. Stockholm, Sweden. Available at: http://www.wmdcommission.org (Accessed 5 February 2013).

Fisher, D. (2000) Decorporation: officially a word. *Health Physics* 78(5), 563–565.

Ford, J. (1998) Radiological dispersal devices – assessing the transnational threat. National Defense University, Institute for National Strategic Studies Strategic Forum, No. 136.

Frykberg, E. (2005) Triage: principles and practice. *Scandinavian Journal of Surgery* 94, 272–278.

Ginzburg, H. (1993) The psychological consequences of the Chernobyl accident – findings from the International Atomic Energy Agency study. *Public Health Reports* 108(2), 184–192.

Glasstone, S. and Dolan, P. (1977) *The Effects of Nuclear Weapons,* 3rd edn. US Department of Defense, Washington, DC.

Goans, R. and Waselenko, J. (2005) Medical management of radiological casualties. *Health Physics* 89(5), 505–512.

Goans, R., Holloway, E., Berger, M. and Ricks, R. (2001) Early dose assessment in criticality accidents. *Health Physics* 81, 446–449.

Gusev, I., Guskova, A. and Mettler, F. (2001) *Medical Management of Radiation Accidents,* 2nd edn. CRC Press, Boca Raton, Florida.

Hafer, N., Maidment, B. and Hatchet, R. (2010) The NIAID radiation countermeasures program business model. *Biosecurity and Bioterrorism: Biodefense Strategy, Practice and Science* 8(4), 357–363.

Hick, J., Weinstock, D., Coleman, N., Hanfling, D., Cantrill, S., Redlener, I., Bader, J., Murrain-Hill, P. and Knebel, A. (2011) Health care system planning for and response to a nuclear detonation. *Disaster Medicine and Public Health Preparedness* 5(suppl. 1), S73–S88.

Hodgson, A., Stradling, N., Menetrier, F., Berard, P., Paile, W., Joussineau, S., Holt, D., Morcillo, M., Cebrian, D. and List, V. (2007) Dose assessment of inhaled radionuclides in emergency situations. Commission of the European Communities PASR-SEC4-SA-014100. Health Protection Agency, Chilton, UK.

Horan, J. and Gammill, W. (1963) The health physics aspects of the SL-1 accident. *Health Physics* 9(2), 177–186.

Hyams, K., Murphy, F. and Wessely, S. (2002) Responding to chemical, biological, or nuclear terrorism: the indirect and long-term health effects may present the greatest challenge. *Journal of Health Politics, Policy and Law* 27(2), 273–292.

IAEA (2000) *Generic Procedures for Assessment and Response during a Radiological Emergency.* IAEA-TECDOC-1162. IAEA, Vienna, Austria.

IAEA (2001) *Cytogenetic Analysis for Radiation Dose Assessment – a Manual.* Technical Report Series No. 405. IAEA, Vienna, Austria.

IAEA (2002a) *Preparedness and Response for a Nuclear or Radiological Emergency.* Safety Standard Series No. GS-R-2. IAEA, Vienna, Austria.

IAEA (2002b) *Planning and Preparing for Emergency Response to Transport Accidents Involving Radioactive Material.* Safety Guide No. TS-G-1.2 (ST-3). IAEA, Vienna, Austria.

IAEA (2005) *Generic Procedures for Medical Response during a Nuclear or Radiological Emergency.* IAEA-EPR-Medical-2005. IAEA, Vienna, Austria.

IAEA (2006a) *Nuclear Forensics Support – Reference Manual.* Nuclear Security Series No.2. IAEA, Vienna, Austria.

IAEA (2006b) *Manual for First Responders to a Radiological Emergency.* IAEA-EPR-First Responders-2006. IAEA, Vienna, Austria.

IAEA (2009) *INES – The International Nuclear and Radiological Event Scale User's Manual, 2008 Edition.* IAEA, Vienna, Austria.

International Commission on Radiological Protection (ICRP) (2003)*Basic Anatomical and Physiological Data for Use in Radiological Protection: Reference Values.* ICRP Publication 89. ICRP, Vienna, Austria.

Jacocks, J., Danley, R., Green, L. and Gavin, M. (2008) Consequence management – What do we do with the contaminated dead? *Joint Center for Operational Analysis Journal* 11(1), 53–60.

Jasper, E., Miller, M., Sweeney, B., Feuer, E. and Reganato, D. (2005) Preparedness of hospitals to respond to a radiological terrorism event as assessed by a full-scale exercise. *The Journal of Public Health Management and Practice* 11(6), S11–S16.

Jensen, R. (1999) *Mass Fatality and Casualty Incidents – a Field Guide.* CRC Press, Boca Raton, Florida.

Koenig, K., Bey, T., Bradley, D., Kahn, C. and Schultz, C. (2008) The RADPACK: a new concept for stockpiling medical countermeasures for a radiation disaster at the local level. *The Western Journal of Emergency Medicine* 9(3), S34.

Koenig, K., Boatright, C., Hancock, J., Denny, F., Teeter, D., Kahn, C. and Schultz, C. (2008) Health care facility-based decontamination of victims exposed to chemical, biological and radiological materials. *American Journal of Emergency Medicine* 26(1), 71–80

Kollek, D. and Karawowska, A. (2009) Populations and risk – paediatrics. *Radiation Protection Dosimetry* 134(3–4), 191–192.

Lake, J., Sanders, R. and Cross, B. (2008) *A Simulation Learning Approach to Training First Responders for Radiological Emergencies – a Continuation of Work.* Oak Ridge National Laboratory Pub-11173, Oak Ridge, Tennessee.

Lanoix, R., Wiener, D. and Zayas, V. (2002) Concepts in disaster triage in the wake of the World Trade Center terrorist attack. *Topics in Emergency Medicine* 24(2), 60–71.

Lemyre, L., Gibson, S., Zlepnig, J., Meyer-Macleod, R. and Boutette, P. (2009) Emergency preparedness for higher risk populations: psychosocial considerations. *Radiation Protection Dosimetry* 134(3–4), 207–214.

Leon, G. (2004) Overview of the psychosocial impact of disasters. *Prehospital and Disaster Medicine* 19(1), 4–9.

Liland, A., van der Meer, K., Rojas-Palma, C., Østreng, A., Hodgson, A., Youngman, M., Etherton, G., Rahola, T., Muikku, M., Pellow, P., Jaworska, A., Pérez, M., Carr, Z. and Aaltonen, H. (2009) *TMT Handbook* – Triage, Monitoring and Treatment of People Exposed to Ionising

Radiation Following a Malevolent Attack. In: Rojas-Palma, C., Liland, A., Næss Jersted, A., Etherington, G., del Rosario Perez, M., Rahola, T. and Smith, K. (eds) *TMT Handbook*. Østerås, Norway. Available at: http://www.tmthandbook.org (Accessed 5 February 2013).

Loper, H. (1951) *Radiological Defense, Vol. II – the Principles of Military Defense against Atomic Weapons*. Armed Forces Special Weapons Project, Naval Radiological Defense Laboratory, San Francisco, California.

Ménétrier, F., Bérnard, P., Joussineau, S., Stradling, N., Hodgson, A., List, V., Morcillo, M., Paile, W., Holt, D. and Eriksson, T. (2007) TIARA: treat initiatives after radiological accidents. *Radiation Protection Dosimetry* 127(1–4), 444–448.

Mettler, F. (2005) Medical resources and requirements for responding to radiological terrorism. *Health Physics* 89(5), 488–493.

Moulder, J. (2004) Post-irradiation approaches to treatment of radiation injuries in the context of radiological terrorism and radiation accidents: a review. *International Journal of Radiation Biology* 80(1), 3–10.

Musolino, S. and Harper, F. (2006) Emergency response guidance for the first 48 hours after the outdoor detonation of an explosive radiological dispersal device. *Health Physics* 90(4), 377–385.

National Council on Radiation Protection and Measurements (NCRP) (2001) *Management of Terrorist Events Involving Radioactive Material*. NCRP Report No. 138. NCRP, Bethesda, Maryland.

NCRP (2008) *Management of Persons Contaminated with Radionuclides: Handbook*. NCRP Report No. 161. NCRP, Bethesda, Maryland.

Nuclear News (NN) (2011) Special report: Fukushima Daiichi after the earthquake and tsunami. *Nuclear News* 54, 17–18b, 83–84b.

Okie, S. (2008) Dr. Pou and the hurricane – implications for patient care during disasters. *New England Journal of Medicine* 358, 1–5.

Organisation for Economic Co-operation and Development/Nuclear Energy Agency (OECD/NEA) (2010) *Comparing Nuclear Accident Risks with those from other Energy Sources*. NEA No. 6861. OECD/NEA, Washington, DC.

Perry, R. (2003) Incident management systems in disaster management. *Disaster Prevention and Management* 12(5), 405–412.

Phelps, S. (2006) Mission failure: emergency medical services response to chemical, biological, radiological, nuclear and explosive events. *Prehospital and Disaster Medicine* 22(4), 293–296.

Powell, S., Plouffe, L. and Gorr, P. (2009) When ageing and disasters collide: lessons from 16 international case studies. *Radiation Protection Dosimetry* 134(3–4), 202–206.

Remick, A., Crapo, J. and Woodruff, C. (2005) U.S. national response assets for radiological incidents. *Health Physics* 89(5), 471–484.

Richardson, R. (2009) Factors that elevate the internal radionuclide and chemical retention, dose, and health risks to infants and children in a radiological-nuclear emergency. *Radiation Protection Dosimetry* 134(3–4), 167–180.

Schleipman, A., Gebaudo, V. and Castronova, F. (2004) Radiation disaster response: preparation and simulation experience at an academic medical center. *The Journal of Nuclear Medicine Technology* 32, 22–27.

Schuster, M., Stein, B., Jaycox, L., Collins, R., Marshall, G., Elliot, M., Zhou, A., Kanouse, D., Morrison, J. and Berry, S. (2001) A national survey of stress reactions after the September 11, 2001 terrorist attacks. *New England Journal of Medicine* 345(20), 1507–1512.

Severa, J. and Bár, J. (1991) *Handbook of Radioactive Contamination and Decontamination*. Elsevier Science Publishing Company, New York.

Shapira, S. and Shemer, J. (2002) Medical management of terrorist attacks. *Israel Medical Association Journal* 4, 489–492.

Simon, S., Bouville, A., Kleinerman, R. and Ron, E. (2006) Dosimetry for epidemiological studies: learning from the past, looking to the future. *Radiation Research* 166(1), 313–318.

Simon, S., Bailiff, I., Bouville, A., Fattibene, P., Kleinerman, R., Lloyd, D., McKeever, S., Romanyukha, A., Sevan'kaev, A., Tucker, J. and Wieser, A. (2007) BiodosEPR-2006 consensus committee report on biodosimetric methods to evaluate radiation doses at long times after exposure. *Radiation Measurements* 42(6–7), 948–971.

Stradling, G., Hodgson, S. and Pearce, M. (1998) Recent developments in the decorporation of plutonium, americium and thorium. *Radiation Protection Dosimetry* 79(1–4), 445–448.

Stradling, G., Henge-Napoli, M., Paquet, F., Poncy, J., Fritsch, P. and Taylor, D. (2000) Approaches for experimental evaluation of chelating agents. *Radiation Protection Dosimetry* 87(1), 19–28.

Sullivan, H. and Häkkinen, M. (2006) Disaster preparedness for vulnerable populations: determining effective strategies for communicating risk, warning, and response. *3rd Annual MaGrann Research Conference on the Future of Disasters in a Globalizing World*. Rutgers University, New Brunswick, New Jersey.

Tan, G. and Fitzgerald, M. (2002) Chemical-biological-radiological (CBR) response: a template for hospital emergency departments. *Medical Journal of Australia* 177, 196–199.

Taylor, D., Stradling, G. and Henge-Napoli, M. (2000) The scientific background to decorporation.*RadiationProtection Dosimetry* 87(1), 11–17.

Turai, I., Veress, K., Günalp, B. and Souchkevitch, G. (2004) Medical response to radiation incidents and radionuclear threats. *British Medical Journal* 328, 568–572.

United Nations Scientific Committee on the Effects of Atomic Radiation (UNSCEAR) (2000) *Sources and Effects of Ionizing Radiation, Volumes I and II*. United Nations, New York.

UNSCEAR (2006) *Effects of Ionizing Radiation, Volume I*. UNSCEAR Report A/61/46. UNSCEAR, New York.

UNSCEAR (2008) *Sources and Effects of Ionizing Radiation, Volume I*. UNSCEAR Report A/63/46. UNSCEAR, New York.

Unterweger, M. and Pibida, L. (2005) Advances in radiation detection technologies for responders. *Health Physics* 89(5), 485–487.

Voelz, G. (1969) Excretion measurements for internal exposure to radionuclides – a general discussion. US Atomic Energy Commission, Idaho Operation Office, Idaho Falls, Idaho.

Voelz, G. and Bushberg, J. (1994) Medical management of internal contamination accidents. In: Raabe, O. (ed.) *Internal Radiation Dosimetry*. Medical Physics Publishing, Madison, Wisconsin.

Wagner, P. and Curran, P. (1984) Health beliefs and physician identified 'worried well'. *Health Psychology* 3(5), 459–474.

Waller, E. (2010a) Combined hardware-software considerations for triage of internally contaminated personnel. *Radiation Protection Dosimetry* 142(1), 24–28.

Waller, E. (2010b) First response considerations for children exposed to a radiological dispersal device. *Radiation Protection Dosimetry* 142(1), 63–67.

Waller, E. and Wilkinson, D. (2010c) MEDECOR – a MEdical DECORporation tool to assist first responders, receivers and medical reach-back personnel in triage, treatment and risk assessment after internalization of radionuclides. *Health Physics* 99(4), 581–590.

Waller, E., Millage, K., Blakely, W., Ross, J., Mercier, J., Sandgren, D., Levine, I., Dickerson, W., Nemhauser, J., Nasstrom, J., Sugiyama, G., Homann, S., Buddemeier, B., Curling, C. and Disraelly, D. (2009) Overview of hazard assessment and emergency planning software of use to RN first responders. *Health Physics* 97(2), 145–156.

Waselenko, K., MacVittie, T., Blakely, W., Pesik, N., Wiley, A., Dickerson, W., Tsu, H., Confer, D., Coleman, N., Seed, T., Lowry, P., Armitage, J. and Dainiak, N. (2004) Medical Management of the Acute Radiation Syndrome: Recommendations of the Strategic National Stockpile Radiation Working Group. *Annals of Internal Medicine* 140, 1037–1051.

Weiss, W. (1997) Strategies for monitoring and for the assessment of the radiological situation in an emergency. *Radiation Protection Dosimetry* 73(1–4), 7–10.

Wells, M., Stearns, L., Davie, A. and Day, E. (2007) Challenges for early responders to a nuclear/radiological terrorism incident. Waste Management '07 Conference,25 February – 1 March 2007, Tucson, Arizona.

Wilkinson, D. (2009) Dealing with at-risk populations in radiological/nuclear emergencies. *Radiation Protection Dosimetry* 134(3–4), 136–142.

Wood, C., DePaolo, F. and Whitaker, R. (2007) Guidelines for handling decedents contaminated with radioactive materials. Centers for Disease Control and Prevention, Atlanta, Georgia. Available

at: http://www.bt.cdc.gov/radiation/pdf/radiation-decedent-guidelines.pdf (Accessed 5 February 2013).
World Nuclear Association (WNO) (2011) Safety of nuclear power reactors. World Nuclear Association. Available at: http://www.world-nuclear.org/info/inf06.html (Accessed 5 February 2013).

Section 7

Defeating Emerging Health Threats:

Managing by Prophylactic and Therapeutic Approaches

Chapter 20

Superhumanized Antibodies for Biodefence: The Example of Anthrax

Philippe Thullier, Michael Hust and Thibaut Pelat

Introduction

Today the development of recombinant antibodies, mostly in the form of whole G immunoglobulins, is a burgeoning class of therapeutics. Their main benefit lies in the fact that genetic engineering allows the construction of antibody molecules very similar to human antibodies and which do not have the drawbacks of xenogenic antibodies of, for example, equine origin, which are used in serum therapy and can be a source of accidents like serum disease and anaphylactic shock. Engineering of recombinant monoclonal antibodies has emerged recently and has revolutionized the treatment of many diseases such as auto-immune diseases or cancer. Today it offers new prospects for treatment and prevention in military medicine. First isolated in mice but not well tolerated in humans, therapeutic antibodies have become chimeric (70% human) by fusion of the genes encoding the variable regions of a murine antibody with the human genes encoding the remainder of the antibody. By further reducing the murine component, a new class of so-called humanized antibodies (90% human) appeared, and then recently, entirely human antibodies have been obtained. Currently more than 20 therapeutic antibodies have received their approval from the US Food and Drug Administration (FDA); more generally, recombinant antibodies account for half of the molecules undergoing clinical trials (Reichert, 2011). Furthermore it appears that the success rate of recombinant antibodies at the end of phase I is very high thanks to their good tolerance levels, especially if these antibodies are of human nature; this situation is to be compared with small synthetic molecules, which are rejected nine times out of ten for reasons of bioavailability or tolerance.

Among the advantages of recombinant antibodies, it should be noted that they are effective immediately after administration, they can be used both prophylactically and as treatment, possibly in synergistic combination with other molecules. In addition, the length of their half-life allows for sustained protection over time because the half-life of a human antibody in humans is estimated to be about 1 month. Faced with scarce pathogens for which no human donors of serum and antibodies are available, animals can be immunized and then, antibodies can be reconstituted from their lymphocytes. Those will be modified, if necessary, to make them very close to human antibodies. This is particularly true in the context of specific medical countermeasures: in the face of the intentional biological risks posed by bioterrorism and biological weapons, it is of great benefit to develop a prophylactic method and a post-exposure treatment with recombinant antibodies for victims who are potentially exposed or already suffering from the disease.

Anthrax and Bioterrorism

Anthrax is an anthropozoonosis affecting livestock and sometimes humans who are in contact with animal products in the context of occupational or industrial diseases, or food poisoning. It is still present in Africa, central and South-east Asia, China, India, the Middle East and southern and eastern Europe (Mock and Fouet, 2001; Turnbull, 2002). Human cases are rare in industrialized countries and in France, the departmental veterinary laboratories record about ten sporadic outbreaks each year that correspond to 'cursed fields', formerly known to have been contaminated with anthrax spores (Savoie, Pyrenees, Jura, Massif Central). The disease takes different forms: cutaneous anthrax, which is easily treated by antibiotics; digestive forms that are more difficult to diagnose, and are therefore more serious; inhalational anthrax, which is deadly, with a banal influenza-like phase followed by a phase of sudden deterioration with respiratory distress (Holty *et al.*, 2006) and meningeal complications. The anthrax cycle involves a telluric sporulated form and an encapsulated vegetative form producing anthrax toxins in the host.

The pathogenicity of *Bacillus anthracis* is based on the presence of two virulence plasmids, pXO1 and pXO2, which control the synthesis of two toxins and the capsule, respectively. These toxins involve three proteins: the protective antigen (PA), the edema factor (EF) and the lethal factor (LF). PA and LF form the lethal toxin and PA and EF, which are the two major toxins in the physiopathology of anthrax, form the edema toxin. The PA role is to allow EF or LF to be internalized. EF is a calmodulin- and calcium-dependent adenylate cyclase (Shen *et al.*, 2005), which causes an increase in intracellular AMPc, whereas LF is a metallo-protease that cleaves the mitogen-activated protein kinase kinases (MAPKK) and deregulates cytokine expression (Duesbery *et al.*, 1998; Tournier *et al.*, 2005). These toxins are the cause of the toxaemia developed in the course of infection. The *B. anthracis* capsule, consisting exclusively of poly-D-glutamic acid, protects the bacteria from the host's defences and, through its antiphagocytic power, promotes dissemination of the bacteria (Candela and Fouet, 2005). Thus the disease manifests itself with two physiopathological mechanisms: one related to the multiplication and dissemination of the bacteria in the organism of the infected host, and the other is related to the production of toxins by these vegetative bacteria.

Anthrax represents a high-level threat among the potential bioweapons agents owing to its pathogenicity, which is driven by the toxins and the capsule, and to its ability to sporulate, which lends it exceptional resistance to heat, desiccation and ultraviolet radiation (Inglesby *et al.*, 2002; Sylvestre *et al.*, 2005). Several countries have studied the military use of anthrax from the 1930s (Japan, UK, USA) until the years 1970–1990 (Soviet Union and Iraq). Finally, the attacks with envelopes containing anthrax spores in the USA in September and October 2001 caused 22 cases of anthrax, 11 cases of cutaneous anthrax and 11 cases of inhalational anthrax with five deaths. Genotyping studies have clearly identified the US origin of the strain involved, the Ames strain, which is the anthrax reference strain in American laboratories (Jernigan *et al.*, 2001; Baggett *et al.*, 2005). These attacks were followed by a wave of bioterrorism-type alerts in Europe with, as a result, an unprecedented crisis situation and a considerable cost to society. In France, in the absence of an approved vaccine, prophylaxis and treatment of anthrax depend on antibiotics, the use of which has some limits, however, antibiotic prophylaxis has to be extended for 60 days after the risk of exposure to spores, due to late germination of the spores. This duration was not always respected in the USA in 2001. Antibiotic therapy must be started very soon after infection, otherwise the toxic shock is lethal even in the presence of antibiotics.

Method of Obtaining the Recombinant Antibodies

The first recombinant antibodies were historically obtained by grafting variable regions of murine monoclonal antibodies on constant regions of human antibodies. While certain of these 'chimeric' antibodies are still commercialized, the following generations of recombinant antibodies are intended to be closer to human antibodies. The second generation of recombinant antibodies has thus been that of 'humanized' antibodies, where only the hypervariable regions are still of murine origin (Fig. 20.1). Currently, totally human antibodies are becoming the norm for recombinant antibodies. However, the naturally occurring process of affinity maturation induces mutations in human antibodies, and these mutations are not always useful for improving this affinity. Moreover, these mutations can be immunogenic.

Germline humanization, so called because this type of humanization is done with the germline sequences encoding the antibodies as template, or super-humanization, aims at eliminating such mutations without impairing affinity and thus aims at perfect tolerance.

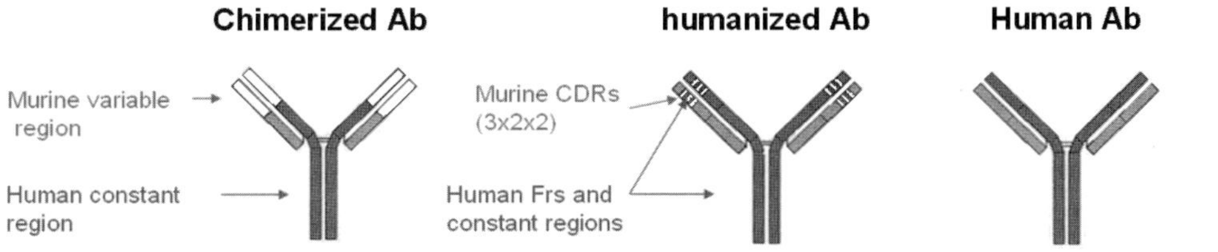

Murine	30%	10%	0%
Human	70%	90%	100%

Fig. 20.1. Recombinant antibody. Chimeric antibodies were obtained by grafting variable regions of murine monoclonal antibodies (in white) on human constant regions (in grey); the murine part still represents around 30% of the whole molecule. Only the hypervariable regions (10% of the whole molecule) of humanized antibodies have a murine origin (in white). Fully human antibodies are 100% of human origin (self drawn).

Recombinant Antibodies Directed Against Anthrax Toxins

Antibodies (Ab) neutralizing the lethal toxin of *B. anthracis* are likely to improve prevention and treatment of the anthrax disease. It has been shown in particular that such Ab synergize with antibiotherapy so that together, both types of molecules remain effective for several hours after infection, by blocking the induction of toxic shock (Mohamed *et al.*, 2005; Peterson *et al.*, 2006; Vitale *et al.*, 2006). Several recombinant anti-PA Ab, neutralizing the lethal toxin, have been developed in the USA for this purpose (Sawada-Hirai *et al.*, 2004; Albrecht *et al.*, 2007; Steiniger *et al.*, 2007).

Our team developed an anti-PA antibody neutralizing the lethal toxin of anthrax, by using the technology of immune libraries exposed to the surface of phages, constructed from an immunized non-human primate (*Macaca fascicularis*) (Laffly *et al.*, 2005). A Fab Ab fragment, called $35PA_{83}$, with high affinity for PA (3.4 nM) and which effectively neutralizes the lethal toxin (IC_{50} = 5.6 nM, in the standardized neutralization test) was obtained (patent FR0706744). The $35PA_{83}$ antibody was engineered in its hypervariable regions and in its framework regions, and it was expressed in the form of whole IgG so as to be tested *in vivo*.

The hypervariable regions of $35PA_{83}$ are directly involved in the interaction with the antigen. They have been mutated so as to increase the affinity of the Fab with PA by a factor of 20, and to improve the neutralization capacity (Laffly *et al.*, 2008). In the standardized neutralization test, this improvement of affinity results in a 40% decrease of the IC_{50} compared with the parental Fab.

The framework regions maintain the three-dimensional structure of the hypervariable regions. They are much less mutated, during affinity maturation, than the hypervariable regions and are considered to be directly involved in antibody tolerance. The framework regions of $35PA_{83}$ (178 amino acids in total) have 22 amino acids different from the human framework regions, encoded by the closest (unmutated) germline genes and retrieved using the IMGT/VQUEST tool (Brochet *et al.*, 2008). We have called the percentage of identity between the FRs of any immunoglobulin, and the most similar FRs encoded by human, germinal V(D)J genes the 'germinality index' (GI) (Pelat *et al.*, 2008). For $35PA_{83}$, the GI is 87.6%, lower than the mean GI of human IgGs (95%). These differences may correspond to differences between the human and the non-human primate NHP species, or to mutations introduced during the affinity maturation of the NHP antibody, but the origin of these differences is of no practical importance because both types of differences are possibly immunogenic and should be suppressed. We have engineered the Fab $35PA_{83}$ by mutating macaque residues into their human counterpart, encoded by the closest human germline genes. Thanks to this 'superhumanization' work, this number was reduced from 22 to 4, without impairing the affinity of the Fab. These four last unmutated macaque residues were showed to be so scattered at the surface of the Ab that they could not form a B epitope, at risk of being immunogenic in humans. Thus, 97.7% of the framework regions of the germinalized variant are encoded by human germline genes, a result that can be regarded as predicting an excellent tolerance (Pelat *et al.*, 2008). This putative tolerance was then evaluated positively with the G-score predictive tool, which compares the sequences of an IgG with a pool of expressed IgG (Thullier *et al.*, 2010). Interestingly, the GI of the superhumanized variant of $35PA_{83}$ was superior to the GI of a fully human antibody, having similar affinity and neutralization properties (Wild *et al.*, 2003). IMGT Colliers de Perles of the VH and VK domains of the Fab 35PA83 superhumanized variant are presented in Fig. 20.2.

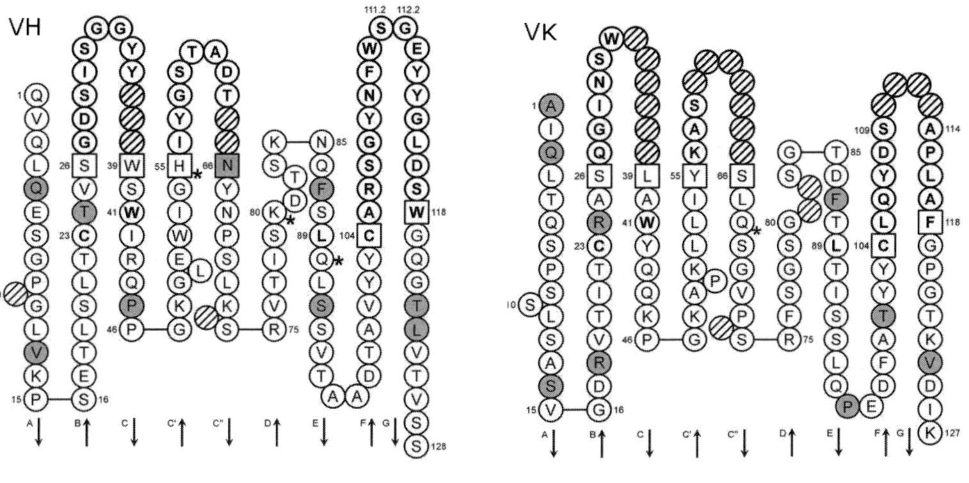

Fig. 20.2. IMGT Colliers de Perles of the VH and VK domains of the Fab $35PA_{83}$ superhumanized variant. IMGT Colliers de Perles representations are displayed according to the IMGT unique numbering (Lefranc *et al.*, 2003). The macaque residues which have been mutated into their human germline counterparts are shown in grey, and the four unmutated macaque residues are indicated by an asterisk (*). The CDRs (in bold) are limited by amino acids shown in squares (anchor positions).

In parallel, the full-sized IgG deriving from $35PA_{83}$ was obtained through an industrial collaboration (Laboratoire Français de Fractionnement et des Biotechnologies, Les Ulis). We tested it in the model of anthrax caused by intraperitoneal infection of A/J mice by the Sterne strain of *B. anthracis* (Flick-Smith *et al.*, 2005; Harvill *et al.*, 2005). We showed that $35PA_{83}$ IgG can improve the management of anthrax in both the clinical situations initially envisaged:

- When antibiotic prophylaxis using doxycycline was performed for only 7 days after exposure to anthrax, the mice died soon after this treatment was stopped. When the $35PA_{83}$ IgG was added to the antibiotic prophylaxis on the seventh and final day, all the mice survived.
- When a treatment using ciprofloxacin alone was started 12 or 24 h after exposure to anthrax, no animal survived. When $35PA_{83}$ IgG was added to ciprofloxacin, 80% of the animals survived if the combined treatment was given at the 12th hour.

These results are currently being confirmed in other models of experimental infection, especially after nasal instillation of spores of a lethal strain of anthrax (9602) in rabbits. Clinical development of this antibody is envisioned.

In accordance with the anthrax experts' recommendations, an antibody directed against LF was obtained (Pelat *et al.*, 2007). It aims at preventing any risk of the lethal toxin escaping the anti-PA antibody, by natural or induced mutation. Synergies with the anti-PA will be sought, because such synergies between anti-PA and anti-LF have already been observed (Brossier *et al.*, 2004). Engineering of this anti-LF antibody is underway, according to the same method as that for the anti-PA.

Conclusion

The isolation of anti-anthrax antibodies is an example of the search for anti-biowarfare antibodies, which is an active field of research. For instance, a team has recently shown the advantage of antibodies directed against the light chain of botulinum toxin A (BoNTA/L) for the neutralization of this toxin (Cheng *et al.*, 2009). We participated in this field by isolating a ricin-neutralizing antibody (Pelat *et al.*, 2009) and, thanks to European funding, we are currently looking for antibodies that neutralize botulinum toxins (www.antibotabe.com). Antibodies directed against other agents posing an intentional threat, such as pox viruses or the viruses of haemorrhagic fevers and forms of encephalitis, could also be eventually developed. In the highly competitive market of anti-infective drugs, the search for antibodies is developing rapidly: for example, an anti-CCR5 allows viraemia to be reduced in patients suffering from AIDS; an anti-West Nile antibody has been produced; antibodies directed against the secretion systems that ensure the virulence of bacteria such as *Pseudomonas aeruginosa* and *Yersinia pestis* (Hill *et al.*, 2006); anti-influenza antibodies, which would generally be used in the form of oligoclonal associations of antibodies to counter the mutations of the virus. Our strategy to obtain NHP antibody fragments of high affinity and high protective potency, which may later be superhumanized, is effective to isolate potential therapeutic molecules against biological warfare agents and might be of more general interest.

References

Albrecht, M.T., Li, H., Williamson, E.D., LeButt, C.S., Flick-Smith, H.C., Quinn, C.P., Westra, H., Galloway, D., Mateczun, A., Goldman, S. *et al.* (2007) Human monoclonal antibodies against anthrax lethal factor and protective antigen act independently to protect against *Bacillus anthracis* infection and enhance endogenous immunity to anthrax. *Infection Immunity* 75, 5425–5433.

Baggett, H.C., Rhodes, J.C., Fridkin, S.K., Quinn, C.P., Hageman, J.C., Friedman, C.R., Dykewicz, C.A., Semenova, V.A., Romero-Steiner, S., Elie, C.M. *et al.* (2005) No evidence of a mild form of inhalational *Bacillus anthracis* infection during a bioterrorism-related inhalational anthrax outbreak in Washington, D.C., in 2001. *Clinical Infectious Diseases* 41, 991–997.

Brochet, X., Lefranc, M.P. and Giudicelli, V. (2008) IMGT/V-QUEST: the highly customized and integrated system for IG and TR standardized V-J and V-D-J sequence analysis. *Nucleic Acids Research* 36, W503–W508.

Brossier, F., Levy, M., Landier, A., Lafaye, P. and Mock, M. (2004) Functional analysis of *Bacillus anthracis* protective antigen by using neutralizing monoclonal antibodies. *Infection Immunity* 72, 6313–6317.

Candela, T. and Fouet, A. (2005) *Bacillus anthracis* CapD, belonging to the gamma-glutamyltranspeptidase family, is required for the covalent anchoring of capsule to peptidoglycan. *Molecular Microbiology* 57, 717–726.

Cheng, L.W., Stanker, L.H., Henderson, T.D., 2nd, Lou, J. and Marks, J.D. (2009) Antibody protection against botulinum neurotoxin intoxication in mice. *Infection Immunity* 77, 4305–4313.

Duesbery, N.S., Webb, C.P., Leppla, S.H., Gordon, V.M., Klimpel, K.R., Copeland, T.D., Ahn, N.G., Oskarsson, M.K., Fukasawa, K., Paull, K.D. *et al.* (1998) Proteolytic inactivation of MAP-kinase-kinase by anthrax lethal factor. *Science* 280, 734–737.

Flick-Smith, H.C., Waters, E.L., Walker, N.J., Miller, J., Stagg, A.J., Green, M. and Williamson, E.D. (2005) Mouse model characterisation for anthrax vaccine development: comparison of one inbred and one outbred mouse strain. *Microbial Pathogenesis* 38, 33–40.

Harvill, E.T., Lee, G., Grippe, V.K. and Merkel, T.J. (2005) Complement depletion renders C57BL/6 mice sensitive to the *Bacillus anthracis* Sterne strain. *Infection Immunity* 73, 4420–4422.

Hill, J., Eyles, J.E., Elvin, S.J., Healey, G.D., Lukaszewski, R.A. and Titball, R.W. (2006) Administration of antibody to the lung protects mice against pneumonic plague. *Infection Immunity* 74, 3068–3070.

Holty, J.E., Bravata, D.M., Liu, H., Olshen, R.A., McDonald, K.M. and Owens, D.K. (2006) Systematic review: a century of inhalational anthrax cases from 1900 to 2005. *Annals Internal Medicine* 144, 270–280.

Inglesby, T.V., O'Toole, T., Henderson, D.A., Bartlett, J.G., Ascher, M.S., Eitzen, E., Friedlander, A.M., Gerberding, J., Hauer, J., Hughes, J. *et al.* (2002) Anthrax as a biological weapon, 2002: updated recommendations for management. *Journal of the American Medical Association* 287, 2236–2252.

Jernigan, J.A., Stephens, D.S., Ashford, D.A., Omenaca, C., Topiel, M.S., Galbraith, M., Tapper, M., Fisk, T.L., Zaki, S., Popovic, T. *et al.* (2001) Bioterrorism-related inhalational anthrax: the first 10 cases reported in the United States. *Emerging Infectious Diseases* 7, 933–944.

Laffly, E., Danjou, L., Condemine, F., Vidal, D., Drouet, E., Lefranc, M.P., Bottex, C. and Thullier, P. (2005) Selection of a macaque Fab with framework regions like those in humans, high affinity, and ability to neutralize the protective antigen (PA) of *Bacillus anthracis* by binding to the segment of PA between residues 686 and 694. *Antimicrobial Agents Chemotherapy* 49, 3414–3420.

Laffly, E., Pelat, T., Cedrone, F., Blesa, S., Bedouelle, H. and Thullier, P. (2008) Improvement of an antibody neutralizing the anthrax toxin by simultaneous mutagenesis of its six hypervariable loops. *Journal of Molecular Biology* 378, 1094–1103.

Lefranc, M.P., Pommie, C., Ruiz, M., Giudicelli, V., Foulquier, E., Truong, L., Thouvenin-Contet, V. and Lefranc, G. (2003) IMGT unique numbering for immunoglobulin and T cell receptor variable domains and Ig superfamily V-like domains. *Development Comparative Immunology* 27, 55–77.

Mock, M. and Fouet, A. (2001) Anthrax. *Annual Review of Microbiology* 55, 647–671.

Mohamed, N., Clagett, M., Li, J., Jones, S., Pincus, S., D'Alia, G., Nardone, L., Babin, M., Spitalny, G. and Casey, L. (2005) A high-affinity monoclonal antibody to anthrax protective antigen passively protects rabbits before and after aerosolized *Bacillus anthracis* spore challenge. *Infection Immunity* 73, 795–802.

Pelat, T., Hust, M., Laffly, E., Condemine, F., Bottex, C., Vidal, D., Lefranc, M.P., Dubel, S. and Thullier, P. (2007) High-affinity, human antibody-like antibody fragment (single-chain variable fragment) neutralizing the lethal factor (LF) of *Bacillus anthracis* by inhibiting protective antigen-LF complex formation. *Antimicrobial Agents Chemotherapy* 51, 2758–2764.

Pelat, T., Bedouelle, H., Rees, A.R., Crennell, S.J., Lefranc, M.P. and Thullier, P. (2008) Germline humanization of a non-human primate antibody that neutralizes the anthrax toxin, by in vitro and in silico engineering. *Journal of Molecular Biology* 384, 1400–1407.

Pelat, T., Hust, M., Hale, M., Lefranc, M.P., Dubel, S. and Thullier, P. (2009) Isolation of a human-like antibody fragment (scFv) that neutralizes ricin biological activity. *BMC Biotechnology* 9, 60.

Peterson, J.W., Comer, J.E., Noffsinger, D.M., Wenglikowski, A., Walberg, K.G., Chatuev, B.M., Chopra, A.K., Stanberry, L.R., Kang, A.S., Scholz, W.W. *et al.* (2006) Human monoclonal anti-protective antigen antibody completely protects rabbits and is synergistic with ciprofloxacin in protecting mice and guinea pigs against inhalation Anthrax. *Infection Immunity* 74, 1016–1024.

Reichert, J.M. (2011) Antibody-based therapeutics to watch in 2011. *MAbs* 3, 76–99.

Sawada-Hirai, R., Jiang, I., Wang, F., Sun, S.M., Nedellec, R., Ruther, P., Alvarez, A., Millis, D., Morrow, P.R. and Kang, A.S. (2004) Human anti-anthrax protective antigen neutralizing monoclonal antibodies derived from donors vaccinated with anthrax vaccine adsorbed. *Journal of Immune Based Therapy Vaccines* 2, 5.

Shen, Y., Zhukovskaya, N.L., Guo, Q., Florian, J. and Tang, W.J. (2005) Calcium-independent calmodulin binding and two-metal-ion catalytic mechanism of anthrax edema factor. *Embo Journal* 24, 929–941.

Steiniger, S.C., Altobell, L.J., 3rd, Zhou, B. and Janda, K.D. (2007) Selection of human antibodies against cell surface-associated oligomeric anthrax protective antigen. *Molecular Immunology* 44, 2749–2755.

Sylvestre, P., Couture-Tosi, E. and Mock, M. (2005) Contribution of ExsFA and ExsFB proteins to the localization of BclA on the spore surface and to the stability of the *Bacillus anthracis* exosporium. *Journal Bacteriology* 187, 5122–5128.

Thullier, P., Huish, O., Pelat, T. and Martin, A.C. (2010) The humanness of macaque antibody sequences. *Journal Molecular Biology* 396, 1439–1450.

Tournier, J.N., Quesnel-Hellmann, A., Mathieu, J., Montecucco, C., Tang, W.J., Mock, M., Vidal, D.R. and Goossens, P.L. (2005) Anthrax edema toxin cooperates with lethal toxin to impair cytokine secretion during infection of dendritic cells. *Journal of Immunology* 174, 4934–4941.

Turnbull, P.C. (2002) Introduction: anthrax history, disease and ecology. *Current Topics Microbiology Immunology* 271, 1–19.

Vitale, L., Blanset, D., Lowy, I., O'Neill, T., Goldstein, J., Little, S.F., Andrews, G.P., Dorough, G., Taylor, R.K. and Keler, T. (2006) Prophylaxis and therapy of inhalational anthrax by a novel monoclonal antibody to protective antigen that mimics vaccine-induced immunity. *Infection Immunity* 74, 5840–5847.

Wild, M.A., Xin, H., Maruyama, T., Nolan, M.J., Calveley, P.M., Malone, J.D., Wallace, M.R. and Bowdish, K.S. (2003) Human antibodies from immunized donors are protective against anthrax toxin *in vivo*. *Nature Biotechnology* 21, 1305–1306.

Chapter 21

Medical Support in the Case of Chemical and Biological Incidents

Kamen Kanev, Christophor Dishovsky and Stoian Tonev

Introduction

Medical support of the population is a complex of interrelated organizational, medical-evacuation, hygienic and anti-epidemic activities. In the case of emergency situations (ES) it is based on the existing healthcare system and an organized approach is required to adapt to a new mode of work with the available personnel and material-technical base. Medical support in disasters and accidents has some common characteristics including simultaneous occurrence of mass casualties and a large percentage of medical losses, discrepancy between acute need for medical forces and lack of means for carrying out triage and providing medical care, insufficient number of hospital beds for injured patients, insufficient sanitary transport for evacuation, an aggravated medical situation in the case of patients contaminated by dangerous substances and secondary injuries of the casualties and medical staff. Regardless of these common characteristics, the medical support required in cases of chemical and biological accidents should be distinguished from that required in other types of accidents.

Chemical Incidents

The past century, especially the second half, has been characterized by rapid development of the chemical industry, in particular the synthesis of new chemical compounds. In industry, agriculture and households more than 10 million chemical compounds are used, 60,000 of which are produced in large quantities, and 500 are intermediate or final toxic substances dangerous to humans. Many of them have high toxicity and ability under certain conditions (during storage or accidents) to cause massive damage to humans and animals. Data from the United Nations Awareness and Preparedness for Emergencies at the Local Level (APELL), chemical accident database (information for about 300 major chemical accidents between 1970 and 1998) showed that:

- 38% of the accidents occurred with hydrocarbons (fuel gases, fuel liquids, oil or refined petroleum products);
- 15% explosive industrial chemicals;
- 8% chlorine;
- 6% ammonia;
- 6% industrial acids and bases;
- 3% pesticides and chemical intermediates;
- 21% polychlorinated biphenyls
- 5% unspecified chemicals and other.

Hydrocarbon production, storage, transportation and distribution facilities are at the top of the list of potential targets.

In Bulgaria there are over 300 companies, factories, businesses and warehouses that are potential sources of major industrial accidents. Accidents have occurred, for example, in Burgas (1973), Devnya (1974), Alen Mak – Plovdiv (1983) and Montana (1986). The causes of industrial accidents can be subjective and objective. The subjective include terrorism, war, design or construction faults, technological problems, or problems with equipment, transportation, storage and outdated equipment, as well as poorly qualified workers. Natural disasters can also lead to the occurrence of industrial accidents.

Definitions and characteristics

Highly toxic substances are chemicals or compounds used in industry and agriculture, which in accidents are released into the atmosphere or on to the surface of the ground, and can cause massive damage to people, animals and plants. They could also have a detrimental effect on the ecosystem. Highly toxic industrial substances with the potential to produce a zone of chemical contamination (ZCC) are: chlorine, ammonia, sulphur oxides, nitrogen oxides, phosgene, hydrogen cyanide, hydrochloric, sulphuric and nitric acid and their anhydrides, carbon monoxide, dioxins and others. Of those industrial toxic substances the most likely to produce ZCC are chlorine and ammonia. According to the 'Rules of the Organization and Procedure for Prevention and Liquidation of Consequences of Disasters and Catastrophes 1998', 'risk sites' (Tonev, 2008a) are those where highly flammable or explosive materials and substances are stored, or which are used for materials processing, manufacturing or transporting highly toxic, pathogenic or radioactive materials, or where activities are engaged in that pose a potential danger to workers, employees, the population and the environment. There are many risk sites. These include chemical plants, refineries, metallurgical and textile factories, etc. In the warehouses of many factories located near cities hundreds of tonnes of hazardous substances such as chlorine and ammonia are kept – some not in accordance with the regulations. Accidents and disasters in high-risk sites (hazardous chemical sites) are a common phenomenon these days.

Airtight containers, tankers and tanks in which toxic substances are transported are also considered to be risk sites. Toxic substances may be in gaseous, liquid or solid form. Dispersal of gaseous toxic substances in an accident leads to rapid contamination of the air. In the case of spillage of liquid toxic substances on surfaces (ground, concrete or other coatings) they begin to evaporate with a rate that is determined by the volatility of the substance (its ability to transfer into gas) and meteorological conditions (air temperature, wind speed, etc.) at the time of accident. The speed of evaporation of toxic substances can significantly increase in the case of a fire. In the case of explosions solids and liquids are dispersed in the air, forming aerosols – solid form (smoke) and liquid (cloud). In assessing the hazard risk of highly toxic chemicals their physicochemical properties mainly determine their toxic effect: the relative density of their vapour, their stability, solubility and speed of their impact action.

Relative vapour density

If the vapour density of any substance is less than 1, it is lighter than air and quickly disperses. High hazard industrial chemicals are those that have a relative vapour density more than 1 as they are retained longer on the earth's surface, accumulate in different places and their impact on humans is more prolonged. Stable chemicals are those with a boiling temperature of more than 130°C. Unstable ones are those with boiling temperature of less than 130°C. Unstable chemicals remain in the area for minutes to tens of minutes. The impact of the stable ones persists for several hours to several weeks and months.

Solubility

The solubility of highly toxic substances greatly determines their ability to penetrate the body and their distribution in various tissues. In addition, solubility is important for the ability of these substances to enter into water reservoirs.

Speed of development of impact effect

Toxic industrial chemicals (TICs) are divided into two categories, fast acting and slow acting. Following impact with slow-acting TICs, the clinical picture of intoxication develops quickly within tens of seconds to 10 min. In contrast, with a slow-acting TIC, symptoms develop after a latent period of several hours up to 10–12 h.

All toxic substances contaminating the air enter the body through the respiratory system (inhalation route). Most of them can also cause intoxication by penetrating through unprotected skin surfaces (percutaneous route) and also through the mouth (oral route) via contaminated food and water. In an accident at a risk site inhalation intoxication is probably the most common. The actions of toxic substances on the body are very diverse. This is for many reasons, the main of which are: the structure, physicochemical and toxic characteristics of the toxin, its quantity, the biological characteristics of the affected organism and external factors at the time of impact of the agent. There is a close relationship between chemical structure and the biological activity of the toxic substance. For example, toxic compounds with similar molecular structures ultimately present with the same or a similar clinical picture of intoxication.

Characteristics of TICs

Highly toxic substances have the following characteristics:

- They are easily taken by the wind and can contaminate large areas.
- Quantities of TIC-contaminated air can penetrate into non-sealed areas and intoxicate people located there.
- The wide variety of highly toxic compounds excludes the possibility of producing a universal gas mask.
- Most of the highly toxic substances cause intoxication as a result not only of their direct effect on humans, but also through contaminated water, food and surroundings.

Classifications of highly toxic industrial substances

Depending on the characteristics of toxic effects on the body and the leading syndromes, highly toxic substances are divided into the following six groups:

1. Highly toxic substances with an asphyxiating effect.

   - With a strong asphyxiating effect (chlorine, etc.).
   - With a weak asphyxiating effect (phosgene, sulphur chloride, etc.).

2. Highly toxic substances with a general toxic effect.

   - Blood poisons (hydrogen arsenide, carbon monoxide, sulphur dioxide).
   - Tissue poison (cyanide, dinitrophenol, etilenchlorhidrin).

3. Highly toxic substances with asphyxiating and general toxic effect.

   - With a strong asphyxiating effect (acrylonitrile, nitric acid).
   - With a weak asphyxiating effect (sulphur dioxide, nitrogen oxide, hydrogen sulphide, etc.).

4. Neurotoxic poisonous substances (organophosphorus compounds, hydrogen sulphide, tetraethyl lead, etc.).

5. Highly toxic substances with neurotoxic and asphyxiating effect (ammonia, hydrazine, etc.).

6. Metabolic poisons.

   - With alkylating effect (methyl bromide, ethylene oxide).
   - With influence on the metabolism (dioxins and furan).

In Bulgaria for practical purposes the classification of TICs shown in Table 21.1 is used.

Table 21.1. Classification of TICs. (Adapted from Tonev, 2008b.)

Indicators	Extremely toxic	Highly toxic	Toxic	Less toxic
	Class 1	Class 2	Class 3	Class 4
Maximum permitted concentration in the air at work place (mg/m^3)	<0.1	0.1–1.0	1.1–1.0	>10
LD_{50} oral exposure (mg/kg)	<15	15–150	151–5,000	>5,000
LD_{50} dermal exposure (mg/kg)	<100	100–500	501–2,500	>2,500
LC_{50} inhalation (mg/m^3)	<500	50–5,000	5,001–50,000	>50,000

Types of industrial accidents

Depending on the scale (size) of the territory, industrial accidents are categorized as:

1. Local accident with air contamination. These are accidents that affect only a single section of the production and contaminate air with TICs. These accidents are accompanied by leakage of small amounts of TICs from gas transportation equipment (pipe, equipment, vessels), which can easily be repaired. They affect only some individuals and there is no need for the plant to stop production.

2. Aerial accident contamination of air. In these accidents, TICs are released in large amounts. They produce a high level of contamination that spreads to the work unit, but there is no danger of contamination of the entire site. Production is partially or temporarily suspended.

3. Major industrial accidents with air contamination. These industrial accidents lead to sudden cessation of production and cause human casualties, losses of infrastructure and equipment, as well as contamination of the air not within the factory but also outside it. These accidents are often accompanied by explosions, fires and dispersion of large amounts of TICs. Large ZCCs are produced, resulting in the formation of toxic clouds spreading miles away, which cause many casualties and contamination of livestock and plants.

Major industrial accidents with contamination of air can be divided into two groups:

- Major industrial accidents that cause contamination of air with TICs over large areas.
- Major industrial accidents, accompanied by explosions, fires, destruction and contamination of large areas.

The second group of major industrial accidents are the most dangerous. In addition to the large number of casualties there is destruction of property, and in some cases, whole plants. This type of accident is also the most common because most TICs form explosive mixtures with air.

Organization of medical support

The organization of medical support is a part of the overall organization of the relief operations. Training of medical personnel is essential as well as their interaction with other professionals. The principles of organization of medical care for those intoxicated with highly toxic substances in the zone of mass destruction are determined by the medical and tactical situation. This depends on the characteristics of the toxic substance, the characteristics of the zone of impact and the specificity of the situation.

When organizing medical support the following should be taken into account:

- The high level of contamination of the environment;
- The possibility of highly toxic substances entering the body through inhalation and in some cases through the skin;
- Mass casualties with acute intoxication;
- Combined and multiple injuries;
- Difficulties in carrying out complete emergency detoxication activities;
- Negative moral and psychological impact of the disaster;
- Possible occurrence of adverse epidemiological situation;
- Difficulties in management of the relief activities in the zone.

Characteristics of medical support

The organization of medical support in the case of mass casualties intoxicated with TICs has the following basic features:

- The need to conduct activities related to chemical protection in the ZCC;
- The need for providing first medical aid fast (no more than 30 min from the time of zone formation) and quick evacuation from the area of impact;
- The need for decontamination of all people contaminated with stable TICs;
- It is essential that the first medical aid is provided as close as possible to the ZCC (no more than 1 h away from its formation);
- The need to provide quickly qualified and specialized medical aid (not more than 2 h from the time of formation of the ZCC).

These characteristics and practical experience show that crucial to the effective medical care is immediate ‘on the spot’ treatment. Although this is the oldest system of medical support, in chemical accidents this model can provide help to a maximum number of the intoxicated as with some TICs the intoxication is very fast (from seconds to 10 min). The essence of this system lies in the provision of the fastest possible first aid as close to the zone as possible. In general the system for 'on the spot' treatment in the occurrence of a ZCC includes the following.

First medical aid

This depends on the current situation and the qualifications of the rescuers. It could be extended from first aid to first medical aid. The volume of first medical aid depends on the type of the toxic substance, but generally and chronologically the on-going activities are the following:

1. Active search for the casualties;
2. Interruption of the contact with the poison (donning a gas mask);
3. Antidote administration;
4. Partial decontamination;
5. Maintaining basic life processes (breathing, blood circulation);
6. Triage and removal of the casualties on a stretcher.

The first medical aid provided in the disaster zone is in the form of self and buddy aid. It is also provided by the emergency rescue teams, units from Civil Protection and medical personnel from unaffected health centres. The teams that will enter the zone should be equipped with personal protection. Artificial breathing apparatus is provided outside the borders of the zone, and if provided within, it can be used only if there is the technical means to enable it to be used safely – the 'mask to mask method'. Owing to the risk of developing pulmonary oedema in intoxication with chlorine, ammonia, phosgene and other TICs, the use of artificial breathing apparatus is contraindicated.

Casualties of asphyxiating substances should not leave the area on foot in case of chemical damage to the lung tissue and due to the risk of developing pulmonary oedema (Tonev, 2008a).

Behaviour and activities of the residents after accidents with TICs

The behaviour and activities of residents depend on the concentration, type and characteristics of the TICs, weather conditions, etc. Staff and residents living near industrial facilities need to be acquainted with the characteristics, properties and hazards from the TICs that are used there, the opportunities for personal protection and how to provide first medical aid to the contaminated.

In the event of an accident with the release of highly toxic substances, once the alarm has been raised (via radio, TV or loudhailers), the population living near a hazardous chemical plant should put gas masks on. They should close the windows, and get out of the house quickly and without panic in the specified direction or in a cross-wind direction. If possible, they should stay on higher ground at a distance not less than 5 km from the centre of the gas release (for NH_3, and 2–10 km for Cl) until further instructions.

In the absence of a gas mask, gauze or handkerchiefs soaked with water and vinegar (in the case of accidents with ammonia and alkali vapours and gases), water and baking soda (for accidents with chlorine and acid vapours and gases), or with water only may be used to protect the respiratory system. When moving in a contaminated area it is necessary to observe strictly the following rules:

- Move quickly, without running or raising dust;
- Do not hide behind buildings or touch surrounding objects;
- Do not step on liquids or powders of unknown origin;
- Do not take off personal protective equipment (PPE) until ordered;
- If there are drops on the skin, clothing, footwear or PPE they should be removed with swabs;
- If possible, provide medical aid to the casualties.

After leaving the ZCC a decontamination procedure is a must. All the people (population, medical personnel, emergency rescue groups, etc.) who were in the ZCC must be hospitalized and monitored for 24 h, regardless of their general condition.

Those who are contaminated must go to the medical establishments for treatment. It is therefore necessary to conduct targeted training for medical personnel and to provide specific support for the required minimum (from the expected aetiopathogenetic factor) antidotes and medical devices at the healthcare facilities in and around the potentially hazardous sites. In all cases, entry to residential premises, industrial buildings and warehouses in the territory of the ZCC should be allowed only after sanitary control of the air. In the general complex of measures to combat large-scale industrial accidents, measures for preventive protection are essential. This requires a risk assessment of the potentially hazardous chemical sites to ensure flawless operation as well as consequence mitigation in the ZCC (Tonev, 2008a).

Chemical Weapons

Chemical weapons could be used as a terrorist act or could provoke accidents in peace time in their production, transfer or destruction. Medical treatment of accidents involving chemical weapons is described separately because of the existence of important specific characteristics.

Definitions, basic concepts and classification of chemical weapons

According to the Convention on the Prohibition of the Development, Production, Stockpiling and Use of Chemical Weapons and on their Destruction Article 2 (1): ‘chemical weapons’ can be defined as the following, together or separately:

> (a) toxic chemicals and their precursors except those intended for purposes not prohibited under this Convention as far as the types and quantities are consistent with such purposes; (b) munitions and devices specifically designed to cause death or other harm through toxic properties of toxic chemicals specified in subparagraph (a) which are released as a result of the use of such a device; (c) any equipment specifically designed for use directly or indirectly, in connection with such munitions or devices specified in subparagraph (b).

In military circles the following definition is accepted: 'chemical weapons' (CWs) are weapons employing different chemicals and methods for their use for military purposes. In most cases, the term chemical weapons refers only to chemical warfare agents (CWAs), as they involve highly toxic chemicals with physicochemical properties allowing them to inflict high numbers of casualties and/or destroy living organisms, to contaminate the environment, food, water and technical facilities, and render their use impossible for a long time.

Classification

Depending on their physicochemical properties and tactical characteristics, destructive effects, methods and storage, transport and dispersion, different authors classify CW agents differently, but the most widely used classification is the following:

1. Lethal agents

1.1. Nerve agents

- Tabun (GA)
- Sarin (GB)*
- Soman (GF)
- V-gas (VX)

1.2 Blister agents

- Mustards: distilled mustard (HD), technical grade (H), Distilled and oxygen mustard (HT), Nitrogen mustard (HN3)
- Lewisite (L)
- Phosgene oxime (CX)

1.3. Choking agents

- Chlorine (Cl)
- Phosgene (CG)
- Diphosgene (DP)

1.4. Blood agents

- Hydrogen cyanide (AC)
- Cyanogen chloride (CK)

2. Incapacitating agents

2.1. Psychotomimetics

- BZ
- LSD

2.2. Irritants

2.2.1. Tear gas (lacrimators)

- Chloroacetophenone (NC)
- Brombenzylcyanide (CA)
- CS
- CR

2.2.2. Sneezing (sternites)

- Adamsite (DM)
- Diphenylchlorarsine (DA)
- Diphenylcyanarsine

3. Slow acting (phytotoxins)

- Agent orange (2,4,5 T)
- Agent white (4:1 mixture 2,4, –D and Picloram)
- Agent blue $(CH_3)_2AsO.\cdot OH$.

From a tactical perspective, CWAS are classified into two main groups:

- Stable (nerve agents: soman, VX; skin agents: psychomimetics and irritants);
- Unstable (nerve agents: sarin, generally toxic and asphyxiating).

Stability of CWAs is defined as the duration of retention of their toxic effect after use. It depends on the physicochemical parameters of the specific CWA, and the meteorological conditions and geography of the area at the time of the attack with the CWA.

Organization of medical care in an area of chemical contamination (ACC)

In the organization of medical care the following circumstances should be taken into account:

- Most of the CWAs are able to intoxicate via every possible entry route.
- The environment will be contaminated and medical teams will have to work with protective suits on.
- There will be mass casualties with severe symptoms of poisoning and possible combined injury.
- Various decontamination procedures will need to be observed for both victims and assistance teams.
- There is a need for rapid evacuation of a large number of people, in most cases severely injured, to a medical facility for qualified medical aid.
- There will be problems with leadership because of the negative psychological impact of the CWA, sometimes to the extent of a loss of control.

Each one of the military or civilian personnel must be equipped with individual technical and medical means for protection, and be trained to use them.

Military gas masks and skin protective suits (protective clothing, gloves and socks) are used for prevention. Medical protection consists of Pyridostigmin tablets (30 mg) administered orally, 3 × 1 tablet daily if there is a threat of nerve agent attack (good protection is achieved 2 h after taking the first tablet, but at the occurrence of the first symptoms of poisoning intake should be terminated immediately – danger of synergism. No medical prevention has been found yet for the rest of the CWAs.

First aid

The signs of intoxication with CWAs are presented in Table 21.2.

Table 21.2. Signs of intoxications with CWA. (Adapted from USAMRICD, 2000.)

Agents	Signs	Symptoms	Beginning	Diagnosis and differential diagnosis
Nerve: Sarin (GB) Tabun (GA) Soman (GD) Cyclosarin (GF) VX Other phosphoro-organic substances (carbamates and pesticides)	Myosis Broncho-constriction Acute respiratory failure Hypersecretion Hypersalivation Diarrhoea Loss of memory Loss of consciousness	**Medium to serious:** Rhinorrhoea, shortness of breath, sweating, eye pain, blurred vision, muscular cramps and tremor **Serious:** To the above symptoms is added sudden loss of consciousness	**Aerosol:** Seconds to minutes **Liquid:** Minutes to hours	Clinical picture: Serum ChE **DD:** Carbamates Pesticides Cyanides Myasthenia gravis
Cyanides: Hydrogen cyanide (HCN) Cyanogen chloride	**Medium to serious:** Pink skin Increased blood oxygenation	**Medium to serious:** Headache, dizziness, vertigo, palpitations, eye irritation, nausea, vomiting, drowsiness,	Seconds to minutes	Clinical picture: Smell of bitter almonds Measuring cyanide blood level

	Metabolic acidosis Hypotension **Serious:** The above symptoms worsening; coma and fits follow leading to cardiac respiratory failure	hyperventilation **Serious:** Immediate loss of consciousness, convulsions leading to death within 1–15 min		Thiocyanates in blood and urea **DD:** Nerve agents: CO, H_2S
Choking: Chlorine, Phosgene Diphosgene Nitrogen oxides Sulphur dioxide Chlorpicrin	Irritation of the airways ARDS Lung consolidation	Laryngospasm Rapid, snoring respiratory efforts Oppression in the chest Irritated skin and mucosa	1–24 h After exposure seldom 72 h Possible latent period of several hours	History Clinical picture **DD:** Non-toxic pulmonary oedema
Blistering: Mustards Lewisite Mixture of mustard and lewisite Phosgenoxim	Skin rash Severe conjunctivitis Irritation of the upper airway and pulmonary oedema Neutropenia	Rash on skin and mucosa, subjective feelings with some agents burning and itching Vomiting Difficulty breathing	Lewisite: Minutes Mustards: Hours to days	Smell of garlic, horseradish, mustard Clinical picture: Urine-thiodiglycol levels **DD:** Chemical burning with acids or bases

First aid is performed as self and buddy aid immediately by the troops within the ACC or by the first ones who enter it. This consists of (Tonev, 2003):

- Cleaning the face with a multipurpose decontamination solution from the personal medical kit.
- Donning a gas mask or replacing a faulty gas mask with a reliable one.

- Applying the antidote – autoinject the antidote with 'Combopen' for nerve agent poisoning, inhalation of amyl nitrite beneath the gas mask for cyanide poisoning and inhalation of anti-smoke mixture beneath the gas mask after contact with irritants.
- Partial decontamination of the exposed parts of the body with the multipurpose decontamination solution from the personal protective kit. If there is difficulty breathing, provide ventilation through masks, using the 'mask to mask' method.
- Evacuation outside the ACC (if there has been contact with a choking CWA, regardless of the confidence of the casualty the evacuation must be carried out in prone position on a stretcher!).

First aid outside the ACC is as follows (Tonev, 2003):

- Ensure rest and warmth of the casualty if necessary.
- Immobilization of the casualty if necessary.
- Respiratory resuscitation continues if the condition of the casualty requires it (in intoxication with choking agents the artificial breathing is contraindicated!).
- Control of symptoms of poisoning and if necessary reapplication of the antidote (combopen for nerve agents; amyl nitrite beneath the gas mask for cyanides; an ampoule with anti-smoke mixture beneath the gas masks for irritating agents).
- Full decontamination and change of clothing, the gas mask is removed last. Wash the eyes, nose and mouth with clean water or use an appropriate solution for CWA removal (2% solution of sodium bicarbonate for intoxication by choking and nerve agents, 0.2% chloramine, 0.05% potassium permanganate for eye flushing, 0.5% and 0.1% for other mucous membranes in impact with skin agents, with subsequent treatment of the eyes with 5–10% synthomycine ointment or unitol ointment, and in the case of an attack with lewisite, 3.5% dimercaprol ointment). Symptomatic treatment as necessary.

When the impact is with nerve agents:

- Full sanitary care if for some reason it has not been done before and if the status of the casualty allows it.
- Injecting of cholinolytics until improvement of the condition or atropinization (atropine in the common antidotal doses of im/iv according to the condition of the casualty).
- Injecting of cholinesterase reactivators or their extensive application if applied beforehand, with the dose depending on degree of intoxication (toxogonin/obidoxim, Ln H, 6/25% sol. amp 1 ml iv/s depending on the degree of intoxication; pralidoxim/2 PAM/1% sol. 50 ml for iv administration; Hi-6 in autoinjectors (toxidin, 200 mg, 10% sol. 2 ml, im/iv slow, Bulgarian ampoule form; Dishovsky, 2005).
- Other important measures: oxygen therapy, medications affecting the cardiovascular system, anticonvulsants, symptomatic drugs, etc.

The antidote activity of reactivators of cholinesterase activity is different against the different organophosphorus compounds (OPCs), which is why new antidotes continue to be investigated (Dishovsky, 1989). At the moment in Bulgaria there is a new complex antidote against OPCs called 'Lekatod' and a decontamination gel, 'Tolekatod' (Kanev, 2009).

When the impact is with blistering agents:

- On the skin – the affected skin areas are decontaminated and dressed with gauze soaked in 1–2% sol. monochloramin. Large blisters (bullae) are only treated in hospital!
- Gastrointestinal tract – immediately swallow an aqueous suspension of charcoal (25 g charcoal in 1000 ml water), followed by gastric lavage with 0.05% aqueous solution of potassium permanganate. It is necessary to cause multiple vomiting, so 400–500 ml of this solution needs to go into the stomach 10–20 times.
- Inhalation hazard – treat with recommended antibiotic, cardiovascular and oxygen therapy in a hospital.

When the impact is with blood agents:

- Antidote therapy (iv, 50 ml of a 25% sol. (12.5 g) of sodium thiosulphate over a 10-min period hydroxocobalamin (via injection);
- Artificial breathing and oxygen therapy;
- Respiratory and cardiovascular analeptics;
- Venesection 250–300 ml in cases of cyanogen chloride intoxication;
- Calcium gluconate in cases of pulmonary oedema/10% 10 ml in cases of cyanogen chloride intoxication;
- Atropine if pulse is slow, until normal pulse frequency is reached.

Intoxication with blood agents:

- Oxygen therapy with a 40–50% mixture of air and oxygen, prolonged with short breaks, or a helium–oxygen mixture, 30% He and 70% O_2, oxygen with pressure 3–6 cm H_2O.
- In grey hypoxia a good effect is obtained with carbogen, a mixture of oxygen and carbon dioxide, given briefly so as not to agitate the respiratory centre.
- Injection of 40% glucose.
- Artificial breathing must not be applied!

Qualified medical care is best accomplished in a hospital! All moderate and seriously affected casualties are best treated in specialized toxicology wards and other clinics to allow complete healing and final or partial restoration of health and performance. The medical care should include the following:

- Full decontamination if for some reason it was not carried out at one of the previous stages.
- Final revision of the initial treatment and detoxification activities.
- Continue the specific antidotal therapy or immediately begin therapy if it has not been done so far, according to the type of chemical agent and following the above regimens.

- Continuation of respiratory and cardiovascular resuscitation if necessary.
- Surgical treatment by a specialist in the case of combined injury.
- Adequate symptomatic therapy.
- Organization and conduct of rehabilitation and restoration procedures.
- Expertise on fitness for military service and return to duty or transfer to the reserve.

Organization of medical support in the case of terrorist acts with chemical weapons

The last instance of such an act was the sarin attack in the Tokyo subway in 1995. The main 'lesson' from this was that although the amounts used of the CWA were small, the social and medical authorities were unprepared and the consequences were serious! The reasons for this have proved to be mainly as follows (Tonev, 2008a):

- In a terrorist act the surprise factor is at the heart of the effect. Citizens are not supplied with personal protection equipment and are not trained to recognize the signs of an attack, nor have they mastered the basic algorithm of the behavioural reaction that reduces damage, as predominantly severe and lethal cases are expected.
- Usually civil healthcare is not well enough prepared to cope with the medical aid required for those affected by CWAs. It is possible that due to lack of protective equipment or unpreparedness for their use, there may be casualties among the medical staff.
- Urbanization, high population and building density and widespread use of air conditioning favour the dispersion of CWAs and increase the number of injuries to dimensions that are difficult to predict, which puts the health system in an extremely difficult position.
- Often panic confuses rescue and medical-evacuation events, and there can be problems with leadership.

Planning and preparation of anti-terrorist action should be focused on the following specific points (Dishovsky, 2004, 2006):

- Inventory and assessment of the available means for medical treatment of chemical intoxication. Assessment of the required amounts and types of antidotes (in view of the broader range of potentially toxic agents) and their update with the development and introduction of new compounds.
- Modernization and optimization of individual protection with a particular focus on respiratory protection and protective clothing.
- Creation of a new national pharmaceutical stockpile, which ensures the availability of medicines, antidotes, medical supplies and medical equipment necessary to counter the effects of biological pathogens and chemical agents.
- Creation of an effective system of information and supply to the area where a terrorist act has taken place.
- Assessment of the available means for indication and control of chemical contamination and the effectiveness of decontamination. This should consider the broader range of potentially toxic agents and the available state-of-the-art technologies.

- The preparation of all levels of civil institutions and the army to counteract chemical terrorism. This should incorporate and implement the latest developments in computer simulation and virtual reality technologies.
- Intensive education and training of first responders and physicians is needed to meet the medical challenges imposed by chemical and other weapons of terror.

To ensure a successful outcome it is necessary that all government institutions and departments are prepared, and the population educated and trained. Every citizen must be prepared, with minimal supplies of food and water in reliable packaging and some medicines, and, in case of the need to seal their homes, with useful tools. When in need he or she must be able to recognize the danger signals, to keep calm, to follow the instructions given by the competent authorities through the media without being susceptible to panic and fear.

In the case of CWA attack by terrorists the area is isolated by the police, and the hot, warm and cold zones are determined (Fig. 21.1), the population is alerted through the media and the evacuation of people at risk is organized.

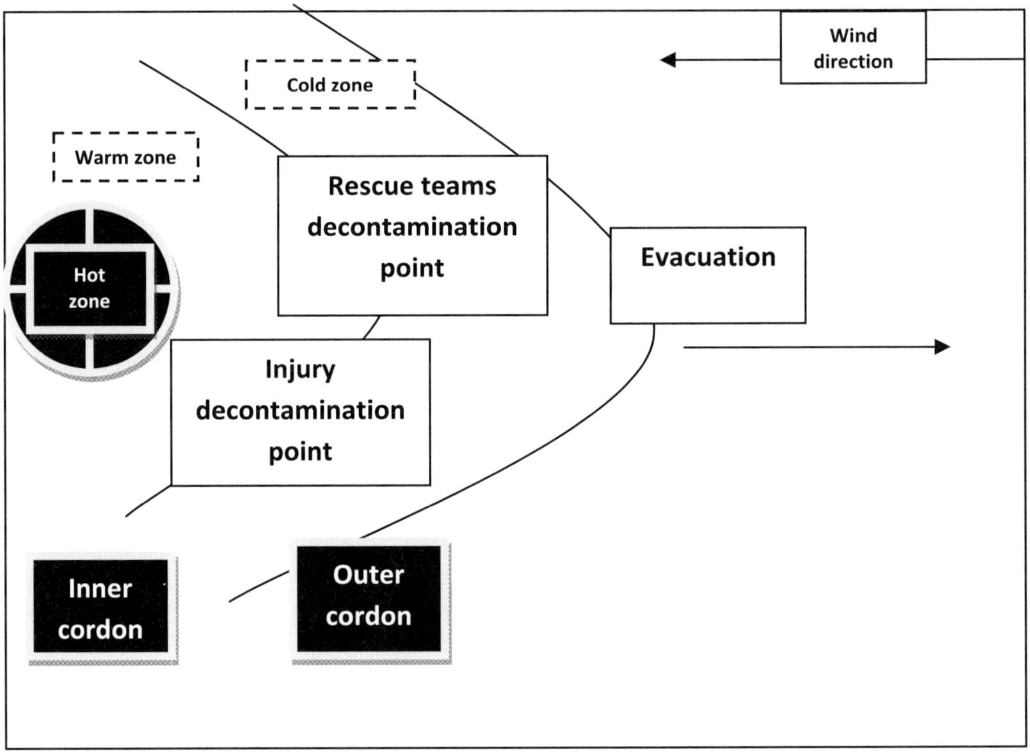

Fig. 21.1. ACC in CWA terrorist attack. (Adapted from Tonev, 2008b.)

When required, civil protection teams, equipped with a full set of personal protective equipment and supported by the fire and police services should move out the casualties, conduct decontamination and first therapeutic procedures. Rescue teams equipped with complete personal protective equipment should administer first aid and assist with evacuation to the nearest hospital outside the ACC where treatment should continue to enable final recovery or stabilization of the patient and transfer to a specialized clinic.

Biological Incidents

Biological weapons are bioagents and the means for their transmission and distribution (equipment or live vectors). The term bioagents includes microorganisms and/or their toxins that cause illness or death in humans, animals and plants and infect the environment. The number of bioagents that may be included in the arsenal of biological weapons is extremely high. Some have a naturally high strike effect (plague, botulism, cholera, etc.); for others virulence has been increased artificially.

According to the classification of the International Society of Disaster Medicine (Tonev, 2008a), bioagents can be grouped as follows:

- Group I (Class A)
  - *Bacillus anthracis* – anthrax;
  - *Clostridium botulinum* – toxin – botulism;
  - *Variola major* – smallpox;
  - *Fransiella tularensis* – tularaemia;
  - *Pasteurella pestis* – plague;
  - Viruses causing haemorrhagic fever – haemorrhagic fever.
- Group II (Class B)
  - *Coxiella burneti* – Q fever;
  - *Brucella* species – brucellosis;
  - *Burkholderia mallei*;
  - *Ricinus communis* – ricin intoxication;
  - *Clostridium perfringens* – Σ toxin;
  - *Staphylococcal enterotoxin* B – enterotoxin GI intoxication;
  - *Vibrio chollerae* – cholera
- **Group III (Class C)**
  - Nipah virus – Nipah virus infection;
  - Hantavirus – Hantavirus infections;
  - Viruses spread by ticks – haemorrhagic fever;
  - Viruses spread by ticks – encephalitis – tick encephalitis, yellow fever;
  - Multi-drug resistant tuberculosis.

Characteristics of biological weapons

Biological weapons include agents of infectious diseases and toxins, which are intended for intentional contamination of humans and animals. In its present form, a biological weapon has features different from those of other weapons of mass destruction and the causative agents of natural epidemics.

- Identification of biological agents is relatively slow and difficult (sampling, transportation in microbiology laboratories, culture). Moreover, exotic agents are difficult to diagnose if they are genetically modified.
- It is possible to differentially use bioagents on humans, animals or plants, and to vary the degree of injury.
- The effects of biological weapons begin after a certain incubation period (the shortest is in toxins), leading to a possibility of remote secondary outbreaks.
- Biological weapons have the ability to induce long-term illness requiring long treatment and care, which is determined by:
  - natural or artificially increased resistance in the environment;
  - some intrinsic ability to cause atypical course of the disease.
- Production of biological formulations is cheap and easy.
- They are easy to conceal, transport and spread.
- There is an unclear clinical picture at the time of infection with biological weapons.

Medical casualties in a biological outbreak

Medical casualties in an outbreak are those people who fall ill after a biological weapons attack. They are designated as primary casualties when the sickness caused is due to inhalation of contaminated air, intake of contaminated food and water and through vectors; and secondary casualties when the infection is transmitted from sick people.

The medical casualties have clinical symptoms or biochemical changes observed in the laboratory. However, all persons who were in the area during the dispersal of the biological agents are considered to be contaminated until the neutralization of the agent and specification of their health status. The number of medical casualties in the outbreak depends on the type of agent, the dose, the duration of exposure in the affected zone, the degree of protection and individual susceptibility, and can be 25–50% of the population. For estimation of the possible casualties it is important to have some information on the number of people living in the area. After assessment of the expected number of medical casualties we can estimate the number of medical teams and resources needed. Correct and reasonable decisions in terms of the organization of medical support in a mass epidemic situation can only be accomplished if there is extensive knowledge about the nature of bioagents, their characteristics, modes of emergence and development of the epidemic process (spontaneous or artificially induced).

Medical support in a disastrous epidemic situation comprises the organization and application of a number of measures for protecting people from infectious diseases and rapid eradication of epidemic outbreaks, occurring naturally or artificially after use of biological weapons. In general, the measures that are taken are not significantly different for both types of crisis situation. The experience of the healthcare system in the neutralization of spontaneous epidemics serves as a basis for planning and implementing measures after use of biological weapons.

Protective measures against biological weapons

Protection from biological weapons is a difficult and complex problem. There are two stages: protection preparedness and protection after the immediate impact of the biological weapons.

Protection preparedness is a continuous process and is accomplished in peaceful times. It is determined by the state of the country's economy, science, healthcare, etc. Protection preparedness requires general organizational and also some specific measures for the prevention of epidemics. Seeking knowledge of the special characteristics of biological weapons and methods for their use is also necessary.

In a military conflict and a classic attack the emphasis is on the use of protective equipment.

In a concealed attack or sabotage, the most important measures are to eliminate the consequences. In essence, these activities are complementary and are conducted in the following sequence:

- Determination of the biological weapons used by specialized facilities. This is based on direct and indirect evidence or aerosol formation after explosion, excessive amounts of rodents or insects, presence of containers, etc.
- Announcement of the on-going attack – this is done immediately, as soon as signals have been received from the civil protection authority or other institution.

As soon as possible personal and collective protection equipment should be used. Apart from that, improvised equipment in order to protect the airway and body could be used. Measures should be taken for further protection of food, drinking water, property, etc.

Hygiene and anti-epidemic measures in epidemiological disaster situations

In the event of infectious disease outbreak there is a real risk of the development of an epidemic. An epidemic is a process with three main elements: a source of infection, healthy contact persons and the external environment (within certain limits), where the infection circulates. Measures for epidemic disaster prevention are carried out in the following three directions.

Measures on the sources of contamination

- Early detection of possible sources of contamination. This is realized through active inquiry based on suspected signs and symptoms. Until the involvement of the specialized experts, this is a duty of doctors from all areas.
- Early clinical and aetiological diagnosis. In the first cases of disease a working diagnosis is made based on even scant clinical findings and epidemiological data. As soon as possible aetiological diagnosis should be made by the microbiological laboratory. Express testing methods are of great value given the huge importance of rapid response and targeted implementation of the disaster response plans.
- Isolation of infectious patients. Generally, isolation is carried out in cases of contagious infection and it has value when it is done as early as possible. To meet this requirement it is not necessary to have an aetiological diagnosis. It is done on the basis of clinical syndromes and the epidemiological situation. This isolation is a primary and a temporary measure and the patients must be hospitalized for definite isolation and specific treatment.
- Transportation of patients with infectious diseases. Usually this is done with sanitary transport, including sanitary trains or aircraft. In large-scale disasters

transport for general use could be used. In both cases, evacuation is carried out in conditions of isolation from other sick and wounded persons. Disinfection of vehicles is mandatory and it is done by the hospitals where the patients are admitted.

- Hospitalization and specific treatment. As a rule, this takes place in the nearest infectious hospital. If there are mass casualties, in many cases it is possible to convert public buildings or general medical wards into infectious therapeutic wards. In other types of disaster, hospitalization would be in different medical and surgical wards, according to the main injury. In these cases there is a risk of contracting secondary diseases due to in-hospital infections. In both cases infection control working practices should be introduced. Adequate and specific treatment is carried out when needed, depending on the aetiology, and considering the duration of isolation.
- Epidemiological investigation. This is a mandatory activity that starts with the consultations of the first patients. It should clarify the reasons and circumstances relating to the origins and evolution of the epidemic situation, its characteristics and prognosis, with a view to prompt and adequate measures for its eradication. For these reasons, an epidemiological study should not be one-act, but continuing and creative work that include different methods and stages.

Measures to trace the contact persons

- Tracing the contacts. This is a labour-intensive, responsible activity with two aspects: on the one hand to carry out some preventive measures; and on the other, to discover possible potential sources of infection (infected, healthy and contacts). Contact persons are registered and undergo medical observation, preferably isolated. Diagnosed carriers are admitted to infectious wards or units where they are isolated.
- Extreme prevention of contact. This applies to epidemics in general, particularly those developing with high dynamics or those leading to high mortality. It is used in individuals who are possibly infected to prevent the occurrence of an infectious process (infectious disease). In other words, they are treated in the incubation period. Usually, antibiotics or specific gamma-globulins are used.
- Specific prophylaxis of the contacts. Vaccine prophylaxis has little value in an epidemic situation because of the relatively slow formation of specific protection. However, some have some value, for example, the tetanus anatoxin and antibotulin anatoxin, especially when the patients have so-called background immunity. The use of vaccines would be appropriate in some infections with a long incubation period (e.g. rabies), and also to protect individuals indirectly at risk from those close to the outbreak.

Sanitary measures for the environment

- Additional hygienic measures should take place. In the background of the on-going preventive measures in different directions, in particular effort should be focused on sanitizing environmental factors associated with the emergence of epidemics, such as water, food and utility projects.

- Disinfection and pest control. These are measures carried out in the local area on epidemic indications. Their purpose, means and methods depend on the risk factors that contribute to the spread of the infection. When the role of insects and rodents in spreading the infection is clear, the necessary measures to control their populations should be taken. In the case of excessive workloads, formation of teams equipped with the necessary disinfection technology and tools may be needed.
- Prevention of the spread of infection outside the outbreak area. During the epidemic investigation the territory of the outbreak of the epidemic is determined and, depending on the type of infection, the period of time for which it could spread further. These are the most important criteria for the introduction of restrictive measures to prevent spread of infection outside the outbreak area.

Recovery operations

The use of biological weapons is a prerequisite for the artificial creation of an epidemic outbreak. It is expected that such an outbreak will possess specific characteristics and dynamics, which are more likely to lead to a serious epidemic. There is no particular difference in the approaches of the recovery operations for natural outbreaks and for outbreaks caused by biological contamination. To mitigate the consequences the events are conducted sequentially or in parallel fashion, in different orientation and with certain specificity.

- Defining the boundaries of the outbreak. That is necessary in order to specify all the details and objects which come under the impact. This determines the scope and orientation of the next counter-epidemic events.
- Sampling of contaminated sites. Samples from food, water, surfaces, insects, rodents, etc. are sent immediately to the appointed fixed or mobile microbiology laboratories for identification of the biological agent.
- Observation of the infected individuals. In this case the observation has a broader meaning. It is a collective form of isolation, which aims to prevent the spread of infection outside as well as the occurrence of infections among the contaminated. The observation takes place after the attack and includes limitation of entry and exit of the infected, except for those involved in the recovery operations.
- Sanitary procedures. A thorough sanitary procedure includes clothes decontamination, shower and chamber (chemical) disinfection (decontamination). If this not possible it is recommended that a partial procedure – brushing (using gas masks) and decontamination of the skin with a decontaminator – is carried out.
- Initiation of extra prophylaxis. As a rule a broad-spectrum antibiotic is administered (total extra prophylaxis), and when the antibiogram is available to carry out accordingly.
- Intensive medical supervision. This is carried out by medical workers to enable early detection.
- Hygiene control and health awareness. The aim is to prevent the consumption of contaminated food and drinking water and to avoid the risk of secondary infections.

Specific identification of the biological agent

The use of rapid laboratory methods is recommended, in order to obtain quick results giving information on the nature of the biological agent. The possible answers could be: toxin or non-contagious infection, contagious infection or agent of particularly hazardous infections. Based on this information the relevant measures are taken. In particularly dangerous infections or other rapidly spreading infections the observation is replaced with quarantine.

Quarantine of the area and the contaminated individuals

The measures taken during the observation period are adapted and further developed. The strictest quarantine regime needs to be introduced:

- It is absolutely prohibited for infected individuals to leave the contaminated area, for property to be moved without prior disinfection, and for people to enter the site other than those engaged in the recovery operations.
- Isolation of the contaminated area by armed guards should be introduced.
- The supply of goods, medicines and other resources should take place at preliminary planned areas at the border of the outbreak.
- In residential areas internal isolation should be carried out and restrictive measures for families, neighbourhoods, etc. should be introduced.
- Organization of the supply and implementation of prophylaxis for each residence.
- Medical surveillance. The quarantined patients should measure their temperature twice daily. When there is fever or other suspected symptoms medical staff should be notified.
- The ill are hospitalized in general or specialized hospitals/wards. Evacuation of infectious patients is not permitted.
- Quarantine is cancelled in accordance with accepted criteria and guidances for fighting communicable diseases.

Specific prophylaxis

Specific prophylaxis is done once the causative agent of the contagious disease is known. Initiation of treatment is mandatory for vulnerable populations, such as children, students, managers and health personnel, military personnel, etc.

Counter-epidemic measures

The diseased patients, who are directed to outpatient and hospital units, represent a potential contamination hazard (for medical personnel and other people). Generally this category of patients is admitted to infectious wards, which have routine practices for working with infections. The situation is more complicated when the infected, before or after onset of symptoms, receive another form of injury such as traumatic or somatic injuries that require hospitalization to non-infectious hospital units. In this case the danger of intra-hospital infections is even greater. In either case, the involved hospitals need to initiate counter-epidemic measures. These include isolation and movement restriction, therapeutic, preventive measures and decontamination procedures aimed to prevent the spread of the infection among the medical personnel, the patients and outside the hospital area.

Anti-epidemic procedures include: movement restriction, preventive and disinfecting measures aimed at preventing the spread of the infection among medical staff, the ill hospitalized and those outside the hospital.

Sanitary control

The infectious disease control authorities organize and conduct enhanced sanitary control on nutrition, water supply and essential goods. They also ensure strict compliance with established rules for observation and quarantine. Particular attention is paid to children and public establishments, shelters, transportation, etc.

Decontamination

Decontamination is performed by sanitizing and disinfecting units from the civil defence and infectious disease control authority teams. Generally, the criteria adopted to eliminate epidemic outbreaks are as follows:

- Elimination of the sources of infection.
- Final decontamination measures, lack of new cases from an infection within the maximum incubation period.

Any outbreak that is considered to be managed is the subject of epidemic monitoring. The duration of this observation depends primarily on the maximum incubation period of the disease. In infections with known carriers and an established role of insects and rodents, the period of epidemic control can not be fixed and a reasonable approach is needed.

The creation of an adequate organization of anti-epidemic efforts and resources to promptly and effectively neutralize the effects of the use of biological agents in a terrorist act is one of the main tasks of chief recovery managers. For this purpose in Bulgaria, three teams are formed, based at the Centre for Military Epidemiology and Hygiene (CMEH) in the Military Medical Academy (MMA) – Sofia (Tonev, 2008a; Kanev, 2009):

- The first team is a group that works in the epidemic outbreak zone and is dispatched in the alleged attack area.
- The second team is a diagnostic group, equipped with necessary laboratory and diagnostic supplies, which is ready to act immediately after the return of the first team.
- The third team is a recovery group, which is the last activated and enters the area after receiving the preliminary laboratory diagnosis.

The groups are assembled and act on an assigned territory with teams from CMEH – Sofia and the Preventive Medicine Boards in Plovdiv, Pleven, Varna and Sliven within the structure of the Ministry of Defence.

The first team performs the following tasks:

- Determination of the boundaries of the infected area;
- Sampling and sample transportation;
- Epidemiological survey;
- Analysing collected data;
- Preliminary epidemiological diagnosis;
- Provide analysed data to the crisis staff of the MMA.

The second team operates to:

- Make epidemiological diagnosis;
- Propose specific counter-epidemic and sanitary measures with respect to diet, water supply, accommodation, garbage transportation;
- Submit the analysed data to the crisis quarter of the MMA.

The third team will:

- Receive, record and process the submitted samples of food, water and wastewater, soil, air, vectors and specimens;
- Make a preliminary diagnosis for bacterial, viral and parasitic infections;
- Package and submit the suspected infectious materials and isolated strains to MMA for a definitive diagnosis.

The organization, the announcement, team management and the coordination for implementing the measures is accomplished by the Crisis Centre of MMA and the National Military Coordination Centre. During training and exercises, guidelines created in 2004 have repeatedly proved their role and importance for the implementation of the measures to mitigate the consequences of biological agent misuse. In specific situations, when needed, it is possible to use the NBC defence module of Military Medical Detachment for Emergency Response (MMDER) from MMA. It is appropriate to create a joint organization to achieve maximum efficiency and collaboration of the activities of specialized units within the Ministry of Defence, Ministry of Health and Ministry of State Policy for Disasters and Accidents in the Republic of Bulgaria.

Nowadays, the organization of healthcare of each country towards rapid and effective protection of biological weapons is a top priority due to the increased threat of terrorist attacks. The importance of knowledge about the nature of bioagents, the presenting symptoms and syndromes of infectious diseases, and the mechanism of outbreaks can not be overemphasized. Information about modes of transmission of communicable diseases, and basic knowledge of medical support in accidents will ensure the timely implementation of effective measures. The main purpose of these measures is to protect people and minimize health consequences after the use of biological weapons.

Conclusion

The organization of medical treatment in chemical and biological incidents is highly complex and requires a common state strategy against chemical and biological traumatism and terrorism. The most important principles of this strategy must include improvement of the national organizational and medical programmes with implementation of universal programmes for diagnosis and treatment, preparedness of medical facilities, well-organized stockpiles of antidotes and vaccines, and increased skills and training of all units included in medical treatment. Working social information systems and effective international collaboration are also very important points in this area.

References

Dishovsky, C. (1989) Contemporary antidote therapy of organophosphorus intoxications. MSc work, MMA, Sofia, Bulgaria (in Bulgarian).

Dishovsky, C. (2004) Problems of chemical and biological terrorism. In: Monov, A. and Dishovsky, C. (eds) *Medical Aspects of Chemical and Biological Terrorism and Traumatism.* Publishing House of Union of Scientists of Bulgaria, Sofia, Bulgaria, pp. 11–22.

Dishovsky, C. (2005) Some aspects of the mechanisms of action of oxime reactiors of cholinesterase. In: In: Monov, A. and Dishovsky, C. (ed.) *Medical Aspects of Chemical and Biological Terrorism and Traumatism.* Publishing House of Union of Scientists of Bulgaria, Sofia, Bulgaria, pp. 209–226.

Dishovsky, C. (2006) Problems of chemical terrorism and ways of its overcoming. In: Dishovsky, C., Pivovarov, A. and Benshop, H. (eds) *Medical Treatment of Intoxication and Decontamination of Chemical Agents in the Area of Terrorist Attack.* NATO Science Series, Springer, Dordrecht, the Netherlands, pp. 3–11.

Kanev, K. (2009) Medical support in case of chemical and biological threat. In: Tonev, S., Kanev, K. and Dishovsky, C. (eds) *Medical Management of Chemical and Biological Casualties.* MMA, Publishing House IRITA, Sofia, Bulgaria, pp. 34–39.

Tonev, S. (ed.) (2003) *First Aid Handbook.* MMA, Publishing House IRITA, Sofia, Bulgaria (in Bulgarian).

Tonev, S. (ed.) (2008a) *Terrorism, Valuation and Management of Medical Risk.* MMA, Publishing House IRITA, Sofia, Bulgaria, pp. 210–331 (in Bulgarian).

Tonev, S. (ed.) (2008b) *Medical Support in Crises.* MMA, Publishing House IRITA, Sofia, Bulgaria, pp. 149–182, 259–271 (in Bulgarian).

USAMRICD (2000) Field Managementof Chemical Casualties Handbook. Available at: https://www.rke.vaems.org/wvems/Libraryfiles/Dis/E_04.pdf (Accessed 6 February 2013).

Chapter 22

Gearing up Paraphernalia for the Management of CBRN Emergencies: A Multi-stakeholder Approach is the Need of the Hour

Rajesh Arora, Raman Chawla, Preeti Arora, Pallavi Thakur, Ayush Chowdhary, Rajeev Goel and Rakesh Sharma

Introduction

The term CBRN (chemical, biological, radiological and nuclear) emergencies has evolved from previous terms nuclear, biological and chemical (NBC) (Cold War era) and atomic, biological and chemical (ABC) (pre-Cold War era) due to the spectral changes in the definition and terminology of warfare. Today, in the present scenario, the economic wars and short-impact wars for capitalizing on energy resources are on the rise rather than conventional wars between two countries. However, the rogue states have initiated a new era of state-sponsored terrorism to resolve issues of conflict of interests. The advent of technology has further added value to such attacks. The earlier terms NBC/ABC were used in terms of probable use of the nuclear option by one country against another. However, the present situation is different as due to continuous dialogue between countries, multilateral trade, common resource-related economic investment issues, United Nations with their varied peace-keeping forces, international collaborative intelligence, extreme space exploration by various countries and awareness/closeness among world communities due to increased tourism, the usage of such options directly has been significantly reduced. On the other hand, the rise of chemical warfare agents (CWAs), availability of precursors as dual chemicals for pesticides and other industries, an exponential increase in knowledge of gene play and recombinants has placed 'Chemical' and 'Biological' in the forefront of probability of usage as a part of a possible terrorist attack (Grace *et al.*, 2007).

In the case of terrorism to achieve immediate attention, chemical (a category of explosives only) attacks remain the weapons of choice for inflicting widespread impact, while to cause extensive damage by a state-sponsored agency particularly on the global economy, a bioterrorism attack could be planned. The likelihood of the latter being severely lethal is less, due to increased air travel between nations and reversal of impact. A potent combination of panic with no worry that the impact of the event will bounce back can be achieved by employing 'dirty' bomb attacks using a radiological source referred to as 'R' – Radiological – or using a nuclear option. The probability of an accident in a nuclear reactor is higher than the probability of usage of a nuclear bomb in today's scenario, where conventions, treaties and self-imposed restrictions and disarmament strategies dissuade the usage of nuclear weapons, e.g. the Fukushima incident is an example of a disaster despite having all safety mechanisms in place, highlighting that human technology can become powerless in the face of nature's fury. The 'e' component referred to as Explosives is now widely being used to terrorize people. Another associated term, referred to as 'cyber' – 'C' – is a low-cost panic bomb that can jeopardize the economy and is always associated with the probability of occurrence of secondary disasters. It may lead to extreme loss of lives and property in the wrong hands (Fig. 22.1).

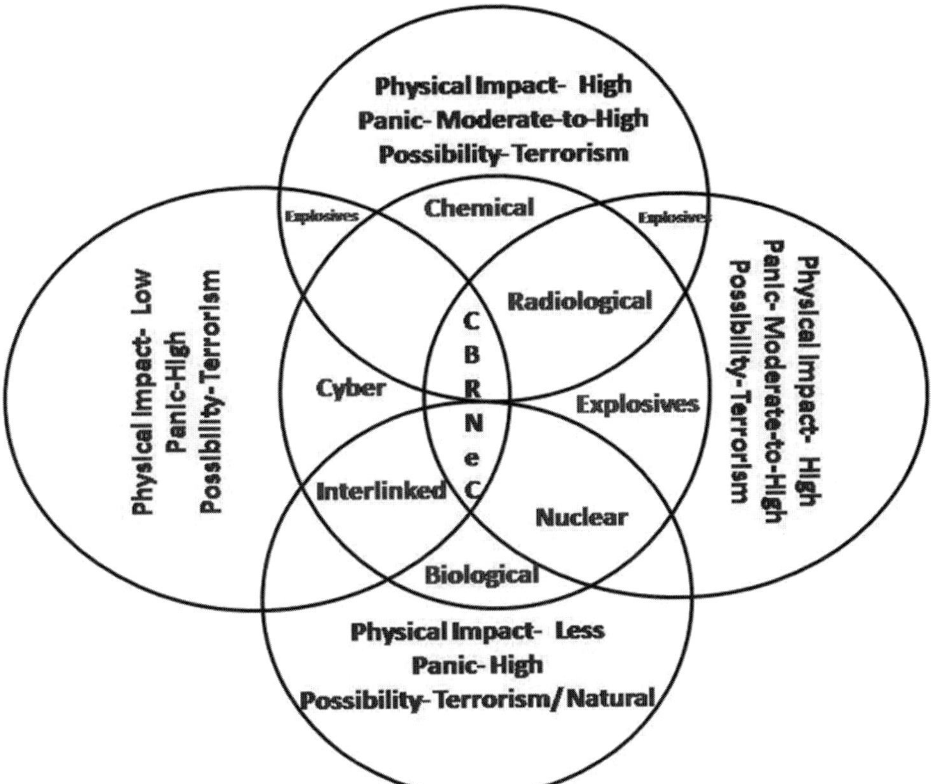

Fig. 22.1. CBRN emergencies: a proposed model multicentric approach to mitigate their effects.

A messenger-based attack to terrorize a particular community has recently been observed in various parts of the South Asian region. The combination of these CBRN attacks could potentially be a trigger for a war-like situation. Threat analysis of the plausible occurrence of such events can lead to a cascade of reactions, which might lead to disruption of societal internal security structure. It is essential to understand that such incidences will accompany contamination and the possibility of exposure in the case of attack with radioactive chemicals.

With respect to enhanced threat, it is essential to develop specialized human resources with appropriate levels of expertise, logistics and resources in order to be able to safeguard the responding agencies from contamination. The motivation to work in and manage contaminated scenarios presents an important challenge. Utilization of resources in an optimal manner requires a robust management structure in place.

CBRN emergencies and their management

Chemical emergencies

A chemical emergency can be an accident, as in the case of an unintentional industrial accident, e.g. the Bhopal gas incident, or could be planned, as in the case of a terrorist attack with a chemical weapon inflicting damage to defence personnel and/or civilians. Many hazardous chemicals are used in modern day industries or are found in nature that can be used for impairment of health and economy by people with nefarious designs. Specific measures to handle an incident involving a CWA includes immediate administration of antidotes, preparation of hospital emergency preparedness plans, hazardous materials (HAZMAT) response vehicles, etc., trauma care facilities and specialized treatment care facilities.

Agents of chemical origin, synthetic or natural, aimed at incapacitating enemies, disrupting military or civilian operations or for any other malicious intent are termed as CWAs. Most CWAs are toxic, corrosive and irritants that excel at rapidly impeding services at the defined area of dispersal. Their chemical, heat labile properties hinder their dispersal via explosive force, requiring other dispersal methods such as aerosolization. These agents are specific in their outcomes, for example defoliants, which destroy vegetation, are specifically employed to reveal densely vegetative area to gain strategic advantage or for elimination of agriculture and livestock to cause famine resulting in enemy starvation.

Currently, on record, about 70 chemicals have been used or stockpiled during the course of the past century as CWAs. Possession of CWAs by nearly 25 nations worldwide and by certain terrorist groups, owing to the involvement of some politically instable nations, has raised global concerns. Most responsible countries are against the offensive use of CWAs. However, being surrounded by hostile neighbours and owing to the involvement of nefarious elements, active monitoring and surveillance of CWAs becomes imperative.

Such precarious conditions increase the probability of clandestine chemical weapon attacks by potential adversaries, necessitating beefing up of defensive measures. By utilizing appropriate personal protective equipment (PPE) and donning personal protective clothing, trained personnel can decontaminate the affected areas, largely overcoming the primary effects of chemical weapons.

Biological emergencies

Agents of biological origin, encompassing viruses, bacteria, fungi, toxins, etc., which are intentionally introduced into a population, aiming to incapacitate or disrupt the functioning of states/regions are termed as biological warfare agents (BWAs). The expected outcome of BWA release is dependent on a multitude of variables starting from agent dispersal method, formulation, meteorological and terrain conditions, natural immunity in the targeted population and size of inoculum received/required for disease establishment. This variability also affects the incubation period prior to disease initiation from as little as 2 days to weeks.

Bacteria, viruses and toxins can be disseminated into the air, used to contaminate food and drinking water, and can be transmitted by person-to-person contact to cause biological emergencies. To combat biological emergencies, there is a need to ensure the development of mechanisms for prompt detection of incipient outbreaks, isolation of the infected persons and making use of therapeutic countermeasures.

Toxins merit a special mention here owing to their defined chemical structure and biological origin, thereby putting them in a grey area between CWAs and BWAs. This is further supported by their intermediate properties of incubation period, also lying between CWAs and BWAs.

The Second World War brought along with it extensive research in the field of biological weapons. A secret research branch of the Japanese Army Unit 731 initiated a plague epidemic by dropping plague-infected fleas over highly populated areas of Manchuria, China. The plague bacilli remained viable as an aerosol for about 1 h over about 10 km. This saw the beginning of the BWA race with tularaemia, anthrax, smallpox, etc. being stockpiled rapidly by various countries. The numerous BWAs are categorized as lethal, sub-lethal and incapacitating, and incapacitating only.

The recent scenario of a novel H1N1 pandemic exhibited the deleterious effects of a possible biological agent being used as a weapon demonstrating rapid worldwide spread in a matter of few weeks (Arora *et al.*, 2010b).

Radiological and nuclear emergency

Weapons that result in dispersal of radioactive material or radiation or energy associated with radiological decay in an uncontrolled way, with the intent of causing widespread death and destruction, fall under the category of radiological and nuclear emergencies.

Radiological threats/emergencies arise from radiation exposure, which may further be accompanied by internal or external contamination. Radiological accidents such as the incidents at Goiania, San Salvador, Lilo, Istanbul, Yanango, Tammiku, Panama and the recent accident at Mayapuri, India have highlighted the importance of a pre-prepared plan of action for rapid mitigation of radiological accidents. The absence of appropriate preparedness may lead to mass exodus and chaos resulting in huge socioeconomic losses. Radiological threats pose a grave concern given the current political scenario, with reference to acquisition and deployment by terrorist organizations (Coleman and Parker, 2009).

Nuclear emergencies arise from the energy released from a nuclear chain reaction or from the decay of toxic radiological products of the reaction, for example the Chernobyl incident, Tokamura, Kystym, etc. (Mettler and Voelz, 2002). The long-term effects of such incidents are disastrous, with continued exposure to radiation of the general public from external sources such as contaminated soil, buildings, etc. or internal sources via intake of contaminated food, water or by direct inhalation of radioactive nuclei. On the other hand a nuclear weapon explosion leads to mass destruction, contamination and management of such an incident requires adequate preparedness and capacity development at the hospital level (Arora *et al.*, 2008; Sharma *et al.*, 2008).

Any hazard caused by radiation exposure resulting from a radiological exposure device (RED)/radiological dispersal device (RDD)/improvised nuclear device (IND) comes under the category of radiation emergencies. A plethora of sources of radiation are used in various fields, including industry and research, particularly in medicine and, therefore, radiological emergencies may occur anywhere (Arora *et al.*, 2008; Pradeepkumar, 2008).

Medical management of radiation-induced health impact

Radiation-induced damage can be manifested as either local radiation injury (LRI) or acute radiation syndrome (ARS). LRI may cause skin burns, erythaema, pigmentation, epithelitis, fibrosis, necrosis and skin atrophy, and ARS can cause haematopoeitic, gastrointestinal, central nervous system and cutaneous syndromes, thereby leading to functional impairment (Arora *et al.*, 2010a,c). Severity of radiation-induced damage depends on the dose, type of radiation, location and size of the area exposed. On the other hand, the effect of radiation depends on three guiding factors, i.e. time, distance and shielding (TDS). The concept of TDS can be effectively used for protection against radiation effects.

Regimens that should be used against radiation-induced damage include radiation mitigators, which may be administered prior to exposure, radiation prophylactics/protectors, which can be given immediately after exposure to restore homeostatic levels of metabolic enzymes, and therapeutic regimens that include decontamination agents, decorporation agents and symptomatic care drugs (Arora *et al.*, 2008, 2010a,c).

Radiation exposure causes damage to DNA, lipids and proteins within the body via generation of reactive oxygen species (ROS) and reactive nitrogen species (RNS), thereby causing oxidation and peroxidation of biomolecules (Grace *et al.*, 2010). Hence to counteract the deleterious effects imposed by radiation, drugs comprising antioxidants, oncogene targeting agents, immunomodulators and growth factors are often administered. Radioprotectivepharmacologics include agents like amifostine, phosphorothioates, phosphoenol, nitroxides, 5-androstenediol (5-AED), etc. (Whitnall*et al.*, 2001; Arora *et al.*, 2005, 2008, 2010a,c). Aside from the conventional approaches, chemical engineering of drug analogues and alternative medicinal approaches are also being explored (Christie *et al.*, 2010).

Radiation treatment modalities includes stem cell transplantation, platelet infusion, growth factor therapy, bone marrow transplantation and supportive therapies like anti-emetic, analgesic, brain oedema management, adapted nutrition and other modalities (Xiao *et al.*, 2007). Radiation treatment modules differ for every victim depending upon the lymphocyte count of the exposed victim in the first week. If the levels are 200–500 cells/μl, antibiotics and platelet infusion should be given and as the levels increase, growth factor therapy is advocated. If they increase further, bone marrow transplantation is the final option (Davis *et al.*, 2007).

Decontamination aims towards reducing the contamination levels to at least twice that of the background level, i.e. 0.05 mR/h. Decontamination should be executed giving priority to skin areas, eyes, hair, mouth, nose and wounds. Precautionary measures should be kept in mind while decontaminating a victim and this includes changing gloves and surveying hands, performing decontamination with a circular motion so as to contain the contaminant in the central portion of the exposed area and wiping off the contaminant carefully from the centre thereafter. Tepid water, specific solutions of 3% citric acid/hydrogen peroxide, mild shampoo, nail clippers and isotonic saline water may be used for decontamination.

Once radioactive materials cross cell membranes they are said to be incorporated and their management requires decorporation agents, which need to be administered so as to remove the incorporated radioactive material from the body. Examples of decorporating agents include potassium iodide, which is used to protect the thyroid glands by decorporating radioactive iodine, and Prussian blue, which acts as a sequestering agent against cations with one unit of positive charge and is commonly used to decorporate heavy metal ions. In addition to these decontamination and decorporation agents, several plants have also been found to show immense potential as radioprotectors, e.g. *Podophyllum hexandrum*, *Mentha* spp., *Hippophae rhamnoides*, *Rhodiola imbricata*, *Tinospora cordifolia*, *Ocimum sanctum* etc. (Arora *et al.*, 2005, 2012; Arora, 2008; Chawla *et al.*, 2006; Arora and Selvamurthy, 2012).

Managing CBRN emergencies

CBRN emergencies can be considered as a combination of sequential activities especially with respect to the new face of terrorism emerging globally. Explosions at vulnerable locations all across the globe due to local conflicts, state-sponsored terrorism and technology-intensive terrorism crimes can include CBRN agents. Such terrorism activities are initially primed by extensive communication exchange through the cyber world; a misuse of this technology is an essential component of planning terrorism strategies in today's world. Thus, adequate cybercrime prevention and monitoring technologies are important preventive tools against CBRN emergencies. Specialized preparedness for CBRN emergencies requires mitigation strategies for contamination control in addition to general preparedness. Expected emergencies are unlikely to be mass casualty events; however, due to the associated panic and management of a large population a large number of problems can be anticipated.

Final Comments

In the developed world, management structure is designed to be resilient against such attacks. Adequate in-built mitigation strategies within existing infrastructure provide a plausible framework to control unprecedented events. In addition, the present-day fact is that most countries are unlikely to use such agents directly or in a wartime scenario due to responsive international military action, condemnation and alienation of the attacking country and consequent crippling of the socio-economic structure. Management of CBRN emergencies requires the coordinated efforts of a number of service/stakeholders providers, while they need to perform secondary functions in addition to their primary mandatory function by law. Such functions are enumerated in Table 22.1.

Table 22.1. Secondary functions of primary stakeholders/service providers for CBRN emergency management.

Stakeholder/service provider/responder	Primary function	Secondary function
Police	Maintenance of law and order	a. Protection b. Detection and impact assessment c. Basic first aid/pre-hospital trauma care d. Perimeter control and cordoning off e. Medico-legal/forensic investigation f. Recovery operations g. Management of contaminated dead
Fire and emergency services	Fire control and its management HAZMAT response mechanism	a. Detection and impact assessment b. Field level decontamination c. Dynamic quantitative assessment of fire hazards/mitigation measures d. Chemical neutralization/prevention of on-site becoming off-site emergencies e. Mop-up operations

Medical services at field site	Medical response at incident site and evacuation	a. Resuscitation, triage and life care b. Management of serious contaminated victims in hot zones c. Incident level decontamination d. Antidote administration e. Water intoxication management
Transport department	Evacuation to relief camps	a. Specialized provisions for self-protection and vehicle support b. Evacuation (air, road, rail, water etc.) c. Heli-ambulance integrated services d. Transportation support to rescue, relief, recovery process, relocation, rehabilitation and reconstruction
Emergency medical services at hospitals	Hospital care	a. Hospital level decontamination b. Definitive care against health effects of CBRN agents c. Care of care providers d. Follow-up healthcare e. Public health issues
National disaster response force/state disaster response force	Specialized force for management of natural disasters and CBRN emergencies	a. Protection, detection, decontamination and impact assessment b. Field-/hospital-level decontamination c. Basic trauma care d. Hot/warm/cold zone management e. Specialized care provision f. Medical care at incident site Basic Life Support (BLS) g. Long-term relief and recovery operations

Home guards and civil defence	a. Supporting and community care concerns b. Auxillary to police (internal security)	a. Support to police and specialized forces b. Community evacuation c. Traffic management, if necessary d. Filler functionary system
Communication department	Maintain connectivity	Self protection and business continuity of operations
Water supply	Ensure safe water supply	a. Additional provision for drinking water, mass decontamination, mop-up operations and fire fighting/prevention of compressed gas release b. Business continuity operations
Power supply	Power back-up and continued supply	a. Mitigation of power failures due to mechanical and human errors b. Alternative power options for long-term crisis – an inbuilt approach c. Business continuity planning for contaminated scenarios
Relief and recovery department	Disaster management recovery and mitigation	a. Funding and compensation strategies b. Restoration of civic amenities and maintainance of minimum standards of food, water, health and sanitization
Public health	Management of public health issues	a. Psychosocial support to affected communities b. Community resilience c. Personal hygiene d. Follow-up care of victims
Defence, paramilitary and other aided forces	Primary function as mandated by law	Contingent force if the emergency is level 3 and not manageable by state-level resources

The primary distinguishing factor of CBRN emergencies from non-CBRN emergencies is the presence of contaminant, the removal of which is paramount. Medical preparedness also varies depending upon the type of agent employed/present as a contaminant. For example, chemical emergency casualties require immediate trauma care, burn care and acute health management practices within the golden hour due to the unlikely transmission of the contaminating factor, while biological emergencies require isolation and quarantine and other preventive measures prior to treatment/invasive operations due to the ease of transmission of the contaminating factor (Arora *et al.*, 2010a,c; Chawla *et al.*, 2011a,b). Management of radiological emergencies is largely dependent on exposure dose and site of contamination (internal or external), with the first hour (golden hour) or the first few minutes (platinum minutes) after the accident being the most critical for medical intervention. Therefore, preparation of a CBRN casualty management strategy, particularly from a medical perspective highlights the need for a multidisciplinary approach to mitigate the deleterious consequences arising from the deliberate use of such agents.

Acknowledgements

The authors are grateful to Dr W. Selvamurthy, Distinguished Scientist and Chief Controller, Research and Development (Life Sciences and International Cooperation) Director, INMAS for help and support in multifarious ways. Thanks are also due to the Defence Research and Development Organization (DRDO), Government of India for providing resources and funding support.

References

Arora, R. (ed.) (2008) *Herbal Radiomodulators: Applications in Medicine, Homeland Defence and Space*. CAB International, Wallingford, UK, pp. 321.

Arora, R. and Selvamurthy, W. (2012) Development of Radiation Countermeasure Agents through Harnessing High-Altitude Cold Arid Region Bioresource. In: Srivastava, R.B. and Selvamurthy, W. (eds) *Innovations in Agro Animal Technologies*. Satish Serial Publications House, New Delhi, pp. 319–348.

Arora, R., Chawla, R., Prasad, J., Singh, S., Kumar, R., Sharma, A. *et al.* (2005) Radioprotective activity of *Rhodiolaimbricata* – a high altitude medicinal plant. *Molecular and Cellular Biochemistry* 273, 209–223.

Arora, R., Sharma, A., Kumar, R. and Tripathi, R.P. (2008) Herbal radiation countermeasure agents: Promising role in the management of radiological/nuclear exigencies. Proceedings of the 28th IARP National Conference. Focal Theme: Management of Nuclear and Radiological, Emergencies, 19–21 November 2008, Dr S.N. Medical College and Defence Laboratory (Defence Research and Development Organization), Jodhpur, India. *Radiation Protection and Environment* 31(1–4), 304–306.

Arora, R., Basu, M., Chawla, R., Goel, R., Kaushik, A., Kaushik, V., Ravishanker, L., Syed Raza, K., Rakesh, K.S., Silambarasan, M., Tripathi, R.P. and Vijayaraghavan, R. (2010a) In: Sharma, R.K., Chawla, R. and Tripathi, R.P. (eds) *Management of CBRN Casualties in Hospitals*. A publication of the Division of Chemical, Biological, Radiological and Nuclear Defence (CBRN). Institute of Nuclear Medicine and Allied Science (INMAS), Defence Research and Development Organization (DRDO), Delhi, pp. 177.

Arora, R., Chawla, R., Marwah, R., Arora, P., Sharma, R.K., Kaushik, V., Goel, R., Kaur, A., Silambarasan, M., Tripathi, R.P. and Bhardwaj, J.R. (2010b) Potential of complementary and alternative medicine in preventive management of novel H1N1 flu (swine flu) pandemic: thwarting potential disasters in the bud. *Evidence Based Complementary and Alternative Medicine* Epub 13 October 2010.

Arora, R., Chawla, R., Marwah, R., Kumar, V., Goel, R., Arora, P., Jaiswal, S. and Sharma, R.K. (2010c) Medical radiation countermeasures for nuclear and radiological emergencies (NREs): current status and future perspectives. *Journal of Pharmacy and Bioallied Sciences* 2(3), 202–212.

Arora, R., Sharma, J., Sharma, A., Baliga, M.S. and Selvamurthy, W. (2012) *Mentha* species: A pharmacological perspective vis-à-vis biological and behavioral radiation protection. In: Govil, J.N. (ed.) *Recent Progress in Medicinal Plants: Ethnomedicine and Therapeutic Validation*, Vol. 32. Astral International, Delhi, pp. 357–375.

Chawla, R., Arora, R., Singh, S., Sagar, R.K., Sharma, R.K., Kumar, R. *et al.* (2006) *Podophyllumhexandrum* offers radioprotection by modulating free radical flux: role of aryl-tetralinlignans. *Evidence-based Complementary and Alternative Medicine* 3(4), 1–9.

Chawla, R., Goel, R., Silambarasan, M., Kumar, V., Arora, R. and Sharma, R.K. (2011a) *CBRN Glossary: Abbreviations and Some Common Terms.* A publication of the Division of Chemical, Biological, Radiological and Nuclear Defence (CBRN), Institute of Nuclear Medicine and Allied Science (INMAS), (DRDO), Delhi.

Chawla, R., Kumar, V., Goel, R., Silambarasan, M., Arora, R. and Sharma, R.K. (2011b) *CBRN casualty management at incident site.* A Publication of the Division of Chemical, Biological, Radiological and Nuclear Defence (CBRN), Institute of Nuclear Medicine and Allied Science (INMAS), (DRDO), Delhi.

Christie, D.H., Chu, M.C. and Carr, Z. (2010) Global networking for biodosimetry laboratory capacity surge in radiation emergencies. *Health Physics* 98, 168–171.

Coleman, C.M. and Parker, G.W. (2009) Radiation terrorism: what society needs from the radiobiology–radiation protection and radiation oncology community. *Journal of Radiological Protection* 29, A159–A169.

Davis, T.A., Clarke, T.K., Mog, S.R. and Landauer, M.R. (2007) Subcutaneous administration of genistein prior to lethal irradiation supports multilineage, hematopoietic progenitor cell recovery and survival. *International Journal of Radiation Biology* 83, 141–151.

Grace, M.B., Blakelya, W.B. and Landauer, M.R. (2007) Genistein-induced alterations of radiation-responsive gene expression. *Radiation Measurements* 42, 1152–1157.

Grace, M.B., Moyer, B.R., Prasher, J., Cliffer, K.D., Ramakrishnan, N., Kaminski, J., Coleman, C.N., Manning, R.G., Maidment, B.W. and Hatchett, R. (2010) Rapid radiation dose assessment for radiological public health emergencies: roles of NIAID and BARDA. *Health Physics* 98, 172–178.

Mettler, F.A. and Voelz, G.L. (2002) Major radiation exposure – what to expect and how to respond. *The New England Journal of Medicine* 346, 1554–1561.

Pradeepkumar, K.S. (2008) Nuclear and radiological threats and emergency: preparedness at national level. *Radiation Environment and Protection* 31, 48–53.

Sharma, R.K., Chawla, R., Goel, R., Silambarasan, M. and Kumar, V. (2008) Nuclear and radiological emergency preparedness: decontamination issues. *Radiation Protection and Environment* 31, 1–4.

Whitnall, M.H., Elliott, T.B., Harding, R.A., Inal, C.E., Landauer, M.R., Wilhelmsen, C.L., McKinney, L., Miner, V.L., Jackson, W.E. 3rd, Loria, R.M., Ledney, G.D. and Seed, T.M. (2001) Androstenediol stimulates myelopoiesis and enhances resistance to infection in gamma-irradiated mice. *International Journal of Immunopharmacology* 22, 1–14.

Xiao, M., Inal, C.E., Parekh, V.I., Chang, C.M. and Whitnall, M.H. (2007) 5-Androstenediol promotes survival of γ-irradiated human hematopoietic progenitors through induction of nuclear factor-κB activation and granulocyte colony-stimulating factor expression. *Molecular Pharmacology* 72, 370–379.

Chapter 23

Prophylactic Possibilities in Case of High Risk of Exposure to Nerve Agents

Jiri Bajgar

Introduction

Disasters have the potential to occur at any time, including those accompanied by the release of toxic chemicals. The release of toxic chemicals can be intentional or unintentional, however, a basic precondition for release is the existence of a toxic agent, i.e. the necessary conditions are production, processing, storage or transport of toxic substances, either for intentional or unintentional use. Unintentional release can be caused either by a natural disaster (volcanic eruption, earthquake, etc., release of H_2S or other toxic gases) or by a coincidence of negative factors. These factors are, in general, technical fault or human error. Intentional release or use is mostly realized in the case of military or local conflict, and terroristic or sabotage action. It can take the form of an attack on a storage or production facility (indirect release) or direct use of a toxic chemical synthesized with the aim of being used against humans (Bajgar *et al.*, 2009a).

There are thousands of highly toxic chemicals in existence; one group of the present agents is the organophosphates (OPs) (more precisely organophosphonates), especially nerve agents. They are highly toxic chemicals and they represent a potential threat to the civilian population, as evident from recent terrorist attacks in Japan (Yoshida, 1994; Morita *et al.*, 1995; Ohtomi *et al.*, 1996; Nagao *et al.*, 1997; Ohbu *et al.*, 1997; Okomura *et al.*, 1998; Yokoyama *et al.*, 1998; Vale *et al.*, 2007). Therefore, research on their effect, diagnosis, treatment and the prophylaxis of intoxication by these compounds has been one of the main topics within the programme of various laboratories.

Exposure to nerve agents can occur owing to their release during terrorist attacks or some disasters. Terroristic use of nerve agents can be characterized by exposure of many people requiring adequate treatment (Rotenberg and Newmark, 2003; Vale *et al.*, 2007). Treatment is given by medical (or other) personnel using antidotes and other (life-saving) countermeasures. The personnel will be protected by masks and protective clothes; generally, these countermeasures prevent the penetration of nerve agents into the organism, however, it is possible to use pharmacological prophylaxis, too. Thus, in this special case, prophylactic countermeasures are needed (Fig. 23.1).

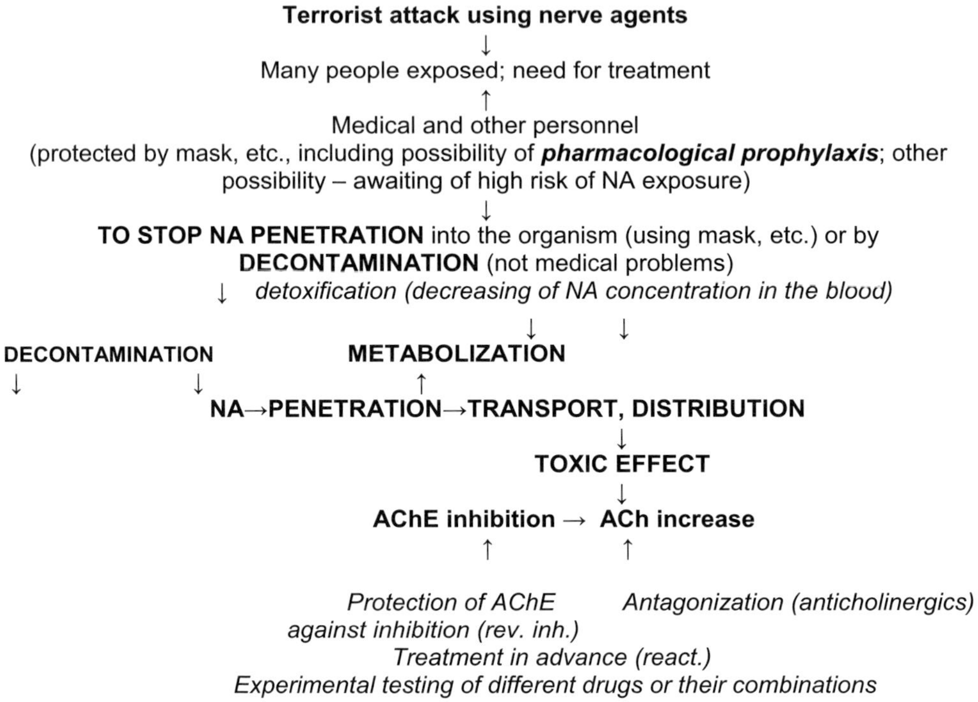

Fig. 23.1. Scheme characterizing the use of prophylactics in a terrorist attack using nerve agents and possible targets/drugs for prophylaxis. (Modifed from Bajgar *et al.*, 2009b.)

Effective prophylaxis is based on a good knowledge of the agents and their mechanism of action.

Nerve Agents

OPs/nerve agents comprise a large variety of compounds with various physical, chemical and biological properties including different toxicities – from practically non-toxic chemicals (e.g. malathion) to highly toxic agents such as nerve agents. They are compounds containing the phosphorus atom with various different radicals. OPs are liquids of different volatility, soluble or insoluble in water, organic solvents, etc.

The most important group, the members of which have a significant biological effect contains compounds of the general formula:

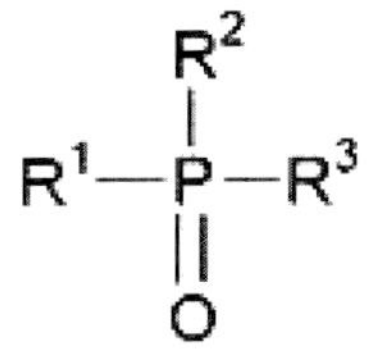

where R^{1-2} are alkyl-, alkoxy, alkylthio- amino- groups; R^3 is a dissociable group, e.g. halogens, cyano- or thio- groups; the rest is made up of an inorganic or organic acid, O-R or maximally one undissociable group such as hydrogen, alkyl (including cyclic), aryl and others.

Nerve agents can be divided into G-compounds (sarin, soman, etc.) and V-compounds (VX, Russian VX, Chinese VX, model VX, etc.) (Marrs *et al.*, 1996; Bajgar, 2004, 2011). There is a large group of OPs with the same basic structure; they are not toxic in comparison with the nerve agents and they are used in veterinary and human medicine (e.g. parathion), in research (e.g. enzyme synthesis – soman) or in agriculture (OP insecticides, e.g. dichlorvos, malathion, etc.). Because of their very similar basic structure, the principles of pharmacodynamics, prophylaxis and treament are the same as for the nerve agents described below.

Prophylaxis against the effects of nerve agents is an interesting and complicated problem. For its effective solution, it is necessary to have good knowledge of the action of nerve agents (pharmacodynamics).

Mechanism of Action of Nerve Agents (Pharmacodynamics)

The mechanism of action of nerve agents is based on irreversible acetylcholinesterase (AChE, EC 3.1.1.7) inhibition at cholinergic synapses. However, before action on the synapses, the nerve agent is absorbed according to the route of administration. Thus, four basic actions (absorption, transport, metabolization and the toxic effect) are in motion following nerve agent exposure (Bajgar, 2004, 2011) (Fig. 23.1). Except for intravenous administration when the agent is directly injected into the blood stream, all other routes are characterized by the losses occurring during penetration and absorption.

Absorption is accomplished by penetration of OP through biological barriers into the blood representing the transport system. In the transport system, the losses originate from detoxification and non-specific binding to proteins and enzymes – esterases, AChE in erythrocytes and butyrylcholinesterase in plasma (BuChE, EC 3.1.1.8). AChE belongs to the group of hydrolases catalysing hydrolysis of choline esters to choline and a relevant acid. They are distinguished into two classes, differing in their enzymatic properties and physiological function (Massoulié *et al.*, 1993; Darvesh *et al.*, 2003) – AChE and BuChE. However, there are other types of cholinesterases such as benzoylcholinesterase, propionylcholinesterase, etc. AChE splits neuromediator acetylcholine at the cholinergic synapses. It has also been observed in erythrocytes but its function here is not yet known in detail, though there is evidence that this enzyme has an important role in cholinergic neurotransmission and could be involved in other nervous system functions and in neurological diseases (Darvesh *et al.*, 2003), similar to the function of BuChE activity in plasma where it is connected to lipid metabolism (Annapurna *et al.*, 1991; Van Lith *et al.*, 1991; Van Lith and Beynen, 1993).

In the molecular structure of AChE is contained a catalytic triad called the esteratic site Ser_{200}-His_{440}-Glu_{327}, at the bottom of a deep and narrow cavity, known as the 'aromatic gorge'. Acetylcholine must pass down into this gorge and bind to the active site within. Ligands binding to the esteratic site are called acylating (OPs, carbamates, alkylsulphonates). Non-acylating ligands are bound to sites other than the esteratic site (anionic sites) and comprise a large group of chemicals including tetralkylammonium, coumarine, tacrine, gallantamine, etc. These anionic sites can be responsible (in a complex with the enzyme structure) for allostericity of AChE (Sussmann *et al.*, 1991; Soreq *et al.*, 1992).

AChE possesses one or more additional binding sites for ACh and other quaternary ligands. Such peripheral anionic binding sites are at the lip of this gorge. In BuChE, Trp_{279}, an important component of the peripheral binding site in AChE, is missing. This site is believed to be responsible for substrate inhibition (Radic *et al.*, 1991), which is one of the features that distinguishes AChE from BuChE. Current knowledge on the structure, role and inhibition of cholinesterases (AChE and BuChE) was published by Bosak *et al.* (2011) in an excellent review.

Nerve agents are bound to plasma proteins (albumin) but the binding is not specific. Inhibition of cholinesterases in the blood is practically the first target for nerve agents according to the principle 'first come, first served' (Benschop and de Jong, 2001).

Activity of cholinesterases is of fundamental importance for diagnosis of intoxication with cholinesterase inhibitors, including OPs/nerve agents and carbamates (Bardin *et al.*, 1994; Cowan *et al.*, 1996; Marrs *et al.*, 1996; Bajgar, 2004). On the other hand, the activity depends on many other factors and, therefore, cholinesterase determination is of diagnostic importance in different pathological states, i.e. not only intoxication (Kutty, 1980; Brimijoin and Rakonczay, 1986; Rakonczay, 1988; Lotti, 1995; Bajgar, 2004, 2005). Activity of other enzymes (AChE and BuChE) is influenced by sex, age, nutrition, hormonal factors, irradiation, etc. (Herink *et al.*, 1975, 1980; Whittaker, 1980; Brown *et al.*, 1981; Skopec *et al.*, 1981; Skau, 1986; Darvesh *et al.*, 2003). The variation in BuChE activity is greater than that of AChE (Kutty, 1980; Brown *et al.*, 1981; Bajgar, 1991, 2005) and it is genetically determined (Whittaker, 1980; Brown *et al.*, 1981).

There are also differences in the detoxification of highly toxic nerve agents: G-compounds like sarin and soman are detoxified but compounds containing the P-S bond (V-compounds) are not detoxified (Bajgar, 2004, 2011). The OP is carried out at the sites of metabolic and toxic effects. The toxic effect sites are the central and peripheral nervous systems and OPs react here with AChE and BuChE. Inhibition of cholinesterases is a trigger mechanism for the toxic action of nerve agents. Different affinities of various nerve agents to central and peripheral compartments are observed. Important nerve agents, soman and sarin are rapidly absorbed via all routes of administration including inhalation, percutaneous and oral administration (Bajgar, 2004; Cabal *et al.*, 2009) and inhibit cholinesterases (preferably AChE) in the central and peripheral nervous system. Because of soman's high lipophility, it possesses a high affinity to brain AChE (Cabal *et al.*, 2009). Sarin is less lipophilic, however, its affinity to brain AChE is also very high (Fusek *et al.*, 2009).

Both groups of nerve agents (G- and V-compounds) are potent inhibitors of cholinesterases *in vitro* and *in vivo* (Marrs *et al.*, 1996; Cabal *et al.*, 2009; Fusek *et al.*, 2009). From the point of view of pharmacodynamics and therapeutic possibilities, soman represents the most serious poison. Its toxicity is comparable with that of sarin and VX (Shih *et al.*, 1990; Bajgar, 2004; Bajgar *et al.*, 2007a,b, 2011) but the therapeutic efficacy of the antidotal treatments with current and perspective drugs is not good enough (Kassa, 2002; Bajgar, 2004, 2011). This is probably a reason for the research dealing with soman intoxication and treatment.

In general, G-compounds are detoxified in the liver, plasma and, according to some authors, also in the lungs (Shapira *et al.*, 1990); and therefore these areas are excluded from the toxic effect. The parent compounds can be monitored in the blood stream as well as their metabolites, which are excreted in urine (van der Schans *et al.*, 2003; Bajgar, 2005; Jokanovic, 2009). Binding to non-specific esterases also causes losses of G-compounds in the organism and this part of soman and sarin does not have a toxic effect. It has been assessed that only 1–3% of the dose administered inhibited AChE in the brain, i.e. 1–3% of the dose administered caused the basic toxic effect (Bajgar, 2004, 2011). Another factor (up to now not very elucidated) influencing soman and sarin poisoning is the existence of a depot in the organism from where the nerve agent can be released causing a new attack of intoxication. This depot has been described for the skin, erythrocytes, muscles and lungs (Kadar *et al.*, 1985; Rotenberg and Newmark, 2003). Bearing in mind the very low portion of the dose administered that causes the basic toxic effect, it is clear that the release of a very small quantity of sarin and soman can significantly influence the survival or death of the intoxicated organism independently of the treatment. V-compounds are not detoxified in the organism (Bajgar, 1991). This is probably the reason for the higher toxicity of V-compounds in comparison with G-compounds. The effect of V-compounds (especially VX) is prolonged in comparison with sarin and soman (Vachek *et al.*, 1996). The toxicokinetics of different nerve agents including stereoisomers have also been described (Benschop and de Jong, 2001). The mechanism of action for VX is inhibition of AChE preferably in the peripheral nervous system. However, inhibition of AChE in the brain parts has been described as being selective and most marked in the pontomedullar area of the brain (Bajgar *et al.*, 2007b; Hajek *et al.*, 2009). Detoxification of OPs with lower toxicity is also important. Moreover, for some OPs especially those containing the P=S bond, oxidation giving rise to more toxic products is observed (P=S → P=O). This reaction, called 'lethal synthesis', is typical, e.g. for malathion (oxidized to malaoxon) or parathion (oxidized to paraoxon). Oxo-derivatives (more toxic) are released into the transport system and can cause new attacks of intoxication. A similar reaction can be observed after releasing the OP from the depot, mostly from fat tissue. In place of the toxic effect (nervous system), the reaction with enzymes is important though some other direct interactions with receptors have been described and non-specific reactions (the stressogenic effect) have also been observed. Depending on the target, acute, intermediate, chronic or delayed effects are manifested (Marrs *et al.*, 1996; Lotti, 2000; Bajgar, 2004).

As was described previously, nerve agents inhibit AChE via phosphorylation/phosphonylation of the esteratic site. The rate of spontaneous dephosphorylation is very low and can be increased by reactivators (oximes). The efficacy of oxime reactivation is dependent on both oxime and conjugated phosphonate structure (Taylor *et al.*, 1999). Simultaneously, the microenvironment of the gorge plays a significant role in determining selectivity of substrate and inhibitors for cholinesterases (Saxena *et al.*, 1999). In the case of some OPs after phosphorylation of the active site, the complex enzyme inhibitor (which is able to be reactivated) is changed to a non-reactivatable complex, resistant to reactivators. The molecular mechanism is explained by splitting of the complex forming the alcohol and unreactivatable enyzme. This reaction, called ageing or dealkylation, is very fast for soman-inhibited AChE (the half-life is about 10 min) and it is less expressed for sarin (the half-life is about 10 h) (Fleisher and Harris, 1965; Talbot *et al.*, 1988; Bajgar, 1991, 1992). This is one of the reasons for the difficulty with therapeutic interventions of soman intoxication (Wolthuis *et al.*, 1994; Bajgar, 1996). Peripheral site ligands may have selective effects on AChE phosphorylation (Rosenberry *et al.*, 1999).

Following AChE inhibition, the acetylcholine level at cholinergic synapses is increased. The resulting accumulation of acetylcholine at synaptic junctions in the central and peripheral nervous system overstimulates cholinergic pathways and subsequently desensitizes cholinegic receptor sites. However, a variety of data have documented that AChE inhibition is not the only important biochemical change during the intoxication. Many other changes have been described that accompany the development of intoxication and might contribute to OP toxicity, including changes in other enzymes, neurotransmitters, immune changes, anaphylactoid reaction, behaviour, etc. The evidence includes data indicating that prophylactic/therapcutic drugs also might have multiple sites of action similar to those observed during intoxication (Bajgar, 1991, 1992; Bardin *et al.*, 1994; Cowan *et al.*, 1996; Kassa, 1998).

Prophylaxis

Prophylaxis, in medical terms, is prevention of disease, preventive measures such as immunization or vaccination (against infectious diseases) or mechanical measures (prevention of venereal diseases). It also comprises teeth cleaning (dental prophylaxis). Prophylaxis against poisoning with different chemicals can be understood as preparing an organism to be protected/resistant or less sensitive to health disturbance/death caused by chemicals. From this point of view, prophylaxis against poisoning could cover the use of protective measures such as protective masks or clothes, or decontamination, etc. They are measures preventing/lowering the penetration of a nerve agent into the organism. However, the term prophylaxis used in this article is limited to medical countermeasures applied relatively shortly before penetration of a toxic agent into the organism. The question now arises of what will happen after the administration of a prophylactic drug. When the treatment is unnecessary, it can be described as prophylaxis. When the treatment occurs after exposure, the term pre-treatment has come to be accepted. However, though successful prophylaxis can be observed for some nerve agents, there are questions around the ability of prophylaxis to fully protect the organism without post-exposure treatment, particularly in the case of soman poisoning.

From a practical point of view, it is obvious that when a drug is administered prior to intoxication (either prophylaxis or pre-treatment) with the aim of protecting the organism against a toxic drug, the exposure to these agents is expected and therefore, post-exposure therapy can very probably be used, i.e. pre-treatment could be used as the right term. For reasons of simplicity, the term prophylaxis is used in this chapter.

General

The basic mechanism of action of OPs/nerve agents is known: it is based on irreversible AChE inhibition at cholinergic synapses. The resulting accumulation of acetylcholine at synaptic junctions overstimulates cholinergic pathways and subsequently desentisizes cholinergic receptor sites. The evidence supporting AChE as the primary site of OP agents' action has been based on a number of observations such as a correlation between AChE inhibition *in vivo* and *in vitro*, good therapeutic efficacy of anticholinergics and cholinesterase reactivators, and on the possibility of preventing intoxication (and cholinesterase inhibition) using reversible cholinesterase inhibitors, e.g. carbamates and others. Nevertheless, the first reaction of the OP is interaction with cholinesterases, first in the blood stream in accordance with the first come, first served principle (Benschop and de Jong, 2001) and then in the target tissues – the peripheral and central nervous system (Bajgar, 1991, 2004; Bardin *et al.*, 1994; Marrs *et al.*, 1996). From this basic mechanism (enzyme inhibition) it appears that prophylaxis should be focused on *protection of AChE against inhibition* or diminishing the level of OPs using enzymes hydrolysing these agents or enzymes binding the agents (to specific proteins or to antibodies) and thus reducing OP level (and inhibition of cholinesterases) in the organism. The first group of drugs can be considered as detoxicants, the second as 'scavengers'. In general, this approach seems to be described as *detoxification*. Another approach to prophylaxis is based on the use of current antidotes. The standard treatment for OPs is combined administration of anticholinergics (preferably atropine) and reactivators. Anticholinergics block the effect of accumulated acetylcholine, while reactivators repair the inhibition of AChE via dephosphorylation thus obtaining normal enzyme. For the treatment of convulsions, benzodiazepines (diazepam) are used. Unlike other nerve agents, treatment of soman poisoning is very difficult and unsatisfactory. This is the reason for intensive studies on pre-treatment/prophylaxis to enable the survival and increase the resistance of organisms exposed to soman.

The administration of present antidotes (anticholinergics, reactivators and others) to prevent the effects of OP is described as *simulation of treatment or treatment in advance.* Standard antidotes have been studied in this respect, i.e. anticholinergics, reactivators, anticonvulsants and others. The problem with their use is the timing, duration and achievement of sufficient levels of these antidotes after administration. Combinations of these approaches are also possible (Fig. 23.1) (Bajgar, 2004, 2011; Layish *et al.*, 2005; Patočka *et al.*, 2006; Bajgar *et al.*, 2009b,c).

Protection of AChE against Inhibition

The conservation of intact AChE is a basic requirement for effective prophylaxis, i.e. to change the enzyme in a way to enable it to be resistant to OPs. This can be attained with the use of reversible inhibitors, which are able to reversibly inhibit AChE and after spontaneous recovery of the activity, normal AChE serves as a source of the active enzyme.

There are many inhibitors of cholinesterases diminishing both AChE and BuChE activities to a comparable extent as has been described by Aldridge (1969). Carbamates belong to the group of inhibitors with a large variation in their effectiveness. They are biologically active because of their structural complementarity to the active surface of AChE and their consequent reaction as substrates with very low turnover numbers (Aldridge, 1969).

It appears from toxicodynamics of nerve agents that prophylactic countermeasures can bring about two main actions: protection of AChE against inhibition and antagonization of the action of accumulated acetylcholine. In general, protection of AChE against inhibition can be focused on the use of reversible cholinesterase inhibitors. AChE that has been reversibly inhibited by carbamates (carbamylated AChE) is resistant to the OP/nerve agent inhibition effect. Carbamylated AChE is spontaneously decarbamylated and serves as a source of a native enzyme (Fig. 23.2).

nerve agents – not affecting

↓

E + C → carbamylated E,

resistant to nerve agents;

spontaneous decarbamylation → free E (source of active E)

+ products

Fig. 23.2. Schematic representation of AChE protection using reversible inhibitors (carbamates). AChE (E) reacts with carbamate (C) to form a carbamylated enzyme (EC) and is spontaneously decarbamylated to free E (normal AChE) and products. Carbamylated AChE is resistant to inhibition by OPs/nerve agents. This reaction can be applied to other reversible inhibitors, e.g. acridines, huperzine A (in these cases, it is not carbamylation). It is clear that higher levels of reversibly inhibited AChE indicate greater protection, however, the effect (inhibition) causes toxic symptoms similar to those observed for nerve agents. Therefore the dose of reversible inhibitor must be as high as possible but too low to cause toxic effects. This is the limiting factor for prophylactic use of reversible inhibitors (Modifed from Bajgar *et al.*, 2009b,c).

The mechanism of the prophylactic action of reversible inhibitors can be explained as follows: after exposure to a nerve agent, a part of AChE (central and peripheral) is irreversibly inhibited. Higher inhibition causes more pronounced symptoms of poisoning.

The reversible inhibitor (preferably carbamate pyridostigmine – C – or other) inhibits (carbamylates) AChE in the non-intoxicated organism at peripheral sites (some inhibitors depending on their structure also act on the central nervous system) in a reversible manner; this part of AChE is then resistant to nerve agents. After spontaneous decarbamylation releasing AChE serves as a source of normal enzyme. A higher dose of the reversible inhibitor leads to higher prophylactic efficacy (but if inhibition is too high, it leads to toxic side-effects). Thus, effective prophylaxis is a compromise: inhibition must be as high as possible for (prophylaxis and, simultaneously, as low as as possible to exclude side-effects). Pyridostigmine bromide was the first prophylactic antidote introduced into different armies, e.g. in the USA, UK, France, Switzerland, etc.

The ability of some carbamates to protect organisms poisoned with OPs has been known about for many years (Koelle, 1946; Koster, 1946). Physostigmine and neostigmine have been used to protect animals against diisopropyl fluorophosphate (DFP). The number of OPs studied for protection was enlarged as well as the number of carbamates studied. These studies were performed both *in vitro* and *in vivo*.

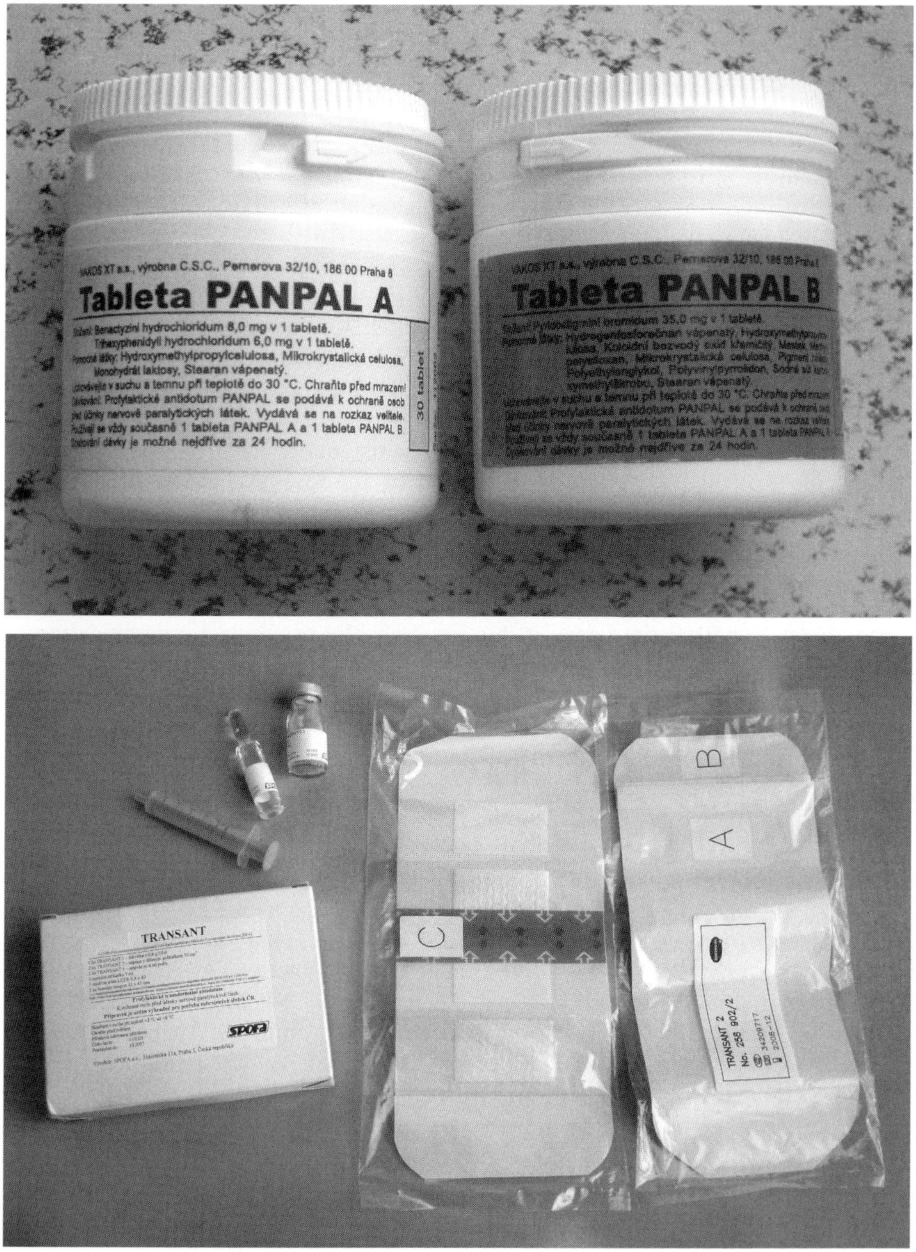

(a)

(b)

Fig. 23.3. Prophylactic means PANPAL (a) and TRANSANT (b) (personal archive of the author).

The results are very dependent on experimental conditions, nevertheless, the protective effect of physostigmine, aminostigmine, pyridostigmine and others against AChE inhibition caused by different OPs (mostly soman) was demonstrated (Patočka, 1989; Marrs *et al.*, 1996; Tonkopii, 2003).

Important contributions based on modelling of different inhibition processes in OP-intoxicated organims were described by Ellin (1982), Green (1983) and Maxwell *et al.* (1987). There have been numerous studies demonstrating effectivity of carbamate pre-treatment/prophylaxis against intoxication with OPs.

From the results published (and unpublished) it appeared that pyridostigmine was the most promising prophylactic drug especially against soman poisoning (Bajgar, 1991, 1996, 2004; Patočka *et al.*, 1991; Anderson *et al.*, 1992; Koplovitz *et al.*, 1992; Maxwell *et al.*, 1993; Wolthuis *et al.*, 1994; Marrs *et al.*, 1996; Kassa *et al.*, 1997, 2001a,b; Kassa, 1998; Tuovinen, 1998; Koupilova and Kassa, 1999; Fusek *et al.*, 2000, 2006; Kassa and Vachek, 2002; Layish *et al.*, 2005). On the basis of these results, pyridostigmine was introduced into some armies as a prophylactic against nerve agents. Its prophylactic effect (like effects of other carbamates) is limited by its dose. At higher doses, higher efficacy was observed but side-effects were more severe too.

This problem can be solved by the addition of pyridostigmine antagonizing drugs – anticholinergics not substantively inhibiting cholinesterases. Many anticholinergics have been tested for the possibility of protecting organisms from intoxication with soman (and other nerve agents) and, on the basis of this research, the prophylactic combination of pyridostigmine with trihexyphenidyle and benactyzine (Bajgar, 1991; Kassa and Bajgar, 1996; Kassa, 1998; Kassa and Fusek, 1998; Kassa *et al.*, 2001a,b; Kassa and Vachek, 2002) was introduced into the Czech and Slovak Army. The presence of two anticholinergics allows the increase of the pyridostigmine dose, which increases its prophylactic efficacy. This combination (and following therapy) is not limited to soman, sarin and VX poisoning but has been observed to have high efficacy against tabun (Kassa and Vachek, 2002), GV (Bajgar, 2004) and cyclosarin (Kassa and Cabal, 1999) intoxication. The aforementioned nerve agents are known to be resistant to common antidotal treatment. The prophylactic antidote called PANPAL (Fig. 23.3a) has no side-effects, as has been demonstrated on volunteers: no statistically different changes in actual psychic state as well as no negative changes in dysfunction time were observed. An improvement of hits by reaction velocity, following PANPAL administration was demonstrated. A reduction in heartbeat frequency 60 min following PANPAL administration lasting 480 min and returning to normal values within 24 h was demonstrated (Fusek *et al.*, 2000, 2006). On the basis of the results for prophylactic efficacy of different carbamates, aminostigmine was chosen as the most effective (Tonkopii, 2003). Its ability to protect cholinesterase to a sufficient extent has been demonstrated but not sufficiently documented. Probably (according to personal discussion), aminostigmine is a prophylactic composed of aminostigmine, antioxidant, diazepam and anticholinergic drug, and its efficacy is very high and long lasting. However, without further information (composition, doses of drugs, form, etc.) it cannot be considered relevant for serious discussion.

Other carbamates also have good prophylactic efficacy, especially physostigmine (in contrast to pyridostigmine, due to its central effect) (Sket, 1993; Wolthuis *et al.*, 1994; Tuovinen and Hanninen, 1999; Kim *et al.*, 2001, 2002). Human studies with transdermal physostigmine suggest serious interest in prophylactic use of this drug (Levy *et al.*, 1992; Walter *et al.*, 1995). Mobam and decarboxyfuran were also experimentally considered as potential candidates for prophylaxis. From other inhibitors, aminophenols and OPs were tested but their effects were lower in comparison with pyridostigmine (Marrs *et al.*, 1996).

Structurally different inhibitors from carbamate and OP groups were also studied. From these compounds (preferably binding to the AChE anionic site), tacrine, methoxytacrine and huperzine A were considered and experimentally studied with respect to prophylaxis *in vitro* and *in vivo* (Freeman and Dawson, 1991; Ashani *et al.*, 1992; Lau, 1992; Raves *et al.*, 1997; Patočka, 1998; Patočka and Kassa, 1999; Lallement *et al.*, 2002). The most interesting results were obtained with huperzine A, which is an inhibitor of rat brain AChE (mixed linear competitive type) (McKinney *et al.*, 1991). Very similar results were obtained with enzymes from other sources (Saxena *et al.*, 1994). Huperzine A was tested as a potential candidate on OP for its long-lasting efficacy and relatively low toxicity (Grunwald *et al.*, 1994). However, the results obtained do not support replacement of pyridostigmine by these drugs.

Detoxification

This principle can be applied in two different ways: administration of the enzymes hydrolysing OP (catalytic scavengers) or evaluating specific binding enzymes (cholinesterases) (stoichiometric scavengers).

Stoichiometric and Catalytic Scavengers

In stoichiometric scavengers, the nerve agent is bound to the exogenously administered enzyme and thus its level in the organism is decreased (it acts as a 'scavenger'). Enzymes hydrolysing OPs/nerve agents – catalytic scavengers – are under research (Raveh *et al.*, 1992; Li *et al.*, 1995). These enzymes display a turnover with OPs/nerve agents as substrates, allowing rapid and efficient protection (Masson *et al.*, 1998). Paraoxonase seems to be very promising (Aharoni *et al.*, 2004; Rochu *et al.*, 2008; Valiyaveettil *et al.*, 2011a,b). On the other hand, many studies have been carried out on cholinesterases as scavengers. BuChE and AChE were observed to be very effective in protection against OP intoxication (Doctor *et al.*, 1991, 1997, 2002; Maxwell *et al.*, 1993, 1998; Marrs *et al.*, 1996; Moore, 1996; Saxena *et al.*, 1997; Clark *et al.*, 2002; Bajgar *et al.*, 2007a,b). The administration of enzymes as scavengers seems to be very promising: the enzyme acts at the very beginning of toxic action, without interaction with target tissues and without side-effects (Clark *et al.*, 2002; Doctor *et al.*, 1997, 2002). All these features are of great interest and they are leading towards practical results (Saxena *et al.*, 2004; Huang *et al.*, 2007). Some problems remain to be solved such as examination for lack of an autoimmune response and establishment of pharmacokinetic and pharmacodynamic properties (Saxena *et al.*, 2002). Recombinant human BuChE can be produced from the milk of transgenic goats (Cerasoli *et al.*, 2005). Moreover, BuChE pre-treatment also showed protective effects on AChE inhibition in the brain parts following low-level sarin inhalation exposure (Sevelova *et al.*, 2004). According to the latest research in bioengineering and biotechnology, connection between two enzymes will be possible, with the aim of obtaining a modified enzyme splitting OP and simultaneously reacting with AChE as a scavenger (Broomfield *et al.*, 1997). Antibodies against OPs are in the stadium of research with the aim to detect different types of OPs.

Pseudocatalytic Scavengers

Simultaneous administration of BuChE and reactivators is also an interesting approach to prophylaxis: BuChE acts as a scavenger binding the nerve agent; the reactivator acting as a pseudocatalytic bioscavenger reactivating BuChE simultaneously, and then reactivated enzyme serves as a new scavenger (Jun *et al.*, 2008).

This approach was tested on human BuChE with the aim of finding a potent oxime, suitable to serve as a pseudocytalytic bioscavenger in combination with this enzyme (Jun *et al.*, 2011). According to their results, the best broad-spectrum AChE reactivators were trimedoxime and obidoxime in the case of paraoxon, leptophos oxon and methamidophos-inhibited AChE. Methamidophos and leptophos oxon were quite easily reactivatable by all tested reactivators. In the case of methamidophos-inhibited AChE, the lower oxime concentration (10^{-5} M) had higher reactivation ability than the 10^{-4} M concentration. Therefore, it was considered that the reactivation ability of obidoxime was in a concentration range of 10^{-3}–10^{-7} M. The reactivation of methamidophos-inhibited AChE with different obidoxime concentrations resulted in a bell-shaped curve with maximum reactivation at 10^{-5} M. In the case of BuChE, no reactivator exceeded 15% reactivation ability and therefore none of the oximes can be recommended as a candidate for pseudocatalytic bioscavengers with BuChE (Jun *et al.*, 2011).

Simulation of Treatment

It appears from therapeutic approaches to OP poisoning that currently used antidotes can be considered and tested as prophylactics. Standard antidotes have been studied in this respect, i.e. anticholinergics, reactivators, anticonvulsants and others (Patočka *et al.*, 1991; Samnaliev *et al.*, 1997; Marrs *et al.*, 1996). The problem with their use is timing and duration and achievement of sufficient levels of these antidotes after administration. However, the prophylactic efficacy is good as is demonstrated in studies of treatment – administration of antidotes is mostly very shortly (minutes) after intoxication. The prolongation of the duration of the antidote effect by ensuring their sufficient levels in the blood by oral administration is not possible (especially reactivators) and therefore is excluded. This was a reason for searching for other routes of administration. Transdermal administration of one of the most effective reactivators (HI-6) was shown to be the most realistic proposition (Dolezal *et al.*, 1988). The final result was a new prophylactic transdermal antidote TRANSANT (Fig. 23.3b) (Bajgar, 2004, 2009; Fusek *et al.*, 2007; Bajgar *et al.*, 2010a,b).

This preparation was clinically tested (including dermal sensitivity) without any harmful effects and field testing was also successful. Final reports are finished and TRANSANT has been prepared for approval and introduction into the Czech Army. Transdermal administration is very promising and this type of administration has also been experimentally studied. There are some examples in clinical practice: transdermal scopolamine for the prevention of operative nausea and vomiting (not for prophylaxis) has been used (Nachum *et al.*, 2006; Apfel *et al.*, 2010). The dosing is not simple, as documented by Lin *et al.* (2011): they observed delirium due to a scopolamine patch in a 4-year-old child. Other anticholinergics (hyoscine) have also been studied as potential prophylactic drugs. Transdermal physostigmine as a reversible inhibitor of cholinesterase in combination with procyclidine was studied in dogs in experimental intoxication with soman (Levy *et al.*, 1992). Sustained release of the same compound (physostigmine) in combination with scopolamine (to combat the side-effects of physostigmine) was described by Meshulam *et al.* (2001). Prophylactic efficacy of other drugs has also been studied – benodiazepines (diazepam, midazolam, alprazolam, triazolam, clonazepam) have been studied to explore their effects as anticonvulsant drugs, but isolated prophylactic administration has not had very good results (Herink *et al.*, 1990, 1991; Kubova *et al.*, 1990; Marrs *et al.*, 1996).

Combination and Different Drugs

Calcium antagonists (nimodipine), neuromuscular blockers (tubocurarine), adamantanes (memantine) and opiate antagonist meptazinol (Galli and Mazri, 1988; Marrs *et al.*, 1996; Karlsson *et al.*, 1998; Stojiljkovic *et al.*, 1998) were also tested with different results but they were not suitable for practical use. On the other hand, positive prophylactic effects have been demonstrated with procyclidine (antimuscarinic, antinicotinic and anti-NMDA receptor drug) (Myhrer *et al.*, 2003). Special attention should be focused on suramine (a protease inhibitor). Administration of this compound prior to soman intoxication (and followed by administration of atropine) showed a good prophylactic effect (Cowan *et al.*, 1996). However, all these studies are experimental studies and have not led to practical output.

Aerosolized scopolamine protects against inhalation toxicity of sarin in guinea pigs Che *et al.* (2011). These combinations can be of very different character. They can be used simultaneously (combination of different drugs) or as pre-treatments and following treatment with different antidotes. Administration of pyridostigmine (or other inhibitors) prior to intoxication and treatment with different drugs is a typical example (Anderson *et al.*, 1992; Kassa and Bajgar, 1996; Tuovinen and Hanninen, 1999; Kim *et al.*, 2001, 2002, 2005; Bajgar, 2009). There are other combinations such as the administration of triesterase (Tuovinen, 1998), procyclidine (Kim *et al.*, 2001, 2002), clonidine (Loke *et al.*, 2001) and sustained release of physostigmine and scopolamine (Meshulam *et al.*, 2001). The results are very dependent on experimental conditions but this approach – administration of different drugs – has yielded some good results though they are until now on an experimental level only.

Summarizing these results, the following drugs have been tested as potential prophylactics: pyridostigmine, aminostigmine, physostigmine, huperzine A, acridines – 7-methoxytacrin and tacrin from the group of reversible cholinesterase inhibitors; benactyzine, biperidene, scopolamine, atropine and trihexyphenidyle from anticholinergics; HI-6, 2-PAM, obidoxime, trimedoxime and methoxime from the reactivators. Suramine, benzodiazepines, memantine, procyclidine, nimodipin and clonidine are other drugs that have been tested. Acetylcholinesterase, butyrylcholinesterase, mutants, triesterase and paraoxonase are other prophylactics based on enzymatic nature. Though the choice of prophylactics is relatively large, only a small number of prophylactic drugs have been chosen for medical military practice. At present, pyridostigmine seems to be a common prophylactic antidote; prophylactics PANPAL (tablets with pyridostigmine, trihexyphenidyle and benactyzine) and TRANSANT (transdermal patch containing HI-6) are other means introduced into different armies as prophylactics. Future development will be focused on scavengers (cholinesterases and other enzymes) acting before the binding of the nerve agent to the target sites, and on drugs such as reversible cholinesterase inhibitors (e.g. huperzine A, physostigmine, acridine derivatives, etc.) or other compounds. Simultaneously, new routes of administration favouring transdermal application (e.g. Levy *et al.*, 1992; Meshulam *et al.*, 2001; Kim *et al.*, 2005; Bajgar *et al.*, 2009b, 2010b, 2011) are of interest.

These and many other studies have been performed to improve prophylaxis of nerve agent/OP poisoning. They contribute to elucidation of nerve agent action on the nervous system. This approach could lead to improvement of our knowledge of mechanisms of action of nerve agents and other inhibitors and of the poisoning caused by these chemicals and their treatments. Simultaneously, it could contribute to better understanding of cholinergic nerve transmission and thus to biochemistry, pharmacology and neuropharmacology in general.

Conclusions

- A very small number of prophylactics studied are in regular use by the military medical service – only three prophylactic antidotes have been introduced into different armies: pyridostigmine alone, PANPAL composed of pyridostigmine, benactyzine and trihexyphenidyle, and TRANSANT (transdermal administration of HI-6).Simple prophylaxis (without post-exposure treatment) is not sufficient to treat OP intoxication.
- Pyridostigmine is an important prophylactic drug especially when it is combined with post-exposure antidotal treatment.
- Prophylaxis with a combination of different drugs is of special importance.
- For further development, it is necessary to research new drugs for prophylaxis.
- New routes of administration of prophylactics are of interest for further evaluation.
- Preparations of cholinesterases are of special importance for development of more effective prophylactics.

References

Aharoni, A., Gaidukov, L., Yagur, S., Toker, L., Silman, I. and Tawfik, D.S. (2004) Directed evolution of mammalian paraoxonases PON1 and PON3 for bacterial expression and catalytic specialization. *Proceedings of the National Academy of Sciences USA* 101, 482–487.

Aldridge, W.N. (1969) Organophosphorus compounds and carbamates, and their reactions with esterases. *British Medical Bulletin* 25, 236–239.

Anderson, D.R., Harris, L.W., Woodard, C.L. and Lennox, W.I. (1992) The effect of pyridostigmine pretreatment on oxime efficacy against intoxication by soman and VX in rats. *Drug and Chemical Toxicology* 15, 285–294.

Annapurna, V., Senciall, I., Davis, A.J. and Kutty, K.M. (1991) Relationship between serum pseudocholinesterase and triglycerides in experimentally induced diabetes mellitus in rats. *Diabetologia* 34, 320–324.

Apfel, C.C., Zhang, K., George, E., Shi, S., Jalota, L., Hornuss, C., Fero, K.E., Heidrich, F., Pergolizzi, J.V., Cakmakkaya, O.S. and Kranke, P. (2010) Transdermal scopolamine for the prevention of postoperative nausea and vomiting: a systematic review and meta-analysis (November, p. 1987, 2010). *Clinical Therapeutics* 32, 2502.

Ashani, Y., Peggins, J.O. and Doctor, B.P. (1992) Mechanism of inhibition of cholinesterases by huperzine A. *Biochemical and Biophysical Research Communications* 184, 719–726.

Bajgar, J. (1991) The influence of inhibitors and other factors on cholinesterases. *Sbornik Vedeckych Praci Lekarske Fakulty UK (Hradec Kralove)* 34, 3–75.

Bajgar, J. (1992) Biological monitoring of exposure to nerve agents. *British Journal of Industrial Medicine* 49, 648–653.
Bajgar, J. (1996) Present views on toxidynamics of soman poisoning. *Acta Medica (Hradec Kralove)* 39, 101–105.
Bajgar, J. (2004) Organophosphates/nerve agent poisoning: mechanism of action, diagnosis, prophylaxis and treatment. *Advances in Clinical Chemistry* 38, 151–216.
Bajgar, J. (2005) Laboratory diagnosis of organophosphates/nerve agent poisoning. *Klinicka Biochemie a Metabolismus* 13(34), 40–47.
Bajgar, J. (2009) Development of antidotes against nerve agents in the Czech Republic. *ASA Newsletters* 09-06, No 135, 1, 7–9.
Bajgar, J. (2011) Chemical warfare agents misuseable in the civilian sector, history and misusing of CWA (in Czech). In: Klement, C. (ed.) *Extraordinary Events in the Public Health Service* (Mimoriadne události vo verejnom zdravotníctve, in Slovak). Vydavatelstvo PRO, Banská Bystrica, pp. 206–257.
Bajgar, J., Bartosova, L., Kuca, K., Jun, D. and Fusek J. (2007a) Changes of cholinesterase activities in the rat blood and brain after sarin intoxication pretreated with butyrylcholinesterase. *Drug and Chemical Toxicology* 30, 351–359.
Bajgar, J., Hajek, P., Slizova, D., Krs, O., Fusek, J., Kuca, K., Jun, D., Bartosova, L. and Blaha, V. (2007b) Changes of acetylcholinesterase activity in different brain areas following intoxication with nerve agents: biochemical and histochemical study. *Chemico-Biological Interactions* 165, 14–21.
Bajgar, J., Fusek, J., Kassa, J., Kuca, K. and Jun, D. (2009a) Global impact of chemical warfare agents used before and after 1945. In: Gupta, R.C. (ed.) *Handbook of Toxicology of Chemical Warfare Agents*. Elsevier/AP, Amsterdam, pp. 17–24.
Bajgar, J., Fusek, J., Kassa, J., Kuca, K. and Jun, D. (2009b) Pharmacological prophylaxis against nerve agent poisoning: experimental studies and practical implications. In: Gupta, R.C. (ed.) *Handbook of Toxicology of Chemical Warfare Agents*. Elsevier/AP, Amsterdam, pp. 877–886.
Bajgar, J., Fusek, J., Kassa, J., Kuca, K. and Jun, D. (2009c) Chemical aspects of pharmacological prophylaxis against nerve agent poisoning. *Current Medicinal Chemistry* 16, 2977–2986.
Bajgar, J., Kuca, K., Fusek, J., Jun, D. and Bartosova, L. (2010a) Cholinesterase reactivators as prophylactics against nerve agents. *Current Bioactive Compounds* 6, 2–8.
Bajgar, J., Kassa, J., Kuca, K., Fusek, J. and Stetina, R. (2010b) Antidotes against chemical warfare agents (CWA) in the Czech Army (in Czech). *Urgentni Medicina* 13, 12–14.
Bajgar, J., Kassa, J. and Kuca, K. (2011) Medical countermeasures in case of threat or use of nerve agents. Presented at CBMTS Industry VII, World Congress on CBRN Threat and Terrorism. Cavtat-Dubrovnik, 10–15 April 2011. Technical Program, p. 22.
Bardin, P.G., van Eeden, S.F., Moolman, J.A., Foden, A.P. and Joubert, J.R. (1994) Organophosphate and carbamate poisoning. *Archives of Internal Medicine* 154, 1433–1441.
Benschop, H.P. and De Jong, L.P.A. (2001) Toxicokinetics of nerve agents. In: Somani, S.M. and Romano, J.A. (eds) *Chemical Warfare Agents: Toxicity at Low Levels*. CRC Press, Boca Raton, Florida, pp. 25–81.
Bosak, A., Katalinic, M. and Kovarik, Z. (2011) Cholinesterases: structure, role, and inhibition (in Croatian). *Archives of Industrial Hygiene and Toxicology* 62, 175–190.
Brimijoin, S. and Rakonczay, Z. (1986) Immunocytology and molecular histology of cholinesterases: current results and prospects. *International Review of Neurobiology* 28, 353–410.
Broomfield, C.A., Lockridge, O., Millard, C.B. and Lenz, D.E. (1997) Design and construction of butyrylcholinesterase mutants that have organophosphorus acid anhydride hydrolase activity. Mini CB Medical Treatment Symposium, Hradec Kralove, Czech Republic.
Brown, S.S., Kalow, W., Pilz, W., Whittaker, M. and Woronick, C.L. (1981) The plasma cholinesterases: a new perspectives. *Advances in Clinical Chemistry* 22, 1–123.
Cabal, J., Kuca, K., Jun, D., Musilek, K., Marek, J., Soukup, O. and Pohanka, M. (2009) Structure-activity relationship of nerve agents. In: Bajgar, J. (ed.) *Central and Peripheral Nervous System: Effects of Highly Toxic Organophosphates and Their Antidotes*. Research Signpost, Kerala, India, pp. 101–117.

Cerasoli, D.M., Griffiths, E.M., Doctor, B.P., Saxena, A., Fedorko, J.M., Greig, N.H., Yu, Q.S., Huang, Y., Wilgus, H., Karatzas, C.N., Koplovitz, I. and Lenz, D.E. (2005) *In vitro* and *in vivo* characterization of recombinant human butyrylcholinesterase (Protexia) as a potential nerve agent bioscavenger. *Chemico-Biological Interactions* 157: 363–365.

Che, M.M., Chanda, S., Song, J., Doctor, B.P., Rezk, P.E., Sabrieka, P., Perkins, M.W., Sciuto, A.M. and Nambiar, M.P. (2011) Aerosolized scopolamine protects against microinstillation inhalation toxicity to sarin in guinea pigs. *Toxicology Mechanisms and Methods* 21, 463–472.

Clark, M.G., Saxena, A., Anderson, S.M., Sun, W., Bansal, R., Myers, T.M. and Doctor, B.P. (2002) Behavioral toxicity of purified human serum butyrylcholinesterase in mice. The 4th International CBMTS, 28 April–3 May 2002, Spiez, Switzerland, Abstract No 19.

Cowan, F.M., Shih, T.M., Lenz, D.E., Madsen, J.M. and Broomfield, C.A. (1996) Hypothesis for synergistic toxicity of organophosphorus poisoning-induced cholinergic crisis and anaphylactoid reactions. *Jornal of Applied Toxicology* 16, 25–33.

Darvesh, S., Hopkins, D.A. and Geula, C. (2003) Neurobiology of butyrylcholinesterase. *Nature Reviews Neuroscience* 4, 131–138.

Doctor, B.P., Raveh, L., Wolfe, A.D., Maxwell, D.M. and Ashani, Y. (1991) Enzymes as pretreatment drugs for organophosphate toxicity. *Neuroscience and Behavioral Review* 15, 123–128.

Doctor, B.P., Maxwell, D.M. and Saxena, A. (1997) Preparation and characterization of bioscavengers for possible use against organophosphate toxicity. M-CB Medical Treatment Symposium, 26–30 May 1997, Hradec Kralove, Czech Republic, Abstracts, pp. 17–18.

Doctor, B.P., Saxena, A., Clark, M.G., Bansal, R., Luo, C., Rosenberg, Y., Lenz, D. and Ashani, Y. (2002) Scavenger protection against organophosphates by human serum butyrylcholinesterase. The 4th International CBMTS, 28 April–3 May 2002, Spiez, Switzerland, Abstract No 24.

Dolezal, P., Vachek, J. and Hrabalek, A. (1988) In vitro transdermal permeation of a cholinesterase reactivator HI-6. In: Brain, R.K. and Walters, K.A. (eds) *Perspectives in Percutaneous Penetration.* Vol. 6A, STS Publishing, Cardiff, UK, p. 84.

Ellin, R.I. (1982) Anomalies in theories and therapy of intoxication by potent organophosphorus anticholinesterase compounds. *General Pharmacology* 13, 457–456.

Fleisher, J.H. and Harris, L.W. (1965) Dealkylation as a mechanism for ageing for cholinesterase after poisoning with pinacolyl methylphosphonofluoridate. *Biochemical Pharmacology* 14, 641–650.

Freeman, S.E. and Dawson, R.M. (1991) Tacrine: a pharmacological review. *Progress in Neurobiology* 36, 257–277.

Fusek, J., Bajgar, J. and Vachek, J. (2000) The prophylactic antidote against nerve paralytic agents – PANPAL. Working Group TG 003, 11–13 September 2000, The Hague, the Netherlands.

Fusek, J., Bajgar, J. and Merka, V. (2006) Prophylaxe von Vergiftungen mit Nervenkampfstoffen (Ergebnisse einer klinischen Studie). *Koordinierter Sanitatsdienst* 24, 48–53.

Fusek, J., Bajgar, J. and Merka, V. (2007) Medikamentose Prophylaxe bei Vergiftungen mit Nervenkampfstoffen. *Koordinierter Sanitatsdienst* 25, 41–47.

Fusek, J., Bajgar, J., Kassa, J., Hajek, P., Slizova, D. and Krs, O. (2009) Differences in the action of G- and V-agents. In: Bajgar, J. (ed.) *Central and Peripheral Nervous System: Effects of Highly Toxic Organophosphates and Their Antidotes.* Research Signpost, Kerala, India, pp. 9–17.

Galli, A. and Mazri, A. (1988) Protection against diisopropylfluorophosphate intoxication by Meptazinol. *Toxicology and Applied Pharmacology* 95, 388–396.

Green, A.L. (1983) A theoretical kinetic analysis of the protective action exerted by eserine and other carbamate anticholinesterase against poisoning by organophosphorus compounds. *Biochemical Pharmacolology* 32, 1717–1722.

Grunwald, J., Raveh, L., Doctor, B.P. and Ashani, Y. (1994) Huperzine A as a pretreatment candidate drug against nerve agent toxicity. *Life Sciences* 54, 991–997.

Hajek, P., Bajgar, J., Slizova, D., Krs, O., Kuca, K., Capek, L. and Fusek, J. (2009) Intoxication with VX and Russian VX: different inhibition of acetylcholinesterase in selected parts of the rat brain. *Drug and Chemical Toxicology* 32, 1–8.

Herink, J., Bajgar, J. and Patočka, J. (1975) Changes of acetylcholinesterase activity in some parts of the limbic system following septal lesions in rats. *Journal of Neurochemistry* 25, 187–188.

Herink, J., Bajgar, J. and Hrdina, V. (1980) Participation of cholinergic mechanisms in the propagation of after-discharges in the limbic system. *Electroencephalography and Clinical Neurophysiology* 48, 56–57.

Herink, J., Koupilova, M. and Hrdina, V. (1990) Effect of alprazolam on pentylentetrazol convulsions. *Activitas Nervosa Superior (Prague)* 32, 297–298.

Herink, J., Koupilova, M. and Bajgar, J. (1991) Effect of triazolam on convulsions induced by pentylentetrazol. *Homeostasis* 33, 181.

Huang, Y.-J., Huang, Y., Baldassarre, H., Wang, B., Lazaris, A., Leduc, M., Bilodeau, A.S., Bellemare, A., Cote, M., Herskovits, P., Touati, M., Turcotte, C., Valeanu, L., Lemée, N., Wilgus, H., Bégin, I., Bhatia, B., Rao, K., Neveu, N., Brochu, E., Pierson, J., Hockley, D.K., Cerasoli, D.M., Lenz, D.E., Karatzas, C.N. and Lagermann, S. (2007) Recombinant human butyrylcholinesterase from milk of transgenic animals to protect against organophosphate poisoning. *Proceedings of the National Academy of Sciences USA* 104, 13603–13608.

Jokanovic, M. (2009) Current understanding of the mechanisms involved in metabolic detoxification of warfare nerve agents. *Toxicology Letters* 188, 1–10.

Jun, D., Musilova, L., Kuca, K., Kassa, J. and Bajgar, J. (2008) Potency of several oximes to reactivate human acetylcholinesterase and butyrylcholinesterase inhibited by paraoxon in vitro. *Chemico-Biological Interactions* 175, 421–424.

Jun, D., Musilova, L., Musilek, K. and Kuca, K. (2011) *In vitro* ability of currently available oximes to reactivate organophosphate pesticide-inhibited human acetylcholinesterase and butyrylcholinesterase. *International Journal of Molecular Sciences* 12, 2077–2087

Kadar, T., Raveh, L., Cohen, G., Oz, N., Baraness, I., Balan, A., Ashani, Y. and Shapira, S. (1985) Distribution of 3H-soman in mice. *Archives of Toxicology* 58, 45–49.

Karlsson, B.M., Koch, M. and Koskinen, L.O.D. (1998) Effects of soman in animals pretreated with nimodipine. Proceedings from 6th CBW Protection Symposium, Stockholm, 15–19 May 1998, pp. 181–184.

Kassa, J. (1998) Non-specific effects of organophosphorus inhibitors of cholinesterases. *Vojenske Zdravotnicke Listy* 67, 15–19.

Kassa, J. (2002) Review of oximes in the antidotal treatment of poisoning by organophosphorus nerve agents. *Journal of Toxicology Clinical Toxicology* 6, 803–816.

Kassa, J. and Bajgar, J. (1996) The influence of pharmacological pretreatment on efficacy of HI-6 oxime in combination with benactyzine in soman poisoning in rats. *Human and Experimental Toxicology* 15, 383–388.

Kassa, J. and Cabal, J. (1999) A comparison of the efficacy of acetylcholinesterase reactivators against cyclohexyl methylphosphonofluoridate (GF agent) by *in vitro* and *in vivo* methods. *Pharmacology and Toxicology* 84, 41–45.

Kassa, J. and Fusek, J. (1998) The positive influence of a cholinergic-anticholinergic pretreatment and antidotal treatment on rats poisoned with supralethal doses of soman. *Toxicology* 128, 1–7.

Kassa, J. and Vachek, J. (2002) A comparison of the efficacy of pyridostigmine alone and in the combination of pyridostigmine with anticholinergic drugs as pharmacological pretreatment of tabun-poisoned rats and mice. *Toxicology* 177, 179–185.

Kassa, J., Fusek, J. and Bajgar, J. (1997) The importance of PANPAL pretreatment for survival of rats poisoned with supralethal dose of soman. Mini-CB Medical Treatment Symposium, 26–30 May 1997, Hradec Kralove, Czech Republic, Abstracts, pp. 21–22.

Kassa, J., Vachek, J., Bajgar, J. and Fusek, J. (2001a) A combination of pyridostigmine with anticholinergic drugs: effective pharmacological pretreatment of soman-poisoned mice. *ASA Newsletter* 84, 16–19.

Kassa, J., Vachek, J., Bajgar, J. and Fusek, J. (2001b) A comparison of the efficacy of pharmacological pretreatments against soman in mice. *Vojenske Zdravotnicke Listy* 70, suppl., 22–25.

Kim, Y.B., Cheon, K.C., Hur, G.H., Phi, T.S. and Yeon, G.B. (2001) Prophylactic effect of physostigmine and procyclidine against nerve-agent poisoning. Seventh International Symposium on Protection against CBWA. Stockholm, Sweden, 15–19 June 2001, Abstracts, p. 158.

Kim, Y.B., Cheon, K.C., Hur, G.H., Phi, T.S., Choi, S.J., Hong, D. and Kang, J.K. (2002) Effects of combinational prophylactics composed of physostigmine and procyclidine on soman induced lethality, seizures and brain injuries. *Environmental Toxicology and Pharmacology* 11, 15–21.

Kim, W.S., Cho, Y., Kim, J.C., Huang, Z.Z., Park, S.H., Choi E.K., Shin, S. and Kim, Y.B. (2005) Protection by a transdermal patch containing physostigmine and procyclidine of soman poisoning in dogs. *European Journal of Pharmacology* 525, 135–142.

Koelle, G.B. (1946) Protection of cholinesterase against irreversible inactivation by DFP in vitro. *Journal of Pharmacology and Experimental Therapeutics* 88, 323–327.

Koplovitz, I., Harris, L.W., Anderson, D.R., Lennox, W.J. and Stewart, J.R. (1992) Reduction by pyridostigmine pretreatment of the efficacy of atropine and 2-PAM treatment of sarin and VX poisoning in rodents. *Fundamental and Applied Toxicology* 18, 192–206.

Koster, R. (1946) Synergisms and antagonisms between physostigmine and diisopropyl fluorophosphate in cats. *Journal of Pharmacology and Experimental Therapeutics* 88, 39–46.

Koupilova, M. and Kassa, J. (1999) The influence of Panpal pretreatment on the elimination of soman-induced neurotoxicity by antidotes in rats. *Homeostasis* 39, 133–135.

Kubova, H., Herink, J. and Mares, P. (1990) Effects of clonazepam on epileptic activity induced by local application of atropine into the septum. *Activitas Nervosa Superior (Prague)* 32, 211.

Kutty, K.M. (1980) Biological function of cholinesterase. *Clinical Biochemistry* 13, 239–243.

Lallement, G., Baille, V., Baubichon, D., Carpentier, P., Collombet, J.M., Filliat, P., Foquin, A., Four, E., Masqueliez, C., Testylier, G., Tonduli, L. and Dorandeu, F. (2002) Review of the value of huperzine as pretreatment of organophosphate poisoning. *Neurotoxicology* 23, 1–5.

Lau, W.M. (1992) Protection by tacrine and atropine against the depressant effects of soman in guinea pig atrium. Proceedings of the 4th International Symposium Protection Against Chemical Warfare Agents, Stockholm, 8–12 June 1992, suppl., p. 182.

Layish, I., Krivoy, A., Rotman, E., Finkelstein, A., Tashma, Z. and Yehezkelli, Y. (2005) Pharmacologic prophylaxis against nerve agent poisoning. *Israel Medical Association Journal* 7, 182–187.

Levy, A., Brandeis, R., Meshulam, Y., Shapira, S. and Levy, D. (1992) Human studies with transdermal physostigmine. Proceedings of the 4th International Symposium Protection Against Chemical Warfare Agents, Stockholm, 8–12 June 1992, pp. 277–284.

Li, W.F., Furlong, C.E. and Costa, L.G. (1995) Paraoxonase protects against chlorpyrifos toxicity in mice. *Toxicology Letters* 76, 219–226.

Lin, Y.G., Chen, P.H., Chang, F.Y., Wu, L.T., Liao, K.Y. and Wu, T.C. (2011) Delirium due to scopolamine patch in a 4-year-old baby. *Journal of the Formosan Medical Association* 110, 208–211.

Loke, W.K., Chua, E., Loo, H.P., Tan, S.H. and Teo, C. (2001) Anticonvulsant effects of post-intoxication administered atropine-clonidine drug combination in soman-poisoned rats. Seventh International Symposium on Protection against CBWA. Stockholm, 15–19 June 2001, Abstracts, p. 160.

Lotti, M. (1995) Cholinesterase inhibition – complexities of interpretation. *Clinical Chemistry* 41 (part 2, Suppl.), 1814–1818.

Lotti, M. (2000) Organophosphorus compounds. In: Spencer, P.S. and Schaumburg, H.H. (eds) *Experimental and Clinical Neurotoxicology*, 2nd edn. Oxford University Press, New York, pp. 898–925.

Marrs, T.C., Maynard, R.L. and Sidell, F.R. (1996) *Chemical Warfare Agents. Toxicology and Treatment*. John Wiley and Sons, Chichester, UK.

Masson, P., Josse, O., Lockridge, O., Viguie, N., Taupin, C. and Buhler, C. (1998). Enzymes hydrolyzing organophosphates as potential catalytic scavengers against organophosphate poisoning. *Journal of Physiology (Paris)* 92, 357–362.

Massoulié, J., Pezzementi, L., Bon, S., Krejci, E. and Vallette, F.M. (1993) Molecular and cellular biology of cholinesterases. *Progress in Neurobiology* 41, 31–91.

Maxwell, D.M., Lenz, D.E., Groff, W.A., Kaminskis, A. and Froehlich, H.L. (1987) The effect of blood flow and detoxification on *in vivo* cholinesterase inhibition by soman in rats. *Toxicology and Applied Pharmacology* 88, 66–76.

Maxwell, D.M., Brecht, K.M., Doctor, B.P. and Wolfe, A.D. (1993) Comparison of antidote protection against soman by pyridostigmine, HI-6 and acetylcholinesterase. *Journal of Pharmacology and Experimental Therapeutics* 264, 1085–1089.

Maxwell, D.M., Brecht, K., Saxena, A., Feaster, S. and Doctor, B.P. (1998) Comparison of cholinesterases and carboxylesterase as bioscavengers for organophosphorus compounds. In: Doctor, B.P. *et al.* (eds) *Structure and Function of Cholinesterases and Related Proteins*. Plenum Press, New York, pp. 387–392.

McKinney, M., Miller J.H., Yamada, F., Tuckmantel, W. and Kozikowski, A.P. (1991) Potencies and stereoselectivities of enantiomers of huperzine A for inhibition of rat cortical acetylcholinesterase. *European Journal of Pharmacology* 203, 303–305.

Meshulam, Y., Cohen, G., Chapman, S., Alkalai, D. and Levy, A. (2001) Prophylaxis against organophosphate poisoning by sustained release of scopolamine and physostigmine. *Journal of Applied Toxicolology* 21 (Suppl. 1), S75–S78.

Moore, D.H. (1996) Bioscavengers as antidotes for organophosphorus (OP) agents. Proceedings of the 2nd CBMTS, 7–12 July 1996, Spiez, Switzerland, pp. 330–349.

Morita, H., Yanagisawa, T., Nakajima, M., Shimizu, M., Hirabayashi, H., Okudera, H., Nohara, M., Midorikawa, Y. and Mimura, S. (1995) Sarin poisoning in Matsumoto, Japan. *Lancet* 346, 290–293.

Myhrer, T., Enger, S. and Aas, P. (2003) Soman-induced seizures in rats: possible treatment and prophylaxis. In: Laihia, K. (ed.) *Symposium Proceedings*, NBC 2003, pp. 136–137.

Nachum, Z., Shupak, A. and Gordon, C.R. (2006) Transdermal scopolamine for prevention of motion sickness – clinical pharmacokinetics and therapeutic applications. *Clinical Pharmacokinetics* 45, 543–566.

Nagao, M., Takatori, T., Matsuda, Y., Nakajima, M., Iwase, H. and Iwadare, K. (1997) Definitive evidence for the acute sarin poisoning in diagnosis in the Tokyo subway. *Toxicology and Applied Pharmacology* 144, 198–203.

Ohbu, S., Yamashina, A. and Takasu, N. (1997) Sarin poisoning in Tokyo subway. *South Medical Journal* 90, 587–593.

Ohtomi, S., Takase, M. and Kunagoi, F. (1996) A clinical experience in Japan Self Defence Force (JSDF) Central Hospital. *International Review Armed Force Medical Service* 69, 97–102.

Okomura, T., Suzuki, K. and Fukuda, A. (1998) The Tokyo subway sarin attack. Disaster management. Part 2: hospital response. *Academical Emergency Medicine* 5, 618–624.

Patočka, J. (1989) Effect of pyridostigmine and syntostigmine pretreatment on the inhibition of acetylcholinesterase by O-pinacolyl-methylphosphonofluoridate. In vitro experiments with rat tissues. *Biomedica Biochimica Acta* 48, 715–720.

Patočka, J. (1998) Huperzine A – an interesting anticholinesterase compound from the Chinese herbal medicine. *Acta Medica (Hradec Kralove)* 41, 155–157.

Patočka, J. and Kassa, J. (1999) Huperzine A – prospective prophylactic antidote against organophosphate warfare agent poisoning. *ASA Newsletter* 99(2), 16–19.

Patočka, J., Jakl, A., Bajgar, J. and Fusek, J. (1991) Efficacy of various pretreatment and therapy regimens against soman lethality in mice. *Sbornik Vedeckych Praci Lekarske Fakulty UK (Hradec Kralove)* 34, 243–247.

Patočka, J., Jun, D., Bajgar, J. and Kuca, K. (2006) Prophylaxis against nerve agent intoxications. *Defence Science Journal* 56, 775–784.

Radic, Z., Reiner, E. and Taylor, P. (1991) Role of the peripheral anionic site on acetylcholinesterase: inhibition by substrates and coumarin derivatives. *Molecular Pharmacology* 39, 98–104.

Rakonczay, Z. (1988) Cholinesterase and its molecular forms in pathological states. *Progress in Neurobiology* 31, 311–330.

Raveh, L., Segall, Y., Leader, H., Rothschild, N., Levanon, D., Henis, Y. and Ashani, Y. (1992) Protection against tabun toxicity in mice by prophylaxis with an enzyme hydrolyzing organophosphate esters. *Biochemical Pharmacology* 44, 397–400.

Raves, M.L., Harel, M., Pang, Y.P., Silman, I., Kozikowski, A.P. and Sussman, J.L. (1997) Structure of AChE complexed with the nootropic alkaloid, (-) huperzine A. *Natural Structures in Biology* 4, 57–63.

Rochu, D., Chabriere, E. and Masson, P. (2008) Human paraoxonase: a promising approach for pre-treatment and therapy of organophosphorus poisoning. *Neurochemical Research* 33, 348–354.

Rosenberry, T.L., Mallender, W.D., Thomas, P.J. and Szegletes, T. (1999) A steric blockade model for inhibition of acetylcholinesterase by peripheral site ligands and substrate. *Chemico-Biological Interactions* 119–120, 85–97.

Rotenberg, J.S. and Newmark, J. (2003) Nerve attacks on children: diagnosis and management. *Pediatrics* 112, 648–658.

Samnaliev, I., Draganov, D. and Dishovski, C. (1997) Cholinesterase reactivators as prophylactics against OP intoxication. Mini CB Medical Treatment Symposium, 26–30 May 1997, Hradec Kralove, Czech Republic, Abstract, pp. 27–28.

Saxena, A., Qian, N., Kovach, I.M., Kozikowski, A.P., Pang, Y.P., Vellom, D.C., Radic, Z., Quinn, D., Taylor, P. and Doctor, B.P. (1994) Identification of aminoacid residues involved in the binding of huperzine A to cholinesterases. *Protein Sciences* 3, 1770–1778.

Saxena, A., Maxwell, D.M., Quinn, D.M., Radic, Z., Taylor, P. and Doctor, B.P. (1997) Mutant acetylcholinesterases as potential detoxification agents for organophosphate poisoning. *Biochemical Pharmacology* 54, 269–274.

Saxena, A., Redman, A.M.G., Jiang, X., Lockridge, O. and Doctor, B.P. (1999) Differences in active-site gorge dimensions of cholinesterases revealed by binding of inhibitors to human butyrylcholinesterase. *Chemico-Biological Interactions* 119–120, 61–69.

Saxena, A., Luo, C., Bansal, R., Sun, W., Clark, M.G., Lenz, D.E., Ashani, Y. and Doctor, B.P. (2002) Scavenger protection against organophosphate agents by human serum butyrylcholinesterase. The meeting of NATO TG 004 Task Group on Prophylaxis and Therapy of Chemical Agents, 4–7 November 2002, Oslo, Norway.

Saxena, A., Doctor, B.P., Sun, W., Luo, C., Bansal, R., Naik, R.S., Fedorko, J.M., Koplovitz, I., Maxwell, D.M., Lenz, D.E. and Ross, M.C. (2004) HuBChE: a bioscavenger for protection against organophosphate chemical warfare agents. *US Army Medical Department Journal* 7, 22–29.

Schans, van der, M.J., Lander, B.J., van der Wiel, H., Langenberg, J.P. and Benschop, H.P. (2003) Toxicokinetics of the nerve agent (+/-)-VX ain anesthetized and atropinized hairless guinea pigs and marmosets after intravenous and percutaneous administration. *Toxicology and Applied Pharmacology* 191, 48–62.

Sevelova, L., Bajgar, J., Saxena, A. and Doctor, B.P. (2004) Protective effect of equine butyrylcholinesterase in inhalation intoxication of rats with sarin: determination of blood and brain cholinesterase activities. *Inhalation Toxicology* 16, 531–536.

Shapira, S., Kadar, T., Cohen, G., Chapman, S. and Raveh, L. (1990) Effects of CBDP and MEPQ on the toxicity and distribution of /H3/-soman in mice. *Archives of Toxicology* 64, 663–668.

Shih, T.M., Penetar, D.M., McDonough, J.H., Romano, J.A. and King, J.M. (1990) Age-related differences in soman toxicity and in blood and regional cholinesterase activity. *Brain Research Bulletin* 24, 429–436.

Skau, K.A. (1986) Mammalian acetylcholinesterase: molecular forms. *Comparative Biochemistry and Physiology* 83C, 225–227.

Sket, D. (1993) Efficacy of antidotes against soman poisoning in female physostigmine-protected rats. *Pharmacology and Toxicology* 72, 25–30.

Skopec, F., Bajgar, J. and Patočka, J. (1981) Changes of acetylcholinesterase activity in different brain areas of the rat following head irradiation. *Radiobiology and Radiotherapy* 22, 631–634.

Soreq, H., Gnatt, A., Loewenstein, Y. and Neville, L.F. (1992) Excavations into the active site-gorge of cholinesterase. *Trends in Biochemical Sciences* 17, 353–358.

Stojiljkovic, M.P., Maksimovic, M., Bokonjic, D., Kilibarda, V., Tadic, V. and Boskovic, B. (1998) Adamantanes versus carbamatres as prophylactic agents in soman-poisoned rats. Proceedings from the 6th CBW Protection Symposium, Stockholm, 10–15 May 1998, pp. 197–202.

Sussmann, J.L., Harel, M., Frolow, F., Oefner, C., Goldman, A., Toker, L. and Silman, I. (1991) Atomic structure of acetylcholinesterase from Torpedo californica: a prototypic acetylcholine-binding protein. *Science* 253, 872–874.

Talbot, B.-G., Anderson, D.R., Harris, L.W., Zarbrough, L.W. and Lennox, W.J. (1988) A comparison of in vivo and in vitro rates of ageing of soman-inhibited erythrocyte acetylcholinesterase in different animal species. *Drug and Chemical Toxicology* 11, 289–395.

Taylor, P., Wong, L., Radic, Z., Tsigelny, I., Bruggemann, R., Hosea, N. and Berman, H.A. (1999) Analysis of cholinesterase inactivation and reactivation by systematic structural modification and enantiomeric selectivity. *Chemico-Biological Interactions* 119–120, 3–15.

Tonkopii, V. (2003) Structure and efficiency of carbamates as drugs for prophylaxis against OP poisoning. In: Laihia, K. (ed.) *Symposium Proceedings*, NBC 2003. Research Report No. 98, Jyvaskyla 2003, pp. 140–145.

Tuovinen, K. (1998) Comparison of pyridostigmine, physostigmine, heptylphysostigmine and phosphotriesterase treatments in sarin intoxication. Supplementary Proceedings from the 6th CBW Protection Symposium, Stockholm, 10–15 May 1998, p. 254.

Tuovinen, K. and Hanninen, O. (1999) Protection of mice against soman by pretreatment with eptastigmine and physostigmine. *Toxicology* 139, 233–241.

Vachek, J., Gersl, V., Fusek, J., Krs, O., Skopec, F. and Bajgar, J. (1996) Toxicities of O-alkyl S-(2-dialkylaminoethyl) methyl phosphonothiolates (V-compounds). *Acta Medica (Hradec Kralove)* 39, 67–71.

Vale, A., Marrs, T.C. and Rice, P. (2007) Chemical terrorism and nerve agents. *Medicine* 35, 573–575.

Valiyaveettil, M., Alamneh, Y., Rezk, P., Perkins, M.W., Sciuto, A.M., Doctor, B.P. and Nambiar, M.P. (2011a) Recombinant paraoxonase 1 protects against sarin and soman toxicity following microinstuillation inhalation exposure in guinea pigs. *Toxicology Letters* 202, 203–208.

Valiyaveettil, M., Alamneh, Y., Rezk, P., Biggemann, L., Perkins, M.W., Sciuto, A.M., Doctor, B.P. and Nambiar, M.P. (2011b) Protective efficacy of catalytic bioscavenger, paraoxonase 1 against sarin and soman exposure in guinea pigs. *Biochemical Pharmacology* 81, 800–809.

Van Lith, H.A. and Beynen, A.C. (1993) Dietary cholesterol lowers the activity of butyrylcholinesterase (EC 3.1.1.8), but elevates that of esterase-1 (EC 3.1.1.1) in plasma of rats. *British Journal of Nutrition* 70, 721–726.

Van Lith, H.A., van Zutphen, L.F. and Beynen, A.C. (1991) Butyrylcholinesterase activity in plasma of rats and rabbits fed high-fat diets. *Comparative Biochemistry and Physiology* 98A, 339–342.

Walter, K., Muller, M., Barkworth, M.F., Niciecki, A.V. and Stanislaus, F. (1995) Pharmakokinetics of physostigmine in man following a single application of a transdermal system. *British Journal of Clinical Pharmacology* 39, 59–63.

Whittaker, M. (1980) Plasma cholinesterase variants and the anaesthesist. *Anaesthesia* 35, 174–197.

Wolthuis, O.L., Van Helden, H.P.M., Melchers, B.P.C., Busker, R.W. and Degroot, D.M.G. (1994) Search for a therapy against soman-intoxication. *Neuroscience and Biobehavioural Reviews*18, 469–486.

Yokoyama, K., Araki, S., Murata, K., Nishikitami, M., Okomura, T., Ishimatsu, S. and Takasu, M. (1998) Chronic neurobehavioral and central autonomic nervous system effects in Tokyo subway sarin poisoning. *Journal of Physiology* 92, 317–323.

Yoshida, T. (1994) Toxicological reconsideration of organophosphate poisoning in relation to the possible nerve-gas sarin-poison disaster that happened in Matsumoto-city, Nagano. *Japanese Journal of Toxicology and Environmental Health* 40, 486–497.

Section 8

Handling Psychosocial Issues:

A Difference in Perspective (Developed and Developing Nations)

Chapter 24

Collective Resilience versus Collective Vulnerability after Disasters: A Social Psychological Perspective

Chris Cocking

Introduction

Disasters seem to strike with increasing frequency in our global community, especially now that we live in an era of almost instant media coverage of each new emergency. Therefore, emergency management and disaster mitigation strategies appear to be increasingly necessary in this post-9/11 world. However, it is debatable whether the world we inhabit has become a more dangerous place to live in, or whether people are now more aware of disasters and are so more risk averse. This may also be influenced by the extensive coverage that many disasters receive, especially now technology allows those affected to broadcast footage of disasters to a global audience as they happen.

Despite common expectations that 'mass panic' is the dominant response in mass emergencies (Goltz, 1984; Fahy *et al*., 2011), over 50 years of research, and nearly 500 published articles archived by the US-based Disaster Research Center (http://www.udel.edu/DRC/E.L.%20Quarantelli%20Resource%20Collection/Publications.html), have found that communities often cope with disasters and emergencies much better than expected. Rather than fracturing social bonds, disasters can actually bring people together in mutual support and cooperation in ways rarely seen before the disaster. Nevertheless, there is a contrast in perspectives on how people cope with disasters. Firstly, there is the prevailing orthodoxy advocating the concept of 'vulnerability' where it is assumed that people will be traumatized by these events, that their capacity to cope with the pressures of everyday life may be compromised as a result, and therefore clinical interventions should be developed to help those traumatized readjust to normal life afterwards. More recently though, a new perspective has emerged that considers the concept of 'resilience', where it is argued that both people and organizations cope surprisingly well with adversity, and that behaviour during and after mass emergencies is not so divorced from usual social norms as previously expected. Indeed, both sociological (Tierney and Trainor, 2004; Dynes, 2006) and psychological (Drury *et al.*, 2009a,b; Williams and Drury, 2010) evidence suggest that far from clichéd accounts of mass panic, people and organizations are remarkably resilient both during and after mass emergencies. Therefore, it would seem that approaches to stress and trauma can benefit from the study of collective resilience, and that groups can be considered as a psychological resource that professionals can draw upon to inform their interventions. This chapter will explore the development of models that attempt to explain behaviour during and after mass emergencies, and look at how collective approaches to stress and trauma may help with disaster management and mitigation.

Vulnerability – The Panic Model

A common assumption of approaches that consider a vulnerability framework is the idea that because they are prone to mass panic, people cannot be trusted to behave sensibly in mass emergencies, and so paternalistic measures are needed to protect people from themselves. Early psychological approaches to emergency behaviour (e.g. LaPiere, 1938; Strauss, 1944; Smelser, 1962) assumed mass panic would be the dominant response, drawing upon the work of Gustave Le Bon, an aristocrat living in France during the 1870–1871 Paris Commune (Le Bon, 1968). The observations of the revolutionary crowds he recorded portrayed a deeply negative view of crowds. According to Le Bon, crowds were inherently irrational, with crowd members losing their individuality to a collective 'mob mentality' where they were no longer responsible for their actions. Therefore, crowds were either an actual or potential threat to the status quo and so should be treated as such by the authorities, because even if they were not currently violent and/or anti-social, they could become so at a moment's notice. The following quote illustrates the negative view he held of crowds:

> By the mere fact that he forms part of an organised crowd, a man descends several rungs in the ladder of civilisation. Isolated he may be a cultivated individual; in a crowd he is a barbarian (1968, p. 12).

Le Bon's work forms part of the irrationalist tradition in crowd psychology (Zimbardo, 2004), which informs the panic model – an amalgamation of early sociological accounts of emergency behaviour that assume a vulnerable response from the public. The panic model assumes that in emergencies, people's emotional reactions are disproportionate to the actual threat faced, and overwhelm their ability to think rationally (Smelser, 1962). Any collective identity that people may have felt previously breaks down, as they display selfish behaviours in an effort to escape, such as pushing and trampling (Strauss, 1944; Schultz, 1964). Finally, any selfish individual acts spread quickly to the crowd as a whole in a process of behavioural 'contagion' (McDougall, 1920).

Critiques of the panic model

However, the panic model is widely criticized in academic circles. Social psychologists (e.g. Reicher, 1996) reject the theoretical basis that Le Bon and the irrationalist approaches provide for taking a deeply ideological and partisan view of crowds. Reicher

(2001) argues instead that crowds can be a force for positive social change and often behave in normative ways that are governed by the social context and their interactions with other social groups (such as the police). The idea of mass panic occurring in emergencies has also been largely discredited (Sime, 1990), with Quarantelli (2001) debating whether 'panic' is even a useful term to describe how people actually behave in emergencies. For instance, a study of behaviours exhibited by those evacuating the World Trade Center's twin towers on 11 September 2001 (Blake *et al.*, 2004), found that classic 'panicked' type behaviours accounted for less than 1% of those reported by survivors. If panicked or selfish behaviour occurs in emergencies, it is rare, usually confined to individuals and does not tend to spread to the collective as a whole. Indeed, Quarantelli (2001) argued that there is very little evidence to support the notion of contagion of panic behaviour, and that it is usually a media creation, rather than supported by scientific evidence. For instance, Cantril's (1940) investigation of the alleged mass exodus from US cities after the broadcasting of H.G. Wells' 'War of the Worlds' radio play found that most coverage drew from sensationalized media reports, and that very few listeners (about 12%) believed that it was a real news broadcast, with even fewer displaying signs of distress and/or fleeing their homes. Furthermore, definitions of panic are often subjective and contextually dependent. For instance, rapid flight from an imminent and potentially fatal threat may seem like a logical course of action to those present who may not have access to other external information (such as whether the threat is real or not), but such behaviour could be considered as irrational and hence 'panic' by an outside observer who has access to more information about the source and scale of the threat (Canter, 1990). However, the discrediting of the panic model in academic circles has not prevented belief in it being maintained not only in coverage of disasters in popular discourse (Dynes, 2003; Tierney *et al.*, 2006), but also amongst institutions charged with the safe management of crowds and public order situations (Drury *et al.*, 2003; Drury, 2004). This has serious implications for the safe and effective management of crowds in emergencies, which will now be discussed.

Implications of the panic model

Distrust of the public's emergency response

Furedi (2007) suggests there is a possible contradiction in current security policy among national and international organizations as, while the emphasis is on promoting resilience during emergencies, the premises underpinning such policies assume the vulnerability of those affected. Furthermore, recent research (Drury *et al.*, 2011, unpublished data) into views about 'disaster myths' (e.g. mass panic, collective hysteria, etc.), held by those with experience of working with crowds in emergencies has found seemingly contradictory results. Respondents tended to believe that crowds were prone to 'mass panic', and 'civil disorder' in emergencies, but they also believed emergency crowds were resilient, and rejected the notion that they were helpless. There is also a commonly held belief that panic is often the cause of fatalities in emergencies. However, Mawson (2005) argues that in fact, the opposite response is more likely:

> From a public health or safety point of view, the problem in disasters is not that people tend to panic and act precipitously in response to danger, but that people typically delay or fail to take appropriate evasive action when it is needed (p. 107).

Assumptions of vulnerability can also have practical implications for communication with the public during emergencies, because information about the scale of the threat could be withheld, for fear that people may 'panic' and over-react. This could in turn mean that people are not given enough advice on how they should act (such as evacuating themselves away from danger). This strategy could result in a self-fulfilling prophesy of non-resilience, as any potential for endogenous resilience within communities affected by disasters could be stifled, and people's anxieties may be raised by a lack of available information about what they should do (Wessely, 2005a). It is also possible that there could even be an increased risk of casualties, as lack of available information about what they should do may result in people not taking preventative measures or delaying their own evacuation from danger until it is too late. Unfortunately, this belief in withholding information from the public for fear of mass panic is still pervasive amongst emergency planners, despite evidence that providing information about threats actually enables people to act effectively to escape danger and cope with the threats faced (Proulx and Sime, 1991; Glass and Schoch-Spana, 2002).

Fear of social disintegration

A more sinister implication of the vulnerability framework is the fear of social breakdown in the aftermath of disasters, with an expected increase in looting and civil disorder, as previously civilized people descend into barbarism in the absence of law and order. However, this fear is usually unfounded, and crime rates usually drop after disasters. For instance, initial media reports of mass looting, gang rapes and murders in New Orleans after Hurricane Katrina were later found to be grossly exaggerated (Dynes and Rodriguez, 2006). Dynes (2006) also argues that media use of the term 'looting' after disasters is often dependent upon contextual norms of what is considered appropriate behaviour, with the difference in perception between gathering essential supplies for survival and acquisitive looting often a matter of subjective interpretation. Furthermore, Rebecca Solnit's (2009) coverage of a variety of different natural and man-made disasters in the USA (such as the 1906 San Francisco earthquake, 9/11 and Hurricane Katrina in 2005) argues that far from descending into barbarism, communities affected by disasters are often very adept at organizing mutual cooperation and support, but this spontaneous cooperation is often disrupted by the authorities' fear of anarchy, which causes them to impose martial law to 'restore order'. She even cites shocking examples of how the forces of law and order were more likely to behave anti-socially than the victims of disasters, with accounts of looting by soldiers after the 1906 San Francisco earthquake and African Americans being shot on sight as suspected 'looters' by police and racist vigilantes after Hurricane Katrina.

The Resilience Framework

Resilience as a concept emerged initially from a reaction to what some felt was the overemphasis placed on the potential for trauma arising from early childhood experiences, and instead focused on how individuals could cope with adverse situations (Masten, 2001; Hart *et al.*, 2008). However, it has since been broadened to encompass collective resilience and is being increasingly adopted by emergency planners in preference to the vulnerability perspective, in order to explore strategies to promote resilient communities that are better equipped to prepare for and cope with disasters when they strike (e.g. Topping *et al.*, 2010). Relevant theoretical models that explain how psychological resilience develops and endures will now be addressed.

The social attachment model

Mawson (2005) believed that the typical human response to emergencies is not uncontrollable fear and/or flight, but instead, it is usually to seek out familiar other people and places in order to alleviate stress, and that being separated from familiar others was more likely to be a stressor than objective physical danger. Therefore, he proposed a social attachment model of human behaviour in disasters, inspired by the work of Bowlby (1969) into the effects of separation from parental carers during infancy, whereby the importance of attachment bonds during times of stress was recognized. If flight in emergencies did occur then it could be explained better in terms of escape from situations towards places or people that they felt such attachment bonds. For instance, Freud and Burlingham (1945) (cited in Mawson, 2005) studied the effects of the bombing of London during the Second World War, and found children could endure extreme danger without severe distress if they remained with their parents, but would become more distressed if they were separated from them. Furthermore, studies of behaviour during fatal fires in the USA (e.g. Cornwell, 2003) have found that people were very unwilling to break affiliation bonds with others around them, and people tended to evacuate in their affiliate groups without leaving slower members behind.

The social attachment model illustrates the importance of attachment bonds during emergencies – something neglected by the panic model. However, it does have limitations in that it emphasizes the role of existing affiliation bonds, therefore implying that panic in a crowd of strangers is more likely, and neglecting the possibility that strangers may cooperate with each other in an emergency. Given that the vast majority of crowds during emergencies will probably be composed of complete strangers, those affected will not feel existing affiliative bonds to others around them, and so have less reason to behave cooperatively to those around them, perhaps making selfish, ‘panicked’ behaviour more likely. However, as already documented, the majority of evidence does not support this notion, and so there needs to be a broader theoretical framework to explain why mass panic is rare in mass emergencies.

The social identity model of collective resilience

The social identity model of collective resilience (or SIMCR; Drury *et al.*, 2009a,b; Williams and Drury, 2010) is grounded in social psychological theory and was developed to explain the apparent lack of mass panic in emergency situations where the majority of those affected have minimal existing ties to each other. While the panic model suggests that selfish, individualistic behaviour predominates in emergencies, and the social attachment model argues that existing attachment bonds are maintained through helping known affiliates, the SIMCR proposes that disasters may actually create social bonds between people who previously had no (or minimal) connections with each other. Therefore, in direct contradiction to the panic model, rather than seeing the dissolution of social bonds, the threats faced by those in emergencies can actually create new social ties as people feel a sense of shared fate, and so help complete strangers. Furthermore, the greater the shared sense of danger, the greater the sense of social cohesion, as the need for cooperation and hence group survival becomes more important in the face of such a threat.

The SIMCR is derived from self-categorization theory (SCT), which explains social behaviour in terms of self and group categorization processes (Turner *et al.*, 1987). SCT argues that human beings categorize themselves through multiple identities (ranging on a continuum from the personal to the more collective) that become more or less salient depending on the social context. When more collective identities become salient, we find ourselves categorizing with similar others, and so a common purpose and hence shared sense of identification (or shared in-group membership) with others becomes more likely, especially if the salient in-group faces an external threat. Initially evidence supporting this sense of shared identity was presented from studies of crowd disorder (e.g. Reicher, 1996; Drury and Reicher, 2000; Stott *et al.*, 2001), where an out-group was perceived to be imposing their will illegitimately upon the in-group. However, further research (e.g. Cocking *et al.*, 2009; Drury *et al.*, 2009a,b) found that the threat of a mass emergency or disaster can create a common purpose through a sense of shared fate (e.g. 'we are all in this together'), which results in similar self-categorization processes whereby people feel a shared identity with others they may not necessarily know or even personally like.

SIMCR suggests a number of psychological and behavioural consequences once a shared identity develops amongst those affected by a mass emergency. First, a shared social identity encourages trust and the expectation that others will be supportive and cooperate (Drury and Reicher, 1999). Second, a shared identity helps provide a consensual definition of social reality (Haslam *et al.*, 1998), which allows collective coordination and the ability amongst survivors to organize to protect themselves from further trauma (Williams and Drury, 2010). Third, shared social identity encourages commitment to shared goals and hence self-policing of shared norms (Stott *et al.*, 2001). Finally, a shared social identity encourages solidarity both in the form of mundane social cohesion (Reicher and Haslam, 2010) and through helping others in need (Levine *et al.*, 2005). A shared social identity can develop from an existing group membership, but it also can arise within the emergency itself through the perception of a 'common fate' among survivors, which brings them together psychologically (Clarke, 2002; Drury *et al.*, 2009a). This new shared identity allows people to rely on each other and engage in the emotional and practical support necessary for immediate survival, and may be temporarily stronger than existing group memberships (especially if it develops out of the necessity for group survival).

Evidence for models of resilience

While the social attachment model and SIMCR derive from theoretical perspectives grounded in social and developmental psychology, there is also support for them from evidence of disasters and mass emergencies. For instance, in 1961, Fritz produced a groundbreaking study showing how disasters could be beneficial rather than detrimental for social cohesion (although it was not published until 1996). He investigated the effects of wartime aerial bombardment in the UK and Europe during the Second World War. Together with evidence from peacetime disasters in the USA, he collected data from over 16,000 people involved in around 150 different incidents to create one of the most comprehensive reports to date on how civilian populations cope with mass emergencies. He found that far from bringing out the worst in human nature, disasters can actually help overcome the social alienation and atomization often prevalent in modern society, and even help people rediscover a more communitarian perspective as they cooperated with their fellow survivors in a 'community of sufferers' (Fritz, 1996, p. 28). He believed that such emergent communities could continue for months after one-off disasters, and even indefinitely in the face of continuous threats (such as recurrent peacetime disasters, or on-going attacks upon civilian populations in wartime). Fritz catalogued the effects on the civilian population of the UK, and found that despite concerns that aerial bombardments would result in mass hysteria, there was no evidence to justify this fear, and a study by Atlun in 1941 (cited in Fritz, 1996) of psychiatric hospital admissions in London from September 1939 to April 1941 (when the bombing was at its worst) found that they were much lower than had been expected. Indeed, the specialist 'neurosis centres' that were established to deal with the expected psychiatric victims during the 'Blitz' were hardly used by civilian personnel, with the majority of self-admissions being from military personnel on leave from combat duties instead (Stokes, 1945, cited in Fritz, 1996). Furthermore, Fritz suggested that rather than engaging in headlong flight at the first inkling of a threat, people were more likely to either remain in the disaster zone (unless forced to flee), or even approach the disaster area if they were not already there for a variety of possible reasons, such as: to offer help, look for loved ones or even watch the spectacle unfold. This phenomenon has since become known as convergence, and has been supported by evidence from more recent studies of mass emergencies, such as 9/11 in the USA (Tierney, 2002) and 7/7 in the UK (Drury *et al.*, 2009b).

Emergence

Not only does there appear to be an absence of mass panic during disasters and their immediate aftermath, the prediction by SIMCR that disasters can create social cohesion is also supported. For instance, sociologists, such as Dynes (2006) and Tierney and Trainor (2004) suggest the concept of emergence, whereby new social relationships and activities emerge in response to adverse situations, with the greater the disaster, the greater the potential for such emergent networks to operate. Dynes (2006) felt they encouraged resilience in the following ways:

> Emergent networks enhance resilience because they raise the probability that needed information and resources will become available through network ties and because they empower even network newcomers within the context of the overall response. Networks are also thought to foster the development and diffusion of innovations … a key requirement in the crisis environment (p. 167).

Furthermore, Tierney and Trainor (2004) suggest that the response to 9/11 provides a good example of how emergence encourages innovation because the Emergency Operations Center (EOC) for New York was housed in the World Trade Center 7 building, which was destroyed shortly after the twin towers collapsed, meaning that a new operations centre had to be quickly assembled from scratch. However, organizational structures remained intact, and the rescue and recovery effort in the aftermath of 9/11 was not adversely affected.

Social capital

The concept of emergence has been developed further to explain how social networks can be a useful resource to draw upon in post-disaster management and reconstruction. For instance, Dynes (2006) suggested the concept of 'social capital', whereby social relationships and support networks endure in the face of the collapse of physical infrastructure and mass casualties, and this embedded resilience can help guide the relief effort after disasters. For instance, he argues that while 9/11 was clearly a day of tragic loss and destruction, those who were in the Twin Towers when the planes struck managed to organize a remarkably successful evacuation – an example of how social capital can emerge from those the vulnerability model may assume would be least able to do so:

> At the time of impact there were an estimated 17,400 occupants in those buildings and eighty-seven percent of them evacuated successfully. Most of the deaths were on the floors, or above the floors where the planes hit. It is now determined that ninety-nine percent of those below the impact floors successfully evacuated.[1] This successful evacuation was not accomplished by conventional search and rescue groups; it was the result of people on site helping others and themselves to take protective action to get out of the towers and to a safe location. While the loss of property and life occurring on 9/11 is frequently recalled, the protective actions of the other 'victims' in the building are often overlooked (p. 1).

Fritz (1996) also found that survivors provide most of the initial practical help in disasters. More recent evidence shows that survivors can often take the role of medical 'first responders' before outside help arrives (Drury *et al.*, 2009b), and this concept has been incorporated within the Israeli authorities' emergency response to suicide bombings, whereby first aid kits are made available to other survivors by the ambulance crews when they arrive, so they can assist with the relief effort (Cole *et al.*, 2011).

Enduring Benefits in the Aftermath of Disasters?

Resilient rather than vulnerable responses seem to be the norm during the emergency itself, but does this resilience endure in the days and weeks afterwards, as those affected try to rebuild their lives and communities? There does indeed appear to be evidence to support the idea that psychological resilience can endure and in the right circumstances may also shield disaster survivors from stress and trauma after mass emergencies. For instance, Fritz (1996) felt that people could reassess their lives and relationships with others after disasters, as previous personal and/or social conflicts might no longer be considered important and/or relevant in the face of the new emergency. He believed a disaster:

> provides a form of societal shock, which disrupts habitual, institutionalized patterns of behavior and renders people amenable to social and personal change. The essential effect of shock is to arrest habitual repetitive patterns of behavior and to cause a redefinition *and* restructuring of the situation in accordance with present realities… A shock, therefore, always contains the seeds of change, especially when accompanied by a change in the objective conditions of life involving a removal or obliteration of the stimulus support for old habits of action (p. 55).

---

[1] National Institute of Standards and Technology, 'NIST and the World Trade Center', 26 May, 2006. Available at: http://wtc.nist.gov/.

This sense of societal shock that emerges from disasters and helps promote resilience may also provide possible clinical benefits for survivors. For instance, the vulnerability framework assumes that a significant proportion of those affected by disasters will suffer from post-traumatic stress, requiring some form of psychiatric intervention (Wessely, 2005a,b). However, Williams and Drury (2010) argue that after disasters, only a small minority of those affected actually need treatment. For example, after 9/11 it was predicted that up to 0.5 million New Yorkers could develop post-traumatic stress disorder (PTSD) (Booth, 2002), and while PTSD type symptoms were experienced by up to 10% in some samples (Hoven *et al.*, 2005), others found that the scale of psychiatric casualties was much less than expected (Bonanno *et al.*, 2006). There are even those who question use of the term ‘PTSD’ as a psychiatric diagnosis. For instance, Summerfield (2001) argues that PTSD can be considered as being constructed from social and/or political ideas as much as it is from medicalized psychiatric origins. Furthermore, Drury (2011) argues that feeling distressed after disasters can be a perfectly normal response after what are often very *abnormal* events, and should not necessarily be labelled as a disorder.

Therefore, there has been a growing movement that has challenged the prevailing orthodoxy of vulnerability after traumatic events, and instead argues for the concept of post-traumatic growth (Tedeschi and Calhoun, 2004) whereby physical or psychological trauma can actually help people reassess their perspective towards adversity and sometimes their entire outlook on life, leading Joseph and Linley (2006) to conclude:

> stressful and traumatic events may serve as a trigger towards personal growth and positive change (p. 1041).

Joseph and Linley (2006) also believed that not only individual but collective growth can occur after trauma, especially after mass emergencies, when entire communities are brought together through adversity, and it is also possible that the disaster could create new forms of collective coping amongst the community affected that is independent of outside professional approaches to stress and trauma. For instance, Fritz (1996) concluded from his research that people are endogenously resilient after emergencies and so develop their own forms of coping:

> the situational characteristics of disasters and the human adjustments to them produced a therapeutic milieu that gave cognizance to virtually all the therapeutic knowledge acquired by these different doctrinal approaches. In other words, disaster-struck communities and societies naturally develop therapies that quickly and effectively overcome the losses, traumas, **and** privations of disaster – without the intervention of mental health care professionals (pp. 16–17 [emphasis in original]).

Therefore, it should not be assumed that the dominant response to disasters will necessarily be psychological trauma. Furthermore, there is also controversy about the usefulness of psychological interventions in the immediate aftermath of traumatic events. For instance, van Emmerik *et al.*’s (2002) meta-analysis of studies of critical incident stress debriefing (CISD) found that CISD did not improve natural recovery rates. Therefore, intervention strategies to help communities after disasters would benefit from the adoption of a more resilient approach – perhaps providing instrumental support and/or advice in the immediate aftermath, then screening those considered at risk of PTSD over 1 month after the event and target resources as required if intrusive symptoms persist, as is required for a diagnosis of PTSD under the DSM IV criteria (APA, 2000).

Social Identity and Social Support

There appears to be evidence to support the notion that mass emergencies do not necessarily result in trauma and suffering for all affected, and that disasters can help bring people together in mutual support. But how is this explained in terms of the psychological processes involved? The origins for such an answer may lie in evidence from more general studies into stress and trauma, and how groups can provide positive benefits. For instance, Jetten *et al.* (2011) suggest that the positive benefits of collective psychological identification can provide both psychological and physical benefits. This assertion is supported by a wealth of evidence from a variety of different perspectives. For instance, Haslam *et al.* (2005) found that bomb disposal workers reported lower levels of stress if they felt a positive sense of identity and social support from their work colleagues, and Falomir-Pichastor *et al.* (2009) found that nurses were more likely to get vaccinated against influenza if they identified as nurses, because they felt it was their professional duty to do so. Furthermore, a shared group identity can also psychologically shield people who have suffered bereavement from conflict. Kellezi *et al.* (2009) found that Kosovans who had lost loved ones during the 1999 war felt lower levels of depression and anxiety and also reported a higher sense of self-efficacy if they identified with the aims of the war. This evidence led Haslam *et al.* (2009) to conclude that engaging in collective activity could result in improved well-being, rather than just being its by-product:

> It's not just that because we are well we are more likely to participate in group life, but also that because we participate in group life we are more likely to be well… The quality of group life should be a primary focus for health professionals and policy-makers interested in the welfare of their clients (pp. 15–16).

The positive benefits of social identification and support can also play a role in psychological protection after traumatic events, especially disasters. For instance, a meta-analysis of 77 studies of PTSD by Brewin *et al.* (2000) found that lack of social support after the incident was the strongest predictor for increased risk of PTSD. This seems to support the theoretical position suggested by the SIMCR that a collective identity emerges amongst survivors of disasters. So, while lack of social support may place survivors at risk of trauma, those receiving social support may be more psychologically protected, and so less likely to be vulnerable to trauma afterwards. Furthermore, such a collective identity may also allow group members to coordinate their individual efforts more easily, thus facilitating the provision of mutual emotional aid and support amongst individual survivors. This prediction is supported by evidence (Drury *et al.*, 2009b) from studies of survivors of the 7/7 London bombings that found that they benefited from social support from other survivors with whom they felt a sense of shared experience and so empathized with their perspective. This led some to form their own mutual support groups with others who survived the same explosion (such as Kings Cross United[2]), and they would meet to offer guidance and support for others with whom they felt a sense of shared identity and support. Finally, there has been a growing realization post-9/11 that a more collective approach to treating trauma after disasters may be necessary. For instance, Keane and Piwowarczyk (2006) argue that it is not sufficient to implement

---

[2] http://www.newstatesman.com/200607030032

solely individual interventions after mass disasters, as the collective nature of such incidents means that group treatments are often needed as well:

> models that incorporate individual, group, and societal levels of analysis will undoubtedly be more predictive of the cumulative response of communities to the adversity experienced via disaster (p. 5).

Social support – the dark side?

Before proclaiming social identification and support as a panacea for all ills, it is possible that there may be some situations where mutual support may not aid recovery from trauma, and could even delay or prevent such recovery. When considering the role of social identities, one must consider the content of the particular identity concerned, and whether it could promote improved well-being, or may instead be maladaptive. For instance, St Claire and He (2009) found amongst a sample of adults aged over 50 that those who self-categorized as 'elderly people' were more likely to believe that they needed a hearing aid, independently of any objective physiological evidence for hearing loss. It is also possible that mutual support groups may have negative consequences if they encourage a maladaptive social identity, which can be damaging for the physical and/or psychological health of their members. For instance, after a review of pro-anorexia websites (where sufferers of eating disorders often engage in mutual support), Norris *et al.* (2006) concluded that such websites could 'promote and support anorexia nervosa' (p. 443), and there have even been calls for such websites to be banned because of their potentially harmful content.[3] Therefore, mutual support groups that emerge after disasters could actually hinder recovery if they encourage a 'victim' identity, and if the shared experience they have with others is centred around traumatic events and psychological distress. However, this is something that many users of such survivor groups are aware of, and they often prefer to categorize themselves as resilient survivors as opposed to victims.[4] Therefore, it would appear that so long as the social identities and/or mutual support that emerge after disasters promote resilience rather than continued vulnerability, they can provide therapeutic benefits to survivors.

Conclusion

There seems to be abundant evidence from both theoretical and applied perspectives to support a resilient rather than vulnerable approach to disasters and their mitigation, and showing that they do not result in the clichéd accounts of mass panic so prevalent in Hollywood disaster movies. Nor does it appear that disasters necessarily result in a significant increase in psychological trauma – they can instead bring greater social cohesion and perceived benefits to those affected. Furthermore, group processes and the sense of collective identification that communities affected by disasters can experience seem to play a vital part in enabling people and communities to cope with disasters and their aftermath, as Drury (2011) illustrates:

---

[3] http://www.eatingdisordersreview.com/nl/nl_edt_6_2_10.html
[4] http://www.newstatesman.com/200607030032

> Coping in disasters is the norm not the exception, and it is not despite the crowd, it is *because* of the crowd. Therefore, rather than being part of the 'problem' in mass emergencies and disasters (to be remedied by more centralized control and more stifling security practices), the crowd can be understood as part of a 'social cure' – to both the disaster and its (mis)management (p. 17).

Moreover, such resilience in the face of adversity is not necessarily dependent upon isolated heroic acts (which by definition are usually performed by exceptional individuals rather than the majority). It is more likely that the mundane cooperative acts of the many (such as comforting victims, providing food and shelter, etc.) promote social cohesion amongst those with a shared sense of identity (Reicher and Haslam, 2010), and can help explain why resilience and cooperation rather than selfishness and vulnerability predominate after disasters.

A final word of caution is perhaps appropriate here. It is important to remember that disasters can result in significant disruption and casualties and to not downplay the real distress that the people and communities affected by them can suffer in their wake. Moreover, psychological trauma after such disasters (such as PTSD) can have a crippling effect on the lives of those afflicted and their loved ones. Therefore, those in authority need to have adequate disaster preparation and mitigation strategies to cope with their effects.[5] However, assuming that those affected will respond in a vulnerable way may not only result in the ineffective allocation of possibly unnecessary resources, but it could also mean missing out on an opportunity to draw upon the collective resource that could provide valuable help in rebuilding the communities affected. The human spirit has shown itself to be remarkably resilient in the face of innumerable tragedies throughout history, and its ability to overcome adversity is not only inspirational, but also in need of greater recognition if it is to be encouraged and nurtured so we are better equipped to cope in this increasingly uncertain world.

References

American Psychological Association (APA) (2000) *Diagnostic and Statistical Manual of Mental Disorders*, revised 4th edn. American Psychological Association, Washington, DC.

Blake, S., Galea, E., Westeng, H. and Dixon, A. (2004) An analysis of human behaviour during the WTC disaster of 11 September 2001 based on published survivor accounts. *Proceedings of Third International Symposium on Human Behaviour in Fire*, Belfast, 1–3 September 2004, pp. 181–192.

Bonanno, G.A., Galea, S., Bucciarelli, A. and Vlahov, D. (2006) Psychological resilience after disaster: New York City in the aftermath of the September 11th terrorist attack. *Psychological Science* 17, 181–186.

Booth, W. (2002) 9/11 trauma: studies find resilience, worry. 7 September, *The Washington Post.*

Bowlby, A. (1969) *Attachment and Loss, Vol. 1: Attachment.* Hogarth, London.

Brewin, R., Andrews, J. and Valentine, J. (2000) Meta-analysis of risk factors for PTSD in trauma-exposed adults. *Journal of Consulting and Clinical Psychology* 68(5), 748–766.

Canter, D. (1990) Studying the experience of fires. In: Canter, D. (ed.) *Fires and Human Behaviour*. David Fulton, London, pp. 1–14.

---

[5] See Drury and Cocking (2007) for guidance on disaster preparation written for those involved in crowd management and emergency planning.

Cantril, H. (1940) *The Invasion from Mars: a Study in the Psychology of Panic.* Princeton University Press, Princeton, New Jersey.

Clarke, L. (2002) Panic: myth or reality? *Contexts* 1, 21–26.

Cocking, C., Drury, J. and Reicher, S. (2009) The psychology of crowd behaviour in fires: implications for the emergency services. *Irish Journal of Psychology* 30(1), 59–72.

Cole, J., Walters, M. and Lynch, M. (2011) Part of the solution, not the problem: the crowd's role in emergency response. *Contemporary Social Science* 6(3), 361–375.

Cornwell, B. (2003) Bonded fatalities. *The Sociological Quarterly* 44, 617–638.

Drury, J. (2004) No need to panic. *The Psychologist* 17, 118–119.

Drury, J. (2011) Collective resilience in mass emergencies and disasters: a social identity model. In: Jetten, J., Haslam, C. and Haslam, S.A. (eds) *The Social Cure: Identity, Health and Well-being*. Psychology Press, Hove, UK.

Drury, J. and Cocking, C. (2007) The mass psychology of disasters and emergency evacuations: a research report and implications for practice. University of Sussex. Available at: http://www.sussex.ac.uk/affiliates/panic/Disasters%20and%20emergency%20evacuations%20(2007).pdf (Accessed 26 July 2011).

Drury, J. and Reicher, S. (1999) The intergroup dynamics of collective empowerment: substantiating the social identity model. *Group Processes and Intergroup Relations* 2, 381–402.

Drury, J. and Reicher, S. (2000) Collective action and psychological change: the emergence of new social identities. *British Journal of Social Psychology* 39, 579–604.

Drury, J., Stott, C. and Farsides, T. (2003) The role of police perceptions and practices in the development of 'public disorder'. *Journal of Applied Social Psychology* 33, 1480–1500.

Drury, J., Cocking, C. and Reicher, S. (2009a) Every one for themselves? Understanding how crowd solidarity can arise in an emergency: an interview study of disaster survivors. *British Journal of Social Psychology* 48, 487–506.

Drury, J., Cocking, C. and Reicher, S. (2009b) The nature of collective 'resilience': survivor reactions to the July 7th (2005) London bombings. *International Journal of Mass Emergencies and Disasters* 27(1), 66–95.

Dynes, R. (2003) Finding order in disorder: continuities in the 9-11 response. *International Journal of Mass Emergencies and Disasters* 21, 9–23.

Dynes, R. (2006) Social capital: dealing with community emergencies. *Homeland Security Affairs* 2(2), 1–26.

Dynes, R. and Rodriguez, H. (2006) Finding and framing Katrina: the social construction of disaster. Available at: http://understandingkatrina.ssrc.org/Dynes_Rodriguez/ (Accessed 10 July 2011).

Fahy, R.F., Proulx, G. and Aiman, L. (2011) Panic or not in fire: clarifying the misconception. *Fire and Materials* 36(5–6), 328–338.

Falomir-Pichastor, J., Toscani, L. and Huyghues Despointes, S. (2009) Determinants of flu vaccination among nurses: the effects of group identification and professional responsibility. *Applied Psychology: an International Review* 58(1), 42–58.

Fritz, C.E. (1996) Disasters and mental health: therapeutic principles drawn from disaster studies. University of Delaware, Disaster Research Center, Historical and comparative disaster series #10 (original work published 1961).

Furedi, F. (2007) *Invitation to Terror.* Continuum Press, London.

Glass, T.A. and Schoch-Spana, M. (2002) Bioterrorism and the people: how to vaccinate a city against panic. *Clinical Infectious Diseases* 34, 217–223.

Goltz, J.D. (1984) Are the news media responsible for the disaster myths? A content analysis of emergency response imagery. *International Journal of Mass Emergencies and Disasters* 2, 345–368.

Hart, A., Blincow, D. and Thomas, H. (2008) Resilient therapy: strategic therapeutic engagement with children in crisis. *Child Care in Practice* 14(2), 131–145.

Haslam, S.A., Turner, J.C., Oakes, P., McGarty, C. and Reynolds, K. (1998) The group as a basis for emergent stereotype consensus. *European Review of Social Psychology* 28, 203–239.

Haslam, S.A., O'Brien, A., Jetten, J., Vormedal, K. and Penna, S. (2005) Taking the strain: social identity, social support, and the experience of stress. *British Journal of Social Psychology* 44, 355–370.

Haslam, S.A., Jetten, J., Postmes, T. and Haslam, C. (2009) Social identity, health and well-being: an emerging agenda for Applied Psychology. *Applied Psychology: an International Review* 58(1), 1–23.

Hoven, C.W., Duarte, C.S., Lucas, C.P., Wu, P., Mandell, D.J., Goodwin, R.D. *et al.* (2005) Psychopathology among New York City public school children six months after September 11. *Archives of General Psychiatry* 62, 545–552.

Jetten, J., Haslam, C. and Haslam, S.A. (eds) (2011) *The Social Cure: Identity, Health and Well-being*. Psychology Press, Hove, UK.

Joseph, S. and Linley, A. (2006) Growth following adversity: theoretical perspectives and implications for clinical practice. *Clinical Psychology Review* 26, 1041–1053.

Keane, T. and Piwowarczyk, L. (2006) Trauma, terror and fear: mental health professionals respond to the impact of 9/11 – an overview. In: Schein, L. *et al.* (eds) *Psychological Effects of Catastrophic Disasters: Group Approaches to Treatment.* Haworth Press, New York.

Kellezi, B., Reicher, S. and Cassidy, C. (2009) Surviving the Kosovo conflict: a study of social identity, appraisal of extreme events, and mental well-being. *Applied Psychology: an International Review* 58(1), 59–83.

LaPiere, R. (1938) *Collective Behavior.* McGraw Hill, New York.

Le Bon, G. (1968) *The Crowd: a Study of the Popular Mind.* Norman S. Berg, Dunwoody, Georgia (originally published 1895).

Levine, M., Prosser, A., Evans, D. and Reicher, S. (2005) Identity and emergency intervention. How social group membership and inclusiveness of group boundaries shape helping behaviour. *Personality and Social Psychology Bulletin* 31, 443–453.

Masten, A.S. (2001) Ordinary magic: resilience processes in development. *American Psychologist* 56(3), 227–238.

Mawson, A.R. (2005) Understanding mass panic and other collective responses to threat and disaster. *Psychiatry* 68, 95–113.

McDougall, W. (1920) *The Group Mind.* G.P. Putnam's Sons, New York.

Norris, M., Boydell, K., Pinhas, L. and Katzman, D. (2006) Ana and the internet: a review of pro-anorexia websites. *International Journal of Eating Disorders* 39(6), 443–447.

Proulx, G. and Sime, J.D. (1991) To prevent 'panic' in an underground emergency: why not tell people the truth? In: Cox, G. and Langford, B. (eds) *Fire Safety Science: Proceedings of the Third International Symposium*. Elsevier Applied Science, London, pp. 843–852.

Quarantelli, E.L. (2001) Panic, sociology of. In: Smelser, N.J. and Baltes, P.B. (eds) *International Encyclopedia of the Social and Behavioural Sciences*. Pergamon Press, New York, pp. 11020–11023.

Reicher, S. (1996) The Crowd century: reconciling practical success with theoretical failure. *British Journal of Social Psychology* 35, 535–553.

Reicher, S. (2001) The psychology of crowd dynamics. In: Hogg, M.A. and Tindale, R.S. (eds) *Blackwell Handbook of Social Psychology: Group Processes*. Blackwell, Oxford, UK, pp. 182–208.

Reicher, S. and Haslam, S.A. (2010) Beyond help: a social psychology of collective solidarity and social cohesion. In: Snyder, M. and Sturmer, S. (eds) *The Psychology of Helping: New Directions in the Study of Intergroup Prosocial Behavior.* Blackwell, Oxford, UK.

Schultz, D.P. (1964) *Panic Behavior: Discussions and Readings*. Random House, New York.

Sime, J.D. (1990) The concept of 'panic'. In: Canter, D. (ed.) *Fires and Human Behaviour*, 2nd edn. David Fulton, London, pp. 63–81.

Smelser, N.J. (1962) *Theory of Collective Behavior*. Routledge and Kegan Paul, London.

Solnit, R. (2009) *A Paradise Built in Hell: the Extraordinary Communities that Arise in Disaster.* Viking, New York.

St Claire, L. and He, Y. (2009) How do I know if I need a hearing aid? Further support for the self-categorisation approach to symptom perception. *Applied Psychology: an International Review* 58(1), 24–41.

Stott, C., Hutchison, P. and Drury, J. (2001) 'Hooligans' abroad? Inter-group dynamics, social identity and participation in collective 'disorder' at the 1998 World Cup Finals. *British Journal of Social Psychology* 40, 359–384.

Strauss, A.L. (1944) The literature on panic. *Journal of Abnormal and Social Psychology* 39, 317–328.

Summerfield, D. (2001) The invention of PTSD and the social usefulness of a psychiatric category. *British Medical Journal* 322, 95–98.

Tedeschi, R. and Calhoun, L. (2004) Post-traumatic growth: conceptual foundations and empirical evidence. *Psychological Enquiry* 15(1), 1–18.

Tierney, K. and Trainor, J. (2004) Networks and resilience in the World Trade Center Disaster. In: *MCEER: Research Progress and Accomplishments 2003–2004*. Multidisciplinary Center for Earthquake Engineering Research, Buffalo, New York, pp. 157–172.

Tierney, K., Bevc, C. and Kuligowski, E. (2006) Metaphors matter: disaster myths, media frames and their consequences in Hurricane Katrina. *Annals of the American Academy of Political and Social Science* 604, 57–81.

Tierney, K.J. (2002) Strength of a city: a disaster research perspective on the World Trade Center Attack. Available at: http://www.ssrc.org/sept11 (Accessed 6 September 2007).

Topping, K., Hayashi, H., Siembieda, W. and Boswell, M. (2010) Editorial. *Journal of Disaster Research* 5(2) Special Issue on 'Building Local Capacity for Long-term Disaster Resilience' Toward Disaster Resilient Communities, 127–129.

Turner, J.C., Hogg, M.A., Oakes, P.J., Reicher, S.D. and Wetherell, M.S. (1987) *Rediscovering the Social Group: a Self-categorization Theory*. Blackwell, Oxford, UK.

van Emmerik, A., Kamphuis, J., Hulsbosch, A. and Emmelkamp, P. (2002) Single session debriefing after psychological trauma: a meta analysis. *The Lancet* 360(9335), 766–771.

Wessely, S. (2005a) Editorial: don't panic! Short and long term psychological reactions to the new terrorism: the role of information and the authorities. *Journal of Mental Health* 14, 1–6.

Wessely, S. (2005b) Victimhood and resilience. *New England Journal of Medicine* 353, 548–550.

Williams, R. and Drury, J. (2010) The nature of psychosocial resilience and its significance for managing mass emergencies, disasters and terrorism. In: Awotona, A. (ed.) *Rebuilding Sustainable Communities for Children and Their Families after Disasters: a Global Survey*. Cambridge Scholars Publishing, Newcastle-upon-Tyne, UK, pp. 121–148.

Zimbardo, P. (2004) *The Lucifer Effect: Understanding How Good People Do Evil*. Random House, London.

Chapter 25

Community-based Psychosocial Support: An Overview

Joseph O. Prewitt Diaz

Introduction

Psychosocial support has been identified as a positive means to alleviate suffering for disaster-affected people, enhance resiliency and foster psychosocial well-being (Hobfoll *et al.*, 2007; Prewitt Diaz, 2010). This chapter introduces psychosocial support as a platform for the development of integrated community programmes. The chapter is divided into three sections. The first section provides a functional definition of psychosocial support, presents a theoretical overview and introduces the current international standards for support programmes. The second section proposes a schematic for psychosocial support as a platform for community-based programmes. The third and final section integrates theory and practice by providing a case study from the psychosocial support programme implemented in Sri Lanka in response to the 2004 South Asia earthquake and tsunami.

Psychosocial Support: Theories and Standards

Major disasters in the last decade including the tsunami in Japan (2011) and the most recent Hurricane Sandy (2012) in the USA have emphasized the need to satisfy the emotional needs of disaster-affected people in order to reduce tensions and awaken the desire to move ahead with their lives. One method to accomplish this is the use of techniques associated with community-based psychosocial support to assist disaster-affected people while meeting their basic needs, thereby helping them to feel secure and react with calmness. Once these goals are established, the desire to re-establish 'place' and to move ahead in a more resilient manner takes root among the disaster-affected people.

Psychosocial support is an umbrella term that can be applied to community-based interventions that alleviate behavioural and emotional human suffering. It is a tool that mobilizes disaster-affected people, groups and communities to use their dynamic capacity to identify culturally appropriate pathways in response to a disaster and positively respond to stressors. It fosters actions that will allow disaster-affected people to transform themselves so that they can contribute to the development of a psychologically, socially and ecologically sustainable environment. Psychosocial support focuses on individual strengths and provides spaces so that disaster-affected people and communities can enhance their resilience. The objectives of the interventions are as follows: (i) the identification and strengthening of internal coping mechanisms; (ii) the active involvement of community residents in community mapping and identifying problems, and resources; and (iii) the recognition of the skills and competence of community residents.

The Sphere Project (2011) has identified psychosocial support as a cross-cutting issue for every sector of disaster response. Moreover, the section on 'Protection' provided guidance for community-based psychosocial support. The Inter-Agency Standing Committee (IASC) and the Mental Health and Psychosocial Support Network (MHPSS) (2007) provided guidance on the integration of mental health and psychosocial support in disaster response efforts. The following is a summary of the guidance offered by Sphere (Sphere Project, 2011) and IASC/MHPSS (2007).

Community-based approaches

Building on local resources, providing training and capacity building, and upgrading local structures and institutions are critical to the success of a psychological support programme. This approach allows trained community volunteers to share their knowledge with fellow community members. Because the majority of emotions that are typically associated with disaster-affected people (e.g. distress and sorrow) do not require professional treatment, these local resources are often quite instrumental in providing effective relief (Lawson, 1967). A much larger number of people can be helped by working with groups rather than individuals and focusing on strengthening networks in the community. Efforts that involve the community with its knowledge, values and practices are most likely to provide culturally appropriate responses.

Interventions are contextual, and culturally appropriate

Culture influences the way that disaster-affected people view the world. Tapping the ability and building the capacity of community volunteers allows the programme to exploit the volunteers' inside knowledge of the local culture and ensures that they will be able to provide culturally and linguistically appropriate assistance to the affected population.

Activities empower disaster-affected people

Quality psychosocial assistance is based on helping others regain self-respect, autonomy and hope. The interventions should focus on the abilities and strengths of the disaster-affected people as well as on their problems and weaknesses (Paton and Johnston, 2006). Active community participation is generally accepted as one way to encourage empowerment and enhance the resilience of disaster-affected people.

Planning encourages community participation

Participation by community residents in collective decision-making about their needs, and the development and implementation of strategies, will help those strategies to be based on the community's collective strength to meet those needs. Through participation, people gain an increased feeling of control over their lives and the life of their community.

Community-based psychosocial support (Table 25.1) acknowledges that communities are diverse and have unique psychological, social and ecological dimensions. It furthers recognizes the ability of disaster-affected people to organize themselves, and as the interventions unfold the capacity of a disaster-affected community can adapt in terms of the response. This strategy has the capacity to create new spaces for doing new things, for innovation and for development. A resilient community is able to use the experience of change to continually develop, and to reach a higher state of functioning (Folke, 2006).

Table 25.1. Psychosocial support actions during the period that elapses after the disaster.

Action/time	Disaster strikes	Community mobilization	Psychosocial reconstruction
Focus of intervention	Psychological, social and cultural needs	Trust, leadership and networking	Ownership of the process, feelings of 'being settled'
Intervention	Psychological first aid	Re-establishment of place	Resilience enhancement activities
Resulting actions	Initial explorations of the community and the process of disaster-induced changes	Community members are able to provide an understanding of the community and how its resilience to change may be enhanced	Examine community's capacity to take action by mobilizing its resources for adaptation

Two psychosocial support interventions are typically used to assist the disaster-affected people in their journey to reconstruction and well-being: i.e. psychological first aid (PFA) and re-establishment of place.

Psychological first aid

The following five evidence-informed principles guided the development of PFA strategies and techniques: (i) promoting a sense of safety; (ii) promoting calming; (iii) promoting sense of self- and community efficacy; (iv) promoting connectedness; and (v) instilling hope (Hobfoll *et al.*, 2007).

Promoting a sense of safety

This refers to helping disaster-affected people find a secure place, and helping them understand that they are safe and are being safeguarded (Hobfoll *et al.*, 2007).

Promoting a sense of calming

This involves engaging disaster-affected people in activities that may alleviate their concerns and providing psycho-education regarding the typical reactions to disasters, thereby ensuring disaster-affected people are aware that that these reactions are typical and normal (Hobfoll *et al.*, 2007).

Promoting self- and collective efficacy

This can be accomplished by involving disaster-affected people in decision-making activities and rebuilding efforts. Assistance should be provided to community members as they are planning and implementing rebuilding projects, and activities that restore order. The community members must be encouraged to share their hope for the future and facilitate activities where they can volunteer and share their goods, resources and skills (Hobfoll *et al.*, 2007).

Promoting connectedness

In order to promote connectedness, programmes should provide the mechanism for disaster-affected people to identify and establish links with their loved ones. These methods of contact should increase the quantity, quality and frequency of supportive transactions between disaster-affected people and support systems. Negative social influences should be addressed through community-wide activities (Hobfoll *et al.*, 2007).

Instilling hope

Providing services to disaster-affected people such as housing, employment, relocation and replacement of household goods, and clean-up kits can help restore hope amongst community residents. Existing community groups should be engaged in establishing systems that enable those in recovery from such traumas to share their experiences and hope with those struggling with recovery; ultimately, the disaster-affected people must accept that their lives and their environment may have significantly changed in order to build hope for the future (Hobfoll *et al.*, 2007).

Re-establishment of place

The major activities of psychosocial support after a disaster often involve community mobilization activities that re-establish place. The objective is to engage disaster-affected people in a set of exercises that will identify their vulnerabilities, resources and adaptive capacities-oriented process in order to determine how internal conditions impact the response to the disaster.

Activities that enhance a sense of purpose, beliefs and leadership at individual, group and community level are listed in Table 25.2.

Ultimately, disaster-affected people should explore the following: (i) which behavioural components of a community weaken the ability to respond to the destruction caused by disasters; (ii) what behavioural characteristics help the community to respond to the disaster; and (iii) what are the community's abilities to change its behaviours to cope better with actual and anticipated social, psychological and ecological stressors.

Table 25.2. Activities that enhance a sense of purpose, beliefs and leadership.

Activities	Individual	Group	Community
Purpose	Reflect on your values and beliefs Learn new skills, volunteer and lend a hand	As a group develops a vision, define a goal and select programme activities Encourage active participation and achievement of programme outcomes Develop goals and objectives and identify activities to achieve them	Organize community meetings to discuss needs and encourage involvement Organize community-wide gatherings to mark significant events Publicize events through community notice boards, newsletters and word of mouth
Beliefs	Think about your place and what is important to your happiness and that of others Participate in church and in environmental activities that provide a space to connect (e.g. church activities and environmental activities)	Include spaces in your programmes that allow all to practise their spirituality Develop outdoor activities so that people can connect with nature Encourage the development of a wide view of spirituality, to allow diverse groups to identify commonalities	Identify and renew rites of passage Connect with local community lore, stories and culture Organize community walks, sports and picnics
Leadership	Engage in activities that promote leadership and communication with others Share ideas and offer your skills or experiences to help others Follow through and volunteer your time and skills	Activities should promote leadership among the disaster-affected people Encourage others to use their skills in areas that assist the community Encourage community members to assume leadership roles	Develop leadership skills in different groups Organize community walks that include leadership training Support leadership in community organizations

Psychosocial Support as the Platform for an Integrated Community-based Programme

In 1998, Hurricane Mitch hit several Central American countries causing thousands of deaths, loss of property totalling in the millions of dollars and extensive human suffering; in response a psychosocial support model was developed following the (Voluntarios en Servico a Puerto Rico Asociados) VESPRA model. This model required a minimum amount per person cost, and was viewed as a potential mechanism to empower affected communities to organize, protect and reconstruct themselves. This model was unlike the standard models of aid giveaway programmes.

The evolution of psychosocial support programmes has corresponded to the increasing severity of disasters and the emergence of international guidelines (IASC/MHPSS, 2007; Sphere Project, 2011). The American Red Cross International Services adopted the proposed development of psychosocial support programmes and generated draft guidelines to systematize the programme within their repertoire of disaster response options (American Red Cross, 2002). In 1998 in Posoltega, Nicaragua (1998), the psychosocial support programme coordinated the response of 21 local non-government organizations (NGOs) to a major mudslide that killed over 2000 people and left over 13,000 injured (Prewitt Diaz and Saballos Ramirez, 2000). Lessons were learned as a result of this experience and focused on types of intervention and early coordination among stakeholders. In another major disaster, i.e. the 2001 El Salvador earthquakes, the psychosocial support programme focused on developing an immediate psychosocial response mechanism and PFA was used as a tool during the relief and response period (Jaquemet, 2001). In 2003, the Indian Red Cross Society (IRCS) and the American Red Cross defined psychosocial personnel needs during a disaster and designed a course of study for technicians, specialists and professionals (Prewitt Diaz *et al.*, 2004). By 2004, the Indian personnel had developed a systematized approach for community-based psychosocial support that included group training, community participatory assessment, staff development (from the community and the university), and monitoring and evaluation mechanisms.

Community-based psychosocial support was implemented in parts and as an integrated model by the American Red Cross International Services during the 2004 tsunami in the Indian Ocean. Figure 25.1 introduces a schematic of an integrated model, in which psychosocial support is used as a platform to initiate community response immediately after a disaster. The integrated programme is a follow-up to the guidance proposed by the Health Standard of the Sphere Project (2004, pp. 197–199), and the request from the funding agency to utilize the ‘project cycle’ methodology to plan and develop the programme.

The goal of a community-based psychosocial support programme is to improve the capacity of the community so that it becomes ‘physically, mentally healthier and become a better-prepared community’. The following six steps are involved in the process of engaging the community in the project development: (i) assessment and planning; (ii) articulating the strategies; (iii) defining the interventions; (iv) engaging the community in small projects to identify the interest of the existing human capital; (v) the outputs; and the (vi) the impacts.

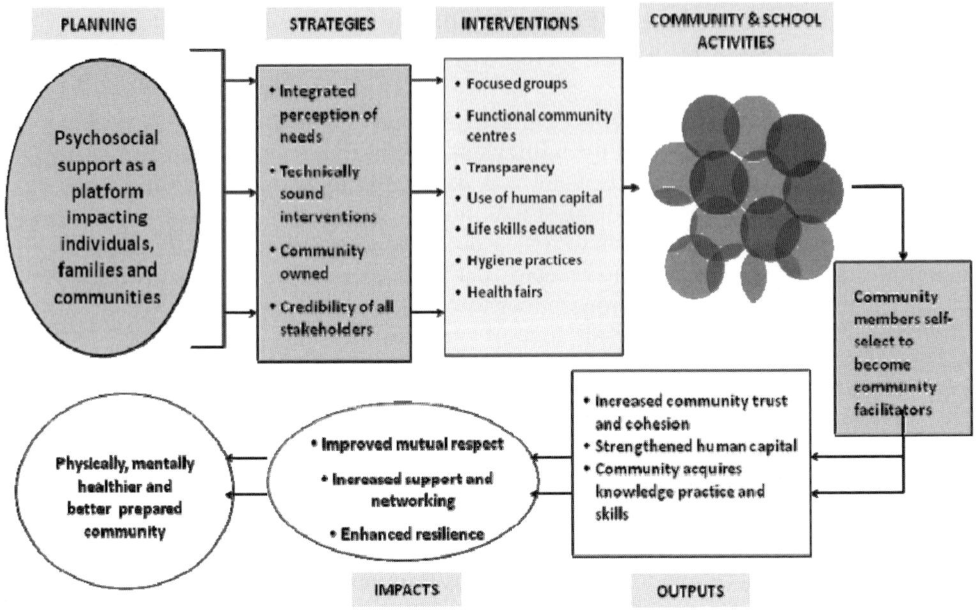

Fig. 25.1. Components of engaging the community in a community-based psychosocial support programme (CBPSP). Each component is explained in the text. (Source: Prewitt Diaz, J.O., Bhadra, S. and Mewari, M. (2007) Psychosocial support as a platform for community development. PowerPoint Presentation, Washington, DC.)

Assessment and planning

Community volunteers are identified and basic training is conducted in PFA topics, participatory assessment and community mapping. The premise for this activity is that disaster-affected people have the most intimate knowledge regarding what their community looked like prior to the disaster, what has happened in their community and what should take place to enable recovery and enhance resilience (Bolton and Tang, 2002).

The activities during this initial phase are designed to encourage disaster-affected people to be active in identifying what activities inspire participation in all segments of the community, to look forward so that they may overcome the initial feelings of hopelessness and helplessness, and take action to plan projects that will shift the power dynamics and foster resilience.

Indeed, disaster-affected people must take an active role in the identification and analysis of needs, project development and decision-making about their priorities and the vision for their future.

Articulating strategies

Community members are encouraged to become engaged in activities that will foster their growth in an inclusive way. These activities may include, but are not limited to the following: (i) providing accurate and timely information about resources, services and common reactions; (ii) providing human capital from among the disaster-affected people; (iii) providing the disaster-affected people with materials, cash and labour, with technical assistance coming from outside stakeholders; or (iv) the disaster-affected people acting independently from external sources.

Defining interventions

Once the broad strategies have been identified then the interventions can be tested. This is the time to experiment with activities and identify the best match between disaster-affected people and broad strategies. For example, some people will engage in sharing information, while others will want to construct, moreover, still others will provide PFA, and yet others will conduct informal educational sessions for children and youth.

In planning the initial interventions the disaster-affected people have to cycle through the following five core interventions of a community-based psychosocial support programme. These interventions are: (i) providing accurate and timely information; (ii) providing formal and informal educational experiences; (iii) identifying and enhancing support and resources; (iv) increasing access for all of the community population; and (v) monitoring and reporting.

Community and school activities

Once the initial response has been initiated the disaster-affected people are busy with the rehabilitation and reconstruction of their respective places and communities. The two settings in which most activities will occur are the community and school. At the community level activities include improving the environment and reconstructing place. In the schools, the efforts focus on re-establishing formal schooling for children and adolescents and on conducting informal schooling activities for youth and adults in the community. The emphasis is on getting everyone engaged in reconstruction. All projects are considered and supported by the coordinating committee of the disaster-affected people. Eventually, the social capital is identified, and small community-wide projects and income-generating activities are initiated. Usually psychosocial support activities serve as the platform for other more concrete projects.

This is a good time to initiate the documentation of community engagement in the rehabilitation and reconstruction process; moreover, specific actions that are taken are documented, and changes made by the disaster-affected people are recorded. The adaptation by the disaster-affected people into the new community life, the institutionalization of changes and capacity building are monitored and reported as a successful step enhancing resilience and well-being.

Outputs

The process to re-establish place and develop the community does not occur in a neat sequential manner. Important actions are taken, based on a given situation. If a community is able to successfully bring about changes, their capacity to create even more community changes related to the group's mission should improve.

Among the important outputs is the generation of trust such that the community works in terms of shared common risks and protective factors. More than one community has formulated a partnership to elicit funds from an outside stakeholder for projects related to new community changes and desired outcomes.

Various initiatives may work well in the disaster-affected community and foster growth, thus remaining flexible in terms of adapting interventions is important. This creates an approach that 'belongs' to community members, and has been modified to fit community needs. Moreover, through changing interventions to fit local needs, community members can improve their ability to take care of their own problems.

Impact

The impact of a community-based psychosocial support programme can be measured by the amount of involvement by the disaster-affected people in the reconstruction activities, the development of trust in the actions by all segments of the community and the desire of volunteers to achieve well-being for the total community. Re-establishment of place as measured by the sharing of cultural activities, problem solving, solution-focused activities, identification of social capital and care for the environment is a second impact. The third impact is an increase in physical and emotional well-being amongst the disaster-affected people.

An Operational Community-based Psychosocial Support Programme Model

This section presents a case study of an actual project that was implemented in Sri Lanka after the 2004 tsunami in that region of the world (Ring *et al.*, 2005). It explains the importance of school and community-based interventions. These types of activities were used throughout this programme in order to facilitate the involvement of the whole disaster-affected community including the elderly, physically handicapped, widows and children in its recovery process. The activities were geared towards assisting the survivors in the process of rediscovering their psychosocial well-being through enhancing their own protective factors. All the activities were planned, executed, monitored and evaluated by the community members alongside personnel from a local NGO to ensure that they are were culturally appropriate and sustainable. An external stakeholder provided financial and technical assistance to conduct interventions in target communities and schools.

Not everyone felt comfortable expressing him or herself verbally after the tsunami. Creative and expressive activities, such as story-telling, art and crafts provided creative ways for disaster-affected people, i.e. often children or older members of the community, to communicate their feelings. Community-based skits and story-telling proved to be a powerful and effective way of venting feelings; it's a simple healing process with enjoyment and togetherness. These types of activities were used in both the school and community-focused activities to facilitate the expression of feelings, to reduce distress and to enhance a sense of belonging. They provided a conduit for disaster-affected people to have a sense of place: (i) by helping them accept responsibility for their place (i.e. village or community); (ii) by developing a knowledge base about their physical, psychological, social and human village; (iii) enabling them to live in the place and enjoy the available facilities; (iv) mapping the place; (v) building the physical infrastructure of the place; and (vi) taking action to preserve the place.

The project goal was to: *Enhance resilience through a community-based psychosocial support programme*. The following objectives and activities supported the development of the project.

Objective 1: *Promote the psychological and social well-being of the community through the schools.*

Resilient schools

In order to recognize and enhance the resilience of the school community, the programme facilitated psychosocial activities in target schools. The objective of these activities was to involve the school community in creating a 'Happy School', which is defined as a school building that is secure, provides space for dialogue between teachers and students, and where students are encouraged to become actively engaged in all activities. Eventually, the activities were channelled towards preparing the school to face a crisis, emergency or disaster. The skills of the students, teachers and volunteers were enhanced in order to develop and implement a 'School Crisis Response Plan', with the help of school mapping and the formation of four school committees composed of students, teachers, other school personnel and parents.

During the first year and a half of the programme the 'resilient schools' programme was implemented in 51 schools in target districts. This model was replicated during the second half of the programme. Each participating school received three school chests, one recreational kit and one large first aid kit per classroom per year, one individual first aid kit per student, and financial support for two school resilience activities and six student–parent activities per year.

Model schools

During their third year of teacher training, pre-service teachers were paired with an in-service teacher, i.e. generally a teacher at a government school, in order to gain practical experience. Working with the National Colleges of Education, the programme selected up to five schools that were designated to receive student teachers in each district to be 'model schools'. Schools that had met the previously established criteria of being partially damaged by the tsunami or acting as a host to internally displaced children were considered for selection into the programme. The programme provided support to these pre-service teachers and their in-service mentors as they implemented aspects of the 'resilient schools' programme in their classroom. Each classroom in these model schools received a first aid kit, a recreational kit and a school educational materials chest. The Educational Specialist in the CBPSP monitored the student teachers and provided them support as they practised their new skills in an effort to organize model schools in target areas.

Within 1 year the model school component was implemented in 40 classrooms as pre-service teachers were trained from January to May 2005. In years two and three, 825 in-service teachers were trained annually. About 40,000 students were served through this programme.

Objective 2: *Strengthen community protective factors.*

Resilient community programme

The objective of the activities under the 'resilient communities' programme was to bring diverse groups within the community together to prepare for, respond to and recover from a crisis, emergency or disaster. This programme began with participatory focus groups each composed of ten families. A community liaison team led these focus groups in planning the activities. During these focus groups, participants were given an overview of the goals of the CBPSP programme and worked together to identify community needs, possible solutions and resources available within and outside the target community. During this period the focus group leader identified those members of the group with an interest in becoming a Community Facilitator.

The 4000 trained Community Facilitators were divided into groups of five. Each group of five worked with 50 family units, which was designated as a village for the purpose of this programme. The Community Facilitators received a variety of support materials to assist their efforts to prepare their 'village' to recognize potential psychological risks among members and to develop a plan to address those issues. They worked with their village to identify two annual 'skills building' activities. The nature of these activities was determined by the village members and included training, tutoring for children or income generation activities. The objective of these activities was to facilitate a sense of security and unity and help community residents to recognize and enhance resilience factors within the village. Villages were required to submit a 'proposal' for these activities to their community liaison for review and approval.

Informal schooling

The CBPSP programme provided informal schooling for children under the age of 5 and out-of-school youth in the target communities. This aspect of the CBPSP programme brought together several marginalized groups including handicapped individuals, the elderly, widows, out-of-school youth and children under the age of 5. Structures were identified within the community that could house the informal schools. These schools were provided with one recreation kit per school and other CBPSP materials. Education within these schools was facilitated by the Community Facilitators and led by the trained informal school teachers. During the morning, the school activities focused on education for children under the age of 5. The Community Facilitators and the informal school teachers included adults and adolescents from a variety of marginalized groups in the process to provide education to and activities for this group. In the afternoon activities focused on education for out-of-school youth and tutoring for children who needed extra attention. In addition, these informal schools served as a venue where community elders came together to educate children about culture and to enhance vocational skills. Breakfast and a fortified snack were served to students and teachers attending the school.

Objective 3: *Assist Community Members to establish a 'sense of place'.*

The programme provided an environment in which disaster-affected people were able to establish a 'sense of place' by providing opportunities to engage in social encounters, encouraging movement between social groups (e.g. individual to social interaction, or small group to large group), providing opportunities for self-expression through creative and expressive activities, and offering opportunities to express a full range of behaviours including exploration, competition and collaboration. All planned activities improved social comfort, collective well-being, social equity and respect, and provided the opportunity to make sense of an environment that had been changed by the tsunami.

In order to facilitate a sense of unity within the community, the programme supported the development of 'community centers'. These centres brought together representatives from all parts of the community to plan and implement activities designed to strengthen community well-being. The centres became the hub for CBPSP activities including planning activities, bringing people together and connecting with external organizations. These day-to-day interactions motivated disaster-affected people to establish a sense of place by: (i) accepting responsibility for their village; (ii) developing knowledge about their village (e.g. watershed, soils, climate, plants and animals); (iii) enjoying the facilities available; (iv) mapping the village; (v) building the physical infrastructure of the village; and (vi) taking action to preserve their village.

Summary and Conclusion

By the beginning of the 21st century the debate over the role of community-based psychosocial support within disaster response had ended. Scholars have agreed that humanitarian actors must address psychosocial support and protection (Sphere Project, 2011). The project described herein is an alternative that proved successful in the amelioration of human suffering and the enhancement of psychosocial well-being via strategies that provided support and protection to all. This chapter has presented: (i) a theoretical justification for psychosocial support as a community integrator; (ii) a practical model for community-based psychosocial support in an integrated programme; and (iii) a case study of using psychosocial support as an intervention in Sri Lanka after the 2004 earthquake and tsunami in the region.

References

American Red Cross (2002) *Psychosocial Support Guidelines*. International Services, American National Red Cross, Washington, DC.

Bolton, P. and Tang, A. (2002) An alternative approach to cross-cultural function assessment. *Social Psychiatry* 37(11), 537–543.

Folke, C. (2006) Resilience: the emergence of a perspective for social-ecological system analyses. *Global Environmental Change* 16, 253–247.

Hobfoll, S.E., Watson, P.E., Bell, C.C., Bryant, R.A., Brymer, M.J., Friedman, M.J. *et al.* (2007) Five essential elements of immediate and mid-term mass trauma intervention: empirical evidence. *Psychiatry: Interpersonal and Biological Processes* 70, 283–315.

Inter-Agency Standing Committee (IASC) (2007) IASC guidelines on mental health and psychosocial support in emergency settings. IASC, Geneva, Switzerland.

Jaquemet, I. (2001) Psychosocial support luxury or necessity? *RCRC – The Magazine of the International Red Cross and Red Crescent Movement* 3(3), 3–11.

Lawson, D.M. (1967) An evaluation of training procedures of the Voluntarios en Servicio a Puerto Rico Asociados. Office of Economic Development, Washington, DC.

Paton, D. and Johnston, D. (2006) (eds) *Disaster Resilience: an Integrated Approach*. Charles C. Thomas Publishers, Ltd, Illinois.

Prewitt Diaz, J. (2010) Participatory community mapping: a tool to enhance psychosocial well being. *Webmedcentral Psychology* 1(9), wmc00585.

Prewitt Diaz, J.O. and Saballos Ramirez, M. (2000) *Salud psicosocial en un desastre complejo: el efecto del huracan Mitch en Nicaragua.* Cruz Roja Nicaraguense y Cruz Roja Americana, Managua, Nicaragua.
Prewitt Diaz, J.O., Srivanasa Murthy, R. and Laksminarayana, R. (2004) *Disaster mental health in India.* Volunteers Health Association of India Press, New Delhi.
Ring, D., Prewitt Diaz, J.O. and Dayal, A. (2005) Community based psychosocial support program for tsunami affected people in Sri Lanka. A proposal submitted to the American Red Cross. American National Red Cross, Colombo, Sri Lanka.
Sphere Project (2004) Humanitarian charter and minimum standards in humanitarian response (2nd edn). Sphere Project, Geneva.
Sphere Project (2011) Humanitarian charter and minimum standards in humanitarian response (3rd edn). Sphere Project, Geneva.

Chapter 26

Disaster Mental Health: A Paradigm Shift from Curative to Preventive Psychiatry

Suresh Bada Math, Naveen C. Kumar, Maria Nirmala Christine and Anish V. Cherian

Introduction

Disasters have been ubiquitously present since antiquity. No one who sees a disaster is untouched by it. Disaster stress and associated grief reactions are normal responses to an abnormal situation. Mental health reactions of disaster survivors stem from the problems of living brought about by the disaster. Developing countries are at a high risk of disaster proneness and also they have to face challenges such as poverty, meagre resources, illiteracy, inadequate infrastructure, a lack of trained manpower, corruption and poor knowledge of disaster mental health (Math *et al.*, 2006). Disasters are known to have a substantial effect on both the physical and mental health of the affected population (Kim *et al.*, 2008). Impact on physical health produces visible and superficial scars on the body, which heal in months but impact on mental health is usually a deep and invisible scar on the mind that takes years to heal. This impact on mental health invariably interferes with the psychosocial rehabilitation of the survivors in the long run. However, psychological reactions to disasters have not received sufficient attention in developing countries, both from service providers and service users. The majority of policy-makers and health professionals do not have knowledge about disaster mental health (Math *et al.*, 2006). Similarly, most of the survivors do not see themselves as needing mental health services following the disaster and will not seek such services (Math *et al.*, 2006). There is a need to understand the effects of disaster on mental health so that precautionary measures can be adopted to prevent and mitigate suffering. The objective of this chapter is to define, classify and elaborate on the various phases of disaster. This chapter also discusses human responses, psychiatric morbidity and management of disasters from a mental health perspective.

In order to meet the above objectives a PUBMED search for all published studies from 1950 to 2010 involving disaster mental health/disaster psychiatry was performed. The following Medical Sub-Headings (MeSH or Keywords) terms from PUBMED were employed to search: 'disasters', 'mental health', 'mental disorders', 'psychiatry', 'post-traumatic stress disorder', 'psychological techniques', 'psychotherapy' and 'drug therapy'. The Boolean operator AND was also used in combinations of the above key words. In addition, the reference sections of major articles and reviews were also screened. We employed the usual hierarchy of evidence to write the review. Systematic reviews and meta-analyses of randomized controlled studies (RCT) were considered the best evidence base followed by RCTs, open-label studies, case series and case reports. In addition, we also considered consensus of clinician and expert guidelines in writing this chapter.

Defining Disaster

What constitutes a disaster? A road traffic accident? Terrorist attack? Suicide bombing? Religious riots? War? Rapid spread of H1N1 virus? Disaster is a very broad term, which implies a diverse set of circumstances from an act of terrorism to natural calamities like tsunamis. This difficulty in defining a disaster has been further accentuated by the inconsistent use of terminology such as calamity, catastrophe, crisis, emergency, misfortune, tragedy, trauma and stress. Defining 'disaster' is inevitable because it poses a real challenge to any country to know what to include and what not to include, for planning, policy making and from a research perspective.

Disasters can be simply defined as violent encounters with nature, technology or humankind (Norris, 1992). In 1978, Lazarus and Cohen defined it as a specific cataclysmic event, that is, a stressor depicted by immense power, large scope, suddenness and placing excessive demands on individual coping (Lazarus and Cohen, 1978). Similarly, in 1992 the World Health Organization defined disaster as 'a severe disruption, ecological and psychosocial, which greatly exceeds the coping capacity of the affected community' (World Health Organization, 1992).

In 1995, the Federal Emergency Management Agency (FEMA) of the USA defined disaster as 'any natural catastrophe, regardless of cause, any fire, flood, or explosion that causes damage of sufficient severity and magnitude to warrant assistance supplementing state, local, and disaster relief organization efforts to alleviate damage, loss, hardship, or suffering' (Young *et al.*, 1998). Similarly, as per the Disaster Management Act 2005 of India(The Disaster Management Act, 2005), disaster is defined as a catastrophe, mishap, calamity or grave occurrence in any area, arising from natural or man-made causes, or due to accident or negligence resulting in substantial loss of life or human suffering or damage to, and destruction of property, or damage to, or degradation of, environment, and is of such a nature or magnitude as to be beyond the coping capacity of the community of the affected area. Some common characteristics across all definitions are: (i) sudden onset; (ii) unpredictability; (iii) uncontrollability; (iv) huge magnitude of destruction; (v) human loss and suffering; and (vi) greatly exceeding the coping capacity of the affected community.

Classification of Disasters

Disasters can be classified as natural and man-made ones (North, 2003). Natural disasters are usually considered as 'acts of God', to punish human beings for their past deeds and are frequently referred to as 'Karma'. This attribution has positive consequences in terms of coping and negative consequences by way of hindering planning and preparedness

(North, 2003). Man-made disasters can occur because of human errors such as the Bhopal gas tragedy or by wilful intention such as an act of terror or war. In terms of evoking mental health morbidity, natural disasters are mild in nature; human errors and technological accidents are moderate in nature; and wilful acts like terrorism are the most severe in nature (Baum and Fleming, 1993). Furthermore, in rare instances these survivors may become perpetrators of a disaster to avenge their sufferings.

Disaster mental health services are based on the principles of 'preventive medicine' (Math *et al.*, 2008a). Earlier, disaster interventions were based more on early identification and treatment at the individual level, but the recent trend is to consider community-level intervention in preventing, planning and mitigating suffering through capacity building (Math *et al.*, 2008a). This principle of 'prevention' has necessitated a paradigm shift from relief-centred post-disaster management to a holistic, multidimensional integrated community approach (Sundram *et al.*, 2008). This can be understood from six (R) basic aspects of disaster management such as readiness (preparedness), response (immediate action), relief (rescue work), rehabilitation (long-term remedial measures using community resources), recovery (returning to normalcy) and resilience (fostering) (Math *et al.*, 2011).

Phases of Disaster Mental Health

The affected community's and individual's reactions to disaster may follow a more or less predictable course as shown in Fig. 26.1. They are the heroic phase, honeymoon phase, disillusionment phase and restoration phase (Young *et al.*, 1998; Math *et al.*, 2006). Immediately after the disaster, the survivors in the community usually demonstrate altruistic behaviour in the form of rescuing, sheltering, feeding and supporting their fellow human beings. Hence this phase is called 'the heroic phase'. This phase usually lasts from a day to weeks depending upon the severity, duration of exposure and availability of the relief sources from various agencies. Once the relief agencies step in, survivors are relocated to safer places like relief camps. Media attention, free medical aid, free food and shelter, VIP visits to the camp, administrations' sympathy and false reassurances of rehabilitation by politicians provide an immense sense of relief and faith in survivors that their community will be restored in no time and their loss will be compensated at least through monetary benefits and a rehabilitation package. Hence this phase is called the honeymoon phase, which usually lasts for 2–4 weeks (Math *et al.*, 2006).

At the end of 2–4 weeks, relief materials and resources start to be reduced. Celebrities' and politicians' visits stop. Media coverage reduces. Administration, relief agencies and non-governmental organizations' (NGO) involvement start fading. This brings the survivors to the ruthless world of post-disaster life (Young *et al.*, 1998; Math *et al.*, 2006, 2008a). The reality of the complex process of rebuilding and rehabilitating appears a distant dream because of administrative hurdles, bureaucratic red tapism, discrimination, injustice and corruption. The harsh reality of the disillusionment phase provides a fertile soil for breeding mental morbidity, which lasts for 2–36 months before the community is restored to harmony. The role of mental health workers is critical during this phase (Math *et al.*, 2006, 2008a).

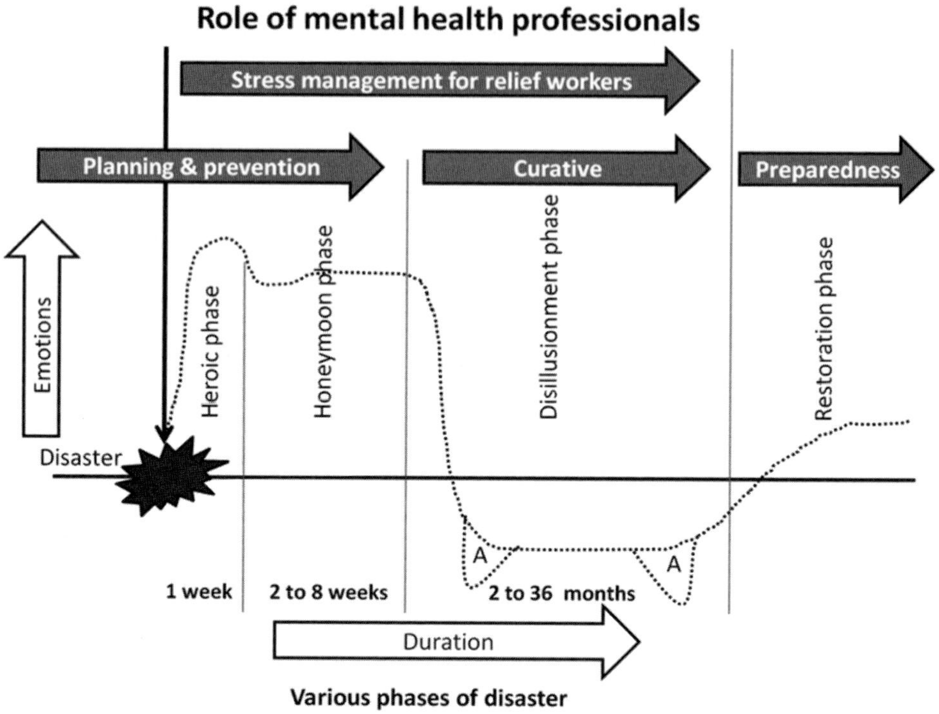

Fig. 26.1. Various phases of disaster and the role of mental health professionals. Immediately after the disaster, the heroic phase sets in. This is followed by the honeymoon phase. The disillusionment phase is the longest and prevalence of mental health morbidity is high during this period. A = Anniversary reactions. This is a modified version of Young *et al.*, 1998, Math *et al.*, 2006 and Math *et al.*, 2011.

Human Responses to a Disaster

Grief is the response to any loss. Grief reactions are normal responses to abnormal situations. Grief's intensity is directly proportional to the severity, duration and intensity of exposure to the disaster. The grief process may comprise various stages such as shock, denial, anger, depression, bargaining and acceptance (Kübler-Ross, 1969). Grief symptoms are often experienced in waves or cycles or episodes with periods of intense and painful emotions. Usually normal grief follows the above phases with a possibility of some variation and resolves over a period of few months. It is to be remembered that survivors are normal people in abnormal situations and each survivor's experience of disaster is unique.

A recent study reported that complicated grief was present in more than two-thirds of the survivors of an earthquake (Ghaffari-Nejad *et al.*, 2007). Complicated grief hinders the healing process and also interferes in the biological, social and occupational functioning (Freedman and Blumenfield, 1986). Resolution of an abnormal grief reaction can be facilitated by fostering the cultural–religious rituals of grieving. Many of the survivors may require trauma/grief-focused interventions within a comprehensive disaster recovery programme (Goenjian *et al.*, 2001). Complicated grief reactions can be grossly classified into delayed, absent, oscillating and exploding types (Math and Chandrashekar, 2003). These complicated grief reactions may require professional help for psychotherapy.

Prevalence of Psychiatric Morbidity in Disaster-affected Population

Prevalence of psychiatric morbidity in disaster-affected population varies from 8.6 to 57.3% (Udomratn, 2008). This magnitude of variation can be attributed to differences in methodology, definition of a 'case', sampling procedure, timing of the study, recall bias, systematic under-reporting, cross-cultural differences and type and severity of the disaster (Norris and Elrod, 2006). Overall, prevalence rates can be approximately estimated to be two to three times higher than that in the general population.

Psychiatric disorders noted during disasters can be classified into those seen in the acute phase (1–3 months) and the long-term phase (> 3 months). The majority of the acute phase reactions and disorders are self-limiting, whereas long-term disorders require assistance from mental health professionals. Along with the diagnosable psychiatric disorders, the affected community also harbours large number of sub-syndromal symptoms. The majority of them report medically unexplained somatic symptoms, and unusual symptom clusters are classically seen (North, 2002). Mental health professionals should be aware of this phenomenon and restrain themselves from labelling this population with a mental disorder and treating them aggressively with medications (Math *et al.*, 2008a). The approach towards management should be conservative in medication and avant-garde in psychosocial approach.

Common Psychiatric Disorders Seen in the Disaster-affected Population

Common psychiatric disorders are: adjustment disorders, depression, post-traumatic stress disorder (PTSD), anxiety disorders, non-specific somatic symptoms and substance abuse (Young *et al.*, 1998; North, 2003; Liu *et al.*, 2006; Tsai *et al.*, 2007; Frankenberg *et al.*, 2008; Hollifield *et al.*, 2008). Researchers have assigned that PTSD is the signature diagnosis amongst the post-disaster psychiatric morbidity (North, 2003). The prevalence of PTSD reported in literature varies from 4 to 60% (Young *et al.*, 1998).

Mood disorders (North *et al.*, 2004; Thienkrua *et al.*, 2006), PTSD (North *et al.*, 2004) and substance use disorders (Pfefferbaum *et al.*, 2002; Reijneveld *et al.*, 2005; Rohrbach *et al.*, 2009) are diagnosed frequently along with other psychiatric disorders. Depression is a well-known co-morbidity and can pose a challenge to any treating team (Basoglu *et al.*, 2004; Salcioglu *et al.*, 2007; Goenjian *et al.*, 2009). Psychiatric disorders continue to be prevalent even after 3–5 years in the disaster-affected community (Liu *et al.*, 2006; Noorthoorn *et al.*, 2010). Most commonly noted psychiatric disorders seen in the Asian tsunami survivors are depicted in Table 26.1 (Math *et al.*, 2006, 2008a,b).

Table 26.1. Psychiatric health morbidity in disaster-affected population.

Common psychiatric disorders among adults

- Relapse of any pre-existing psychiatric disorders
- Adjustment disorders/abnormal grief
- Anxiety disorders like panic disorders, phobic disorders not otherwise specified (NOS), non-specific anxiety symptoms and startle response
- Acute stress reactions
- Insomnia
- Depression/death wishes/suicidal ideas or attempts
- Substance abuse and dependence (monetary relief given is spent on substance abuse)
- Post-traumatic stress disorders
- Non-specific somatic symptoms such as dizziness, headache, body ache, recollection of the disaster events through images and thoughts, nightmares, night terrors and so forth
- Dissociative symptoms
- Somatoform disorders

Common psychiatric disorders among children

- Non-specific symptoms such as dizziness, vertigo, startle response, sleep–wake cycle disturbances, clinging behaviour, excessive crying, withdrawal, fear, anger, irritability, numbing of affect, food refusal and decreased appetite and regressive behaviour
- School refusal, school dropout and academic decline
- Anxiety disorders like panic disorders, phobic disorders NOS, non-specific anxiety symptoms and so forth
- Oppositional defiant disorder (ODD) symptoms
- Conduct symptoms – like truancy, stealing, lying and so forth
- Post-traumatic stress disorders
- Depression
- Somatoform disorders

High Risk Groups for Developing Psychiatric Morbidity

Earlier studies predicted the following high risk variables: severity of the disaster, threat to life, loss of life, loss of family members and duration of exposure (Frankenberg *et al.*, 2008). Recent additions to the list are: female gender, children, elderly, physically disabled, single, ethnic minority, displaced population, poverty, substance use like smoking, loss of economic livelihood, poor social support and family support (Norris *et al.*, 2002a,b; Lubit and Eth, 2003; North, 2003; Bhugra and van Ommeren, 2006; Frankenberg *et al.*, 2008; Math *et al.*, 2008a). Men are at greater risk of developing substance use/dependence disorders and women are at greater risk of developing depression, PTSD and somatoform disorders.

Most children and young people are resilient, but also very vulnerable to the psychosocial effects of disasters (Lubit and Eth, 2003; Williams *et al.*, 2008). People with pre-existing mental disorders are well known to relapse during disasters (Smith *et al.*, 1990; Norris *et al.*, 2002b; Math *et al.*, 2006). Similarly, people with poor coping capacity, substance use and chronic general medical conditions are also at a high risk (Katz *et al.*, 2002; North, 2003; Cepeda *et al.*, 2010). Hence, general physicians practising in the area of disaster should be aware of the high prevalence of mental health disorders in chronic medically ill patients (Yang *et al.*, 2003; Noorthoorn *et al.*, 2010). Similarly, disaster rescue workers are at a high risk of developing psychiatric morbidity (Stellman *et al.*, 2008).

Role of Mental Health Professionals in a Disaster Situation

Contemporary disaster mental health treatment is based on the principles of 'preventive medicine'. This has necessitated a paradigm shift from relief-centred post-disaster management to disaster prevention, preparedness and mitigation. Many mental health professionals themselves do not understand their role in a disaster response effort. They are neither part of a pre-existing nor a post-disaster response team. Unlike other health professionals, mental health professionals have to liaise with the survivors from day one to the restoration phase. They have to play multidimensional roles from educating, training the trainers, negotiating, administration, fund raising, collaborative, skill transferring, treating, advocating and rehabilitating perspectives (see Table 26.2).

In addressing the spectrum of problems during the post-disaster period, mental health clinics in relief camps are useful in identifying and treating moderate-to-severe cases only (Math *et al.*, 2008b). Hence, the role of the specialist as a clinician is very minimal. However, the specialist has a very important role in training local resources in simple community-based interventions. These include: art therapy; informal education; group discussions; drama; structuring of daily activities; engaging in activities such as yoga, meditation, prayers, relaxation, sports and games; spiritual activities; providing factual information; and educating parents and teachers (Math *et al.*, 2008a,b; Kar, 2009). They are intended to provide important components of psychosocial rehabilitation such as normalizing, stabilizing, socializing, defusing of emotions and feelings and restoration of a sense of identification with others and of safety and security (Sundram *et al.*, 2008). These will not only help in the recovery of milder and sub-syndromal symptoms, but also in the prevention of adverse mental health consequences. Such interventions, when feasible, should begin as early as possible, targeting all high-risk populations in the affected area; however, to encourage participation and avoid stigmatization, the 'mental/psychiatric' label needs to be avoided (Math *et al.*, 2006).

Specialized care is required generally only for a small group of the population. The majority of the care occurs informally outside medical settings and is given by community-level workers. Training these community level workers is a highly essential ingredient of disaster management. They also need to be supervised and monitored for development of stress and the mental health impact of the disaster (Thormar *et al.*, 2010). Community level workers need to be trained in identifying severe cases and referring them to mental health professionals.

Table 26.2. Role of mental health professionals in disaster (Math *et al.*, 2011; Math, S.B. and Chaturvedi, 2011, unpublished data).

I. During pre-disaster period (preparedness)

1. Public education activities – life skills education, educating about disaster mental health
2. Disaster response network – to develop collaboration with various existing agencies like governmental agencies, NGOs and community health workers
3. Disaster response training of trainers in
   a. disaster mental health
   b. first aid (both medical and psychological)
   c. counselling skills
   d. stress management
   e. identifying common mental disorders and referral
   f. life skills education
4. Strengthening information, education and communication (IEC) activities

II. Immediately after the disaster (heroic and honeymoon phases)

1. Being part of the multidisciplinary relief team
2. Rapid assessment of
   a. magnitude of the psychological impact
   b. available mental health resources in the affected community
   c. needs assessments
   d. social, cultural and religious perspective of the community
3. Providing healthcare
   a. medical and psychological first aid
   b. treat pre-existing mentally ill patients
   c. substance intoxication and withdrawal in survivors
   d. establishing the referral system
4. Disaster psychiatry outreach teams to provide care
5. Collaborating with administrative and funding agencies
6. Dealing with the victims' and volunteers' stress (stress management)
7. Fostering the mass grieving/mourning
8. Mental health education – 'do's and 'do not's
   a. Educating the administrative personnel, local leaders and public
   b. Utilizing mass media to reach the survivors
9. Initiating collaboration with the local agencies for capacity building and outside agencies for support
10. Planning research

III. During disillusionment phase

1. Providing care for the mentally ill patients
2. Attending to the referrals
3. Continuing and expanding the capacity-building activities; training of resourceful community members like private physicians/doctors, primary healthcare staff, paramedical staffs, school teachers, anganwadi workers, alternative complementary medicine personnel, religious leaders, spiritual leaders and faith healers
4. Community outreach camps
5. Hand-holding of the community health workers
6. Assessment of the interventions and feedback mechanism

There is a need to de-medicalize the survivors' disaster response and also to de-professionalize the service delivery and focus on capacity building of the local community. Community empowerment involves educating and training the local trainers, administration, community leaders, NGOs, faith healers, community level workers and survivors (Aten *et al.*, 2010). The majority of disasters require temporary external aids. These should be culturally appropriate and targeted towards empowering the affected community to enhance their camaraderie and competence to cope with future disasters (Math *et al.*, 2008a; Rosen *et al.*, 2010).

'Foreign disaster relief experts' can be of tremendous value during disasters. Although nobly motivated to help, emergency interventions from them immediately post-disaster can have unintended consequences such as depleting scarce resources (like food and water), duplicating work, fighting with the various relief agencies, criticizing the local administration in the media, poor coordination with other agencies, using culturally inappropriate methods and the presence of a language barrier, which can cause more harm to the affected community (Van Hoving *et al.*, 2010). In this regard, the Sphere Project is an initiative to define and uphold the standards by which the global community responds to the plight of people affected by disasters, principally through a set of guidelines that are set out in the Humanitarian Charter and Minimum Standards in Disaster Response to promote accountability and share standards of good practice (Sphere Project, 2004). All the relief agencies need to adhere to these minimum standards.

Psychological Interventions

Psychological first aid

Survivors may exhibit a range of physical, emotional and cognitive symptoms. This heightened emotional state is similar to the classic fight/flight/freeze reaction of stress. The affected person may not be in a position to think and act rationally during the disaster. This can be explained by the fact that the amygdala has taken over from the frontal lobe. These reactions to disasters are often viewed as analogous to medical emergencies and thus believed to merit the most immediate interventions available called 'psychological first aid' (PFA). Similar to medical first aid, PFA techniques can be performed by minimally trained non-professionals within the affected community(Reyes and Elhai, 2004).

More recently, there has been a revived interest in PFA. It was initially described by Raphael (1986) for use in the civilian domain. The main goal of this is to relieve immediate distress and to prevent or minimize the development of pathological sequel (Vernberg *et al.*, 2008). The concept of PFA for individuals exposed to highly traumatic events has been used in the field of crisis management and disaster mental health for many years (Reyes, 2006). PFA was developed to reflect current best practices in disaster mental health based on research, expert consensus and practical experience. However, there are no systematic studies to examine the efficacy and usefulness of PFA.

Debriefing

Debriefing is defined as group discussions that occur within 48–72 h after an event and are often referred to as 'psychological debriefings' (Watson *et al.*, 2003). In general, these sessions encourage participants to describe and share both factual and emotional aspects of their disaster experience (Katz *et al.*, 2002). The principle behind this debriefing is that immediate processing gives an individual the ability to cognitively restructure the perceived disaster event so that it is remembered in a less traumatic way (Young *et al.*, 1998; Watson *et al.*, 2003). There are various modified forms of debriefing such as critical incident stress debriefing (CISD) (Mitchell, 1983) and critical incident stress management (CISM) (Mitchell and Everly, 2000). Debriefing is successfully used and implemented in military combat settings and by relief workers (Armstrong *et al.*, 1998; Knobler *et al.*, 2007). However, effectiveness of debriefing in survivors is controversial, while some studies do suggest that the technique may actually produce harm (Hobbs *et al.*, 1996; Armstrong, 2000; Rose *et al.*, 2003; Raphael and Wooding, 2004; Roberts *et al.*, 2009a). However, debriefing occurring outside the therapeutic setting is infrequent. Many of the survivors and relief workers like to talk about the disaster responses to family members, spouses, friends, colleagues and significant others (Fullerton *et al.*, 2000). The effect of such debriefing has not been explored in a systematic way.

Cognitive behavioural intervention (CBT)

CBT has been found to be effective in reducing subsequent psychopathology after exposure to disaster (Duffy *et al.*, 2007; Layne *et al.*, 2008). There are randomized controlled studies to support the findings that early intervention CBT groups had less PTSD when compared to a control group (Echeburua *et al.*, 1996; Bryant *et al.*, 1998, 1999; Gidron *et al.*, 2001; Shooshtary *et al.*, 2008). Although these studies report positive results, there are no long-term follow-up studies. A review by Roberts and his colleagues (Roberts *et al.*, 2009b) reported that trauma-focused CBT within 3 months of a traumatic event appears to be effective. CBT appears to be promising in mitigating the suffering of the survivors of a disaster. However, in a developing country like India, where the availability of trained manpower is sparse, the use of a computerized version of CBT needs to be explored (Litz *et al.*, 2007).

Other interventions

Recently there has been a re-emergence of interventions such as eye movement desensitization and reprocessing (EMDR) (Hertlein and Ricci, 2004; Seidler and Wagner, 2006; Bisson and Andrew, 2007) and trauma counselling (Jacobs and Prigerson, 2000) in management of disasters. However, the effectiveness of these procedures is yet to be established. In a recent Cochrane review by Bisson and Andrew (2007), there was evidence to demonstrate that individual CBT, EMDR, stress management and group trauma-focused cognitive behavioural therapy (TFCBT) are effective in the treatment of PTSD (Bisson and Andrew, 2007).

The European Network for Traumatic Stress (TENTS) final guideline on post-disaster psychosocial care summarizes the contemporary practices. TENTS recommends general support, access to social, physical and psychological support. Specific mental health interventions are indicated only after a comprehensive assessment. TFCBT is recommended for acute stress disorder or acute PTSD (Bisson *et al.*, 2010).

Pharmacological Interventions

Prophylactic use of psychotropic medications is discouraged in disaster management due to popular notions like: (i) disaster reactions are generally normal people in abnormal situations; (ii) the majority of the symptoms are self-limiting; and (iii) there are no well-controlled studies to say that prophylactic use of medicine decreases psychiatric morbidity. Various medications have been tried such as propranolol (Cahill *et al.*, 1994; Vaiva *et al.*, 2003), clonidine (Kinzie and Leung, 1989), guanfacine (Horrigan, 1996), prazosin (Raskind *et al.*, 2003), amitriptyline (Lavie, 2001), imipramine (Robert *et al.*, 1999) and risperidone (Stanovic *et al.*, 2001). Use of benzodiazepines such as clonazepam (Gelpin *et al.*, 1996) and temazepam (Mellman *et al.*, 1998) for a longer duration has been considered to prevent development of PTSD. No medication has been found to be effective in preventing psychiatric morbidity in well-controlled studies.

The majority of the studies were open label trials with small sample sizes and from different populations such as combat veterans, accident victims and burn victims. Extrapolation of data from these studies cannot be used as justification to use medication in disaster settings. However, use of prophylactic psychotropic medications may be justified in pre-existing mental illness to avoid relapse, acute substance withdrawal to avoid complications, suicidal attempt and severe depression. Considering the paucity of evidence it is difficult to recommend prophylactic psychotropic medication in a disaster setting.

To summarize, post-disaster mental healthcare needs to be evidence based. This is well documented and analysed in a recent review on post-disaster psychological care (Figueroa *et al.*, 2010). This review article recommended five echelon levels of care according to the best evidence available. The psychological supports in five echelon levels are: diffusion, social support, general medical care, general psychiatric care and psychiatric care provided by experts. Only victims with well-established formal psychiatric disorders should receive psychotherapy or psychotropic medication. The rest should only receive PFA (Figueroa *et al.*, 2010).

Resilience Factors

Resilience means the speed with which homeostasis is achieved after disaster (Norris *et al.*, 2008). This concept of resilience has been applied to describe the adaptive capacities of individuals or communities in response to an adversity like disaster.

The majority of the research on disaster is on psychopathology rather than on resilience factors that protect people from developing psychiatric morbidity (North *et al.*, 2008). There are no systematic studies, however, preliminary research has yielded the following resilience factors: a cohesive community, adequate community resources, minimal displacement, absence of risk factors and good social support (Lopez-Ibor *et al.*,

2005), preserved family system and support, altruistic behaviour of the community leaders, minimal materialistic needs, religious faith and spirituality have been associated with positive outcome and community resilience. This was noted in the native population of the Andaman and Nicobar islands of India (Math *et al.*, 2008a). However, these resilience factors need to be studied systematically in a well-controlled disaster population. Simple steps as mentioned in Table 26.3 may be initiated to foster resilience.

Table 26.3. Simple and effective methods that can be adopted in relief camps.

- If possible avoid displacement of the survivors from their locality
- Foster family, cultural and religious rituals
- Validate the emotions of the survivors' experience and also survivors' guilt
- Provide accurate information about the disaster event, relief work and so forth
- Normalize the daily activities of children and adults
- Engage children in various informal education methods with innovative ideas like drawing, sketching, singing, miming and so forth by using available community resources
- Engage the adult survivors in camp activities like cooking, cleaning and assisting in relief work
- Start schools in the disaster-affected area at the earliest opportunity so that normalization and structuring of the daily activities occurs in children
- Simple sleep hygiene techniques to be taught
- Educating survivors about harmful effect of substance use is essential
- Encourage children to ask as many questions as they want, and be ready to answer them truthfully
- Educate survivors
- Community-based group (CBG) interventions can be planned like art therapy (painting/drawing), informal education, group discussions, dramas, story-telling, structuring their day, engaging in activities, yoga, relaxation and sports/games
- Stress management of the relief worker is essential
- Involving the survivors in rebuilding their community (empowerment) is essential

Conclusions

Disasters are an inevitable truth of life. Planning and preparedness is highly essential to meet challenges. Disaster management is a continuous and integrated cyclical process of planning, organizing, coordinating and implementing measures to prevent and to manage the problems associated effectively. Thinking from 'when' the disaster strikes to 'if' the disaster strikes has necessitated a paradigm shift from relief-centred post-disaster management to a holistic, integrated and preventive approach based upon principles of disaster prevention, preparedness and mitigation. Community-based group interventions should begin as early as possible, targeting all high-risk populations in the affected area; however, to encourage participation and avoid stigmatization, the 'mental health/psychiatric' label needs to be avoided with disaster mental health programmes.

Disaster-related interventions need to be conservative from a medication perspective and predominantly psychosocial in approach. There is a need to de-medicalize the survivors' disaster response and also to de-professionalize the service delivery through local community-level workers. Involving the local affected community not only helps in capacity building but also in community participation. Rehabilitation efforts planned should be culturally appropriate and targeted towards empowering the affected community to enhance their camaraderie and competence to cope with future disasters.

References

Armstrong, K. (2000) Multiple stressor debriefing as a model for intervention. In: Raphael, B. and Wilson, J. (eds) *Psychological Debriefing: Theory, Practice and Evidence*. Cambridge University Press, New York, pp. 290–301.

Armstrong, K., Zatzick, D., Metzler, T., Weiss, D.S., Marmar, C.R., Garma, S., Ronfeldt, H. and Roepke, L. (1998) Debriefing of American Red Cross personnel: pilot study on participants' evaluations and case examples from the 1994 Los Angeles earthquake relief operation. *Social Work Health Care* 27, 33–50.

Aten, J.D., Topping, S., Denney, R.M. and Bayne, T.G. (2010) Collaborating with African American churches to overcome minority disaster mental health disparities: what mental health professionals can learn from Hurricane Katrina. *Professional Psychology: Research and Practice* 41, 167–173.

Basoglu, M., Kilic, C., Salcioglu, E. and Livanou, M. (2004) Prevalence of posttraumatic stress disorder and comorbid depression in earthquake survivors in Turkey: an epidemiological study. *Journal of Traumatic Stress* 17, 133–141.

Baum, A. and Fleming, I. (1993) Implications of psychological research on stress and technological accidents. *American Psychologist* 48, 665–672.

Bhugra, D. and van Ommeren, M. (2006) Mental health, psychosocial support and the tsunami. *International Review of Psychiatry* 18, 213–216.

Bisson, J. and Andrew, M. (2007) Psychological treatment of post-traumatic stress disorder (PTSD). *Cochrane Database Syst Rev*, CD003388.

Bisson, J.I., Tavakoly, B., Witteveen, A.B., Ajdukovic, D., Jehel, L., Johansen, V.J., Nordanger, D., Garcia, F.O., Punamaki, R.L. and Schnyder, U. (2010) TENTS guidelines: development of post-disaster psychosocial care guidelines through a Delphi process. *The British Journal of Psychiatry* 196, 69–74.

Bryant, R.A., Harvey, A.G. and Dang, S.T. (1998) Treatment of acute stress disorder: a comparison of cognitive-behavioral therapy and supportive counseling. *Journal of Consulting and Clinical Psychology* 66, 862–866.

Bryant, R.A., Sackville, T. and Dang, S.T. (1999) Treating acute stress disorder: an evaluation of cognitive behavioral therapy and supportive counseling techniques. *American Journal of Psychiatry* 156, 1780–1786.

Cahill, L., Prins, B., Weber, M. and McGaugh, J.L. (1994) β-Adrenergic activation and memory for emotional events. *Nature* 371, 702–704.

Cepeda, A., Saint Onge, J.M., Kaplan, C. and Valdez, A. (2010) The association between disaster-related experiences and mental health outcomes among drug using African American Hurricane Katrina evacuees. *Community Mental Health Journal* 46(6) 612–620.

Duffy, M., Gillespie, K. and Clark, D.M. (2007) Post-traumatic stress disorder in the context of terrorism and other civil conflict in Northern Ireland: randomised controlled trial. *British Medical Journal* 334, 1147.

Echeburua, E., de Corral, P. and Sarasua, B. (1996) Treatment of acute posttraumatic stress disorder in rape victims: an experimental study. *Journal of Anxiety Disorders* 10, 185–199.

Figueroa, R., Marín, H. and González, M. (2010) Psychological support for disaster victims: an evidence-based care model. *Revista médica de Chile* 138, 143–151.

Frankenberg, E., Friedman, J., Gillespie, T., Ingwersen, N., Pynoos, R., Rifai, I.U., Sikoki, B., Steinberg, A., Sumantri, C., Suriastini, W. and Thomas, D. (2008) Mental health in Sumatra after the tsunami. *American Journal of Public Health* 98, 1671–1677.

Freedman, A.M. and Blumenfield, M. (1986) Recognizing the role of bereavement and reactive depression in modern psychiatry. *Psychopathology* 19 Suppl 2, 37–46.

Fullerton, C.S., Ursano, R.J., Vance, K. and Wang, L. (2000) Debriefing following trauma. *Psychiatric Quarterly* 71, 259–276.

Gelpin, E., Bonne, O., Peri, T., Brandes, D. and Shalev, A.Y. (1996) Treatment of recent trauma survivors with benzodiazepines: a prospective study. *Journal of Clinical Psychiatry* 57, 390–394.

Ghaffari-Nejad, A., Ahmadi-Mousavi, M., Gandomkar, M. and Reihani-Kermani, H. (2007) The prevalence of complicated grief among Bam earthquake survivors in Iran. *Archives of Iranian Medicine* 10, 525–528.

Gidron, Y., Gal, R. and Freedman, S.A. (2001) Translating research findings to PTSD prevention: results of a randomized-controlled pilot study. *Journal of Traumatic Stress* 14, 773–780.

Goenjian, A.K., Molina, L., Steinberg, A.M., Fairbanks, L.A., Alvarez, M.L., Goenjian, H.A. and Pynoos, R.S. (2001) Posttraumatic stress and depressive reactions among Nicaraguan adolescents after hurricane Mitch. *American Journal of Psychiatry* 158, 788–794.

Goenjian, A.K., Walling, D., Steinberg, A.M., Roussos, A., Goenjian, H.A. and Pynoos, R.S. (2009) Depression and PTSD symptoms among bereaved adolescents 6(1/2) years after the 1988 Spitak earthquake. *Journal of Affective Disorders* 112, 81–84.

Hertlein, K.M. and Ricci, R.J. (2004) A systematic research synthesis of EMDR studies: implementation of the platinum standard. *Trauma Violence Abuse* 5, 285–300.

Hobbs, M., Mayou, R. and Harrison, B. (1996) A randomized trial of psychological debriefing for victims of road traffic accidents. *British Medical Journal* 313, 1438–1439.

Hollifield, M., Hewage, C., Gunawardena, C.N., Kodituwakku, P., Bopagoda, K. and Weerarathnege, K. (2008) Symptoms and coping in Sri Lanka 20–21 months after the 2004 tsunami. *British Journal of Psychiatry* 192, 39–44.

Horrigan, J.P. (1996) Guanfacine for PTSD nightmares. *Journals of the American Academy of Child and Adolescent Psychiatry* 35, 975–976.

Jacobs, S. and Prigerson, H. (2000) Psychotherapy of traumatic grief: a review of evidence for psychotherapeutic treatments. *Death Studies* 24, 479–495.

Kar, N. (2009) Psychological impact of disasters on children: review of assessment and interventions. *World Journal of Pediatrics* 5, 5–11.

Katz, C.L., Pellegrino, L., Pandya, A., Ng, A. and DeLisi, L.E. (2002) Research on psychiatric outcomes and interventions subsequent to disasters: a review of the literature. *Psychiatry Research* 110, 201–217.

Kim, S.C., Plumb, R., Gredig, Q.N., Rankin, L. and Taylor, B. (2008) Medium-term post-Katrina health sequelae among New Orleans residents: predictors of poor mental and physical health. *Journal of Clinical Nursing* 17, 2335–2342.

Kinzie, J.D. and Leung, P. (1989) Clonidine in Cambodian patients with post-traumatic stress disorder. *Journal of Nervous and Mental Disorders* 177, 546–550.

Knobler, H.Y., Nachshoni, T., Jaffe, E., Peretz, G. and Yehuda, Y.B. (2007) Psychological guidelines for a medical team debriefing after a stressful event. *Military Medicine* 172, 581–585.

Kübler-Ross, E. (1969) *On Death and Dying*. Macmillan, New York.

Lavie, P. (2001) Sleep disturbances in the wake of traumatic events. *New England Journal of Medicine* 345, 1825–1832.

Layne, C.M., Saltzman, W.R., Poppleton, L., Burlingame, G.M., Pasalic, A., Durakovic, E., Music, M., Campara, N., Dapo, N., Arslanagic, B., Steinberg, A.M. and Pynoos, R.S. (2008)

Effectiveness of a school-based group psychotherapy program for war-exposed adolescents: a randomized controlled trial. *Journals of the American Academy of Child and Adolescent Psychiatry* 47, 1048–1062.

Lazarus, R.S. and Cohen, J.B. (1978) Environmental stress. In: Altman, I. and Wohlwill, J.F. (eds) *Human Behavior and the Environment: Current Theory and Tesearch*. Plenum, New York.

Litz, B.T., Engel, C.C., Bryant, R.A. and Papa, A. (2007) A randomized, controlled proof-of-concept trial of an internet-based, therapist-assisted self-management treatment for posttraumatic stress disorder. *American Journal of Psychiatry* 164, 1676–1683.

Liu, A., Tan, H., Zhou, J., Li, S., Yang, T., Wang, J., Liu, J., Tang, X., Sun, Z. and Wen, S.W. (2006) An epidemiologic study of posttraumatic stress disorder in flood victims in Hunan China. *Canadian Journal of Psychiatry* 51, 350–354.

Lopez-Ibor, J.J., Christodoulou, G., Maj, M., Sartorius, N. and Okash, A. (2005) *Disaster and Mental Health*. John Wiley & Sons Ltd, Chicester, UK.

Lubit, R. and Eth, S. (2003) Children, disasters, and the September 11th World Trade Center attack. In: Ursano, R.J. and Norwood, A.E. (eds) *Trauma and Disaster, Responses and Management, Review of Psychiatry Series*. Vol 22(1). American Psychiatric Publishing, Washington, DC, pp. 63–96.

Math, S.B. and Chandrashekar, C.R. (2003) Adjustment disorder. In: Isaac, M.I. and Mudrak, S.N. (eds) *Anxiety and Depression in Clinical Practice*. Abbott India Ltd, Mumbai, India.

Math, S.B., Girimaji, S.C., Benegal, V., Uday Kumar, G.S., Hamza, A. and Nagaraja, D. (2006) Tsunami: psychosocial aspects of Andaman and Nicobar islands. Assessments and intervention in the early phase. *International Review of Psychiatry* 18, 233–239.

Math, S.B., John, J.P., Girimaji, S.C., Benegal, V., Sunny, B., Krishnakanth, K., Kumar, U., Hamza, A., Tandon, S., Jangam, K., Meena, K.S., Chandramukhi, B. and Nagaraja, D. (2008a) Comparative study of psychiatric morbidity among the displaced and non-displaced populations in the Andaman and Nicobar Islands following the tsunami. *Prehospital Disaster Medicine* 23, 29–34; discussion 35.

Math, S.B., Tandon, S., Girimaji, S.C., Benegal, V., Kumar, U., Hamza, A., Jangam, K. and Nagaraja, D. (2008b) Psychological impact of the tsunami on children and adolescents from the Andaman and Nicobar islands. *Primary Care Companion for Journal of Clinical Psychiatry* 10, 31–37.

Math, S.B., Kumar, N.C. and Maria, C.N. (2011) Disaster mental health and public health: an integrative approach to recovery. In: Stein, D.J., Friedman, M.J. and Blanco, C. (eds) *Post Traumatic Stress Disorder*. John Wiley & Sons, Ltd, Chichester, UK

Mellman, T.A., Byers, P.M. and Augenstein, J.S. (1998) Pilot evaluation of hypnotic medication during acute traumatic stress response. *Journal of Traumatic Stress* 11, 563–569.

Mitchell, J.T. (1983) When disaster strikes: the critical incident stress debriefing. *Journal of Emergency Medical Services* 8, 36–39.

Mitchell, J.T. and Everly, G.S. (2000) Critical incident stress management and critical incident stress debriefings: evolutions, effects and outcomes. In: Raphael, B. and Wilson, J. (eds) *Psychological Debriefing: Theory, Practice and Evidence*. Cambridge University Press, New York.

Noorthoorn, E.O., Havenaar, J.M., de Haan, H.A., van Rood, Y.R. and van Stiphout, W.A.H.J. (2010) Mental health service use and outcomes after the Enschede fireworks disaster: a naturalistic follow-up study. *Psychiatric Services* 61, 1138–1143.

Norris, F. (1992) Epidemiology of trauma: frequency and impact of different potentially traumatic events on different demographic groups. *Journal of Consulting and Clinical Psychology* 60, 409–418.

Norris, F.H. and Elrod, C.L. (2006) Psychosocial consequences of disaster: a review of past research. In: Norris, F.H., Galea, S., Friedman, M.J. and Watson, P.J. (eds) *Methods for Disaster Mental Health Research*. The Guilford Press, New York.

Norris, F.H., Friedman, M.J. and Watson, P.J. (2002a) 60,000 disaster victims speak: Part II. Summary and implications of the disaster mental health research. *Psychiatry* 65, 240–260.

Norris, F.H., Friedman, M.J., Watson, P.J., Byrne, C.M., Diaz, E. and Kaniasty, K. (2002b) 60,000 disaster victims speak: Part I. An empirical review of the empirical literature, 1981–2001. *Psychiatry* 65, 207–239.

Norris, F.H., Stevens, S.P., Pfefferbaum, B., Wyche, K.F. and Pfefferbaum, R.L. (2008) Community resilience as a metaphor, theory, set of capacities, and strategy for disaster readiness. *American Journal of Community Psychology* 41, 127–150.

North, C.S. (2002) Somatization in survivors of catastrophic trauma: a methodological review. *Environmental Health Perspective* 110, Suppl 4, 637–640.

North, C.S. (2003) Psychiatric epidemiology of disaster responses. In: Ursano, R.J. and Norwood, A.E. (eds) *Trauma and Disaster, Responses and Management, Review of Psychiatry Series*. Vol 22(1). American Psychiatric Publishing, Washington, DC, pp. 37–62.

North, C.S., Kawasaki, A., Spitznagel, E.L. and Hong, B.A. (2004) The course of PTSD, major depression, substance abuse, and somatization after a natural disaster. *Journal of Nervous and Mental Disorders* 192, 823–829.

North, C.S., Hong, B.A., Suris, A. and Spitznagel, E.L. (2008) Distinguishing distress and psychopathology among survivors of the Oakland/Berkeley firestorm. *Psychiatry* 71, 35–45.

Pfefferbaum, B., Vinekar, S.S., Trautman, R.P., Lensgraf, S.J., Reddy, C., Patel, N. and Ford, A.L. (2002) The effect of loss and trauma on substance use behavior in individuals seeking support services after the 1995 Oklahoma City bombing. *Annals of Clinical Psychiatry* 14, 89–95.

Raphael, B. (1986) *When Disaster Strikes. How Individuals and Communities Cope with Catastrophe.* Basic Books, New York.

Raphael, B. and Wooding, S. (2004) Debriefing: its evolution and current status. *Psychiatric Clinics of North America* 27, 407–423.

Raskind, M.A., Peskind, E.R. and Kanter, E.D. (2003) Reduction of nightmares and other PTSD symptoms in combat veterans by prazosin: a placebo-controlled study. *American Journal of Psychiatry* 160, 371–373.

Reijneveld, S.A., Crone, M.R., Schuller, A.A., Verhulst, F.C. and Verloove-Vanhorick, S.P. (2005) The changing impact of a severe disaster on the mental health and substance misuse of adolescents: follow-up of a controlled study. *Psychological Medicine* 35, 367–376.

Reyes, G. (2006) Psychological first aid: principles of community-based psychological support. In: Reyes, G. and Jacobs, G.A. (eds) *Handbook of International Disaster Psychology: Vol. 2. Practices and Programs*. Praeger,Westport, Connecticut, pp. 1–12.

Reyes, G. and Elhai, J.D. (2004) Psychosocial interventions in the early phases of disasters *Psychotherapy: Theory, Research, Practice, Training* 41, 399–411.

Robert, R., Blakeney, P.E., Villarreal, C., Rosenberg, L. and Meyer, W.J. III (1999) Imipramine treatment in pediatric burn patients with symptoms of acute stress disorder: a pilot study. *Journal of the American Academy of Child and Adolescent Psychiatry* 38, 873–882.

Roberts, N.P., Kitchiner, N.J., Kenardy, J. and Bisson, J. (2009a) Multiple session early psychological interventions for the prevention of post-traumatic stress disorder. *Cochrane Database System Review*, CD006869.

Roberts, N.P., Kitchiner, N.J., Kenardy, J. and Bisson, J.I. (2009b) Systematic review and meta-analysis of multiple-session early interventions following traumatic events. *American Journal of Psychiatry* 166, 293–301.

Rohrbach, L.A., Grana, R., Vernberg, E., Sussman, S. and Sun, P. (2009) Impact of hurricane Rita on adolescent substance use. *Psychiatry* 72, 222–237.

Rose, S., Bisson, J. and Wesseley, S. (2003) Psychological debriefing for preventing post-traumatic stress disorder (PTSD) (Cochrane Review). In: The Cochrane Library, Issue 1. Update Software, Oxford, UK.

Rosen, C.S., Greene, C.J., Young, H.E. and Norris, F.H. (2010) Tailoring disaster mental health services to diverse needs: an analysis of 36 crisis counseling projects. *Health and Social Work* 35, 211–220.

Salcioglu, E., Basoglu, M. and Livanou, M. (2007) Post-traumatic stress disorder and comorbid depression among survivors of the 1999 earthquake in Turkey. *Disasters* 31, 115–129.

Seidler, G.H. and Wagner, F.E. (2006) Comparing the efficacy of EMDR and trauma-focused cognitive-behavioral therapy in the treatment of PTSD: a meta-analytic study. *Psychological Medicine* 36, 1515–1522.

Shooshtary, M.H., Panaghi, L. and Moghadam, J.A. (2008) Outcome of cognitive behavioral therapy in adolescents after natural disaster. *Journal of Adolescent Health* 42, 466–472.

Smith, E.M., North, C.S., McCool, R.E. and Shea, J.M. (1990) Acute postdisaster psychiatric disorders: identification of persons at risk. *American Journal of Psychiatry* 147, 202–206.

Stanovic, J.K., James, K.A. and Vandevere, C.A. (2001) The effectiveness of risperidone on acute stress symptoms in adult burn patients: a preliminary retrospective pilot study. *Journal of Burn Care and Rehabilitation* 22, 210–213.

Stellman, J.M., Smith, R.P., Katz, C.L., Sharma, V., Charney, D.S., Herbert, R., Moline, J., Luft, B.J., Markowitz, S., Udasin, I., Harrison, D., Baron, S., Landrigan, P.J., Levin, S.M. and Southwick, S. (2008) Enduring mental health morbidity and social function impairment in world trade center rescue, recovery, and cleanup workers: the psychological dimension of an environmental health disaster. *Environmental Health Perspective* 116, 1248–1253.

Sundram, S., Karim, M.E., Ladrido-Ignacio, L., Maramis, A., Mufti, K.A., Nagaraja, D., Shinfuku, N., Somasundaram, D., Udomratn, P., Yizhuang, Z., Ahsan, A., Chaudhry, H.R., Chowdhury, S., D'Souza, R., Dongfeng, Z., Firoz, A.H.M., Hamid, M.A., Indradjaya, S., Math, S.B., Mustafizur, R.A.H.M., Naeem, F. and Wahab, M.A. (2008) Psychosocial responses to disaster: an Asian perspective. *Asian Journal of Psychiatry* 1, 7–14.

The Disaster Management Act (2005) Available at: http://www.ndmindia.nic.in/acts-rules/DisasterManagementAct2005.pdf (Accessed 20 June 2011).

The Sphere Project (2004) Humanitarian charter and minimum standards in disaster response. WHO Geneva: Sphere Project. Available at: http://www.sphereproject.org/component/option,com_docman/Itemid,203/lang,english/ (Accessed 21 April 2011).

Thienkrua, W., Cardozo, B.L., Chakkraband, M.L., Guadamuz, T.E., Pengjuntr, W., Tantipiwatanaskul, P., Sakornsatian, S., Ekassawin, S., Panyayong, B., Varangrat, A., Tappero, J.W., Schreiber, M. and van Griensven, F. (2006) Symptoms of posttraumatic stress disorder and depression among children in tsunami-affected areas in southern Thailand. *Journal of the American Medical Association* 296, 549–559.

Thormar, S.B., Gersons, B.P.R., Juen, B., Marschang, A., Djakababa, M.N. and Olff, M. (2010) The mental health impact of volunteering in a disaster setting: a review. *The Journal of Nervous and Mental Disease* 198, 529–538.

Tsai, K.Y., Chou, P., Chou, F.H., Su, T.T., Lin, S.C., Lu, M.K., Ou-Yang, W.C., Su, C.Y., Chao, S.S., Huang, M.W., Wu, H.C., Sun, W.J., Su, S.F. and Chen, M.C. (2007) Three-year follow-up study of the relationship between posttraumatic stress symptoms and quality of life among earthquake survivors in Yu-Chi, Taiwan. *Journal of Psychiatric Research* 41, 90–96.

Udomratn, P. (2008) Mental health and the psychosocial consequences of natural disasters in Asia. *International Review of Psychiatry* 20, 441–444.

Vaiva, G., Ducrocq, F. and Jezequel, K. (2003) Immediate treatment with propranolol decreases post-traumatic stress disorder two months after trauma. *Biological Psychiatry* 54, 947–949.

Van Hoving, D.J., Wallis, L.A., Docrat, F. and De Vries, S. (2010) Haiti disaster tourism – a medical shame. *Prehospital and Disaster Medicine* 25, 201–202.

Vernberg, E.M., Steinberg, A.M., Jacobs, A.K., Brymer, M.J., Watson, P.J., Osofsky, J.D., Layne, C.M., Pynoos, R.S. and Ruzek, J.I. (2008) Innovations in disaster mental health: psychological first aid. *Professional Psychology: Research and Practice*, 381–388.

Watson, P.J., Friedman, M.J., Gibson, L.E., Ruzek, J.I., Norris, F.H. and Ritchie, E.C. (2003) Early intervention for trauma-related problems. In: Ursano, R.J. and Norwood, A.E. (eds) *Trauma and Disaster, Responses and Management, Review of Psychiatry Series.* Vol 22(1). American Psychiatric Publishing, Washington, DC, pp. 97–124.

Williams, R., Alexander, D.A., Bolsover, D. and Bakke, F.K. (2008) Children, resilience and disasters: recent evidence that should influence a model of psychosocial care. *Current Opinion in Psychiatry* 21, 338–344.

World Health Organization (1992) Psychosocial consequences of disasters: prevention and management. World Health Organization, Geneva.

Yang, Y.K., Yeh, T.L., Chen, C.C., Lee, C.K., Lee, I.H., Lee, L.C. and Jeffries, K.J. (2003) Psychiatric morbidity and posttraumatic symptoms among earthquake victims in primary care clinics. *General Hospital Psychiatry* 25, 253–261.

Young, B.H., Ford, J.D., Ruzek, J.I., Friedman, M. and Gusman, F.D. (1998) Disaster mental health services: a guide for clinicians and administrators. National Center for Post-Traumatic Stress Disorder, Palo Alto, California. Available at: https://www.hsdl.org/?view&did=441325 (Accessed 8 March 2013).

Chapter 27

Efficient Human Resource Management Contributes to Augmented Societal Resilience in the Aftermath of Disasters: Lessons from the 2011 Tōhoku Earthquake and Tsunami

Preeti Arora, Rupa Gunaseelan and Rajesh Arora

Introduction

Disasters, apart from their direct effects on property, infrastructure, human and animal lives, etc. leave a long trail of effects in the psyche of people, which are often subtle and difficult to recognize (Arora *et al.*, 2013). The societal impact of disasters, especially the psychosocial consequences of disasters has been recorded in history, however, increased attention has been paid to these effects in this century (NIMHANS, 2010). In recent years, the psychosocial consequences of disasters have been studied in enormous detail with a view to improving the quality of lives of innumerable people who are affected by disasters. The most common effects manifested in individuals, responders or the community that has been exposed to either natural or man-made disasters include depression, anxiety, psychosomatic symptoms, stigma, fear of the unknown, post-traumatic stress disorder (PTSD), etc. (Norris *et al.*, 2002; Zimmering *et al.*, 2006; Neria *et al.*, 2008; Ehring *et al.*, 2011; Bromet, 2012). It is increasingly being recognized that not only the general population, but also the responders (civilians, military personnel, first responders, emergency and rescue services personnel, humanitarian aid workers, non-health and welfare employed persons and healthcare staff) are susceptible to disaster-related emotional problems (Benedek *et al.*, 2007; Walsh, 2009; Bromet, 2012; Fushimi, 2012).

Disasters and mass casualty incidents overwhelm the social and political fabric of communities and can also aggravate already existing problems in individuals, of course depending on the individual's capacity to cope, to such an extent that the psychosocial profile is disturbed significantly (Katz *et al.*, 2002). At global level there is a paradigm shift in focus from post-crisis intervention to crisis prevention, therefore, it is imperative that preventive steps be taken to mitigate the psychosocial impact of disasters.

Studying human response to disasters enables disaster professionals to devise strategies for better management of psychological problems in the community in general and susceptible individuals, in particular. Provision of psychosocial care to the community is recognized as a neglected area following any disaster and needs attention (van Ommeren *et al.*, 2005; Mahoney *et al.*, 2006; Prasetiyawan *et al.*, 2006; Williams and Drury, 2009; Herrman, 2012). The ability of individuals and the community to bear the brunt of disasters necessitates resilience to be ingrained in society. This chapter presents an on- and off-ground psychosocial perspective of the 2011 Tōhoku earthquake and the ensuing multiple disasters, and highlights a leveraging systems approach for efficient disaster management.

Disasters in Japan and their Societal Impact

In general, Japanese society is quite resilient to disasters; however, the 2011 Tōhoku earthquake and the ensuing multiple disasters were so overwhelming that despite the nation's resilience, it shook the very framework of society (BBC News, 2011). The Japanese community responded in a brave manner to the unprecedented scale of disasters (Parashar *et al.*, 2011). Such was the impact that countries as far away as the USA prepared themselves to handle the impact, including the preparations for a local public health response to the tsunami threat in coastal California (Hunter *et al.*, 2012).

Ever since the great Kobe (Hanshin-Awaji) earthquake in 1995 in Japan, mental healthcare in the aftermath of disasters has been considered as a major concern by mental health professionals and the general community (van Ommeren *et al.*, 2005; Nishio *et al.*, 2009; Kim and Akiyama, 2011).

Adequate measures have been taken by Japan to provide psychosocial care to the community right from the time since relief and rescue work have been first undertaken. Such interventions go a long way towards minimizing the impact disasters in terms of psychosocial manifestation of problems that develop post-disaster.

The Tōhoko 2011 Earthquake and Multiple Disasters

Psychosocial impact in a disaster-resilient society

It is well established that disasters impact humans physically, psychologically, socially and economically in subsequent phases (Fig. 27.1). The Japan 2011 megadisasters were no different and drastically impacted almost all sections and strata of society, causing immense physical, psychological, mental, social, economic and other losses that were evident in various phases of the disaster (Arora, 2011; Arora *et al.*, 2012).

The psychological component cannot be ignored in any case as has been demonstrated in previous natural disasters (Kato *et al.*, 1996; Chen *et al.*, 2001; Kokai *et al.*, 2004). It has been acknowledged by disaster-affected people that their mental health state is compromised to a great extent in the aftermath of the event (Toyabe *et al.*, 2007). Some researchers acknowledge that the maximum effect of disasters on community mental health usually results immediately after the disaster and persists for about a week. This phase is followed by recovery, which is observed usually after about a month's time and may continue for up to a year and a half. However, according to rough estimates the excess morbidity rate of psychiatric disorders in the first year after a disaster is of the order of 20% (Bromet, 2012) as disasters take a heavy toll on the mental health of the affected population. It is often also observed that populations exhibit signs of mental disorders over a period of years, depending upon the socio-cultural milieu.

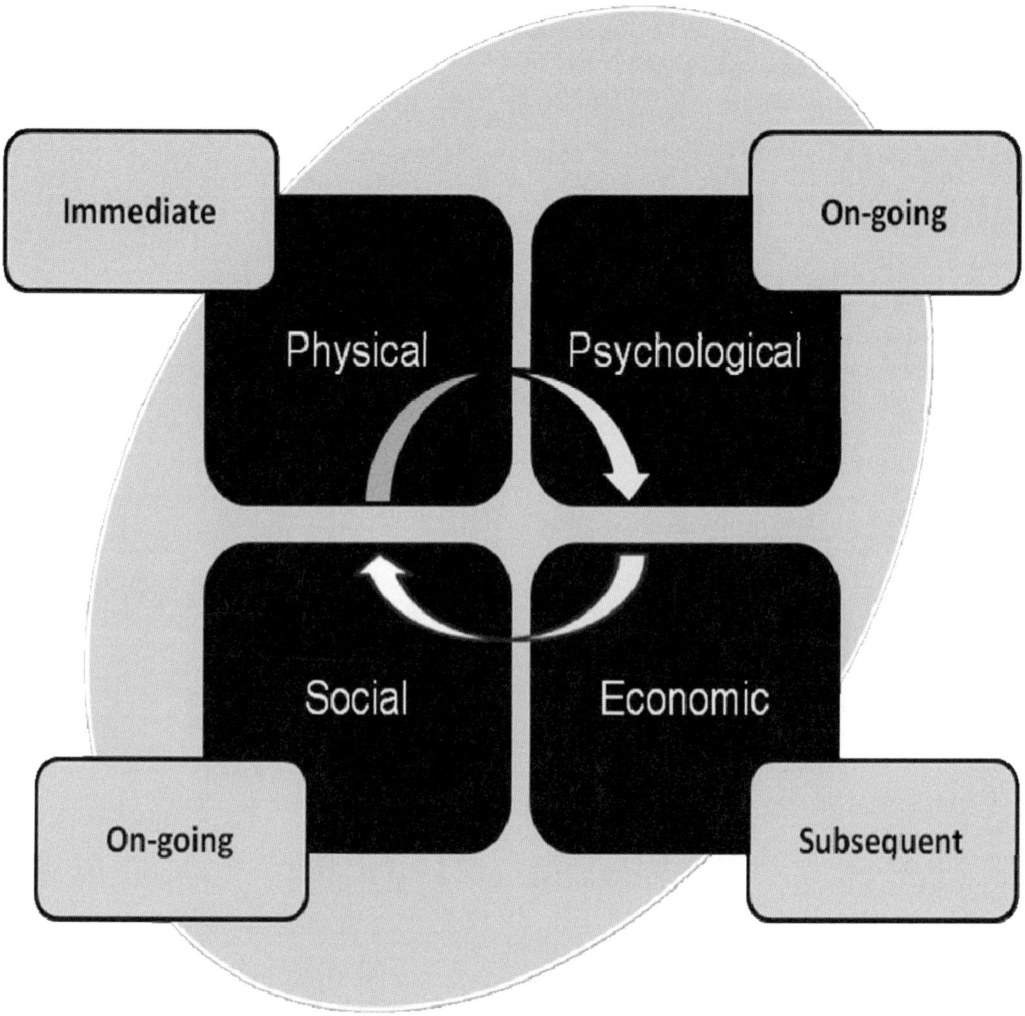

Fig. 27.1. The multitude of factors that impact humans in the event of a disaster.

Wang *et al.* (2000) reported that exposure to an earthquake in China was associated with multidimensional impairment in quality of life, including physical, psychological and environmental domains within 3 months. The victims reported more psychological distress in terms of depression, somatization and anxiety leading the authors of the work to conclude that comprehensive and prospective assessment of disaster effects is imperative for better organization of disaster relief programmes and psychosocial interventions.

In the Japan multiple disasters, besides dead and missing people, a large number of people from all walks of life and belonging to almost all groups were displaced/affected. The number of casualties has been reported to be over 25,000, with over 15,850 dead, over

3250 missing and over 6000 injured. The devastating tsunami created over 300,000 refugees in the Tōhoku region and resulted in partial shortages of food, water, shelter, essential medicines and fuel for survivors. This in itself was a cause of immense stress in the affected community. At official level, in response to this unprecedented crisis, the Japanese government mobilized its highly trained and efficient Self-Defence Forces, which responded very efficiently to the best of its ability. Subsequently, 163 countries and regions too joined, working shoulder to shoulder with 43 international organizations, which extended assistance in various forms, including trained search and rescue teams to help in the search for survivors and salvaging precious items. Non-government organizations (NGOs) and other humanitarian organizations, both in Japan and worldwide, responded with immense care and concern, with the Japanese Red Cross alone contributing US$1 billion in donations.

The economic impact of the disaster was substantial leading to immediate problems, which were felt even the day after the disaster. Industrial production was suspended in several factories and labour was affected in many prefectures. Later on amongst other countries, the threats of radiation in the products manufactured were a cause of major concern. A large number of people were rendered jobless without any earnings in the initial phases. This led to the manifestation of psychological problems in the affected community. The 2011 Tōhoku earthquake and tsunami had a massive socioeconomic impact on the community residing in Japan in the aftermath of the disaster. As per rough estimates, the long-term issue of the cost of rebuilding was estimated at ¥10 trillion (US$122 billion). The colossal population that was affected and also the indirectly affected population were indeed found to be susceptible to psychosocial disorders in the wake of the unprecedented cascade of events.

A further serious impact of the tsunami was the critical damage to the Fukushima Daiichi nuclear power station (Chandler, 2011), resulting in severe radiation leakage (Sharma and Arora, 2011). This event posed a long-term health and environmental hazard and the necessity for an expensive clean-up made conditions appear grim. Several businesses were severely affected. A number of working professionals left Japan due to psychosocial fears associated with continuity of businesses. Business continuity problems arose in the immediate wake of the disaster and this was an important concern. It affected both small businesses and large-scale manufacturers.

Yamazaki *et al.* (2011) reported that on day two after the Great East Japan Earthquake disaster, the Japanese Society for Psychiatry and Neurology had set up a disaster response committee, together with other academic, clinical and medical organizations. The National Centre of Neurology and Psychiatry even launched a website to provide guidelines and manuals for professionals by the third day. This shows the amount of attention paid by Japan to prevent psychosocial disorders in its population. Such was the sensitivity of the government of Japan that within a week's time, the Ministry of Health, Labour and Welfare had organized mental care teams that provided standard care to people with pre-existing mental illness and also to those who needed care in the wake of the disaster, including health workers. Following the disaster, the priorities were mainly to transfer existing psychiatric patients to hospitals outside the disaster-affected area and to re-establish and strengthen mental health services in the disaster-affected region so that the deleterious effects of the disaster could be mitigated.

Yamazaki *et al.* (2011) in the initial phases post-disaster suggested that to make the mental health system sustainable in the Japanese scenario, there is a need to: (i) strengthen the available community mental health services alongside back-up of specialist care (i.e. existing local hospitals and clinics); (ii) mental health services should be integrated into general health services as a large number of people would not seek help at mental healthcare facilities; and (iii) establish a network of self-help groups for survivors as community. Personal as well as family support is important for sharing information about self-care and psychological first aid.

Keio University School of Medicine, Tokyo, Japan also provided mental health and psychosocial support to people living in Soma City in Fukushima prefecture (Kato *et al.*, 2012).

It is important to note that the Japanese culture is very different from cultures prevailing in other countries and societies. The traditional coping mechanism in Japan is not to express grief or anger, but to endure, tolerate and move on, quietly supporting each another (Yamazaki *et al.*, 2011). The resilience of the Japanese community to disasters is worth emulating. The social fabric is so strong that despite unprecedented devastation and despite facing the traumatic experience at close quarters the community exhibited immense courage and the willingness to move on.

We made an attempt to take a broad view of the psychosocial impact of the 2011 multiple disasters of Japan on the directly and indirectly affected population. The population in the affected prefectures formed the basis for the studies. Some of the factors that resulted in psychosocial problems were perceived to be as follows: (i) witnessing the immense destruction as a result of the earthquake and tsunami; (ii) destruction of homes and other infrastructure; (iii) physical injury with disability and pain; (iv) loss of loved ones; (v) exposure to dead bodies; (vi) immediate threat as well as anticipation of another major earthquake and tsunami; (vii) loss of home and belongings; (viii) massive destruction of sites; (ix) loss of jobs and opportunities; (x) physical and sexual abuse and harassment of women; (xi) increased responsibility of family members due to loss of the only working individual in the family; and (xii) increased problems in the aftermath of the disaster and reduced ability to solve them.

Maheshwari *et al.* (2007) have reported in their manual for facilitators various psychosocial reactions. Existing literature points out that psychosocial reactions observed can be classified into four types, namely, emotional reactions, cognitive reactions, physical reactions and interpersonal reactions (Fig. 27.2).

The manifestation of these four types of reactions was also evident in the Japanese population. The elderly, women and children were most affected in the aftermath of the 2011 Tōhoku multiple disasters. Analysis of data revealed manifestations of psychological problems in the Japanese population. Psychological problems were particularly apparent in the bereaved, the widowed and orphaned children. Such symptoms were found to be present in people from the three prefectures hit hardest by the tsunami and earthquake, i.e. Iwate, Miyagi and Fukushima. A number of non-government organizations are still active in this region and are working hard to ameliorate the symptoms manifest in the affected populations. With the passage of time, the degree of symptoms is being reduced; however, there is a lot that remains to be done. Resilience building in the population and training of human resources, particularly responders, families and non-medical professionals, to look for the presence of such symptoms can go a long way in identifying the sufferings and seeking professional medical help before it is too late.

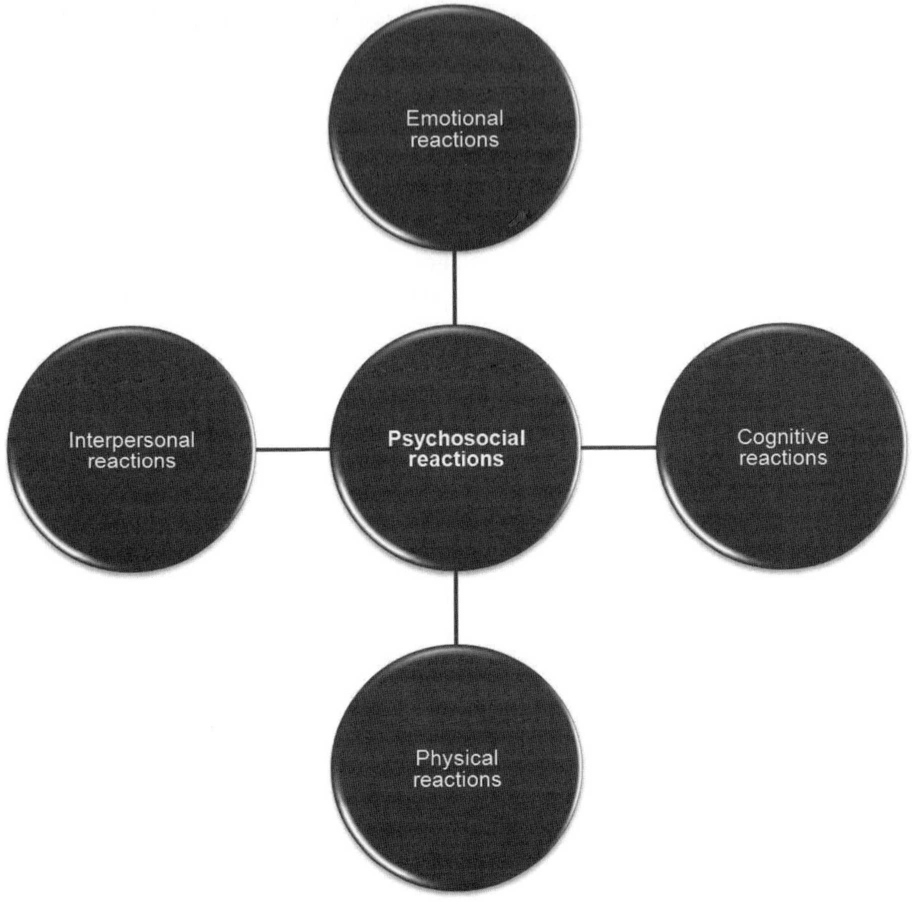

Fig. 27.2. Classification of psychosocial reactions into four types.

However, overall the willpower of Japanese people is very strong. The affected community (especially some women) exhibited signs of anxiety and depression, disturbed sleep, phobia and feeling of helplessness. Similar observations of early psychological distress have been reported among the sufferers after the 2011 Northern Nagano prefecture earthquake (mountainous area), wherein gender and age-specific differences were evident – particularly, females and old people were found to be risk factors for poor psychological outcome (Shindo *et al.*, 2012).

Some of the commonly observed reactions observed in the aftermath of the disasters were also observed in the population of Japan following the 2011 Tōhoku earthquake and are summarized in Fig. 27.3.

Emotional	Cognitive	Physical	Interpersonal
Anger Fear Grief Guilt Helplessness Hopelessness Numbness Resentment Shame Shock	Confusion Difficulty in concentrating Disorientation Indecisiveness Memory loss Self-blame Shortened attention span Unwanted memories Worry	Abnormal heartbeat Appetite changes Body aches/pain Difficulty in sleeping Fatigue Nausea Tension etc.	At school, Work, in friendships, in marriage, as a parent: distrust, irritability, conflict, withdrawal, isolation, feeling rejected or abandoned, being distant, judgemental etc.

Fig. 27.3. Some of the psychological reactions observed in the affected Japanese community.

The overall psychological reactions in the Japanese population were found to be in accordance with the laid-down psychosocial interventions of the World Health Organization (WHO) immediately occurring in four post-disaster phases (WHO, 2006) with defined duration (NIMHANS, 2010), i.e. the rescue phase (2 weeks), the relief phase (up to 6 months), the rehabilitation phase (up to 2 years) and the rebuilding phase (lifelong). Various populations within the community are differentially susceptible to disasters. Depending on age, physical condition, gender, health status, etc. some members of the population are more susceptible than others. The effect of the disaster on some of the vulnerable groups affected in Japan in the 2011 Tōhoku earthquake and the ensuing tsunami are discussed in the following section.

The Vulnerable Populations

Women

Women are considered to be more susceptible to disasters than men. Studies by several workers, including those by Hyodo *et al.* (2010) have indicated that long-term mortality from suicide after an earthquake decreases in men and increases in women, suggesting that post-earthquake suicide mortality is gender-dependent. The authors of this study go on to conclude that post-disaster suicide prevention strategies should more aggressively target women. Sometimes, following disasters suicidal tendencies are precipitated in some patients and they may consume overdoses of medicines or resort to other modes in a suicide attempt. It is important to ensure that medical and psychosocial support is made available to susceptible patients with such tendencies (Ozaki *et al.*, 2007). Support to find employment is also a necessity following disasters (Maheshwari *et al.*, 2007).

Following the 2011 Great East Japan Earthquake, an interview-based analysis was carried out on the community residing in Japan at the time of the disaster. The study was conducted immediately after the disaster and continued up to 9 months after the disaster. The results revealed that out of the interviewed women, 28% exhibited some or all of the following symptoms: sleeplessness, guilt, flashbacks, loneliness and helplessness, stress, fear of the return of the disaster, fear of the unknown, loss of appetite, feelings of doubt, worries related to reconstruction and inability to express their feelings in the family in the immediate aftermath of the disaster. Some women suffered from violence and abuse too, though the percentage was very low. The survivors were thankful to people who empathized with them. The affected were in general helpful towards other members of both genders. Japanese society places a lot of emphasis on the professional front and hence there was a feeling of guilt in the surviving women that they were unable to contribute to their profession in the aftermath of the disaster. The men also exhibited inability to express their feelings (Arora, 2011). The need for a forum or person to talk to about their sadness was felt by the Japanese government, which has taken a lot of steps to support women in disaster situations (Cabinet Office, Japan 2011a,b,c).

Psychological support in action on-ground

Measures taken to specifically address the needs of mothers and women after the Great East Japan Earthquake of 2011

The Japanese Government exhibited an efficient human resource management-based response. Female officers from the National Police Agency were sent to the disaster-affected areas, where they not only heard the problems encountered by the women and children with great empathy, but also instructed them on crime prevention and provided them with a much-needed sense of security. The number of crimes against women following the disaster was very low, though some sporadic incidents were reported. The Japan government's careful and well-planned strategy in this regard went a long way towards reducing the incidences of crimes against women and children.

Disaster response efforts were carefully coordinated and action was taken in such a manner so as to ensure that the needs of mothers and other women were met. The life at the designated shelters was carefully monitored in a manner that catered to and took care of the needs of women. Japan's Ministry of Health, Labour and Welfare funded a grant-in-aid to ensure that help was given to pregnant women and infants residing in shelters in the disaster-affected area. Women were provided women's kits, baby formula, baby food and other items of daily use. The needs of the disaster-affected women were assessed by establishing the continued presence of Gender Equality Bureau staff in the disaster areas, and, based on their needs, appropriate help was extended. In addition, centres were set up for counselling women who faced problems and for helping victims of any form of violence, whether physical, mental or sexual. Efforts were also made to inform people about the existence of such centres in the disaster-affected areas.

In some cases, the most vulnerable populations – small children, the aged, the poor and pets – suffered disproportionately because of the difficulty in evacuating or reaching them, mainly due to impassable roads, evacuations and housing centres where pets were prohibited, and a general reluctance by elderly populations to abandon their homes.

Furthermore, some of the infrastructure that provided care for vulnerable populations was eliminated by the earthquake or by the tsunami.

Based on experience of the Chernobyl nuclear incident, as a precautionary measure the pregnant women and children were shifted from the Fukushima prefecture in particular to avoid them from being exposed to the deleterious effects of ionizing radiation.

Children

After the disaster more than 10,000 children were displaced and faced numerous physical, mental and psychological problems (JNPA, 2012). In several cases, either or both parents were dead or missing, and siblings or other close family members were missing. Some of the children were injured and/or physically/psychologically traumatized. Their homes were destroyed, friends and relatives had disappeared and the destruction witnessed had left them with trails of fear and stress. Some of them were abused and haunted by fears that disaster would strike again. Due to such psychological conditions, children typically were unable to sleep, had problems with bedwetting, and were withdrawn and antisocial. Some of them completely stopped talking and became reticent. These were all signs of distress. It has been emphasized that the psychosocial needs of children need to be addressed through training school teachers in psychosocial cases, using story-telling, games, drawing and group activities (Kelly, 2010; Murray, 2010).

The Japanese Red Cross Society deployed nearly 900 medical teams and hundreds of psychosocial workers to support the relief operation. Since over 300,000 people were living in temporary housing, it was especially stressful for the children who were staying in such shelters.

How children were affected

It is a well-recognized fact that in children who grow up in environments that are troubled or not peaceful, or who have witnessed trauma and bad memories, their character can be distorted and this is manifested in subsequent life. They have adjustment problems when they grow up. Some of the children who witnessed the tsunami and experienced traumatic events accompanying the multiple disasters found it difficult to express their feelings in the way adults would have, leading to deep imprints of such stressful conditions in their subconsciousness. Children often encountered double stress because they experienced not only their own anxiety, but witnessed the stress of their parents or care providers. This led to accentuation of their stress. In addition, in some cases they had to bear the brunt of what their families were going through. Stress often resulted in parents being short-tempered and worried about their future (McFarlane, 1988; Winstanley and Whittington, 2002). The children bore the brunt of this and, with their limited ability to cope with and differentiate between the real and the unreal, they were confused. The psychosocial interventions made in Japan by the government, various national and international NGOs and universities were steps aimed at reducing the incidence of PTSDs, and included support to face their situation, feeling empathy for others as well as recognizing differences, coming to terms with the disaster events and the death or loss of family members, developing a sense of self-esteem and fearlessness, enabling the candid expression of true feelings, etc. Several exercises were employed in the temporary shelters in the affected prefectures to avoid the onset of PTSD in the children who were exposed to the traumatic events. These included playing and participation in indoor games, writing song lyrics, photography, videography, enacting dramas, crafts involving participation of children, etc. Release of feelings of sadness, grief and negative emotions is definitely known to improve the general well-being of the affected young community. This was observed in the case of children affected by the earthquake and tsunami.

In every disaster response team of the Japanese Red Cross Society, there was at least one nurse who was trained in providing psychological support, while distributing relief materials. They were trained to provide interventions to manage short-, medium- and long-term effects of disaster on children (ReliefWeb, n.d.).

The elderly population

As alluded to earlier, Japan lies in an area highly prone to natural disasters, and disasters occurring in rural areas, where the proportion of elderly adults is quite high, pose immense concern. Although elderly persons are vulnerable members of communities at the time of disaster, the prevalence of mental disorders among this population has not been adequately reported in Japan. Japan has 35% of the population belonging to the elderly category and conversely as compared with children, being aged and prone to pre-existing diseases, many of them suffer from lack of sleep, difficulty in shifting to evacuation centres and inability to adjust to changing dynamics (Zimmering *et al.*, 2006). Several workers have attempted to study the effect of disasters on the aged population. Suzuki *et al.* (2011) aimed to determine the prevalence of mental disorders and suicidal thoughts among the community-dwelling elderly persons 3 years after the Niigata-Chuetsu 2004 earthquake and to identify risk factors associated with their quality of life. During the 3-year period of the study after the earthquake, 1.6% of men and 5.5% of women had received a diagnosis of major depression. Elderly women were reported to be more likely than men to report tendency towards suicide, since women are good at expressing their feelings compared with men. The prevalence of mental disorders was found to be lower than that reported in previous studies. These authors concluded that despite the low prevalence of mental disorders, the percentage of community-dwelling elderly persons with subclinical mental health symptoms was high. The results of this study indicated that appropriate public health and medical interventions are warranted after a natural disaster.

Elderly people are generally reluctant to shift from their homes and even a small change in their routine life can result in aggravation of psychosomatic problems. In the aftermath of the 2011 Japan disaster, it was observed that many elderly people had to shift from their homes. In fact, a large number of members of this population refused to shift despite reassurances. The old people who had pre-existing problems like hypertension, diabetes or who were on regular medication faced problems upon movement due to lack of availability of medication on time, insomnia and emotional insanity.

In the case of the 2011 Japan disaster, after the initial response, it was realized that the impact on the elderly was immense and consequently the focus of the Japanese Red Cross Society, which actively addressed the medical and psychosocial issues, was shifted from evacuation centres to temporary housing settlements where they organized tea parties and massage sessions for the elderly residents to reduce stress. In many cases it was observed that old people with dementia and even their families had to leave shelters to return to partially or half-destroyed houses or to their relatives. This often deprived such people from receiving enough relief items.

Young professionals

Fear psychosis regarding radiation from Fukushima in professionals (Tokyo and Fukushima region)

Fear psychosis was evident in the residents especially of the Tokyo and Fukushima region due to the perceived risks associated with radiocontamination. Concerns regarding contamination with radionuclide especially in vegetables, fish, food and even tap water were observed. Another global concern was about the food exported from Japan to China, Taiwan, India, South Korea and Malaysia. This was seriously addressed by the WHO. Radiation-tainted fava beans, imported from Japan, raised problems in Taiwan due to enhanced radioactive contamination concerns. One of the biggest worries was amongst families, particularly mothers about the existence of radioactive contamination in baby food. Baby food manufacturing companies withdrew several products from the market as they were found to be contaminated with radiation. The fear in the community with respect to what was safe to eat or drink was clearly evident. This psychosocial impact was so strong that several members, particularly foreigners residing in Tokyo city migrated from there as they felt quite vulnerable and unsafe despite government reassurances.

Community apprehension and anti-nuclear protests

The nuclear accident at the Fukushima Daiichi Nuclear Plant after the Great East Japan Earthquake resulted in long-term, on-going anxiety amongst the residents of Fukushima (Yasumura *et al.*, 2012). Japanese protesters in masks protested against nuclear plants in front of the Tokyo Electric Power Co. (TEPCO) headquarters in Tokyo. Similar types of anti-nuclear protests were observed in other countries too. People attended a candlelight vigil organized by Greenpeace in Hong Kong for victims of the Japan earthquake and tsunami following the disaster.

However, with a view to assessing damage to the population, immediately after the disaster, Fukushima prefecture launched the Fukushima health management survey to investigate long-term low-dose radiation exposure caused by the accident. The primary purpose of this survey was to monitor the long-term health of residents, promote their future well-being and confirm whether long-term low-dose radiation exposure has health effects. In this cohort study, all people living in Fukushima Prefecture after the earthquake were enrolled and a basic survey and four detailed surveys were carried out. The basic survey was done to estimate levels of external radiation exposure among all 2.05 million residents and internal radiation levels were estimated using whole-body counters. The detailed surveys comprised a thyroid ultrasound examination for all Fukushima children aged 18 years or younger, a comprehensive health check for all residents from the evacuation zones, an assessment of mental health and lifestyles of all residents from the evacuation zones, and recording of all pregnancies and births among all women in the prefecture who were pregnant as on 11 March. However, the low response rate (< 30%) to the basic survey complicated the estimation of health effects. No cases of malignancy to date have been reported among 38,114 children who received thyroid ultrasound examinations. The importance of mental healthcare was stressed by the mental health and lifestyle survey and the pregnancy and birth survey. It is anticipated that this long-term, large-scale epidemiological study will provide valuable data regarding the health effects of low-dose radiation and disaster-related stress.

Meineke and Dörr (2012) have recently highlighted changed psychosocial factors in the age of the internet and globalization, and the ignorance of the effects of ionizing radiation following a nuclear/radiological emergency in the wake of the Fukushima radiation accident. Ignorance and misinformation are major reasons for a lot of apprehension amongst both the community and healthcare professionals. However, with radiation one needs to be very careful since the deleterious effects can be manifested in subsequent generations.

Special needs population

People with special needs, when affected by a disaster are not in a position to take care of themselves. They need special care and medication and, in the absence of assistance during a disaster and in its aftermath, they are unable to fend for themselves. The special needs population is a category that is now being recognized as a highly vulnerable group and immense attention is being paid to taking care of them in the aftermath of disasters (Olness *et al*., 2005). Following the Japan 2011 disaster, attention was paid to this category also. In the main the help rendered by the community and the Japanese responders in this regard was commendable.

Responders

In the wake of disasters, in the few days immediately following the disaster the need for help and assistance increases substantially overwhelming the available resources and also the capabilities of the responders. Under such circumstances, the rescue and relief teams are unable to provide help to all victims and their relatives/friends in need. It is the innate human nature to care and nurture for others, more so in times of need and it is a motivational force in humans to take care of individuals affected by disasters. Responders are trained for this purpose. However, sometimes for inevitable reasons, rescue and relief personnel have to reject the victims even though they do not wish to. This can lead to the development of guilt feelings or a sense of failing to meet the demands of the situation. This factor does cause problems in the future in disaster relief and rescue personnel in some cases. The mental health of the responders is also immensely affected.

A number of studies have reported an increased level of post-traumatic stress reactions in disaster and emergency rescue personnel (Chang *et al*., 2003; Fullerton *et al*., 2004; Armagan *et al*., 2006; Zimmering *et al*., 2006; Dolce and Riccardi, 2007; Thoresen *et al*., 2009), in police and other first responders (van der Ploeg and Kleber, 2003; Marmar *et al*., 2006), in humanitarian aid workers (Cardozo *et al*., 2005) and in peacekeepers (Unwin *et al*., 1999; Black *et al*., 2004).

It is commonly observed that during and after exposure to an intense, unusual or abnormal disaster incident, certain emergency workers and disaster victims experience reactions that are not ordinarily observed. The event may create a stress response, which can result in disruption of physical and psychological processes. These reactions are normal. Often, these reactions occur immediately after the event, but they can appear hours, days, weeks or months later.

To quote an example, the liquidators who worked in the spring and summer of 1986 following the Chernobyl reactor incident had long-term mental health consequences and reports indicated excess suicide cases in a cohort from Estonia (Rahu *et al*., 2006) and significantly higher rates of depression, suicide ideation, PTSDs and severe headache in the cohort from the Ukraine (Loganovsky *et al.*, 2008).

The effect of the 2011 Japan disaster on psychosocial parameters in an international responder team that participated in relief and rescue operations in Japan, has also been investigated by us (results to be published separately).

Trained Human Resource is Critical to Developing Societal Resilience

Human resources (HR) are the mainstay of any organization and the nation. Some of the key HR functions are depicted in Fig. 27.4.

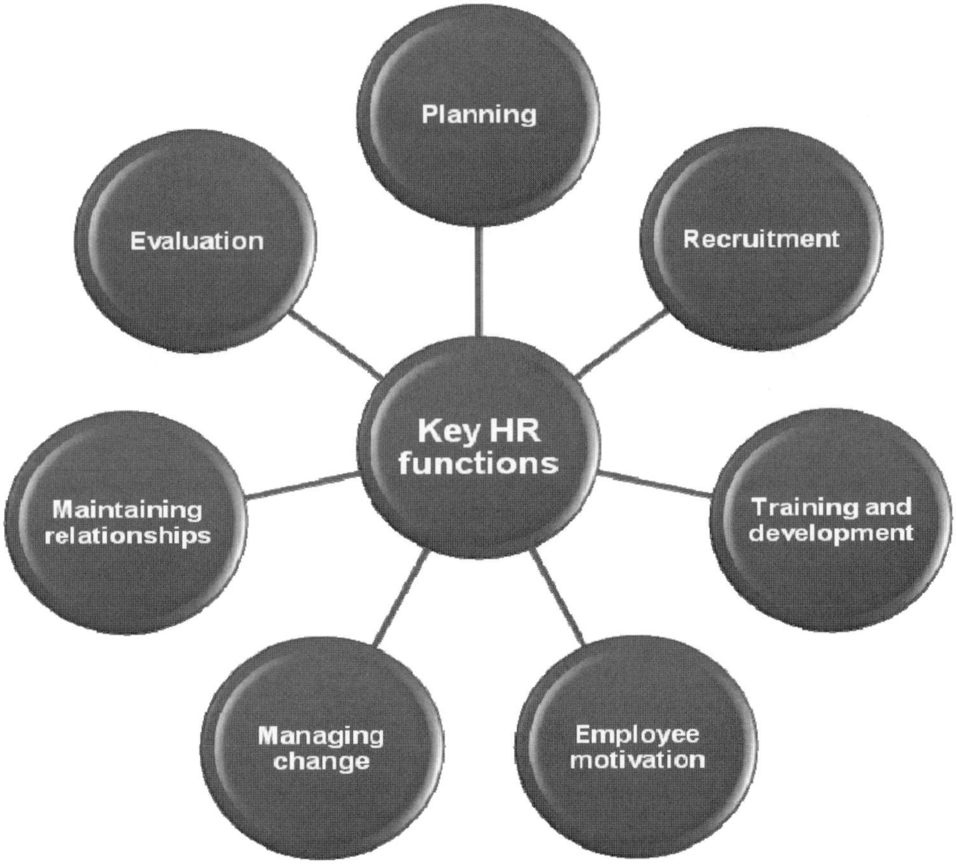
Planning
Recruitment
Training and development
Employee motivation
Managing change
Maintaining relationships
Evaluation
Key HR functions

Fig. 27.4. Key HR functions.

The Human Resource Management (HRM) system in the government milieu can be seamless or a very complex system, often involving a lot of red tape and intricate rules and procedures. In some countries, the rules and procedures are functionally simple and do not present hindrances prior to or in times of disasters; while in other countries they are so multifarious that they may even hinder initial rescue operations and inordinately delay post-disaster recovery. The HRM system takes care of two main functions: pre- and post-disaster service delivery through an integrated system with separate and unique HR planning (estimation of type, number and nature of people needed to work in an organization, e.g. one that is borderless and has a global presence), HR procurement (recruitment and selection of HR specifically for disaster management purposes, who are prepared to work anywhere in the globe), HR development (training and placing in the field with specific skills), HR maintenance (appropriate remuneration, generating funds and compensation for the employees of the organization; possessing international pay structures and suitably compensating the employees for risking their lives for the cause of mankind; also their family security needs to be included as a point of concern); and changes and system improvement are supposed to be in-built. Examination of the integration or fit among HRM practices, and other features for macro applications like disaster management, etc. are the need of the hour.

The role of HR in disaster management cannot be overemphasized. Each of the key functions of HR can change the outcome of disasters and are in turn adversely affected during disasters. This was evident in the wake of the 2011 Japan multiple disasters. The need to leverage crucial HR cannot be understated. There is a need for countries to learn from Japan, where disaster management has been integrated well within the HR policies. One of the major lessons learnt from the Japanese is the ability to handle a disaster of such magnitude, which was only possible due to the inherent building of disaster resilience in organizations (including the crucial human resource) over a period of several years.

It is apparent that particularly in disaster-prone countries, disaster management should be ingrained in business policies/government organizational functioning and should be an integral part of key HR functions so that in the event of a disaster there is better capability to handle such events. While carrying out planning, recruitment, training and development and other key functions, the need for building resilience to disasters should be kept in mind and strategies worked out in advance not only to ensure business continuity, but also to tackle disasters, their psychosocial impact amongst employees and the society at large as an effort in the direction of corporate social responsibility.

The Japan case in point shows that there is a need for very strong leadership in order to plan in advance for the consequences of disasters. Strong leadership ensures that businesses are well organized to face disasters, without affecting the business continuity in the aftermath of disasters, at the same time serving society in multifarious ways. The strong leadership and inculcation of a culture of preparedness and resilience engrained in Japanese society ensured that most business operations were functional within days of the unprecedented 2011 triple disaster.

Experience from Japan shows that relationship building is an essential component of HR. There were approximately 2 million foreign permanent residents in Japan before 2011. In the aftermath of the 2011 triple disasters, several young professionals from foreign countries either left their jobs to move temporarily further south, or left Japan altogether. This was perhaps the first time that such an exodus was seen in the history of Japan in the initial stages post-disaster. The shortage of such workers posed a major challenge to recovery. Mass exodus of young professionals can pose a great concern to the economy. Building good relationships is also important from a disaster management perspective, since during times of disasters it is essential for the professionals to have faith in the business operations and they need to be not only reassured, but their interests should be taken care of in the event of such emergencies since this is a part of the overall corporate social responsibility. Usually it is also seen that if business operations are affected following disasters, a large number of employees are laid off. Such trends can have immense psychosocial impact and should best be avoided by responsible companies. Business enterprises should aim towards sustainable operations. Uplifting of the morale of the employees, community and responders is of prime importance.

A shortage in HR is almost always encountered at some stage following an unprecedented disaster, despite the best preparedness. Trained HR to handle disasters is even less available for deployment in various affected zones. The HR planning cycle can be effectively used for planning for disaster management (Fig. 27.5).

Psychologists, mental health professionals and first responders, especially trained in the area of psychosocial issues, are in demand in times of disasters. It is often not possible to provide specialized and professional psychological care to one and all in need following a disaster and, consequently, the health professionals, namely doctors, nurses, emergency medical response personnel and first responders (anyone who reaches the site first) too should be trained (at least minimally) to identify and handle psychosocial issues in remote locations as, in the absence of professional help (for obvious reasons like restricted access to the disaster site, non-availability of sufficient trained HR, etc.), they have to fulfil the responsibility towards the affected community.

Business continuity becomes a problem following disasters and terror events. In recent years it has been recognized that business organizations need to be prepared to handle any eventuality. Business continuity plans have been made by several companies. Due to the globalization of economy, despite the disaster situation customers expect that supplies and/or services will continue as if nothing has happened or resume as soon as possible, shareholders expect management control to remain operational through any crisis, employees expect their livelihoods to be protected, suppliers expect that they will continue to receive revenue, regulatory agencies expect their requirements to be met. The burden on the company increases to immediately come into operation or else they might lose business. The HR of the company can play an important role in mitigating the effects of disaster. In the immediate aftermath of the 2011 Japan disaster, a large number of foreign professionals working in Japan began moving out due to the obvious fears that surrounded the disaster, despite assurances from the government and all measures to allay fears. Interviews with several such professionals led to the conclusion that there was a great deal of fear amongst them despite reassurances by the government and media. As a result of government support and assurances, the professionals soon returned to ensure business continuity. However, such instances have raised the emergence of problems that can affect business continuity and countries need to be prepared to handle such issues in a balanced, clear and transparent manner. The loss of crucial HR can severely jeopardize business operations following disasters and the economy can be persistently affected.

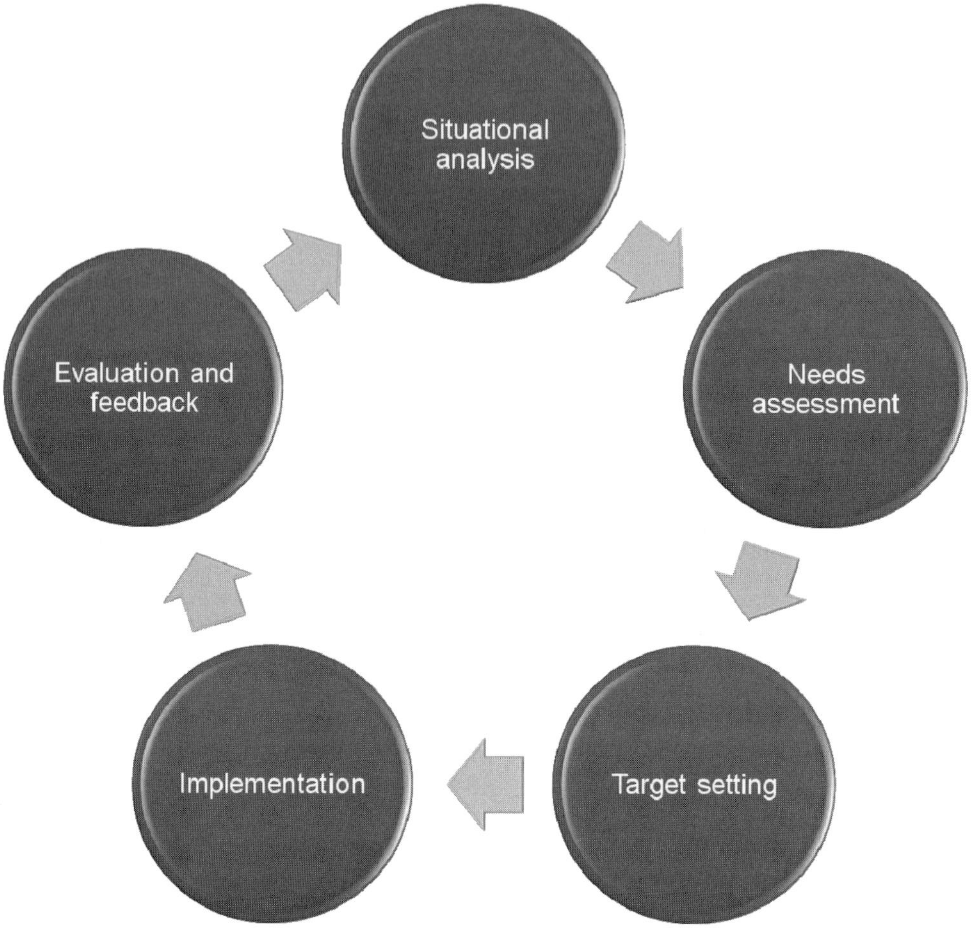

Fig. 27.5. The HR planning cycle can be effectively used for designing effective disaster management programmes.

Recently in 2012, the ILO and the government of Japan signed a new Framework for Cooperation agreement aimed at lending a helping hand to the Asia Pacific countries in dealing with the effects of natural disasters and strengthening the role of employment in early recovery and reconstruction. The agreement known as the 'Framework for Cooperation by ILO/Japan Fund for Dissemination of Employment and Labour Measures for Recovering from the Great East Japan Earthquake as International Public Resources' has been allocated approximately US$1.5 million in funding. The agreement aims to bring together the expertise of the ILO with the experience and know-how gained by Japan in dealing with the 2011 multiple disasters. Some of the outcomes expected are improvements in the compiling, analysis and distribution of information on how employment and labour measures can support disaster recovery and capacity building for governments in Asia Pacific to improve their ability to respond to natural disasters in a better manner. This is a welcome step in the direction of reducing the impact of disasters in the Asia Pacific region, which is prone to disasters.

Japan's Ministry of Health, Labour and Welfare (MHLW) estimated that nearly 841,000 workers and 88,000 businesses were located in the regions directly affected by the Great East Japan Earthquake (International Monetary Fund Report, 2011). The IMF reported a significant rise in national bankruptcies and applications for employment assistance subsidies in the months following the 2011 earthquake.

1. In developing countries where a clear-cut policy is lacking, there is a need to formulate an appropriate policy for psychosocial care and mental health problems particularly to handle post-disaster issues in a coherent manner giving due emphasis to HR development.
2. The policy should be linked directly to HR planning in consultation with health programme managers and training institutions.
3. Training should be reviewed and continuously improved (Kaizen). Continuing education, training and supervision should be developed for the provision of the best quality care that meets users' needs.

With respect to psychosocial care, the primary healthcare professionals should be able to identify the manifestation of psychosocial problems in individuals, administer basic medications and psychosocial interventions, recommend referrals to specialist mental healthcare facilities, facilitate family and community psycho-education, provide interventions during crises and provide post-disaster counselling to the directly and indirectly affected populations. Since in many cases the elderly and special needs population are either left alone or do not wish to move post-disaster for feeling of security, the healthcare professionals should try to reach out to their homes and render all possible help. Networking is essential. The HR in need of training vis-à-vis psychosocial interventions include, but are not limited to: community health workers, primary healthcare nurses, general practitioners, mental health nurses, psychiatrists, psychologists, pharmacists, administrators and information managers.

Recent trends indicate that following a disaster, mental health specialists are often not available or are not available in sufficient numbers to meet the identified psychosocial needs of the community. Specialty mental healthcare is needed to aid survival and recovery at every stage of disaster response and telemental health is being flaunted as an efficient means of bringing sustained mental health best practices to communities following a disaster (Augusterfer, 2013). Telemental health can also have a core role in providing supervision, mentoring and case consultation to first responders and others providing care in the field, especially when there is a shortage of trained HR. Creation of an appropriate HRM framework and adopting a systems approach is the key to achieving effective disaster management across the globe (Fig. 27.6)

Some suggestions on how HRM can be effectively utilized in management of disasters at global level include: a redesigned human resource system at global level free from interference of any country; an independent decision-making body like the United Nations; HR concerns and issues should be heard through an independent law body; identification of the needed HR; creation of new jobs; defined job descriptions and profiles so that HR can be made available from any part of the globe for rescue and relief operations in the event of a disaster; entrust the HR division with human capacity development in coordination with the training institutions to offer effective technical solutions to any sort of disaster problems, in such a way as to ensure that it is well linked to all technical training institutions of disaster management across the globe; and ensure that this HR development responds in quantity and quality to the needs of the disaster management sector.

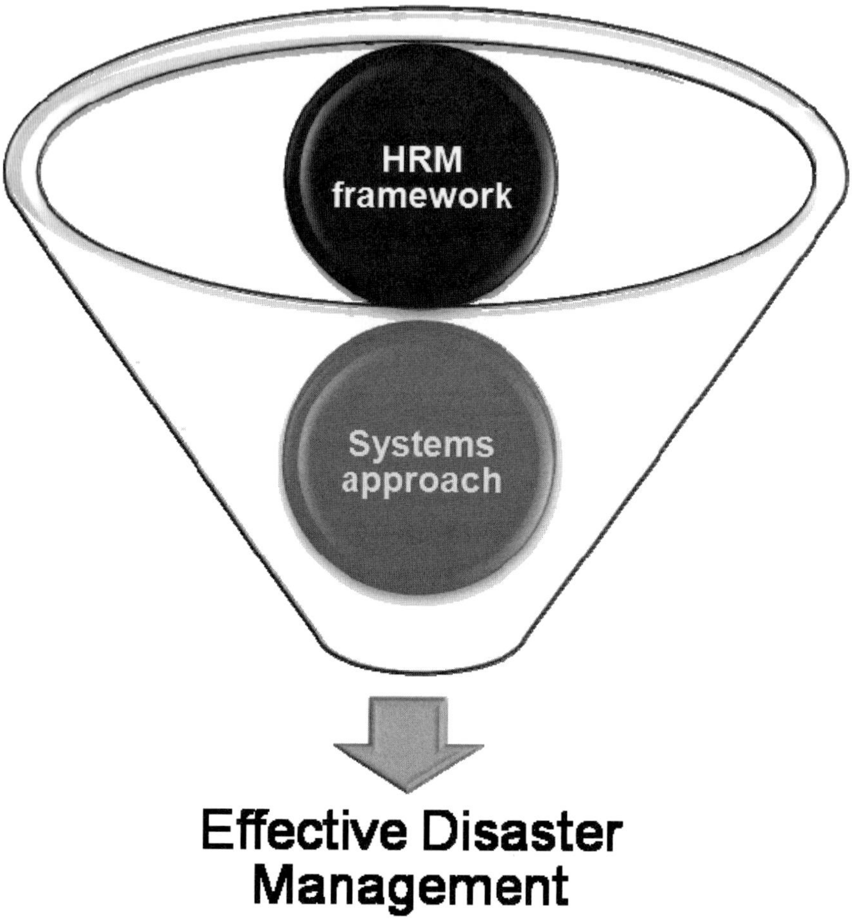

Fig. 27.6. Achieving effective disaster management across the globe through a leveraging systems approach of HRM is a key challenge ahead of all of us.

A model for integrating HR functions and disaster management is proposed (Fig. 27.7). In the proposed model, during implementation, country-specific HR policies, leadership, finance, partnerships, education and training can be included to achieve efficient disaster management.

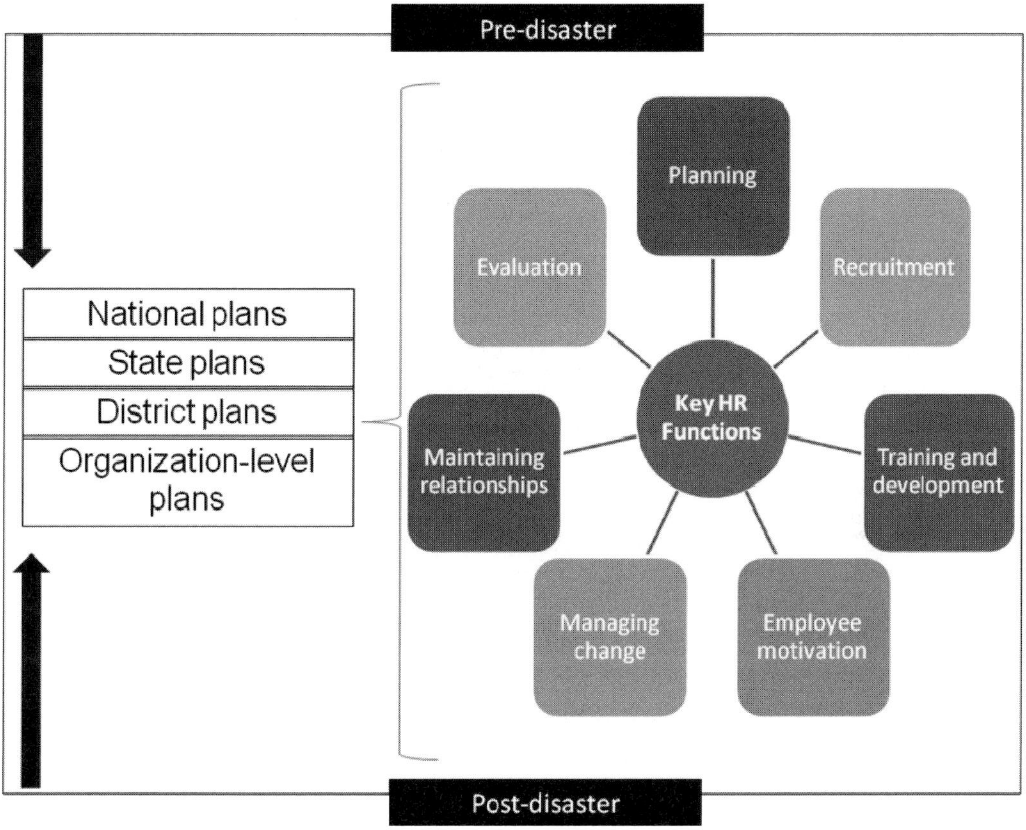

Fig. 27.7. A simplistic model for integrating HR functions and disaster management.

Conclusions

The data collected from the directly and indirectly affected populations, authentic sources (including the Japan Cabinet) and also an international rescue and relief team validated the psychosocial impact on the Japanese population and the residing overseas community. The impact on the directly affected population is likely to take years to recover fully. However, given the spirit of the Japanese people, return to normalcy was only a matter of time. There are a number of lessons to be learnt from the Japanese community.

A cardinal point that emerged from this disaster response was that adequate attention was focused on the needs of the vulnerable populations (women, children, and the sick and elderly population) by mobilizing trained HR in a timely manner. This paradigm shift in relief and response efforts needs to be emulated during future disasters, especially in developing countries. The close-knit community and existence of family and strong social and professional values in the Japanese community, in addition to support from the Japanese government, NGOs and the international community, helped in early recovery from the initial psychosocial problems that would have manifested otherwise to a great extent. Prior experience of the Indian Ocean tsunami in 2004 has evidently shown that community resilience really helps mitigate the effects of the disaster to a great extent in a long-term perspective. Keeping this in mind, there is a need to systematically carry out studies to investigate the medium- and long-term societal impact of the 2011 Japan disaster on the resident population, as the psychosocial impact is felt often for years in the community as well as in responders, however resilient they may be. Such initiatives would help reduce the psychosocial impact of megadisasters to a large extent and calls for support from the academia, medical fraternity, national and international NGOs. The Japan 2011 multiple disasters have brought to the fore the crucial role of leveraging HR functions for alleviating the impact of disasters.

Acknowledgements

Preeti Arora would like to sincerely acknowledge the Japan Institute for Labour Policy and Training (JILPT), Tokyo, Japan for provision of an opportunity to participate in the International Visiting Researcher Program. The authors express their sincere gratitude to innumerable colleagues for their support and cooperation. The authors are also thankful to Prof. Manas K. Mandal, Chief Controller Research and Development and Outstanding Scientist, Defence R&D Organization (DRDO) for useful suggestions for the work.

Disclaimer

The views expressed are entirely those of the authors and do not necessarily reflect the views of their respective organizations, the governments or the sponsoring/funding agencies. Any inadvertent errors are solely the responsibility of the authors.

Dedication

This chapter is dedicated to all those who perished or silently suffered during the 2011 Japan disasters.

References

Armagan, E., Engindeniz, Z., Devay, A., Erdur, B. and Ozcakir, A. (2006) Frequency of post-traumatic stress disorder among relief force workers after the tsunami in Asia: do rescuers become victims. *Prehospital and Disaster Medicine* 21(3), 168–172.

Arora, P. (2011) The 2011 Tōhoku earthquake and tsunami of Japan: Lessons learnt and implications for effective disaster management. Dissertation submitted to the Center for Disaster Management Studies, Guru Gobind Singh University, Kashmere Gate, Delhi, p. 156.

Arora, P., Arora, R. and Bhardwaj, J.R. (2012) Psychosocial impact of 2011 Japan Tōhoku earthquake and ensuing multiple disasters. In: Bhardwaj, J.R. (ed. in chief) *Chemical (Industrial) Disaster Management* (CIDM) 2012. Federation of Indian Chambers of Commerce and Industry (FICCI), New Delhi, pp. 339–369.

Arora, P., Gunaseelan, R. and Arora, R. (2013) Emerging Trends in the Management of Disasters and Mass Casualty Incidents. *CAB Reviews* (in press).
Augusterfer, E.F. (2013) Clinically informed telemental health in post-disaster areas. In: Myers, K. and Turvey, C.L. (eds) *Telemental Health*. Elsevier, London, pp. 347–366.
BBC News (2011) Japan earthquake: tsunami hits north-east. Available at: http://www.bbc.co.uk/news/world-asia-pacific-12709598 (Accessed 11 February 2013).
Benedek, D.M., Fullerton, C. and Ursano, R.J. (2007) First responders: mental health consequences of natural and human-made disasters for public health and public safety workers. *Annual Review of Public Health* 28, 55–68.
Black, D.W., Carney, C.P., Peloso, P.M., Woolson, R.F., Schwartz, D.A., Voelker, M.D., Barrett, D.H. and Doebbeling, B.N. (2004) Gulf War veterans with anxiety: prevalence, comorbidity, and risk factors. *Epidemiology* 15(2), 135–162.
Bromet, E.J. (2012) Mental health consequences of the Chernobyl disaster. *Journal of Radiological Protection* 32, N71–N75.
Cabinet Office, Government of Japan (2011a) Disaster Management Plan of Japan 2011. Cabinet Office, Government of Japan, Tokyo.
Cabinet Office, Government of Japan (2011b) White Paper on Disaster Management 2011. Cabinet Office, Government of Japan, Tokyo.
Cabinet Office, Government of Japan (2011c) Women and Men in Japan. Cabinet Office, Government of Japan, Tokyo.
Cardozo, B.L., Holtz, T.H., Kaiser, R., Gotway, C.A., Ghitis, F., Toomey, E. and Salama P. (2005) The mental health of expatriate and Kosovar Albanian humanitarian aid workers. *Disasters* 29, 152–170.
Chandler, D.L. (2011) What we know, and don't know, about Japan's reactors, MIT News Office. Available at: http://web.mit.edu/newsoffice/2011/nuclear-panel-japan-0136.html (Accessed 11 February 2013).
Chang, C.M., Lee, L.C., Connor, K.M., Davidson, J.R., Jeffries, K. and Lai, T.J. (2003) Posttraumatic distress and coping strategies among rescue workers after an earthquake. *Journal of Nervous and Mental Diseases* 191(6), 391–398.
Chen, C.C., Yeh, T.L., Yang, Y.K., Chen, S.J., Lee, I.H., Fu, L.S., Yeh, C.Y., Hsu, H.C., Tsai, W.L., Cheng, S.H., Chen, L.Y. and Si, Y.C. (2001) Psychiatric morbidity and post-traumatic symptoms among survivors in the early stage following the 1999 earthquake in Taiwan. *Psychiatry Research* 105, 13–22.
Dolce, A. and Riccardi, M. (2007) Impact of psychological risk factors on disaster rescue operation: the case of Italian volunteers. *Disasters* 31, 91–103.
Ehring, T., Razik, S. and Emmelkamp, P.M.G. (2011) Prevelance and predictors of posttraumatic stress disorder, anxiety, depression and burnout in Pakistani earthquake recovery workers. *Psychiatry Research* 185, 161–166.
Fullerton, C.S., Ursano, R.J. and Wang, L. (2004) Acute stress disorder, posttraumatic stress disorder, and depression in disaster or rescue workers. *American Journal of Psychiatry* 161(8), 1370–1376.
Fushimi, M. (2012) Posttraumatic stress in professional fire fighters in Japan: Rescue efforts after the Great East Japan earthquake (Higashi Nihon Dai-Shinsai). *Prehospital Disaster Medicine* 9, 1–3.
Herrman, H. (2012) Promoting mental health and resilience after a disaster. *Journal of Experimental and Clinical Medicine* 4(2), 82–87.
Hunter, J.C., Crawley, A.W., Petrie, M., Yang, J.E. and Aragon, T.J. (2012) Local public health system response to the tsunami threat in coastal California following the Tōhoku earthquake. *PLoS Curr* 4, e4f7285b804.
Hyodo, K., Nakamura, K., Oyama, M., Yamazaki, O., Nakagawa, I., Ishigami, K., Tsuchiya, Y. and Yamamoto, M. (2010) Long-term suicide mortality rates decrease in men and increase in women after the Niigata-Chuetsu earthquake in Japan. *Tōhoku Journal of Experimental Medicine* 220(2), 149–155.

International Monetary Fund Report (2011) Available at: http://www.imf.org/external/pubs/ft/ar/2011/eng/index.htm (Accessed 12 July 2013).

Japanese National Police Agency (JNPA) (2012) Damage situation and police countermeasures associated with 2011 Tōhoku district – off the Pacific Ocean earthquake, 16 May 2012. Available at: http://www.npa.go.jp/archive/keibi/biki/higaijokyo_e.pdf (Accessed 11 February 2013).

Kato, H., Asukai, N., Miyaka, Y., Minakawa, K. and Nishiyama, A. (1996) Post-traumatic symptoms among younger and elderly evacuees in the early stages following the 1995 Hanshin-Awaji Earthquake in Japan. *Acta Psychiatrica Scandinavica* 93, 477–481.

Kato, Y., Uchida, H. and Mimura, M. (2012) Mental health and psychosocial support after the Great East Japan earthquake. *Keio Journal of Medicine* 61(1), 15–22.

Katz, C.L., Pellegrino, L., Pandya, A., Ng, A. and DeLisi, L.E. (2002) Research on psychiatric outcomes and interventions subsequent to disasters: a review of literature. *Psychiatry Research* 110, 201–207.

Kelly, F. (2010) Keeping pediatrics in pediatric disaster management: before, during, and in the aftermath of complex emergencies. *Critical Care Nursing Clinics of North America* 22, 465–480.

Kim, Y. and Akiyama, T. (2011) Post-disaster mental health care in Japan. Correspondence. *Lancet* 378(9788), 317–318.

Kokai, M., Fujii, S., Shinfuku, N. and Edward, G. (2004) Natural disaster and mental health in Asia. *Psychiatry and Clinical Neurosciences* 58, 110–116.

Loganovsky, K., Havenaar, J.M., Tintle, N., Tung, L., Kotov, R.I. and Bromet, E.J. (2008) The mental health of clean-up workers 18 years after the Chernobyl accident. *Psychological Medicine* 38, 481–488.

Maheshwari, S., Varghese, C. and Venkataraman, K. (2007) *Manual for facilitators*. World Health Organization (WHO), Geneva.

Mahoney, J., Chandra, V., Gambheera, H., De Silva, T. and Suveendran, T. (2006) Responding to the mental health and psychosocial needs of the people of Sri Lanka in disasters. *International Review of Psychiatry* 18, 593–597.

Marmar, C.R., McCaslin, S.E., Metzler, T.J., Best, S., Weiss, D.S., Fagan, J., Liberman, A., Pole, N., Otte, C., Yehuda, R., Mohr, D. and Neylan, T. (2006) Predictors of posttraumatic stress in police and other first responders. *Annals of the New York Academy of Sciences* 1071, 1–18.

McFarlane, A.C. (1988) Long-term psychiatric morbidity after a natural disaster. *Medical Journal of Australia* 145(11–12), 561–563.

Meineke, V. and Dörr, H. (2012) The Fukushima radiation accident: consequences for radiation accident medical management. *Health Physics* 103(2), 217–220.

Murray, J.S. (2010) Responding to the psychosocial needs of children and families in disasters. *Critical Care Nursing Clinics of North America* 22(4), 481–491.

Neria, Y., Nandi, A. and Galea, S. (2008) Post-traumatic stress disorder following disasters: a systematic review. *Psychological Medicine* 38, 467–480.

NIMHANS (National Institute of Mental Health and Neuro Sciences), Bangalore (2010) Psychosocial care for survivors of natural disasters. Available at: http://www.nimhans.kar.nic.in/dis_man/bro_disassur.pdf (Accessed 13 February 2013).

Nishio, A., Akazawa, K., Shibuya, F., Abe, R., Nushida, H., Ueno, Y., Nishimura, A. and Shioiri, T. (2009) Influence on the suicide rate two years after a devastating disaster: a report from the 1995 Great Hanshin-Awaji Earthquake. *Psychiatry and Clinical Neurosciences* 63(2), 247–250.

Norris, F.H., Friedman, M.J., Watson, P.J., Byrne, C.M., Diaz, E. and Kaniasty, K. (2002) 60,000 disaster victims speak: Part I. An empirical review of the empirical literature, 1981–2001. *Psychiatry* 65, 207–239.

Olness, K., Sinha, M., Herran, M., Cheren, M. and Pairojkul, S. (2005) Training of health care professionals on the special needs of children in the management of disasters: experience in Asia, Africa, and Latin America. *Ambulatory Pediatrics* 5(4), 244–248.

Ozaki, Y., Nakata, Y., Kameoka, M., Hayashi, N., Nakayama, Y. and Yagi, K. (2007) Clinical analysis of 104 cases of overdose in suicide attempts. *The Japanese Journal of Toxicology* 20(4), 367–374.

Parashar, S., Uy, N., Nguyen, H., Fernandez, G., Mulyasari, F., Joerin, J. and Shaw, R. (2011) Mega disaster in a resilient society, the Great East Japan (Tōhoku Kanto) earthquake and tsunami of 11th March 2011. International Environment and Disaster Management, Graduate School of Global Environmental Studies, Kyoto University, Kyoto, Japan, pp. 81.

Prasetiyawan, V.E., Marmis, A. and Keliat, B.A. (2006) Mental health model of care programmes after the tsunami in Aceh, Indonesia. *International Review of Psychiatry* 18, 559–562.

Rahu, K., Rahu, M., Tekkel, M. and Bromet, E. (2006) Suicide risk among Chernobyl cleanup workers in Estonia still increased: an updated cohort study. *Ann Epidemiology* 16, 917–919.

ReliefWeb (n.d.) Latest updates from various reports. Available at: http://www.reliefweb.int/rw/rwb.nsf/doc106?OpenForm&rc=3&emid=EQ-2011-000028-JPN (Accessed 11 February 2013).

Sharma, R.K. and Arora, R. (2011) Fukushima, Japan: an apocalypse in the making? *Journal of Pharmacy and Bioallied Sciences* 3(2), 315–316.

Shindo, M., Kitamura, H., Tachibana, A., Honma, H. and Someya, T. (2012) Early psychological distress among sufferers after the 2011 Northern Nagano Prefecture earthquake. *Psychiatry and Clinical Neuroscience* 66(5), 454–456.

Suzuki, Y., Tsutsumi, A., Fukasawa, M., Honma, H., Someya, T. and Kim, Y. (2011) Prevalence of mental disorders and suicidal thoughts among community-dwelling elderly adults 3 years after the Niigata-Chuetsu earthquake. *Journal of Epidemiology* 21(2), 144–150.

Thoresen, S., Tonnessen, A., Lindgaard, V., Andreassen, A.L. and Weisaeth, L. (2009) Stressful but rewarding: Norwegian personnel mobilized for the 2004 tsunami disaster. *Disasters* 33, 353–368.

Toyabe, S., Shioiri, T., Kobayashi, K., Kuwabara, H., Koizumi, M., Endo, T., Ito, M., Honma, H., Fukushima, N., Someya, T. and Akazaw, K. (2007) Factor structure of the General Health Questionnaire (GHQ-12) in subjects who had suffered from the 2004 Niigata-Chuetsu Earthquake in Japan: a community-based study. *BMC Public Health* 7, 175.

Unwin, C., Blatchley, N., Coker, W., Ferry, S., Hotopf, M., Hull, L., Ismail, K., Palmer, I., David, A. and Wessely, S. (1999) Health of UK servicemen who served in the Persian Gulf War. *Lancet* 353(9148), 167–178.

Van der Ploeg, E. and Kleber, R.J. (2003) Acute and chronic job stressors among ambulance personnel: predictors of health symptoms. *Occupational and Environmental Medicine* 60(Supplement I), i40–i46.

van Ommeren, M., Saxena, S. and Saraceno, B. (2005) Aid after disasters. *British Medical Journal* 330, 1160–1161.

Walsh, D.S. (2009) Interventions to reduce psychosocial disturbance following disturbance following humanitarian relief efforts involving natural disasters: an integrative review. *International Journal of Nursing Practice* 15, 231–240.

Wang, X., Gao, L., Zhang, H., Zhao, C., Shen, Y. and Shinfuku, N. (2000) Post-earthquake quality of life and psychological well-being: longitudinal evaluation in a rural community sample in Northern China. *Psychiatry and Clinical Neuroscience* 54(4), 427–433.

Williams, R. and Drury, J. (2009) Psychosocial resilience and its influence on managing mass emergencies and disasters. *Psychiatry* 8(8), 293–296.

Winstanley, S. and Whittington, R. (2002) Anxiety, burnout and coping styles in general hospital staff exposed to workplace aggression: a cyclical model of burnout and vulnerability to aggression. *Work and Stress* 16(4), 302–315.

World Health Organization (WHO) (2006) The mental health and psychosocial aspects of disaster preparedness. Report of an intercountry meeting, Khao Lak, Thailand, 20–23 June, WHO, Geneva.

Yamazaki, M., Minami, Y., Sasaki, H. and Sumi, M. (2011) The psychosocial response to the 2011 Tōhoku earthquake. *Bulletin of the World Health Organization* 89(9), 623.

Yasumura, S., Hosoya, M., Yamashita, S., Kamiya, K., Abe, M., Akashi, M., Kodama, K. and Ozasa, K. (2012) Study protocol for the Fukushima health management survey. *Journal of Epidemiology* 22(5), 375–383.

Zimmering, R., Gulliver, S.B., Knight, J., Munroe, J. and Keane, T.M. (2006) Posttraumatic stress disorder in disaster relief workers following direct and indirect trauma exposure to Ground Zero. *Journal of Traumatic Stress* 19(4), 553–557.

Section 9

Bridging the Great Divide:

The Challenge of Managing Disasters and MCIs in Resource-poor Settings

Chapter 28

Managing Disasters from a Health Security Perspective

Nibedita S. Ray-Bennett

Introduction: Disasters and their Impact on Health

Disasters and epidemics have had significantly larger health impacts on developing nations than on developed nations due to the ability of the latter to mitigate the impact. Between 1961 and 1981, natural disasters (drought, earthquakes and floods) claimed 1.1 million lives in low-income countries, 345,000 in middle-income countries and only 11,300 in high-income countries, although the number of disasters experienced by these three groups of countries was similar (Kloos, 2001). The most significant causes of the rise in the number and impact of disasters are poverty, vulnerability, inequality and land shortages, which drive people on to much more marginal territory and increase their exposure to natural hazards (Maskrey, 1989; UN, 1994).

To mitigate the impact of disasters on humans, national and international organizations organized the Hyogo Framework for Action (HFA) in Kobe in 2005 (UN, 2005). One hundred and sixty-eight UN Member States subsequently adopted the Framework for Disaster Risk Reduction (DRR). Yet the question remains as to whether these initiatives are adequate enough to reduce disaster impact on community health, and to promote human security and disaster resilience at household level. The Hyogo Framework recommended the integration of disaster risk reduction into the health sector through the goal of 'hospitals safe from disasters: Reduce risk, protect health facilities and save lives'. This approach is useful for building disaster-resilient infrastructure and yet limited in promoting community health for effective disaster management. I posit that a 'health security' perspective can enhance the effective implementation of HFA because the approach is people-centred and has the potential to reduce disaster vulnerability at household and community levels.

Before delving into the specifics of health security, the ensuing sections discuss the importance of health security and its linkage with the wider literatures on disaster, development and human security. Later I have outlined the components of health security. The concluding section charts out some implications for disaster management from a health security perspective.

Importance of Health and Health Security in Reducing Disaster Risk and Vulnerability

It is predicted that the coastal zones will be particularly at greatest risk due to increased flooding from the sea, sea erosion and in some areas flooding from the rivers (IPCC, 2007). The likely effect of this flooding is that by 2018 particularly in the developing nations there will be: increases in malnutrition, deaths, diseases and injury due to extreme weather events, reductions in crop productivity and exacerbation in current stresses on water resources (IPCC, 2007). Some of these effects are already evident in the Indian subcontinent, with a record level of poverty and malnutrition owing to disasters (GoB, 2003; GoO, 2005; UN, 2011). This indicates that environmental security is closely related to food, health and economic securities.

In this light, I posit that managing disasters through the lens of health[1] and health security could be more effective ways to reduce disaster risks and vulnerability at the household level rather than the approach forwarded by the Hyogo Framework as mentioned above; although I do not undermine the importance of the Hyogo Framework's approach at national and community levels as discussed later in this article.

There is established knowledge amongst health and developmental economists on the importance that health plays in development and this is understood under two overarching paradigms: (i) health as a means to achieve development; and (ii) health as an integral part of good development (Ruger, 2003, 2004). The former is often the view of multilateral organizations like the World Health Organization (WHO) and the United Nations (UN), where health is considered as a means to achieve economic development (Ruger, 2003). A 2001 report by the WHO Commission[2] on macroeconomics and health set specific goals for health investment as a means to promote economic development (Ruger, 2003). Studies have shown an intrinsic link between health and economic progress. Better health contributes to increasing gross domestic product (GDP) per capita growth because healthy workers are more productive, and better incomes raise per capita income by: (i) altering decisions about expenditure (on nutrition, housing and so on) and savings over the life cycle thereby breaking the classical cycle of poverty; and (ii) encouraging foreign direct investment as investors shun environments where the labour force suffers a heavy disease burden (Phillips and Verhasselt, 2001; Bloom *et al.*, 2004).

Viewing good health as a means to promote economic development is a useful strategy though it has limitations, particularly in acknowledging the intrinsic value of health and understanding development more broadly (Phillips and Verhasselt, 2001; Bloom *et al.*, 2004). While there is a strong connection between wealth and opulence, longevity and other achievements, the link may well be extremely contingent on other circumstances like the *capability* to live for a really long time (without being cut off in one's prime years) and to have a good life while alive (rather than a life of misery and lack of freedom) – things that would be strongly valued and desired by nearly all (Sen, 1999a). This expansion towards understanding 'health' is progressive, onward looking, process

[1] Health is the extent to which an individual or group is able to realize aspirations to satisfy needs, and to change or cope with the environment. Health is therefore seen as a resource for everyday life, not the objective of living. Health is a positive concept emphasizing social and personal resources, as well as physical capacities (WHO, 1986, quoted in Naidoo and Wills, 2001, p. 2).

[2] http://www.cmhealth.org/docs/wg1_paper3.pdf.

oriented and considers 'health itself as a valued freedom' (Sen, 1999a), which brings us to the later approach also known as the alternative paradigm to health.

This alternative paradigm considers health as an integral part of good development. As a result health is expanded to include ability to lead a socially and economically productive life, alleviating poverty, reducing social disparities and participating in collective decision making as health is considered as an integral part of good development (Sen 1999a,b; Ruger, 2003, 2004). This paradigm (mostly derived from Aristotelian political philosophy and Amartya Sen's capability approach[3]) sees health as both intrinsically and instrumentally valuable but takes health as an end in itself (Ruger, 2003). In reality both the paradigms operate in developing nations in some form or the other – independently or in combination.

In this light, managing the impact of disasters through the perspective of health will reinvigorate our focus on humans rather than technology,[4] and identify areas that can build people's skills, knowledge, ability to work and good health, which together enable people to pursue different livelihood strategies and achieve their livelihood objectives (UN, 1996; DfID, 1999). This in turn has the potential to reduce poverty as well as disaster vulnerability at the household level. Considering health and health security as an asset of humanity would enable health security to be instrumental as an early warning tool to avoid major environmental or socio-economic events becoming disasters amongst the vulnerable section of the population living with risk.

The health security perspective is therefore people-centred and is derived from a 2-year empirical research study conducted in Bangladesh.[5] The project was funded by the Economic and Social Research Council-Department for International Development (ESRC-DfID) and was conducted between Northumbria University and the International Centre for Diarrhoeal Disease Research (ICDDR), Bangladesh. A 'mixed method' approach, combining quantitative and qualitative methods, was employed to understand the meaning of health security for disaster resilience at a regional and household level in Bangladesh. Fieldwork was conducted over 12 months (September 2007–September 2008) in three communities affected by environmental and non-environmental disasters: Matlab in Chandpur district, Chakaria in Cox Bazaar district and Domar in Nilphamari district (see Nahar *et al.*, 2010; Ray-Bennett, 2010; Ray-Bennett *et al.*, 2010). Using

---

[3] This alternative approach basically rests on three major arguments: first, 'according to Aristotle, society's obligation to maintain and improve health is grounded in the ethical principle of human flourishing, which holds that society is obligated to enable human beings to live flourishing and thus healthy lives. Certain aspects of health, in particular, sustain all other aspects of human flourishing because without being alive no other human functioning, including agency are possible. Therefore, public policy should focus on individual capacity to function, and health policy should aim to maintain and improve this capacity by meeting health needs' (Sen, 1999a; Ruger, 2003, p. 678). Second, the link between health and economic development is a two-way process because health depends on economic development in the same way that economic development depends on health. Third, health improvement and economic development are both linked to individual opportunities to exercise their agency and participate in political and social decision making (Ruger, 2003, p. 678). 'The penalty of inaction and apathy can be illness and death' (Sen, 1999a).

[4] The dominant views on disasters received criticism in the first half of the UN's International Decade for Natural Disaster Reduction (IDNDR), which heavily focused on technology to mitigate disaster impact in the developing nations (Haque and Zaman, 1994; Zaman, 1999).

[5] These are the author's views.

people's knowledge or people's perspective (Antonovsky, 1987; Calnan, 1987) as a method of investigation into health security, it revealed three interrelated components: *health security and capability*, *health security and public health*, and *health security and self-care*. Promoting as well as supporting all these three interrelated components is vital to reduce disaster vulnerability at household level. Currently these components are unaddressed comprehensively by the disaster management policies and programmes in South Asia in general, and India and Bangladesh in particular. I address each component in detail in the next section, which relates the health security perspective to wider disaster, development and security scholarships.

Relationship of Health Security Perspective with Disaster, Development and Security Literatures

The origin of health security can be traced back to the concept of human security proposed by the UN's human security framework in 1994, which added a new dimension to the narrowly defined dominant concept of 'security'.[6] Security was defined as a threat to countries' borders, protection of national interests in foreign policy and security from the threat of nuclear holocaust. The human security framework departed from the nation state's security to individuals and people's security. Therefore the concept is people-centred, and puts an individual's well-being, environment and livelihood central to the development and security discourse (UN, 1994; Commission on Human Security, 2003). The UN's framework acted as a bridge between the dominant/national security and alternative/human security schools and envisaged that human security may be threatened by interconnected and reinforcing aspects of economic, food, health, environmental, personal, community and political insecurities (UN, 1994). In 2003, the Commission on Human Security (CHC) published a report *Human Security Now*, which also defined the meaning of security from the state to the security of people and to human security. The report acknowledged that health security or good health is 'essential and instrumental to achieving human security' (CHC, 2003, p. 96). The report also emphasized human security as being complementary to state security, but with a focus on human development and human rights (CHC, 2003). Therefore, both the UN's Human Development Report and the CHC reinforce health security as instrumental for human security and human development.

Health security has a public health dimension. In 2001, the World Health Assembly's Resolution 54.14 'Global health security: epidemic alert and response' linked the health security concept to a global strategy for prevention of movement of communicable diseases across national borders (Aldis, 2008). This was taken forward when the WHO launched the 'global public health security' designed to 'Invest in Health and Build a Safer Future' (WHO, 2007a). The global debate included emerging

---

6 The dominant security tradition (which came into existence in 1919 after the First World War) is that of realism, which for the most part remains focused on the state and various measures. These include the economy and military strength. In 1983 from within the realist security studies, alternative thinking emerged and argued that focusing only on national security is increasingly inappropriate and could be counterproductive. However, these thoughts were already conceived and continued on by the development studies since the 1970s (Roberts, 2008, p. 13).

and rapidly spreading diseases, environmental change, bioterrorism, humanitarian emergencies caused by natural disasters, chemical spells or radioactive accidents and the impact of HIV/AIDS (WHO, 2007a,b).[7] Furthermore, global public health security as proposed by the WHO is epidemiological in nature. This means the focus is on disease and causation, and is based on the study of groups rather than individual cases.[8] The downside of this approach is the limited scope to understand health security at a household level and the social processes that potentially play an important role in Bangladesh, India or other developing nations given the impact of poverty and ill health most significantly experienced in these countries. However, the health security perspective complements both the human security and public health perspectives by invoking vulnerability analysis.

The vulnerability analysis that emerged in the 1970s in opposition to the dominant view on disasters[9] suggested that disasters (both natural and human-made) unfold when hazards intersect with vulnerable portions of the population. Vulnerability is defined as 'the conditions determined by physical, social, economic, and environmental factors or processes, which increase the susceptibility of a community to the impact of hazards' (UNISDR, 2004). Vulnerability can itself be traced back to quite 'remote' roots and general causes, which entail socio-economic processes and political factors that are requisite for understanding why hazards affect people in varying ways and why people experience disasters differently (Winchester, 1992, 2000; Maskrey, 1989; Bankoff, 2001, 2004; Wisner *et al.*, 2004; Sivakumar, 2005; Ray-Bennett, 2009b). The probability that a particular system or population will be affected or experience losses (deaths, injuries, property, livelihoods, economic activity disrupted or environmental damaged) resulting from interactions between natural or human-induced hazards and vulnerable conditions is known as the 'risk' (PAHO, 2000; UNISDR, 2004). Therefore, risk is a function of the vulnerability and the hazard. Risk is converted into vulnerability by the underlying state of human development, inequality, unequal opportunities and lack of political power that marginalizes people (UN, 2007/2008).

Vulnerability analysis goes beyond vulnerability and builds on people's resilience (Winchester, 2000) and this understanding is particularly relevant because health security

---

[7] However, this approach has invited criticism such as from Lee and Collins (2005) who argued that the overlap between health security and national security can become highly contested and limited by its inconsistencies with current developments. Two key questions arise: 'which issues are considered global health security issues?' and 'whose security is being considered?' (Lee and Collins, 2005). Not all global health issues are considered threats to national security. Some long-term health issues that cause high morbidity and mortality such as chronic diseases are not presently considered national security threats, although the security and economic development nexus has been noted by many development experts (see Vaux and Lund, 2003).

[8] See Antonovsky (1985) (dated but still relevant) for the public health model and criticism on the epidemiology approach.

[9] A dominant mainstream approach, emerged in the post-Second World War period (Kreps, 1998). This conventionally treats a disaster as an accident, triggered solely by natural hazards – an inevitable occurrence in an environment that is physically vulnerable. People need to protect themselves from environmental risks, which have little or less recognized connections to their vulnerability in everyday life. Put simply, 'natural disasters' are attributable to the forces of nature against which technology is seen as a solution. However, this paradigm has evolved as more recently evidenced by the Hyogo Framework, the successor of the UN's IDNDR (Ray-Bennett, 2009a).

is about building people's resilience as well. The health security perspective enables us to address the agentive capabilities of individuals in securitizing health in a vulnerability context. This is explained further through the three interrelated components of health security in the ensuing sections. The degree of people's vulnerability and their ability to recover from disasters in relation to health, are directly related to the forces that govern everyday lives. As such, the health security perspective stands at the intersection of human security, development and public health scholarships. Vulnerability and risk analysis are the threads that bind the three in order to plug gaps in a locally centred analysis by focusing on individuals and households with different socioeconomic status and gender. The disaster impact and the resilience to disaster risk vary with the level of vulnerability of people in a particular place and over time. Tapping the reasons for lesser or greater vulnerability will be the key in promoting health security. Currently cross-over between the disciplines of health, security and disaster is a rarity both at policy and conceptual level, albeit the need for cross-over was identified a long time ago. Recently this has been re-emphasized in the Hyogo Framework (UN, 2005). As a result, the health security perspective is anticipated to advance our practical knowledge on the implementation of the Five Priorities for Action (PoA) outlined by the Hyogo Framework and offer a deeper theoretical understanding that underpin them for effective DRR and human security.

The caveat of the health security perspective is that like the concept of health, it is subjective and multidimensional. This is partly because health security is people-centred and the empirically lived realities of people in relation to health and disaster vulnerability are diverse, dynamic and context specific (Health Security Project, 2009; Ray-Bennett *et al.*, 2010). The subjective element of health security can be challenging for both policy makers and practitioners. Keeping this challenge in mind a conscious effort has been made in the following sections to deduce some operational elements of health security that can directly contribute to effective disaster management whilst discussing the three health security components (capability, public health and self-care) in the *pre-impact*, *impact* and *post-impact* phase of a disaster (Wetterhall and Noji, 1997) including flood and cyclone in general.

Exploring the health security components

Health security and capability

'Capability' is intrinsically connected with the health security perspective. Capability is crucial to promote health security because 77% of people lack basic or minimally essential human capabilities in Bangladesh (GoB, 2003). As health security is primarily about people's knowledge, the emphasis is on promoting their capability and resilience to disasters and other shocks. Unfortunately this has received the least attention from the policy makers and alike in Bangladesh, India or other developing nations.

The analysis of capability stems from the alternative paradigm of health, which considers health as an integral part of good development as discussed earlier (Ruger, 2003, 2004). Capability is a broad concept as proposed by Sen and it incorporates concerns associated with the 'standard of living', but goes beyond it[10] (Dreze and Sen,

[10] Capability primarily relates to the richness of the person's life, whereas a person may also value his or her capability to be socially useful and influential. Secondly, capability is nutrition-related but nutrition related capabilities are defined with reference to the relevance or otherwise of

1989; Sen, 1999a,b). It is a holistic and humanistic approach that places the whole person – what we are able to do or be – at the centre of social analysis and public action. The health security perspective enables one to revisit this noble approach by reassessing poverty as capability deprivation, since low income is considered clearly as one of the major reasons of poverty and ill health (Sen, 1999, p. 87). The capability deprivation is influenced by an individual's everyday vulnerability based on his/her gender, caste, class, race, disability and location (e.g. proneness to flooding or drought). Tackling these inequalities and deprivation should form the central tenet for DRR programmes. I therefore posit that people-centred strategies to promote capability can be achieved in three interrelated ways with the help of disaster, development and health professionals.

First, in the pre-impact phase of a disaster (be it flood, cyclone, drought), protective democracy is fundamental to create income and employment opportunities with the help of government, NGOs and with the market, through small-scale farming, diversification and microenterprise (UN, 1996). The government as well as the NGOs must regulate labour laws that promote unfair wage rates based on caste, gender or other social differences. Social security and safety nets[11] including disaster insurance have to be promoted amongst vulnerable groups to protect their desirable household assets (including bed, chair, table, mobile stove) in order to reduce disaster risks. Households without these assets feel extremely vulnerable to disasters (see Ray-Bennett *et al.*, 2010). The Self Employed Women's Association (SEWA) offers an excellent model in this regard by offering an Integrated Insurance Scheme and SEWA Bank to promote security for its members against disasters in Gujarat (see Vaux and Lund, 2003). Places that do not have cyclone and flood shelters have to be provided with these shelters so that they can protect poor people's assets. The cyclone and flood shelters should also have the provision for cattle shelter along with fodder supply. These shelters have to be sensitive to caste, class, gender and culture (Rashid and Michaud, 2000; Ray-Bennett, 2009b). This is also the phase where contingency plans and context-specific disaster management plans have to be charted out through the devolution of responsibility with the local governmental, non-governmental and community organizations.

Second, in the impact phase of a disaster, contingency plans have to be put in place in a participatory way and resources deployed including boats, temporary tents, potable water, food aid and provision of sanitation in vulnerable pockets. Effective relief policy must also be put into place that goes beyond food aid and includes non-food items (NFI)

---

improved food intake, education, healthcare, sanitation and safe drinking water. Thirdly, capability also represents the various combinations of functioning (being and doing) that the person can achieve, reflecting their freedom to lead one type of life or another. Fourthly, capability is the ability to debate, negotiate, add voice to political process and be an agent of 'social change'. Fifthly, capability is also the ability to avoid morbidity, being informed and educated and being well nourished (Dreze and Sen, 1989; Sen, 1999b). This approach bears some resemblance to the human security approach of the CHC (2003) especially through themes on survival, dignity, livelihood and strategies (Ruger, 2004; Carpenter, 2009).

[11] During our research period, Bangladesh did not have democracy, and an interim government supported by the army was in power. Both the former and current Prime Ministers (Khaleda Zia and Sheikh Hasina) of Bangladesh National Party (BNP) and Awami League as well as the current and shadow cabinets were in jail due to the allegation of high level of corruption. Many elderly respondents informed us that this had resulted in them not receiving their pension, and also a lack of relief management during and after the floods of 2007 and 2009 (Health Security Project, 2007–2009).

through direct cash or voucher transfer or in combination (Harvey and Bailey, 2011) for housing, kitchen garden, cattle, fodder and miscellaneous aid that addresses the needs of affected households.

Third, in the post-impact phase of a disaster, the primary need is to ensure regular income through food for work or cash for work activities,[12] and to conduct needs assessments[13] so that effective health measures can be put into place, and the public distribution system can be supported to ensure food security (Mooij, 2007). The disaster professionals, relevant NGOs and the community should also ensure that disaster prevention and preparedness is continued throughout the year. In all of these phases effective interaction with the media should be explored (Dreze and Sen, 1989; Dynes and Rodriguez, 2007).

Health security and public health

Public health provisions are also intrinsically connected with health security in a disaster context. The importance of disasters as a public health problem is now widely acknowledged (Noji, 1997) due to the:

1. Unexpected number of deaths, injuries or illnesses that they may cause in the affected community, exceeding the therapeutic capacities of the local health services and requiring external assistance.
2. Destruction of local health infrastructures (including hospitals) that they may cause, which will therefore not be able to respond to the emergency. Disasters may also disrupt the provision of routine health services and preventive activities, leading to long-term health consequences in terms of increased morbidity and mortality. The areas that lack these health services will be the worst affected and their likely recovery will also be prolonged.
3. Adverse effects on the environment and the population which may also increase the likelihood of communicable diseases and environmental hazards that will increase morbidity, premature death and diminished quality of life in the future.
4. Unexpected increase in psychological and social behaviour of the stricken community.
5. Shortage of food in some instances with severe nutritional consequences, such as starvation or specific micronutrient deficiencies – vitamin A deficiency (Noji, 1997, pp. 14–15).
6. Lack of safe drinking water, disposal of human excreta and shelter management (Lillibridge, 1997).

The operational element of public health through the health security perspective is then envisaged to involve medical and public health response to anticipate these different medical and health needs at a community level in the pre-impact phase as well as when they emerge during the impact phase of a disaster. Furthermore, delivering the

[12] A good example is the national rural employment scheme in India.

[13] After the impact of a disaster (be it flood, cyclone, drought, earthquake) rapid needs assessments should be conducted in order to determine the health and medical needs of disaster-affected communities (Malilay, 1997).

appropriate interventions at the precise times and places where they are needed most (Noji, 1997) will be key to achieving health security. Potable water is the most immediate relief commodity essential for the survival of the disaster-affected population, particularly for those who have been displaced and where the supporting public health infrastructure is affected (Lillibridge, 1997). The delivery and distribution of safe and clean water in disaster relief is the raison d'être for public health and health security.[14] The availability of clean water is also associated with sanitary and public health including hand washing and the provision of oral rehydration therapy. The following are key measures for effective water management during the impact phase of a disaster:

1. Health and disaster professionals must provide adequate quantities of water for fluid replacement, personal hygiene, cooking and sanitation.
2. Programmes must provide water of sufficient quality to prevent the transmission of disease since the quality and quantity of public water are so closely related to the health status of a disaster-affected population. Therefore, emergency water programmes must form an integral part of DRR measures.
3. Sites with potential sources of water should be evaluated to determine their patterns of surface drainage, proximity to local sewage systems and potential for chemical contamination.
4. In places where the disaster-affected population use surface water, information and resources on how to treat this water need to be shared and taught to the community in the pre-impact and impact phases of a disaster.
5. The provision of drilled wells must be explored where surface water or other sources of water are unsafe to consume.
6. Potable water must be distributed in a place that is accessible to all men and women of different caste, class or ethnicity.
7. Affected populations must also receive appropriate containers to store and transport portable water.
8. The collection of rainwater must also be promoted (Lillibridge, 1997, pp. 66–67).
9. In all the above activities, gender has to be mainstreamed (UNISDR, 2002).

The operational element of public health through the health security perspective should also include emergency waste management. The temporary latrine system should be set up for the displaced population in an emergency shelter. This should be a high priority during the impact phase of a disaster like flood in particular. The maintenance may

[14] The main reason for the increase in life expectancy in the developed countries since 1900 is the improvement in public sanitation and in the quality of public water (Lillibridge, 1997). In the developing nations, water and sanitation is still one of the great human development challenges in the 21st century (UN, 2006). It is estimated that there are 1.2 billion people without access to safe water and 2.6 billion without access to sanitation (UN, 2006). This situation is likely to worsen during disasters. In two of our research locations, Matlab and Chakaria, we observed households consume tube well and untreated pond water in their everyday life. During the time of floods households whose tube wells went underwater consumed rainwater and untreated river water (Health Security Project, 2007–2009). Elsewhere we have discussed the consequences of these on health and humans (Ray-Bennett, 2010).

require effective coordination and collaboration between local officials, NGOs, the community and public health education programmes to ensure their continued use by the population. The temporary sanitation system should also have lighting for night as well as catering to cultural, gender and children's needs. Relief organizations and governments must also provide technical assistance in the form of sanitarians, environmental engineers, hydrologists, material for latrine construction and maintenance and disinfection supplies in the pre-impact, impact and post-impact phases of a disaster (Lillibridge, 1997, pp. 73–74).

Health security and self-care

'Self-care' is also intrinsically interlinked with health security. Taking self-care as a point of analysis, it directs our attention at household levels because we understand self-care as:

> unorganized health activities and health related decision making by individuals, families, neighbours, friends, colleagues at work, etc. It encompasses self medication, self treatment, social support in illness, first aid in a 'natural setting' i.e. the normal context of peoples' everyday lives. Self-care is definitely the primary health resource in the health care system (Hatch and Kickbusch, 1983; quoted in Kickbusch, 1989).

Segall and Goldstein (1989, p. 153) argued self-care is 'the basic level of health care in all societies'. This came to light whilst exploring the meaning of health security in Bangladesh through household monitoring for 4 months (Health Security Project, 2007–2009). Through a myriad of health-related activities, self-care operates at household level, and women, young girls and boys in particular act as gatekeepers of these activities (Ray-Bennett, 2010). Professional healthcare is therefore seen as supplementary to self-care, instead of viewing lay care as residual and supplemental to professional care (Dean, 1989; Segall and Goldstein, 1989). The professional care includes utilization of trained and untrained doctors, homeopathy, home remedies and traditional healing (Amin *et al.*, 1989; Segall and Goldstein, 1989). This therefore suggests that self-care is not restricted to care provided by the lay community, but also the use of professional care is included within the rubric of self-care (Segall and Goldstein, 1989). This is now increasingly acknowledged. The WHO's 'Regional Consultations on Self-care in the Context of PHC' called for a proactive support for self-care as an important intervention in primary healthcare in South-east Asia (Plianbangchang, 2009) indicating its importance in professional healthcare. Self-care is not opposed or in contrast to professional healthcare, rather it is complementary (Bentzen *et al.*, 1989; Edgeworth, 2011) within the health security context. This understanding is important because previously we have discussed that health security intersects the domains of both professional and alternative healthcare practices (Ruger, 2004; Ray-Bennett *et al.*, 2010).

Kickbusch (1989) also argued self-care is a political project. This was partly to do with Ivan Illich's (1976) call for 'self autonomy' and questioning of the 'medicalization' created by the biomedicine model or professional care. Bloem *et al.* (2003) argued that the Millennium Development Goals (MDGs) played an important role in the medicalization process by promoting health policies solely to meet and reduce the burden of disease.[15] The exclusive focus on treatment and cure diverts attention from the role of the health enterprise in providing care and support to people unable to look after themselves, for instance the chronically ill or disabled (ibid). Ruger (2004) argued that the health-related MDGs can be met only through transformation in underlying values and societal structures and democratic systems that are inclusive and publicly accountable. In this light self-care acts as a 'window' to observe what poor households do to maintain health in their everyday life and how they cope and promote health during and after disasters in the absence of health services and basic needs.

The political element of self-care is also connected with the second wave of the feminists' outcry against the medicalization of birth and human reproduction; which in turn led to the perpetuation of capitalism and patriarchal structures (Kichbusch, 1989; Blaxter, 2004; Nettleton, 2006). Studies have also revealed women as agents for change within their own contexts who are in general the custodians of health at the household level through a myriad of productive, reproductive and caring activities before, during and after disasters (Sen, 1999a; Obrist, 2006; Ray-Bennett, 2010; Ray-Bennett *et al.*, 2010). By way of summary, self-care is intrinsically interlinked with health security. In doing so, the corollary is that health security also attains a political slant. This is potentially an enlightening connection as to date health security as a nascent concept has lacked fuller interpretation and locally focused political edge. The securitization of health or human security implies budgetary priorities (UN, 1994) and a kind of 'call and response' process (Roe, 2004) for disaster management, but generally speaking health security (as proposed by the UN and the WHO) lacks a political slant. Self-care in this light acts as a tool towards understanding health security at a household level and also identifying the state's failure in transforming underlying values and societal structures, which are *prerequisites* for promoting health (Kichbusch, 1989; Ruger, 2004).

The operational element of self-care through the lens of health security is then envisaged to include: (i) financial and support-led investment on local preventive and curative infrastructures; and (ii) financial and support-led investment at household level. The 'support-led' process does not operate through fast economic growth, but works through a programme of skilful social support of healthcare, education and other relevant social arrangements (Sen, 1999a).[16]

To implement the former, there is a requirement for detailed plans of implementation, especially a sequence of investments in physical capital (clinics, hospitals, training centres, mobile health), which are disaster resilient (as suggested by the Hyogo Framework) and in health professionals so that they are able to perform their 'business as usual' during the impact and post-impact phases of a disaster. For this there has to be an effective financing plan, combining additional resources from donors, which would help in plugging the national financial gap. Coordination between the health ministry, mission hospitals, NGOs, community centres and the country coordinating mechanisms that bring together all these critical stakeholders should form part of the integrated DRR measures. However, this assumption rests on the premise that the primary barrier to achieving

[15] Out of eight MDGs, three goals focus exclusively on illness and disease. These include: reduce child mortality; improve maternal health; and combat HIV/AIDS, malaria and other diseases (UN, 2010).

[16] This process is exemplified by the experiences of economies such as Sri Lanka, the Indian state of Kerala, Costa Rica and pre-reform China, which have had rapid reductions in mortality rates and enhancement of living conditions without much economic growth (Sen, 1999a, pp. 621–622).

health security is suboptimal government healthcare spending (Ruger, 2004). From a medical or public health perspective, the problem is not a lack of interventions rather that they are not universally available. Redressing this dilemma of universal coverage through primary healthcare[17] (this was promised to be achieved in the 1980s; Braveman and Gruskin, 2003) with access to technology is a problem of collective action and requires an integrated approach, not one of medicine or public health (Phillips, 1990; Phillips and Verhasselt, 2001; Ruger, 2004). Currently this is lacking in practice because the health sector has little or no direct control over most of the underlying conditions required for health, like education, food supply, nutrition, housing and income (Zaidi, 1988; Asthana, 2001; Braveman and Gruskin, 2003). The Hyogo Framework picked up the importance of food security whilst proposing key activities to 'reduce the underlying risk factors' in relation to health and disasters (UN, 2005:13).

To achieve support-led investment in local preventive and curative infrastructures will then require more than scaling up public health investment, strong commitment by national and local leaders as well as transforming the underlying values and societal structures that constrain people to achieve health (Ruger, 2004). In reality, transformation of social structures that produce inequality and inequities may be hard to believe especially in the South Asian nations because they have failed terribly in their redistribution policies (Zaidi, 1988; Kohli, 1994; Islam, 2007). But the countries that have succeeded in implementing their redistributive reforms and invested in health such as Hong Kong, the Republic of Korea and Taiwan (and to some extent Tanzania) 'developed' quite significantly (Zaidi, 1988; Sen, 1999a,b; Ruger, 2004). This is didactic and the national health and disaster managers in India, Bangladesh or South Asia in general must take this as a lesson to invest in health and local infrastructure that supports community health.

To implement the latter support-led investment at household level, the focus has to be on people. Since health security is about people's knowledge, people-centred strategies should promote their agentive capabilities through skills and information and must become central to DRR. Transferring intellectual aid (Schumacher, 1973) on how to maintain health through effective management of water, sanitation and food during the impact and post-impact phases of a disaster should be key for health security. Currently DRR programmes including early warning programmes (EWPs), disaster risk management programmes, relief and shelter programmes (to mention a few) (see GoO, 1996; UN, 2005; GoI, 2007; Ray-Bennett, 2009b) lack the component of health mechanisms that can tap knowledge that exists amongst people to inform policy. At a community level DRR Committees, also known as Community Based Disaster Preparedness Groups supported by the United Nations Development Programme (UNDP) in India and Africa (see IFRC, 2009; Ray-Bennett, 2009b), or the Cyclone Preparedness Programme (CPP) initiated by the British Red Cross Society in Bangladesh, and micro-credit groups in general (Fisher and Sriram, 2002; Pantoja, 2002; Mechler *et al.*, 2006; Ray-Bennett, 2007) can play an important role in managing and promoting community health through the management of water and sanitation in the pre-impact phase. NGOs can act as moderators to initiate effective coordination between the civil society, government and other stakeholders in order to design and implement context-specific disaster management that promotes health security.

---

[17] In all three locations of our research, the local rural dispensary or the primary healthcare was almost non-existent, leaving the people to rely heavily on private and traditional care.

Conclusion: Implications for Disaster Management

Therefore, managing disasters from a health security perspective will have three important implications: (i) it will indicate an inroad to better specify the intersection of disaster and development activities; (ii) it will build the capacity of households and communities living with risk; and (iii) it will prioritize disaster management as a national security concern.

As outlined earlier, health security is people-centred, and to look for health security themes in disasters would involve listening to people and therefore to 'probe, alter, design, solve, decouple, try, peek and poke, talk, disregard, and improvise' (Weick, 1988, p. 314). This will identify actions for disaster management and will also have the potential to construct, constrict or limit the impact on humans of an unfolding crisis or disaster. In this process people's narratives will also identify where disaster and health-related development activities intersect. This will lead to *organic* disaster management, driven by people's everyday life, shaped by the places which they inhabit, and influenced by the narratives of people and the social structures that constrict their capability and freedom. This organic approach to disaster management takes 'household' as a unit of analysis, in which the contingency plans, relief and disaster risk programmes and so on are designed by people. These plans are fluid and vary depending on the health needs of people across different hazards and time. This suggests that organic disaster management is process-oriented, context-specific and must be designed keeping local realities and people's hardships in mind.

This process-oriented approach to disaster management is in direct contrast to the classical top-down, centralized disaster management model. Nevertheless the top-down disaster model is in flux at the moment with the Declaration of Hyogo Framework. Risk management, consequence management, community involvement and the multisectoral approach are some of the key themes of disaster management as part of DRR (Ariyabandu and Wickramasinghe, 2003; Buckle *et al.*, 2003; UN, 2005; Gopalakrishnan and Okada, 2007) and yet household as a unit of analysis has not received adequate attention. The Standing Order on Disaster Management of Bangladesh of 1997 and 2011 (GoB, 1999, 2010) and the Disaster Management Act 2005 of India (GoI, 2007) are some of the important examples in this regard. Furthermore in reality hazard-specific and reactionary disaster management is still the norm in the developing nations (Cannon, 1994; Buckle *et al.*, 2003; Samal *et al.*, 2003; Ray-Bennett, 2009a,b).

Disaster management through the lens of health security would mean building the capacity of households and communities. This implies human investment by increasing their skill levels, heightening their awareness regarding health management, promoting livelihood strategies (through innovation, diversification, technology), supporting men and women's rights to health, land and property, and providing spaces/forum/opportunities where people are able to voice their opinions, constraints and scopes for effective health and disaster management. This in turn has the potential to reduce vulnerability and disaster risks, rather than focusing on programmes that solely promote preparedness and mitigation of hazards leading to inadequate and potentially dangerous situations (Cannon, 1994).

Disaster management from a health security perspective should prioritize disaster management as a national security concern with the potential for improved innovation and securitization. Securitization of disaster management needs to be understood at the level it can have most impact, requiring the spread of know-how, to meet local conditions of disaster avoidance and development. Securitization is also a communicative process to promote a disaster-resilient culture by enhancing people's capability. The key to operationalizing disaster management through health security is underpinned by communication and communicating processes that take place between different institutions and local level day-to-day realities. To understand these communicative processes that are the lynchpins for successful disaster management and health security, I suggest that more sociological and anthropological research is required that can engage with the ever-growing community of scholars, policy makers, practitioners, and civil societies that are engaged with mainstreaming of DRR to explore communicative processes, whilst being grounded in the local experiences of day-to-day adaptation and resilience in pursuit of reduced vulnerability and sustainable development.

Acknowledgements

I would like to thank Dr Matt Qvortrup and Mr Matt Craig at Cranfield University for their comments on the initial draft of this paper. The findings of this research are part of a 2-year ESRC-DFID funded project on the 'Meaning of Health Security for Disaster Resilience in Bangladesh'. This was a joint project between Northumbria University and International Centre for Diarrhoeal Disease Research, Bangladesh. I was a Research Associate for this project. This chapter is based entirely on my own views and analysis and not that of the research team.

References

Aldis, W. (2008) Health security as a public health concept: a critical analysis. *Health Policy and Planning* 23(6), 369–375

Amin, R., Chowdhury, S.A., Kamal, G.M. and Chowdhury, J. (1989) Community health series and health care utilization in rural Bangladesh. *Social Science Medicine* 29(2), 1343–1349.

Antonovsky, A. (1985) *Health, Stress, and Coping.* Jossey-Bass Publishers, London.

Ariyabandu, M.M. and Wicramasinghe, M. (2003) *Gender Dimensions in Disaster Management: a Guide for South Asia.* ITDG South Asia Publication, Colombo, Sri Lanka.

Asthana, S. (2001) Economic crisis, adjustment and the impact on health. In: Phillips, D.R. and Verhasselt, Y. (eds) *Health and Development.* Routledge, London, pp. 50–64.

Bankoff, G. (2001) Rendering the world unsafe: 'vulnerability' as western discourse. *Disasters* 25(1), 19–35.

Bankoff, G. (2004) The historical geography of disaster: 'vulnerability' and 'local knowledge'. In Bankoff, G., Frerks, G. and Hilhorst, D. (eds) *Mapping Vulnerability: Disasters, Development and People.* Earthscan, London, pp. 25–37.

Bentzen, N., Christiansen, T. and Pedersen, K.M. (1989) Self-care within a model for demand for medical care. *Social Science Medicine* 29(2), 185–189.

Blaxter, M. (2004) *Health.* Polity Press, Cambridge, UK.

Bloem, M.W. *et al.* (2003) Urbanisation and the Millenium Development Goals – Insights from nutritional surveillance data. In: Bloem, M.W., Mench-Pfanner, R. and Panagides, D. (eds) *Health and Nutritional Surveillance for Development.* Helen Keller International, Singapore.

Bloom, D., Canning, D.E. and Jamison, D.T. (2004) Health, wealth, and welfare. *Finance and Development* 41, 10–15.

Braveman, P.A. and Gruskin, S. (2003) Poverty, equity, human rights and health. *Bulletin of the World Health Organization* 81(7), 539–545.

Buckle, P., Marsh, G. and Smale, S. (2003) Reframing risk, hazards, disasters, and daily life: a report of research into local appreciation of risks and threats. *The Australian Journal of Emergency Management* 18(2), 81–87.

Calnan, M. (1987) *Health and Illness: the Lay Perspectives*. Tavistock Publications, London.

Cannon, T. (1994) Vulnerability analysis and the explanation of 'natural disasters'. In: Varley, A. (ed.) *Disasters, Development and Environment*. John Wiley & Sons, New York.

Carpenter, M. (2009) The capabilities approach and critical social policy: lessons from the majority world. *Critical Social Policy* 29, 351–373.

Commission on Human Security (2003) *Human Security Now*. 159. UN Publication, New York.

Dean, K. (1989) Conceptual, theoretical and methodological issues in self-care research. *Social Science Medicine* 29(2), 117–123.

Department for International Development (DfID) (1999) Sustainable livelihoods guidance sheets. Available at: http://www.livelihoods.org/info/info_guidancesheets.html (Accessed 22 October 2010).

Dreze, J. and Sen, A. (1989) *Hunger and Public Action*. Clarendon Press, Oxford, UK.

Dynes, R.R. and Rodriguez, H. (2007) Finding and framing Katrina: the social construction of disaster. In: Brunsma, D.L. Overfelt, D. and Picou, J.S. (eds) *The Sociology of Katrina: Perspectives on a Modern Catastrophe*. Rowman and Littlefield Publishers, New York, pp. 23–34.

Edgeworth, R. (2011) Disease resilience in rural Bangladesh: the adoption and practice of curative self-care. *Local Environment* 16(5), 461–472.

Fisher, T. and Sriram, M.S. (2002) *Beyond Micro-Credit: Putting Development Back into Micro-Finance*. New Economics Foundation, London.

Gopalakrishnan, C. and Okada, N. (2007) Designing new institutions for implementing integrated disaster risk management: key elements and future directions. *Disasters* 31(4), 353–372.

Government of Bangladesh (GoB) (1999) Standing order on disaster. Ministry of Food and Disaster Management, Disaster Management Bureau, Dhaka, Bangladesh.

Government of Bangladesh (GoB) (2003) Conceptual Framework of Health, Nutrition and Population Sector Programme (HNPSP) July 2003–June 2006. Planning Wing, Ministry of Health and Family Welfare, Dhaka, Bangladesh.

Government of Bangladesh (GoB) (2010) Standing order on disaster. Ministry of Food and Disaster Management, Disaster Management Bureau, Dhaka, Bangladesh.

Government of India (GoI) (2007) The Disaster Management Act, 2005. Available at: http://www.ndmindia.nic.in/acts-rules/DisasterManagementAct2005.pdf (accessed 12 February 2013).

Government of Orissa (GoO) (1996) *The Orissa Relief Code*. Government of Orissa, Bhubaneswar, India.

Government of Orissa (GoO) (2005) *Orissa Human Development Report 2004*. Government of Orissa, Planning and Coordination Department, Bhubaneswar, India.

Haque, E. and Zaman, M. (1994) Vulnerability and responses to Riverine hazards in Bangladesh: a critique of flood control and mitigation approaches. In: Varley, A. (ed.) *Disasters, Development and Environment*. John Wiley & Sons, New York.

Harvey, P. and Bailey, S. (2011) *Good Practice Review: Cash Transfer Programming in Emergencies*. ODI, London.

Health Security Project (2007–2009) Health Security for Disaster Resilience project document. Disaster and Development Centre and International Centre for Diarrhoeal Disease Research, Bangladesh (ICDDR,B), Research project-2007–2008, funded by ESRC-DFID, Research Grant RES-167-25-0241.

Illich, I. (1976) *Medical Nemesis: The expropriation of Health*. Pantheon Books, New York.

International Federation of Red Cross and Red Crescent Societies (IFRC) (2009) World disaster report: focus on early warning, early action. Available at: www.ifrc.org/en/publications-and-report/world-disasters-report (Accessed 12 February 2013).

Intergovernmental Panel on Climate Change (IPCC) (2007) Climate change 2007. Synthesis report. Contribution of Working Groups I, II and III to the Fourth Assessment Report of the

Intergovernmental Panel on Climate Change. Available at: www.ipcc.ch (Accessed 12 February 2013).
Islam, A.M. (2007) A comparative analysis of socio-economic-political indicators of Bangladesh vis-a-vis its four south Asian neighbours. In: Islam, M.F. and Andaleeb, S.S. (eds) *Development Issues of Bangladesh-III: Human Development and Quality of Life*. The University Press Limited, Dhaka, Bangladesh, pp. 1–36.
Kickbusch, I. (1989) Self-care in health promotion. *Social Science and Medicine* 29(2), 125–130.
Kloos, H. (2001) The poorer third world: health and health care in areas that have yet to experience substantial development. In: Phillips, D.R. and Verhasselt, Y. (eds) *Health and Development*. Routledge, London, pp. 199–215.
Kohli, A. (1994) Introduction: developing a state-in-society perspective. In: Migdal, J., Kohli, A. and Shue, V. (eds) *State Power and Social Forces: Domination and Transformation in the Third World*. Cambridge University Press, Cambridge, UK.
Kreps, G.A. (1998) Disaster as systemic event and social catalyst. In: Quarantelli, E.L. (ed.) *What is a Disaster? Perspectives on the Questions*. Routledge, London, pp. 31–55.
Lee, K. and Collins, J. (2005) *Global Change and Health: Understanding Public Health*. Open University Press, Milton Keynes, UK.
Lillibridge, S.R. (1997) Managing the environmental health aspects of disasters: water, human excreta, and shelter. In: Nojji, E.K. (ed.) *The Public Health Consequences of Disasters*. Oxford University Press, Oxford, UK, pp. 65–78.
Malilay, J. (1997) Floods. In: Nojji, E.K. (ed.) *The Public Health Consequences of Disasters*. Oxford University Press, Oxford, UK, pp. 287–301.
Maskrey, A. (1989) *Disaster Mitigation: a Community Based Approach*. Oxfam, Oxford, UK.
Mechler, R., Linnerooth-Bayer, J. and Peppiatt, D. (2006) Disaster insurance for the poor? A review of micro insurance for natural disasters risks in developing countries. Available at: www.eldis.org/go/country-profiles&id=23423&type=Document (Accessed 17 June 2007).
Mooij, J.E. (2007) Is there an Indian policy process? An investigation into two social policy processes. *Social Policy and Administration* 14(4), 323–338.
Nahar, P., Alamgir, F., Bhuiya, A., Ray-Bennett, N. and Collins, A.E. (2010) Interrelations between water, health and livelihood in disasters. In: Prakash, A., Vs, S. and Chourey, J. (eds) *Water and Health in South Asia*. South Asia Consortium for Interdisciplinary Water Resources Studies. Sage Publications, Delhi.
Naidoo, J. and Wills, J. (2001) Introducing health studies. In: Naidoo, J. and Wills, J. (eds) *Health: an Introduction Studies*. Palgrave, London, pp. 1–8.
Nettleton, S. (2006) *The Sociology of Health and Illness*. Polity Press, Cambridge, UK.
Noji, E.K. (1997) Introduction. In: Noji, E.K. (ed.) *The Public Health Consequences of Disasters*. Oxford University Press, Oxford, UK, pp. xiii–xvii.
Obrist, B. (2006) *Struggling for Health in the City: an Anthropological Inquiry of Health, Vulnerability and Resilience in Dar es Salaam, Tanzania*. Peter Lang, Berlin, Germany.
Pan American Health Organization (PAHO) (2000) *Natural Disasters: Protecting the Public's Health*. Scientific Publication No. 575. PAHO, Washington, DC.
Pantoja, E. (2002) *Microfinance and Disaster Risk Management: Experience and Lessons Learned*. ProVention Consortium, World Bank, Washington, DC.
Phillips, D.R. (1990) *Health and Health Care in the Third World*. Longman Scientific & Technical, New York.
Phillips, D.R. and Verhasselt, Y. (2001) *Health and Development*. Routledge, London.
Plianbangchang, S. (2009) Opening remarks. Regional consultation on self care in the context of PHC, 7–9 January 2009. WHO South-East Asia.
Rashid, F.S. and Michaud, S. (2000) Female adolescents and their sexuality: notions of honour, shame, purity and pollution during the floods. *Disasters* 24(1), 54–70.
Ray-Bennett, N.S. (2007) Environmental disasters and disastrous policies: An overview from India. *Social Policy and Administration: Regional Issue: South Asia* 41(4), 419–424.
Ray-Bennett, N.S. (2009a) Multiple disasters and policy responses pre- and post-independence Orissa, India. *Disasters* 33(2), 274–290.

Ray-Bennett, N.S. (2009b) *Caste, Class and Gender in Multiple Disasters: the Experiences of Women-headed households in an Oriya Village*. VDM Verlag, Saarbrucken.
Ray-Bennett, N.S. (2010) Monitoring household health security for disaster resilience in Bangladesh. Disaster and Development Conference, 23–24 November 2010, Northumbria University, Newcastle-upon-Tyne, UK.
Ray-Bennett, N.S., Collins, A., Edgeworth, R., Bhuiya, A. and Alamgir, F. (2010) Exploring the meaning of health security for disaster resilience: through people's perspectives in Bangladesh. *Health and Place* 16, 581–589.
Roberts, D. (2008) *Human Insecurity: Global Structures of Violence*. Zed Books, London.
Roe, P. (2004) Conditons of desecuritization. *Security Dialogue* 35(3), 279–294.
Ruger, J.P. (2003) Health and development. *Lancet* 362, 678.
Ruger, P. (2004) Millennium Development Goals for health: building human capabilities. *Bulletin of the World Health Organization* 82(12), 9.
Samal, K.C., Meher, S. and Panigrahi, N. (2003) *Beyond Relief Disaster Mitigation, Livelihood Rehabilitation and the Post-cyclone Recovery in Orissa: Village Level Studies in Three Most Cyclone Affected Districts in Orissa*. NCDS, Bhubaneswar, India.
Schumacher, E.F. (1973) *Small is Beautiful: Economics as if People Mattered*. National Book Store Inc., Manila, the Philippines.
Segall, A. and Goldstein, J. (1989) Exploring the correlates of self-provided health care behaviour. *Social Science Medicine* 29(2), 153–161.
Sen, A. (1999a) Health in development. *Bulletin of the World Health Organization* 77(8), 619–623.
Sen, A. (1999b) *Development as Freedom*. Oxford University Press, Oxford, UK.
Sivakumar, M.V.K. (2005) Impacts of natural disasters in agriculture, rangeland and forestry: an overview. In: Sivakumar, M.V.K., Motha, R.P. and Das, H.P. (eds) *Natural Disasters and Extreme Events in Agriculture: Impacts and Mitigation*. Springer, New York, pp. 1–20.
United Nations (UN) (1994) *Human Development Report 1994: New Dimensions to Human Security*. UNDP Publication, New York, Oxford University Press. Available at: http://hdr.undp.org/en/reports/global/hdr1994/ (Accessed 15 July 2013).
United Nations (UN) (1996) *Human Development Report 1996: Economic Growth and Human Development*. UNDP Publication. New York, Oxford University Press. Available at: http://hdr.undp.org/en/reports/global/hdr1996/ (Accessed 15 July 2013).
United Nations (UN) (2005) World Conference on Disaster Reduction, 18–22 January 2005, Kobe, Hyogo, Japan. Hyogo Framework for Action 2005–2015: Building the Resilience of Nations and Communities to Disasters. Available at: http://www.unisdr.org/we/inform/publications/1037 (Accessed 15 July 2013).
United Nations (UN) (2006) *Human Development Report 2006: Beyond Scarcity: Power, Poverty and the Global Water Crisis*. UNDP Publication, Basingstoke, Palgrave Macmillan. Available at: http://hdr.undp.org/en/reports/global/hdr2006/ (Accessed 15 July 2013).
United Nations (UN) (2007/2008) *Human Development Report 2007/8: Human Solidarity in a Divided World*. UNDP Publication, Basingstoke, Palgrave Macmillan. Available at: http://hdr.undp.org/en/reports/global/hdr2007-8/ (Accessed 15 July 2013).
United Nations (UN) (2010) *Human Development Report 2010: The Real Wealth of Nations: Pathways to Human Development*. UNDP Publication, Palgrave. Available online http://hdr.undp.org/en/reports/global/hdr2010/ (Accessed 15 July 2013).
United Nations (UN) (2011) *Human Development Report 2011: Sustainability and Equity: A Better Future for All*. UNDP Publication. New York, Palgrave. Available at: http://hdr.undp.org/en/reports/global/hdr2011/ (Accessed 15 July 2013).
United Nations International Strategy for Disaster Risk Reduction (UNISDR) (2004) Terminology: basic terms of disaster risk reduction. Available at: http://www.unisdr.org/eng/library/lib-terminology-eng%20home.htm (Accessed 15 June 2010).
United Nations International Strategy for Disaster Risk Reduction (UNISDR) (2002) *Gender Mainstreaming in Disaster Reduction*. Presentation at the Commission on the Status of

Women, 6 March 2002, New York. Available at: http://www.eird.org/bibliovirtual/hospitales-seguros/pdf/eng/doc13937/doc13937-contenido.pdf (Accessed 15 July 2013).

Vaux, T. and Lund, F. (2003) Human security of working women: response to crisis. In: Chen, L., Fukudu-Parr, S. and Seidensticker, E. (eds) *Human Insecurity in a Global World.* Global Equity Initiative, London, pp. 137–182.

Weick, K.E. (1988) Enacted sensemaking in crisis situations. *Journal of Management Studies* 25(4), 305–317.

Wetterhall, S.F. and Noji, E.K. (1997) Surveillance and epidemiology. In: Nojji, E.K. (ed.) *The Public Health Consequences of Disasters*. Oxford University Press, Oxford, UK, pp. 37–64.

WHO (2007a) High-level debate tackled need for improved international health security: World Health Day 2007: International health security: Invest in health, build a safer future. WHO, Geneva.

WHO (2007b) A safer future: global public health security in the 21st century. WHO, Geneva.

Winchester, P. (1992) *Power, Choice and Vulnerability: a Case Study in Disaster Management in South India 1977–1988*. Earthscan, London.

Winchester, P. (2000) Cyclone mitigation, resource allocation and post-disaster reconstruction in south India: lessons learnt from two decades of research. *Disasters* 24(2), 18–37.

Wisner, B., Blaikie, P., Cannon, T. and Davis, I. (2004) *At Risk: Natural Hazards, People's Vulnerability and Disasters*, 2nd edn. Routledge, London.

Zaidi, S.A. (1988) Poverty and disease: need for structural change. *Social Science Medicine* 27(2), 119–127.

Zaman, M.Q. (1999) Vulnerability, disaster, and survival in Bangladesh: three case studies. In: Oliver-Smith, A. and Hoffman, S.M. (eds) *The Angry Earth: Disaster in Anthropological Perspective*. Routledge, London, pp. 192–212.

Chapter 29

Management of the 2011 Japan Multiple Disasters (Earthquake, Tsunami and Ensuing Disasters): A View through an International Lens

Preeti Arora, Rajesh Arora, Rupa Gunaseelan, Raman Chawla and J.R. Bhardwaj

Japan: An Introduction from a Disaster Perspective

11 March 2011 brought with it untold devastation and suffering in Japan, which will be remembered by future generations as the day of the worst disaster in the history of this century. The multiple disasters, i.e. the earthquake, the tsunami and the nuclear disaster (Fig. 29.1) caused extensive damage to infrastructure (Fig. 29.2), a large number of deaths (Table 29.1) and a feeling of insecurity, fear of another strike, devastation and a huge loss – physically, economically and emotionally. A disaster of this kind would have left the people in the disaster-struck region shattered, however, it was during these stressful conditions that the people of Japan proved their strong mettle and, through their preparedness and resilience, not only coped but also moved ahead for a better tomorrow.

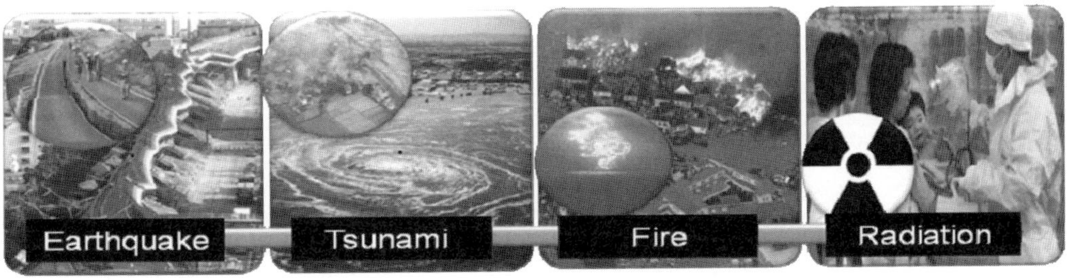

Fig. 29.1. Japan's multiple disasters: a natural catastrophic event of unimaginable magnitude led to a man-made disaster. Never before in the history of human civilization had different types of disasters been encountered simultaneously. This made the 2011 Japan multiple disasters unique in several respects and tested the mettle of a disaster-resilient society to its extremes.

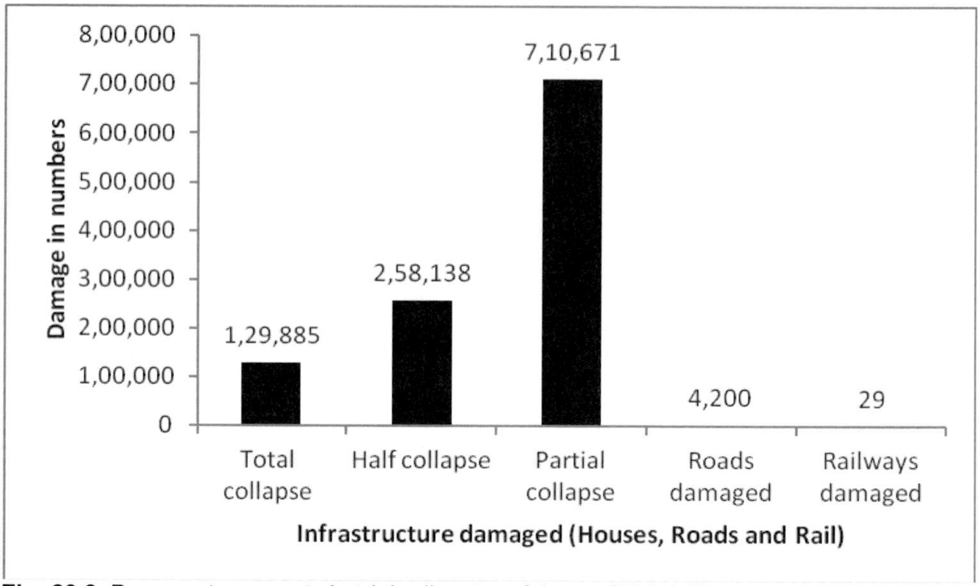

Fig. 29.2. Damage to property in triple disaster of Japan (2011) (Source: JNPA, 2012).

Table. 29.1. Depiction of the losses due to the 2011 Japan multiple disasters. (Data as on 16 May 2012; Source: JNPA, 2012.)

Confirmed deaths	15,858
Injured	6,011
People missing across 18 prefectures	3,021
Property damage Totally collapsed Half collapsed Partially collapsed	 129,885 258,138 710,671
Roads damaged	4,200
Trains damaged	29

Japan is an archipelago of 6850 islands and lies between latitudes 24° and 46°N, and longitudes 122° and 146°E. The total area of Japan is approximately 378,000 km^2 with a coastline of nearly 34,751 km. The archipelago is susceptible to tsunamis and more than 195 tsunamis have been recorded over a period of 1313 years over this coastline, which is home to nearly three-quarters of the population (BBC, 2011). On the other hand, the land area of Japan lies on 'the Pacific ring of fire' (intersection of three major tectonic plates) and, therefore, encounters 90% of the world's earthquakes. These vulnerabilities make Japan a hub for natural disasters.

This chapter describes the severe impact of the sequential multiple disasters that occurred in March 2011 and their physical/psychological impact, interventions practised and lessons learnt to develop resilience among the community. Figure 29.1 shows the March 2011 multiple disasters of Japan. The life expectancy in Japan is 85.90 years for women and 79.44 years for men (Cabinet Office, Government of Japan, 2011c; The Statistical Handbook of Japan (SHJ), 2012). A total of 23% of the population is over the age of 65 years, while 11.5% is above the age of 75 years, which is likely to increase by 40% by 2055. Japan's elderly population makes up about 35% of the world's elderly population, which is the highest in the world. This sector of the population is vulnerable to extreme psychological shock.

The chapter also provides the outcome of the survey carried out on the members of the Japanese community directly or indirectly affected by the multipronged disaster.

The Tōhoku Earthquake/Great East Japan Earthquake

It was early afternoon on 11 March 2011 when the clock struck 14:46 (JST) that a major earthquake of magnitude 9.0 Richter occurred offshore at Sanriku affecting the north-eastern region of Japan. This is commonly referred to as the Tōhoku earthquake. The Tōhoku earthquake's Japanese name is 'Higashi Nihon Dai-Shinsai'. The earthquake lasted for approximately 6 min. The epicentre was 130 km east–south-east of the Ojika Peninsula and approximately 130 km east of Sendai city, Tōhoku, Japan, lying at latitude 38.6°N and longitude 142.52°E. The earthquake occurred at a shallow depth with its hypocentre 24.4 km deep. Honshu, which is Japan's largest island was shifted 2.4 m east by this earthquake. It also shifted the Earth's axis by 10–25 cm, which proves how powerful the earthquake was. According to the White Paper on Disaster Management of Japan (2011b), it was the most massive earthquake ever observed in Japan. On the same day as the earthquake more than 50 aftershocks were recorded out of which three aftershocks were of magnitude 7 or greater. The seismic intensity ranged between 3 and 7 on the Japanese scale of 1–7 (JMA). Several cities and towns in the coastal region of Miyagi, Fukushima, Ibaraki and Tochigi prefectures were severely affected and experienced severe aftershocks of magnitude ranging 6–7 on the Richter scale and seismic intensity of 6 and > 6. In the north of Miyagi prefecture, a seismic intensity of 7 was recorded, which is the maximum according to the Japanese scale. There were more than 650 aftershocks triggered by the earthquake. This earthquake initiated a major tsunami and several fire incidents. The tsunami further worsened the situation by causing damage to the Fukushima nuclear power plant. This was the largest earthquake in the history of Japan, shaking Eastern Japan from Hokkaido down to Kyushu, which means approximately the entire archipelago of Japan was shaken by the earthquake (Kyoto University, 2011).

Fire outbreaks

Every major earthquake is followed by some fire events due to the shaking of the ground. A large number of fire events were recorded following the 11 March 2011 Great East Japan Earthquake. Approximately 325 cases of fire incidents were recorded, out of which 163 cases were in Miyagi prefecture. On 11 March 2011 15:47 JST the Cosmo Oil Company Refinery in Ichihara city, Chiba prefecture, which is 40 km east of Tokyo, was ablaze after the earthquake. It took firefighters until 14 March 2011 to put out the blaze. The liquid petroleum gas (LPG) tanks at the refinery caught fire, shutting down the refinery. The fire extinguishing operation started immediately at 16:04 under the instructions of the Ichihara Fire Department. As the fire was caused by the explosion of the LPG tanks, it was necessary for the entirety of the petroleum gas in the tanks to be burnt to prevent any secondary accidents that could have occurred if the fire were not directly extinguished (www.cosmo-oil.co.jp). On 11 March 2011 alone, there were 44 cases of fire incidents. The Japan Police Agency (JPA) regularly monitored and updated all the fire events. The Fire and Disaster Management Agency deployed 27,373 teams and approximately 103,600 firefighters to take care of the fire outbreaks and other rescue operations.

The ensuing tsunami

The Great East Japan Earthquake of magnitude 9.0 resulted in a devastating tsunami. The tsunami created by the earthquake was an oceanic-trench earthquake. The earthquake struck the boundary of the Pacific plate and the continental plate. Japan had experienced many major earthquakes like the Great Kanto earthquake (1923) and the Kobe earthquake – also known as the Great Hanshin-Awaji earthquake – (1995), which are often used to compare the damages and losses. But the major difference here is that the Great Kanto earthquake and the Kobe earthquake caused damage due to building collapse and secondary fire events, whereas the destruction and the losses caused by the Tōhoku earthquake were more due to the tsunami than to the earthquake itself. This disaster caused the most casualties since the Second World War (Cabinet Office, Government of Japan, 2011b). The devastating tsunami arrived within 30 min in the northern region of Japan impacting the coastal regions of Hokkaido, Iwate, Miyagi and Fukushima, and the Pacific coast of Aomori, Ibaraki and Chiba prefecture. This accounts for the continuous coastal area of Honshu islands, from the Tōhoku to Kanto regions covering > 500 km in length. The maximum wave height recorded in the 2011 Tōhoku earthquake tsunami was 40.38 m, while tsunamis of 3 m or more were recorded in several places in Japan.

The tsunami warning in Japan was so efficient that the earthquake occurred at 14:46, and the tsunami warning was issued at 14:49, and information and advice was on the JMA website at 14:49, i.e. within 3 min of the occurrence of the earthquake. Several aftershocks were also followed by the issuing of tsunami warnings. The regions affected by the tsunami extended over an extremely wide area. The destruction and the scale of inundation caused by the tsunami were so enormous as to be almost unbelievable. The areas of Iwate, Miyagi and Fukushima prefectures were the most affected by the tsunami. Japan has a history of tsunamis and hence they had constructional mitigation measures in place. The frontline defences alone focused on tsunami breakwaters, coastal dykes and tidal barriers. However, these could not effectively protect from the severe effects of the tsunami. In the Taro region of Iwate prefecture, a 10-m-high and 2.5-km-long sea dyke, which was built after the tsunami caused by the Syowa-Sanruku earthquake to prevent tsunami damage, was destroyed by the 2011 tsunami. The dyke could not completely prevent the damage, but it was effective to some extent in reducing the impact of the tsunami in the region.

On 3 March 2011, which was just a few days ahead of the Tōhoku earthquake, evacuation training was conducted in Kamaishi, Japan. It was reported that the training was very effective for the local residents in evacuation and helped to save many lives. Almost all of the elementary and junior high school children of Kamaishi, a small coastal town in Iwate prefecture, survived the tsunami. It was the response capabilities they learned at school that helped them to overcome an unprecedented disaster. Out of a total of 2924 elementary and junior high school children in Kamaishi, only five were reported dead or missing in Japan's disaster. Of the five, four had been absent or had left school early, while one disappeared after being reunited with family following the dramatic escape from the tsunami. The 'sorrowful wisdom', commonly known on the Sanriku coast – the Pacific side of the Tōhoku region – has been passed on from generations and is called 'tsunami tendenko'. It can be summarized as: 'go uphill independently at the time of tsunami caring only for your own safety, not thinking of anyone else, even your family'. This training strategy helped to save the children's lives.

Buildings were severely damaged by the tsunami to such an extent that it was difficult for local people to find their own property. The use of communication systems like mobile phones and the internet was severely constrained due to the tsunami, which made the situation worse, cutting access to cities from the outside world. Train tracks and roads were damaged, further disrupting connectivity to the affected cities. The fishing industry was badly affected as the tsunami struck the coastal areas. Sendai Airport, which is the biggest in the Tōhoku area, was damaged by the disaster.

This disaster has been labelled as the costliest in human history (US$235 billion according to the World Bank). Japan, despite being a developed country, was hit hard by the compound (multiple) disasters. The Japanese community has shown a great sense of resilience in coping with the impact, leading to mitigation of the effect. Table 29.1 shows the losses as per the latest data obtained from the Japanese National Police Agency (JNPA) as on 16 May 2012.

The impact of the disaster on human life and property is given in Figs 29.1 and 29.2, respectively, as per information from the JNPA. Around 4.4 million households in north-eastern Japan were left without electricity and 1.5 million without water for days. The main causes of death in the Tōhoku earthquake in Iwate, Miyagi and Fukushima prefectures was drowning due to the tsunami. According to the data provided by JNPA, 92.4% of deaths were due to drowning, 4.4% due to crush/other injuries, 1.1% due to burns and 2% due to unspecified reasons.

The nuclear crisis (Fukushima incident)

11 March 2011 had some more dark and threatening events in store for the land of Japan. The destructive tsunami was followed by another unbelievable accident at the nuclear power plant at Fukushima. The height of the tsunami of 14–15 m, which was way beyond imagination and the coping capacity of the Japanese, broke the 10-m sea wall. The back-up diesel generators, which were supposed to supply the water pumps with energy to cool down the fuel rods inside the reactors failed (Chandler, 2011). Out of the six reactors, three reactors (Reactors 1, 2, 3) stopped automatically at 04:30 JST, and an emergency situation was declared at the Fukushima Daiichi (no. 1) nuclear power plant and reported to the International Atomic Energy Agency (IAEA) (Sharma and Arora, 2011). The cascade of events is recorded in Table 29.2.

This emergency situation was further reported as having the potential to become an international public health concern. The fuel rods inside the reactors were receiving water as a coolant, which was pumped in by the on-site diesel generators placed in the basement. These diesel generators failed due to the tsunami water gushing in, meaning the fuel rods could not be cooled further, thereby increasing the pressure inside the reactors. The heat generated caused evaporation of water, worsening the situation in the reactors and making it very difficult to cool the spent fuel pools in Reactors 1 and 4.

Table 29.2. Cascade of events in nuclear episode.

Day	Date	Description
Day 1	11 March 2011	A magnitude 9.0 earthquake and tsunami hit Japan's north-eastern coast, knocking out power and swamping the back-up diesel generators needed to cool the six reactors and spent fuel pools at the Fukushima Daiichi nuclear plant
Day 2	12 March 2011	Engineers scrambled to prevent a nuclear meltdown. Some of the reactors began to grow hotter with their cooling systems disabled. A hydrogen explosion rocked Unit 1, causing a radiation leak. Workers furiously pumped seawater into the reactor's core
Day 3	13 March 2011	New problems appeared at Unit 3, where workers vented steam to try to avoid another hydrogen explosion. Seawater was pumped to Units 1 and 3
Day 4	14 March 2011	The crisis deepened at Fukushima Daiichi. The pressure and heat continued to build in Unit 3, resulting in a hydrogen explosion that destroyed the outer containment building. Fuel rods at Unit 2 were fully exposed to air twice, worrying officials. Workers pumped seawater into the cores of Units 1, 2 and 3
Day 5	15 March 2011	Unit 2 became the new focal point as a hydrogen explosion occurred there and its suppression pool was damaged. Explosions and fires also plagued Unit 4, and leaked radiation into the atmosphere. The government evacuated residents from the 12-mile (20-km) radius around the plant
Day 6	16 March 2011	Another fire at Unit 4 hindered efforts to get the reactors and spent fuel pools under control. Steam and smoke rose from Unit 3, due to evaporation of water in the spent fuel pool. Radiation levels surged. The US government advised its citizens within 50 miles of the plant to evacuate
Day 7	17 March 2011	Water levels at Unit 4's spent fuel pool ran low and radiation levels at the plant were high. Workers attempted to spray the spent fuel pool at Unit 3 with helicopters, fire trucks and water cannons. Little water reached the pool. The Tokyo Electric Power Corp. reported that 23 of its workers sustained injuries and 18 were contaminated with radiation from the events at the plant following the tsunami
Day 8	18 March 2011	Unit 2 was connected to a power line. Water spraying continued. The International Atomic Energy Agency raised the International Nuclear and Radiological Event Scale rating from 4 to 5
Day 9	19 March 2011	Water spraying resumed at Unit 3. Elevated radiation levels were detected in milk and spinach from areas around the power plant. Emergency power was restored to the cooling systems for the spent fuel ponds in Units 5 and 6
Day 10	20 March 2011	Seawater was injected into the spent fuel pool at Unit 2. Reactors at Units 5 and 6 went into cold shutdown. Radiation levels higher than the legal limit were detected in spinach in several prefectures near the plant
Day 11	21 March 2011	Smoke was emitted from Units 2 and 3. The US Nuclear Regulatory Commissioner said that the situation at the plant appeared 'to be on the verge of stabilizing'
Day 12	22 March 2011	Smoke was seen at Units 3 and 2. All six reactor units were connected to the power grid. Radioactive materials were detected in seawater near the plant

Day 13	23 March 2011	Smoke was seen again at Unit 3. Tokyo water officials said they had found elevated radiation levels in the city's water supply. Testing found the amount of radioactive iodine was at twice the recommended limit for infants
Day 14	24 March 2011	Two plant workers were hospitalized with injuries to their feet after coming into contact with radioactive water while laying electrical cables in the basement of a turbine building next to reactor No. 3. The two men were subcontractors for TEPCO. Food safety concerns lingered in Japan, as residents began stockpiling clean water with the news that radiation in tap water was above recommended levels for infants
Day 15	25 March 2011	The power plant operators said it was likely that radiation detected in water pooling in the basement of one reactor building came from the reactor's main vessel. This raised concerns that the reactor core may have been breached, but there were conflicting accounts of this. Separately, the Japanese Nuclear Safety Commission widened a voluntary evacuation area around the plant to a radius of 18 miles
Day 16	26 March 2011	The US Navy rushed to deliver fresh water to replace the corrosive saltwater being used to cool the plant's nuclear reactors, as the Japanese government urged TEPCO to be more transparent in sharing information with the public. Radiation had been making its way into milk, seawater and 11 kinds of vegetables, including broccoli, cauliflower and turnips
Day 17	27 March 2011	Workers fled the Unit 2 reactor after TEPCO officials erroneously reported a reading of radiation levels nearly 10 million times above normal. 'The number is not credible,' TEPCO spokesman Takashi Kurita later said. 'We are very sorry.' Officials acknowledged the presence of radioactive water in each of the four most troubled reactors
Day 18	28 March 2011	Plant officials reported that highly radioactive water had filled a series of underground tunnels at the damaged power plant, raising concerns that the contaminated water could start spilling out into the ocean. Experts said that the water was a result of frantic efforts to cool overheated reactors and spent fuel pools
Day 19	29 March 2011	Highly toxic plutonium was detected in the soil outside the nuclear power plant. Safety officials said the amounts were low and did not pose a risk to humans, but the finding supported suspicions that radioactive water was leaking from damaged nuclear fuel rods inside the plant
Day 20	30 March 2011	Japanese officials said seawater outside of the Fukushima Daiichi nuclear power plant contained more than 3300 times the normal amount of radioactive iodine. The country's nuclear safety agency said it was a 'concern' – but not necessarily an immediate threat. Workers at the plant continued to battle large amounts of radioactive water that had flooded parts of the facility; tanks to store contaminated water began to fill up
Day 21	31 March 2011	Radiation levels continued to rise in the ocean, offshore from the nuclear power plant. Officials also evaluated whether to expand the mandatory evacuation area after the report of high levels of radiation in the village of Iitate, 25 miles from the plant. Workers also continued to struggle with pooling radioactive water; they had to keep pumping water to cool the reactors, but storage of contaminated water was becoming problematic

Day 22	1 April 2011	Japan's Nuclear and Industrial Safety Agency ordered TEPCO to review its latest radiation measurements taken in air, seawater and groundwater samples around the disabled Fukushima Daiichi plant, saying they seemed suspiciously high. TEPCO said it may have mis-stated radiation levels in water near the plant, officials said on Friday
Day 23	2 April 2011	Highly radioactive water was leaking into the sea from a crack discovered in a maintenance pit at the facility. Water flowing into the ocean from the 8-inch crack was expected to dissipate quickly and not cause any health hazard, officials said. Soon after discovering the crack TEPCO officials tried to fill the pit with cement
Day 24	3 April 2011	A Japanese safety agency spokesman said it could take several more months for engineers to get the tsunami-ravaged plant under control. Bringing the reactors at the plant under control would require permanently restoring the cooling systems that prevent reactors from dangerously overheating
Day 25	4 April 2011	TEPCO planned to release 10,000 metric tonnes of radioactive water into the ocean in an effort to clear space in a waste storage building for water that was even more highly contaminated than the dumped water. Chief Cabinet Secretary Yukio Edano called it an 'unavoidable' step. Officials said the water must be disposed of before the normal cooling systems could be brought back on line, and intentionally draining some of it into the ocean was the best option
Day 26	5 April 2011	The Japanese government set its first radiation safety standards for fish today after the distressed nuclear power plant reported radioactive contamination in nearby seawater measuring at several million times the legal limit. TEPCO insisted that the radiation would rapidly disperse and that it posed no immediate danger
Day 28	7 April 2011	A magnitude 7.1 earthquake hit off the north-east coast of Japan, near the city of Honshu. TEPCO officials said there was no additional damage to the plant at the time and all workers had been accounted for
Day 29	8 April 2011	The 7.1 magnitude aftershock on 7 April caused blackouts in nearly 1 million homes in north-east Japan. Officials reported that two people were killed
Day 30	9 April 2011	Japan's government announced it would ban farmers from planting rice in soil contaminated by radiation from the tsunami-flooded nuclear power plant, adding another food central to Japanese culture to the list of items raising concerns. The ban applied to any soil found to contain high levels of radioactive caesium, and farmers unable to grow rice would be compensated
Day 32	11 April 2011	Japan's nuclear regulators raised the severity level of the crisis at the stricken nuclear plant. The regulators said the rating was being raised from 5 to 7 – the highest level on an international scale overseen by the International Atomic Energy Agency. However, there was no sign of any significant change at the tsunami-stricken Fukushima Daiichi nuclear plant
Day 33	12 April 2011	INES level 7 confirmed, the Nuclear and Industrial Safety Agency (NISA) estimated 10% of radioactive material had been released as compared with the Chernobyl accident; 20 km point as planned evacuation area; evacuation preparedness area – 20–30 km; reported iodine above threshold; Fukushima power plant 0.6–1.6 μSv/h (1 μSv/h is last line acceptable dose); beta contamination was also reported

Day 34	13 April 2011	Restrictions on consumables in affected regions
Day 35	14 April 2011	Earthquake Hamadori (5.4) 67 km from Fukushima; fresh water injection in Units 1 to 3; nitrogen gas used to prevent explosions; Gamma dose rate 2 μSv/h

The Japanese Government declared the situation at the Fukushima Daiichi nuclear power plant level 4 on the International Nuclear and Radiological Event Scale (INES) – 'accident with local consequences'. This was later upgraded to level 7 (equivalent to Chernobyl on 26 April 1986) (Sharma and Arora, 2011).

The nuclear event spread panic amongst the community despite assurances by Tokyo Electric Power Company (TEPCO) that there was no radiation leakage to be worried about. However, residents as far as Tokyo were quite worried and some of them even showed signs of psychosomatic symptoms as to how they would deal with the contamination. The possibility of small children being affected by the radiation in water and milk products became a cause of immense concern for the residents.

During Chernobyl, 5.2 million terabecquerel (TBq) of radioactivity was released and approximately 0.37–0.63 million TBq radioactivity was released at the Fukushima Daiichi nuclear power plant. Evacuation of people by the Japanese government in the radius of 20 km around the Fukushima Daiichi power plant started immediately after the first hydrogen explosion in Reactor no. 1, which occurred at 15:30 JST on 12 March 2011. Another explosion occurred at Reactor 3 on 14 March at 11:01 JST with a blast sound at Reactor 2 on 15 March at 6:14 JST. On 15 March 2011 a fire breakout at Reactor 4 was reported. Radioactive emissions occurred outside the nuclear power plant due to the water used in extinguishing the fire. The Japanese government took measures by instructing TEPCO to control the pressure inside the containment vessels. An area of 30 km around the Fukushima Daiichi nuclear power plant was declared as a no fly zone. Approximately 99,000 people were evacuated from the Fukushima prefecture. Continuous insufficient cooling problems were experienced at the Fukushima nuclear power plant. The on-site radiation levels were reported to be higher than normal radiation levels. Cooling activities of the overheating reactors were increased by using helicopter water spraying and water canon trucks. TEPCO's efforts towards cooling the overheated reactors were supported by the Japanese Self Defense Force. The evacuation was carried out in an area of 20 km radius from the Fukushima Daiichi nuclear power plant in Liate village, Katsurao village and some parts of Nanmie town and Kawamata town. The crisis became more problematic because of the large amounts of radioactive waste water in Reactors 1, 2 and 3 (approximately 60,000 t) and in Reactors 5 and 6 (approximately 11,500 t) where handling the contaminated water became a problem for the government of Japan. The release of the radioactive contaminated water into the sea raised serious concerns for neighbouring countries like China and Korea, besides concerns for countries as far away as the USA. Traces of radioactive materials were found in tap water, sea water and food products like milk, leafy vegetables and fish. Radiation levels in food products were monitored every day. Sales of food items, milk and other products that failed to meet the provisional regulation levels were banned by the Ministry of Health, Labour and Welfare, Japan. The discrepancy in the design of the Fukushima Daiichi Power plant, i.e. the positioning of the diesel generators in the basement, was not considered to cause particular vulnerability of the plant to the floods and tsunami.

The resident as well as the non-resident community was also in a state of panic (Arora, 2011; Arora *et al.*, 2012). Some do's and dont's are given in Table 29.3, which can help save lives during nuclear disasters.

This nuclear disaster at the Fukushima nuclear power plant has forced the entire world to rethink their nuclear power facilities and safety measures. The need for in-depth research of the entire event is required and there is also a need to incorporate the lessons learnt into mitigation plans.

Table 29.3. Do's and Don'ts during nuclear accidents.

Do's	Don'ts
Fulfil strictly the given instructions regarding radiation protection	Keep calm and don't panic
Pass on received information about the accidents	Do not take action yourself, without instruction from the competent authorities
Reduce time outside to a minimum	Do not take trips, excursions, walks or picnics
Maintain cleanliness, wash hands thoroughly before eating, bathe daily with free-flowing water, wash clothes worn outside frequently	Do not bathe in the water basin or stagnant water (pond, lake, etc.)
Wash foodstuffs thoroughly before consumption	Do not eat food stuffs that have been banned
Select a suitable place where the people affected by the accident can be shifted to	Do not perform wilful and unorganized evacuation without explicit instruction from a competent authority

Emergency response to the multiple disasters

Immediately after the disaster the Japanese government declared an emergency situation. For an organized, speedy response an emergency response team headed by the Prime Minister was activated in the immediate aftermath of the disaster. All the resources of the Japanese Military were deployed by the Ministry of Defence, Japan. Over 307,500 members of the National Police Force and the Fire and Disaster Management Agency were activated by the Japanese government. Various ministries and agencies took active participation in the response. These included the National Police Agency, the Ministry of Defence, the Fire and Disaster Management Agency, the Ministry of Health, Labour and Welfare, the Ministry of Finance, the Ministry of Land and infrastructure, the Ministry of Foreign Affairs and the Ministry of Agriculture, Forestry and Fisheries. Volunteers were also organized and coordinated by the government of Japan on a priority basis. The rescue and relief was done using helicopters and ships. The Japanese Red Cross came into action immediately for disaster relief. The overall coordination between the different civil agencies, government departments and NGOs was carried out by the Japan Civil Network for disaster relief. Japan Self Defence Forces (JSDF) numbering approximately 110,000 troops were deployed. They cleared the roads within 3 days, which improved the response time to the disaster sites. The Japanese response to the disaster was so efficient that at 14:50 JST the response office at the Prime Minister's office convened the Emergency Response Team, within 4 min of the disaster. The Extreme Disaster Management Headquarters and the local headquarters for Disaster Management were set up for a streamlined response. This was the first establishment of the Extreme Disaster Management Headquarters after the enactment of the Disaster Management Law in Japan. Disaster Medical Assistance teams (DMATs) numbering 193 were activated for emergency medical care by the Ministry of Health, Labour and Welfare, Japan. Over US$50 billion was allocated for critical tasks such as debris clearance, temporary shelters, etc. The major transportation network was restored within a few days of the disaster. Here, we take an example of the Tōhoku expressway where 347 km out of the 675 km was damaged on 11 March due to the earthquake. The expressway was restored to working condition. Sendai Airport, which was completely inundated and was in a damaged state after the tsunami, was made serviceable by 29 March and the first passenger flight took off on 13 April. Gradual restoration of electricity, gas supply, water, sewage and telecommunications was done most expeditiously.

Lessons learnt

During the operation of nuclear power plants, the likelihood of an accident with radiation has a very low probability. However, the potential risk in the event of such an accident should be analysed and evaluated in advance considering all possible emergency measures aimed at the prevention of the accident and mitigation to acceptable levels. The important considerations that should be applied from the competent authorities include: (i) planning for emergency preparedness based on the analysis of possible scenarios for the origin and development of various accidents and assessment of the radiation risk to the population; (ii) the developed emergency plans should be approved at national, regional and institutional level for each site; (iii) the emergency plan should be documented for maintenance, protection against radiation, mitigation and liquidation of the accidents; and (iv) define the responsibilities and obligations of the competent authorities.

The emergency plans can be implemented in the following two ways: (i) an off-site emergency plan to protect the population in case of an accident; and (ii) an on-site emergency plan for the corresponding sites. It is essential to maintain emergency preparedness measures during such incidences by way of: (i) establishing emergency teams at the national level; (ii) maintaining a system for notification and early warning to the population; (iii) assuring funds for radiation protection and radiation monitoring, including forecasting emergency rescue and recovery work; (iv) periodical updating of the emergency plans by the relevant institutions and local authorities; (v) educating society to perform actions according the emergency plans; (vi) conducting exercises and training for the implementation of the emergency plans; (vii) informing the public on important issues related to radiation protection and implementation of protection measures in case of accidents; (viii) giving timely notification to the population and submission of appropriate instructions; (ix) providing shelters in appropriate places; (x) restricting and controlling the access to places posing increased radiation risk to the people; (xi) use of protective means to prevent inhalation of radioactive substances; (xii) arrangement of evacuation, temporary or permanent relocation of the affected people; (xiii) implementation of specific requirements for the radiation hygiene of the population; (xiv) restriction of the consumption of radioactively contaminated foodstuffs including water and milk; and (xv) implementation of additional measures for radiation protection of the population based on measurements, forecasts for the development of the accident and estimates of its likely consequences (adapted partly from Cabinet Office, Government of Japan, 2011a).

From the Japan experience, it has been strongly felt that prolonged lack of electrical power must be precluded. While the designers believed their design included sufficient redundancies (diesels, batteries, redundant connections to the electrical grid), the simultaneous extended loss of all sources of power left the operators dependent on creative responses. This lesson is applicable both to the reactor and to fuel pools. In the wake of this disaster, all nuclear installations will probably be required to do a complete review of security to assess their access to electrical power. It may be noted that this lesson is applicable to many more activities than just nuclear power. Extended loss of electrical power in major metropolitan areas can generate a horrible crisis. The loss of power was irrelevant to other activities in the region near the Fukushima plant because they were destroyed by the tsunami. Other lessons learnt that may be expected to impact existing nuclear plants include that better means of control of hydrogen build-up in the case of fuel damage may be required. Some do's and don'ts for such disasters are given in Table 29.3.

Structural/non-structural measures/sensitizing/training community

Japan has taken integrated tsunami mitigation strategies, which consist of structural and non-structural measures: (i) development of tsunami walls: in Japan most of the tsunami walls near beaches were built with the aim of reducing the tsunami risk. These walls are many metres wide and also in some areas they extend several kilometres in length. Tsunami walls are good for the areas that have been identified as being highly vulnerable to tsunamis. (ii) Building of river gates: river gates are built in most of the rivers in Japan to reduce the impact of tsunamis as rivers and other water bodies connected to the sea act as channels for tsunamis to migrate inland. The cost of building river gates, maintenance and impact on the appearance of the natural environment around the location should be considered. (iii) Protecting coastal forests: coastal forests also act as a barrier to tsunamis and, depending on the vulnerable of an area, the length and width of the forest can be decided on the basis of the tsunami threat assessment. Several previous studies have pointed to the role of coastal forests in preventing damage resulting from tsunamis (Forbes and Broadhead, 2007). (iv) Tsunami breakwaters: breakwaters protect the harbours especially, reducing the impact of tsunamis on harbours. This method is advisable in areas identified as high vulnerability areas. (v) Early warnings: during any emergency situation, early warnings are important. The practice of educating people in coastal areas on how to behave during the time of tsunami alerts can be useful. (vi) Displaying tsunami water level height: Japan displays tsunami water level heights of previous tsunamis in many locations so that people can get an idea of high the tsunami can be and in case of a tsunami how vulnerable they are so that they can move to minimum safe-level higher ground. (vii) Evacuation centres: evacuation centres can be built in vulnerable areas. These places are used not only as evacuation centres, but can be used for any other purpose in day-to-day life. The main purpose is to make an evacuation centre with all facilities and all the necessary paraphernalia required in the event of a tsunami. (viii) Signs to display the maps and paths of evacuation centres: in Japan as a pre-emptive measure, action was taken to display signs on the evacuation centres. Moreover, the paths of evacuation are also very important and adequate steps were taken to highlight them so that they could be used during emergencies. It was observed that such paths leading to higher ground were very useful in saving lives. (ix) Memorial plaques: in Japan many areas have memorial plaques in order to remind people that the frequency of tsunamis is high. (x) Hazard mapping: hazard mapping is done in Japan so that everybody can identify the areas that are susceptible to tsunamis. This is important as the vulnerable areas can be identified and adequate tsunami mitigation measures in development programmes can be undertaken in the vulnerable areas. (xi) Educating school children: Japan educates its school children, since education on tsunami helps in effectively facing tsunami hazards. Such best practices should be adopted especially in coastal areas in other parts of the world where there is a likelihood of tsunami. School children can in turn teach others how to behave in a tsunami situation and they can help to guide their parents and other family members. It's a very good method to spread knowledge. (xii) Displaying the height of the floor in buildings: in buildings in coastal areas, displaying the height on the floor so that people get to know at what height they are standing is a good idea. This is not a costly method and also during a tsunami alert it gives a clear idea to people of whether they should move to an evacuation centre or whether they are safe where they are. (xiii) Reserving one floor of tall buildings as a gathering floor: in Japan one floor of taller buildings is reserved as a gathering floor so that at the time of a tsunami people can evacuate to that floor and in case of an emergency be rescued from there. (xiv) Tsunami drills: whatever the frequency, tsunamis can happen anytime and, therefore, preparedness is essential. Tsunami drills help mitigate the impact that tsunamis can have and also it teaches people on how to behave in the event of a tsunami (Cabinet Office, Government of Japan, 2011b).

Assessing on-ground situation

One of the authors (P.A.) had an opportunity to personally visit Japan and assess the on-ground situation. A visit to Japan's Cabinet Office was made on 24 October 2011 under the aegis of the National Women's Education Centre, Japan, wherein knowledge was gained from the Cabinet Office of the disaster management policies in place in Japan. It became evident that Japan pays a lot of attention to inclusion of women in disaster management plans and the Gender Policy Bureau emphasizes gender-related issues since the problems faced by women are quite complex in post-disaster scenarios. Meetings and interviews with disaster management experts and the earthquake/tsunami-affected people were held in Japan. In addition, a survey was carried out on the NDRF Team that visited Japan so as to gain a view from on-ground situations prevailing in the immediate aftermath of the disaster from an international responder perspective.

During the interaction with the officials at the Cabinet Office and experts working in area of disaster management in Japan key points that emerged regarding the 2011 Tōhoku earthquake were that an increased focus was placed on: (i) gender equality; (ii) children; (iii) the elderly; and (iv) the special needs population in Japan. Stress was also laid on studying the psychosocial impact on the affected community. The Japanese government took a lot of care in ensuring that all the basic needs of the vulnerable population were met properly. In the aftermath of a disaster it is imperative that care of the vulnerable population is carried out immediately and with full attention. Despite the fact that the available resources and infrastructure were overwhelmed after the unprecedented earthquake, tsunami and other multiple disasters, the Japanese government took adequate measures to ensure that appropriate care of the people was taken.

International relief and rescue teams in Japan

Relief and help poured in from all the directions of the world. One hundred and sixty-three countries and regions and 43 international organizations offered assistance, while rescue teams from 27 countries, regions and international organizations helped in rescue and relief operations in one form or another.

India's NDRF team in Japan

Following the 11 March earthquake, the Indian government expressed its desire to offer immediate help to the people of Japan. As material assistance, India immediately sent 25,000 blankets, 13,000 bottles of mineral water and 10 metric tonnes of high-calorie biscuits. Since the affected areas at that time were reeling under extremely cold weather conditions, the items provided by India in a timely manner were of great help.

The Government of Japan subsequently requested from the Government India that the NDRF team be deployed for search, rescue and relief in the wake of the 2011 Tōhoku earthquake.

The Government of India immediately despatched a highly trained 46-member NDRF team to Japan on 28 March 2011 to provide disaster relief and rescue assistance (Fig. 29.3). The leader of the NDRF team was Mr Alok Avasthy, Commandant, and the team comprised four officers including a medical officer, six subordinate officers and 36 members of other ranks. Keeping in mind the already overwhelmed situation in Japan, the NDRF team was equipped with the latest state-of-the-art equipment and paraphernalia for radiation monitoring, detection and personal safety. The team sent was in direct operation mode and was self-reliant. They were also in possession of nuclear, biological and chemical (NBC) suits, emergency rations and basic essential medicines to handle any eventuality. They also carried dosimeters to constantly track radiation levels along with other equipment including cutters, life jackets and ration supplies to aid the mission. The team was in possession of advanced satellite phones for international calls and other communication equipment for the purpose of squad-to-squad communication during the period of deployment. In addition, the NDRF team also carried collapsed structure search and rescue (CSSR) equipment and relief materials such as portable shelters, tents, blankets, medicines, water bottles, etc. The NDRF team worked as per the instructions of the Japanese authorities and was supported by the Indian Embassy in Japan, which provided it with translators as well as logistics and fuel supplies. The team was allotted the city of Onagawa for its mission and began operating from its base at Rifu-cho. The team worked hard in sub-zero temperatures. During its mission to Onagawa in Japan, the NDRF team managed to extricate seven bodies and recover cash and valuables worth approximately ¥42 million, which was handed over to the Miyagi Police. The NDRF team was held in high esteem in Japan. The citizens of Onagawa lauded the effort of the Indian NDRF team. The team also won the hearts of Japanese officials and people, who expressed their heart-felt gratitude and appreciation for their dedication and effort through letters in Japanese, which were later translated into English. The local media too appreciated the dedication, commitment and sincerity of the NDRF team and expressed their thanks and gratitude for the work done by the NDRF in Japan. After the conclusion of the operation on 6 April 2011, the Indian team was felicitated by Japan's ex-Prime Minister Mr Mori and other members of the Ministry of External Affairs. The Mayors of Rifo and Onagawa held a meeting and especially thanked the NDRF team for their dedication during this operation.

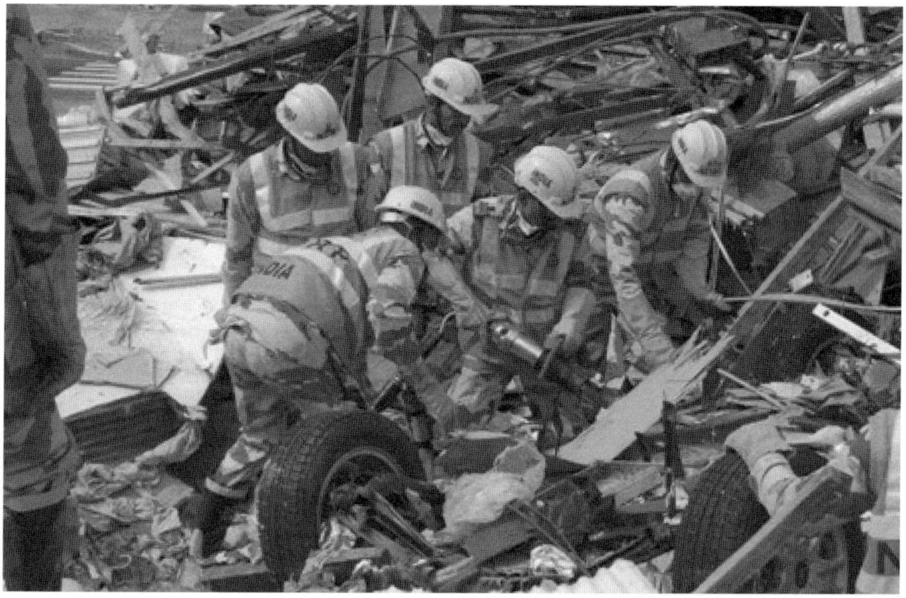

Fig. 29.3. The Indian rescue, relief and rehabilitation team at work in Japan in the aftermath of the massive 2011 tsunami, 28 March–8 April 2011 (source: National Disaster Management Authority, Government of India).

Conclusion

The 2011 Japan disaster has laid bare the gaps that exist in disaster management policies in several countries. There is an urgent need to learn the best practices followed by the Japanese so that the deleterious effects of disasters on humans and other life forms can be averted to the best possible extent. Japan's resilient disaster management systems helped save many lives despite the immense scale of the disaster. It is difficult to predict disaster; however, resilience has to be developed in the response system as well as in the community to cope with disasters. The Japanese nuclear plant authorities did not present a clear picture on the unfolding of the Fukushima crisis in the initial phases. There is a need to effectively and quickly communicate the status to the local, national and global community. In an information era, rapid communication of information helps build better trust and an effective response. In building resilience of national/international communities to disasters, there is an important role that human resources can play. Most developing countries and underdeveloped nations do not have efficient disaster management systems that include early warning systems and other strategies. There is an urgent need to augment human resources for handling disaster scenarios since most of the disaster management planning, relief and rescue operations, etc. are carried out by human resources only. An important lesson learnt from the Japanese experience is that even developed nations can at times be overwhelmed by disasters depending on the scale of the event. It is only through developing proper approaches and making the community resilient to disasters that the goal of a safe community can be achieved.

Acknowledgements

Preeti Arora sincerely thanks the National Women's Equality Center (NWEC), Saitama, Japan for the opportunity to participate in the 2011 Seminar for Gender Equality Officer and Women Leaders in the Asia Pacific Region 'Gender-Responsive Disaster Management' from 20–30 October 2011, which was organized in the aftermath of the Japan 2011 multiple disasters. This enabled us to observe the disaster management framework in Japan closely from a broad perspective. P.A. also visited the Japan Cabinet Office, Tokyo, the Ministry of Education, Sports, Culture, Science and Technology (MEXT) and the Japan and Disaster Reduction Institute, Kobe, where she interacted with a large number of disaster management experts. It also provided an opportunity to interact with people and experts directly or indirectly affected by the disaster. P.A.'s participation in the 2011 NWEC International Symposium: 'Disaster Reconstruction and Gender', held in Tokyo, Japan under the aegis of the Japan International Cooperation Agency (JICA) helped in learning from the Japanese experts and peers working in the area of disaster management. The financial support received from NWEC, Japan for attending the Symposium is duly acknowledged.

Preeti Arora would also like to express gratitude to Professor J.K. Garg, Director, Centre for Disaster Management Studies, Guru Gobind Singh Indraprastha University, New Delhi, and colleagues at the National Disaster Management Authority (NDMA), New Delhi, India and the National Institute of Disaster Management (NIDM), New Delhi, India for their suggestions.

Rajesh Arora would like to thank Dr Manas K. Mandal, Outstanding Scientist and Chief Controller Research and Development and Dr W. Selvamurthy, Distinguished Scientist and Former Chief Controller Research and Development (Life Sciences and International Cooperation), Defence Research and Development Organization, Government of India, New Delhi, for their wholehearted support and constant encouragement.

Disclaimer

The views expressed are entirely those of the authors and do not necessarily reflect the views of their respective organizations, universities, sponsoring or supporting agencies or the Government of India or any other government.

References

Arora, P. (2011) The 2011 Tōhoku earthquake and tsunami of Japan: lessons learnt and implications for effective disaster management. Dissertation submitted to the Center for Disaster Management Studies, Guru Gobind Singh Indraprastha University, Kashmere Gate, Delhi, p. 156.

Arora, P., Arora, R. and Bhardwaj, J.R. (2012) Psychosocial impact of 2011 Japan Tōhoku earthquake and ensuing multiple disasters. In: Bhardwaj, J.R. (ed.-in-chief) *Chemical (Industrial) Disaster Management (CIDM) 2012.* Federation of Indian Chambers of Commerce and Industry (FICCI), New Delhi, pp. 339–369.

BBC News (2011) Japan earthquake: Tsunami hits north-east. Available at: http://www.bbc.co.uk/news/world-asia-pacific-12709598 (Accessed 12 February 2013).

Cabinet Office, Government of Japan (2011a) Disaster Management Plan of Japan 2011. Cabinet Office, Tokyo.
Cabinet Office, Government of Japan (2011b) White Paper on Disaster Management 2011. Cabinet Office, Tokyo.
Cabinet Office, Government of Japan (2011c) Women and men in Japan. Cabinet Office, Tokyo.
Chandler, D.L. (2011) What we know, and don't know, about Japan's reactors. MIT News Office. Available at: http://web.mit.edu/newsoffice/2011/nuclear-panel-japan-0136.html (Accessed 13 February 2012).
Forbes, K. and Broadhead, J. (2007) The role of coastal forests in the mitigation of tsunami impacts. Food and Agriculture Organization of the United Nations, Regional Office for Asia and the Pacific, Bangkok, pp. 30.
Japanese National Police Agency (JNPA) (2012) Damage situation and police countermeasures associated with 2011 Tōhoku district – off the Pacific Ocean earthquake. Available at: http://www.npa.go.jp/archive/keibi/biki/higaijokyo_e.pdf (Accessed 13 February 2013).
Kyoto University (2011) Mega disaster in a resilient society, the Great East Japan (Tōhoku Kanto) earthquake and tsunami of 11th March 2011. Kyoto University, Kyoto, Japan.
ReliefWeb (n.d.) Latest updates from various reports. Available at: http://www.reliefweb.int/rw/rwb.nsf/doc106?OpenForm&rc=3&emid=EQ-2011-000028-JPN (Accessed 11 February 2013).
Sharma, R.K. and Arora, R. (2011) Fukushima, Japan: an apocalypse in the making? *Journal of Pharmacy and Bioallied Sciences* 3(2), 315–316.
Statistical Handbook of Japan (2012) http://www.stat.go.jp/english/data/handbook/c02cont.htm (Accessed 8 June 2013).

Chapter 30

Viewing Mass Casualties from a Hospital Window: Relevant Issues for the Developing World

Shabir Ahmed Dhar, Arshiya Hamid and Tahir Ahmed Dar

Introduction

Mass disasters affect a country at the social, economic and political levels. However, this impact is most immediate and profound on the healthcare system. Even as the world gets to grips with an increasing awareness of mass disaster requirements and challenges, the panacea for such situations is still a mirage. Healthcare providers are confronted with extensive and unique problems in the management of the sick and the injured. In spite of this, major problems in disaster management are reasonably predictable and include communications, authority, command structure, severity and organization (Eiseman, 2001). These problems have to be viewed against the background of inadequate resources to care for the victims in the usual manner (Alexander and Proctor, 1993).

In recent times a great deal of literature concerning mass disasters has been published enriching the vision of the healthcare providers (Langworthy *et al.*, 2004). However, this literature mainly concerns research from areas where healthcare facilities are well equipped and does not necessarily reflect difficulties faced by patients and workers in the developing world.

This chapter focuses on the emerging and established methods and concepts in mass disaster management and the difficulties in applying these to the healthcare dispensation in the developing world.

The Extent of the Challenge

Disasters inflict huge losses on populations in terms of death and disease. The risk of disasters is increasing, with a significant increase in the frequency of recorded disasters since the mid-1950s and over 2 billion people being affected since the mid-1990s (Chamberlain, 2006). Between 1900 and 2006 there were 15,833 reported natural and human-initiated disasters worldwide. One-third of these disasters occurred between 2000 and 2006. A range of causes has been espoused to explain this increase including global warming, population changes, urbanization, civil war and conflict, terrorism, improved technology and improved data collection. A total of 90% of these disasters occurred in countries with a per capita income of less than US$760 per annum. These countries have a limited capacity to plan and prepare and the frequency of disasters means that there is little time to recover (Greaves *et al*., 2009).

The Hospital Viewpoint

A disaster is defined as a sudden massive disproportion between hostile elements of any kind and the survival resources that are available to counterbalance these in the shortest possible time. A disaster at a very basic level produces patients requiring medical management (food poisoning, methyl alcohol poisoning and gas leaks), surgical management (blasts, riots, aviation disasters and earthquakes) or both (Supe and Satoskar, 2008).

The ultimate goal of any mass disaster response, whether to a man-made or a natural event is to obtain the best possible outcome for the greatest number of people. This is not easily applicable from the hospital viewpoint as no one can predict the time, location or complexity of the next mass casualty incident (MCI).

Without a standardized publicly accepted approach to disaster preparedness, physicians will find themselves faced with difficult decisions and in addition fear legal recriminations in the aftermath (Amundson, 2008).

The management process of the patients in an MCI starts as soon as the first information is received. It would make sense to discuss each stage of patient management in sequence. If hospitals are made safe from disasters, it is possible to greatly reduce risk and protect the healthcare facilities, resulting in the saving of lives.

First response

Natural disasters can leave previously functioning public health infrastructure fragmented or destroyed (Galson, 2009). The hospital response can be helped if the on-site management of the casualties is methodical and referral patterns are streamlined. Judgement of the pre-hospital healthcare provider has been found to be effective in accurately predicting triage needs as are many of the tools and scoring systems (Emerman *et al*., 1991).

For an effective response the ideal first response includes the management of the patients at the mass disaster site by Emergency Medical Assistance Teams (EMATs) (Chan *et al*., 2006). However, these teams may take 6–12 h to reach the site. This fact has to be viewed against the sobering truth that traumatic injuries, haemorrhagic shock, crush syndrome and chest and head injuries cannot be treated adequately if help does not arrive within 6 h of an MCI like an earthquake (Safar, 1986).

In addition, for an effective response the following are required:

- An effective Command Centre.
- An excellent communications network.
- Cooperation between the civil and the military establishments.

The transition from the first response teams to the first receivers produces unique challenges in communication, coordination and lines of authority when various agencies are required to coordinate activities with a common goal in a chaotic environment (O'Neill, 2005).

Some issues complicate management of the patients in a disaster:

- In the urban setting a number of patients are transported to the nearby hospitals regardless of the severity of the injury (Ko *et al.*, 2000). A number of these 'walking wounded' have minor injuries that do not require urgent care and they end up overburdening the hospitals.
- As emergency medical services are lacking in vast areas of the developing world, the minimally injured sometimes go 'hospital shopping'. In the World Trade Center attacks St Vincent hospital was swamped by 300 walking wounded within an hour, whereas physicians, nurses and ancillary professionals at St Luke's–Roosevelt hospital, a trauma centre just 3 miles away, sat idle (Simon and Teperman, 2001).
- Absence of emergency medical teams also prevents an orderly transit of patients to pertinent hospitals and a 'scoop and run' methodology is used by private parties and onlookers overburdening the nearby hospitals.

India provides us with a good example of the problems affecting disaster outreach in the developing world. The primary disaster response committee constitutes the Prime Minister, Finance Minister and the Deputy Chairman of the Planning Commission. The pre-hospital care system is nearly absent except in some major cities. Mumbai, which has been affected by repeated mass disaster situations over the past two decades, uses the fire brigade as the first responder. Initially the fire brigade used to transport patients only but recently training has been imparted to the personnel in basic life support and resuscitation protocol (Supe and Satoskar, 2008). In comparison an organized system to deliver medical care to the victims of the disasters developed much earlier in the west (Beary *et al.*, 1982).

The transit period from the disaster scene to the hospital is important in exchanging vital information with hospitals in the vicinity:

- The emergency medical officers in the nearby hospitals can prepare according to the number of patients headed to their hospitals.
- Telephonic triage can be conducted.
- Patients can be redirected to more appropriate locations based on the capabilities and the patient load of a particular hospital.

Pre-hospital management goes through various stages. These stages include rescue, decontamination, sorting and triage, transport and definitive care. At all stages the on-site triage officers and the emergency medical services (EMS) workers should remain in touch with the receiving hospitals.

Unfortunately no dedicated wireless frequency has been allotted exclusively for a disaster. This problem is compounded by the fact that an effective ambulance service is virtually absent.

Our experiences during the Kashmir earthquake of 2005 showed that the documents accompanying the referred patients can be more informative and succinct if line diagrams are used to define wounds and injuries (Dhar *et al.*, 2007). In situations where continuous communication is still a distant possibility, this technique could be useful.

Triage issues

Once patients start arriving at the hospitals and overwhelming the services, the focus shifts from providing care to the sickest to those critically injured patients who are more likely to survive. This is done by means of triage at the reception area of the hospital.

Devereaux *et al.* (2008b) raised certain questions about the problems associated with emergency mass critical care and triage.

- How should resources be allocated?
- Should those at highest risk of mortality receive attention?
- How does one determine prognosis?
- Who takes the final decision?
- What penalties can be levied?

Conventionally the triage officer sorts casualties into management groups (Ashkenazi *et al.*, 2006). The triage process is very exacting and demanding and hence the most experienced trauma physician will work as the triage officer. The triage officer should have exceptional clinical expertise, outstanding leadership qualities and effective communication skills (Baker, 2007).

Triage of multiple victims is difficult as physiological parameters need to be tested and time is scarce. Under such circumstances under-triage and over-triage are likely. This can be avoided by re-triage. This can be achieved by multiple point contacts as the patient travels through the hospital.

Our experience with mass disaster management in Kashmir has underlined a few things that need to be factored into what is a less than perfect scenario. These factors are perhaps experienced across the whole world to a lesser extent but are more pertinent to rural and developing areas (Furbee *et al.*, 2006):

- The public health departments are smaller with less system-wide capacity.
- The resources are limited and the technology is inferior.
- The experts required to conduct critical components of triage are scarce and usually concentrated in teaching hospitals in cities.
- There is an increased reliance on volunteers.

Under these circumstances there is an enormous potential for chaos, confusion and flawed decision making. It is also important to remember that the most widely used mass triage algorithms are not evidence-based. The development of a practical universal triage algorithm that incorporates requirements for decontamination or special precautions for infectious agents would facilitate a more highly organized mass casualty medical response (Jenkins *et al.*, 2008). However, it is important to view the triage process in the context of the system and its deficiencies (Devereaux *et al.*, 2008a). Triage also varies from rural to urban areas (Simon and Teperman, 2001).

Even though triage can be done on the basis of relatively newer scoring systems like the sequential organ failure system (SOFA), it may not be easily applicable in the reception area in a crowded hospital. Onlookers, journalists and police officers mill around the patients making an orderly assessment difficult. Normally triage allows grouping of patients into various categories based on colours. This grouping, even though desirable, results in the creation of several subgroups of patients.

- Red tag – Survival likely if intervention is done in minutes.
- Blue tag – Unlikely to survive and complicated care is needed.
- Yellow tag – Likely to survive if care is given within hours.
- Green tag – Minor injury that can be treated on an outpatient basis.
- Black tag – Treatment is required on an expectant basis.

However, it may be more expedient to use the algorithm used by the Israeli defence forces in situations where space and staff constraints are present.

According to this grouping patients are divided into three groups on the basis of their Injury Severity Score (ISS) (Ashkenazi *et al.*, 2006):

- Mild – Injury does not endanger life, ISS < 9.
- Moderate – Injury does not endanger life immediately, ISS 9–16.
- Severe – Injury endangers life immediately, ISS > 16.

On this basis the emergency department is divided into three distinct divisions. These patients are subsequently categorized as primary and secondary according to the Advanced Trauma Life Support (ATLS) protocol.

Surge capacity

Hospital surge capacity is defined as the ability to provide acute care to both critical and non-critical mass casualties simultaneously and is a marker of the ability to deliver emergency care in a disaster situation (Traub *et al.*, 2007). In essence it is the ability to manage a sudden, unexpected increase in patient volume that would otherwise severely challenge or exceed the current capacity of the healthcare system. Surge capacity in emergency care can be described in technical, scientific terms that are measured by numbers and benchmarks (e.g. beds, patients and medications) or can take on a more conceptual and abstract form (e.g. decisions, authority and responsibility). The former may be referred to as the ‘science’ of surge, whereas the latter, an equal if not more important component of surge systems that is more conceptual and abstract, can be considered the ‘art’ of surge (Tadmor *et al.*, 2006).

Most countries, including those with widely available critical care services, lack sufficient specialized staff, medical equipment and intensive care unit (ICU) space to provide timely, usual critical care for a large influx of additional patients (Rubinson *et al.*, 2008).

A hospital goes through three stages in its management of a large number of casualties:

1. Conventional care – The patient care is achieved without any change in daily practice.
2. Contingency care – The practice of patient care changes a little bit, but there is no impact on the care delivered or the outcomes achieved.

3. Crisis level – There are substantial changes in patient care and outcome may be affected. At this level there is change in caregiver operation, citizen expectation and legal environment.

The ability of a hospital to maintain a conventional and contingency level of patient care is severely constrained in less well-equipped hospitals. According to Tadmor *et al.* (2006), the healthcare system should be able to handle 100–600 patients/million population above the routine capacity. The Israeli healthcare system utilizes a more common and easily applicable measure to calculate surge requirement. Accordingly bed capacity must be augmented by 20% in the affected hospitals. However, this may be an over-simplification as beds are not the only requirement in a mass disaster.

Surge capacity is directly proportional to the time taken by the patients to reach from the disaster site to the hospital. If the disaster occurs very near to a healthcare facility the ability of the administration to increase capacity is seriously compromised. Simon and Teperman (2001) reported that it was possible to provide 20 beds of the intensive care type within 3 h of the World Trade Center attacks and this deployment increased to 100 critical and acute care beds in 4 h.

Critical to the concept of surge capacity is the fact that hospital managers should know about the variables affecting surge capacity. The hospital managers should know about ways and means of harnessing resources and developing surge capacity. Generally the bottlenecks to increased surge are the X-ray machines, operation theatre availability and the intensive care beds. These bottlenecks are greater in the developing world scenario (Fig. 30.1). The emergency department, the bed availability, the staff available and the number of surgeons on duty may all work as a resource ceiling.

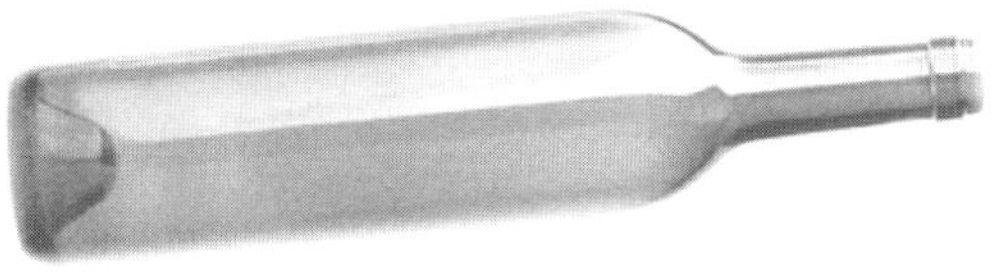

Fig. 30.1. Lack of coordination with other local and regional hospitals increases the number of bottlenecks. Bottlenecks in enhancing surge capacity during a mass disaster situation are greater in hospitals that have no disaster drills.

Surge capacity may be increased via several methods (see Fig. 30.2):

- Early discharge of patients.
- Establishment of a discharge holding area.
- Conversion of outpatient beds into indoor beds.
- Corridors and hallways for placement of beds.
- Partnerships should be developed with other hospitals.
- Non-healthcare areas can be used for holding patients, including stadiums and schools.
- Link the first responders to hospitals in the area.

A team that could initiate rapid discharge of stable patients, for example using the New York rapid discharge tool, would facilitate a more efficient process (Ntuli and Day, 2003–2004).

A proper scalable plan involving local, state, regional or federal healthcare and governmental institutions needs to be evolved for improved management of surge issues.

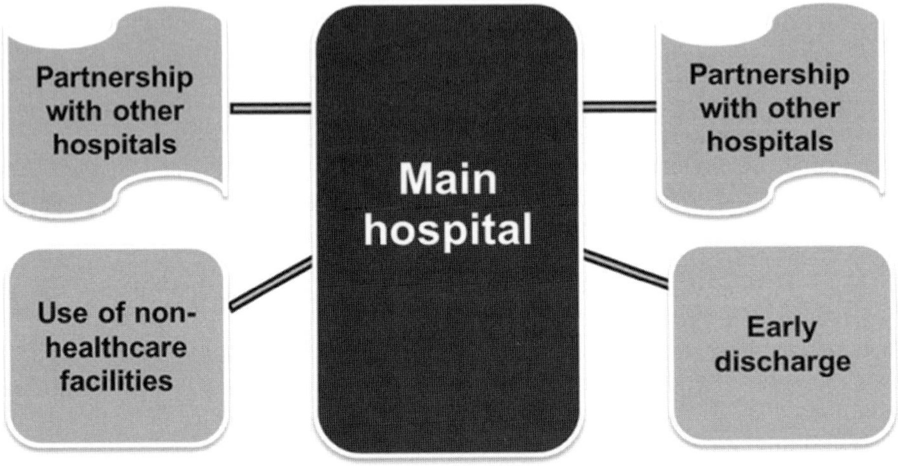

Fig. 30.2. Hospital surge can be enhanced by several methods that allow run-off and prevent overflow and disarray of the main receiving hospital.

Intensive care

Unlike the duration of surge demands on emergency departments, which can be measured in minutes to hours, the critical care response may need to be sustained for days to weeks. Mahoney *et al.* (2005) reported that the emergency department response lasted for hours and the intensive care response lasted for 21 days in the Rhode Island nightclub fire. Similarly in the London bombings of 2005, the emergency department surge lasted for 3 h and 14 min, whereas the intensive care response extended to 12.4 days (Aylwin *et al.*, 2005).

It is possible to increase ICU beds to the maximal extent by expanding ICU capacity and expanding ICUs into other areas (Sprung *et al.*, 2010). This can be done by converting the post-operative area into an intensive care area. In the developing world the availability of intensive care beds is always low. In mass disasters this aspect makes the intensive care area one of the bottlenecks in the management of patients.

Intensive care surge can be increased by several methods (Rubinson *et al.*, 2008).

- Substitution. Replacing a drug in short supply with another one, e.g. morphine with fentanyl.
- Adaptation. Using a less advanced method, e.g. anaesthesia machine for mechanical ventilation.
- Conservation. Changing utilization practices.
- Reuse. Sterilizing things that may in other circumstances be single-use items.

These methods can be used in resource-constrained settings.

Inter-hospital transfer

Inter-hospital and intra-hospital transfer are needed in a disaster situation because the care that the patient can receive elsewhere is better than that which can be received locally. It is important to remember that there is too little work for supraregional specialties such as neurosurgery to justify setting up a specialist service in each acute hospital.

A US Centers for Disease Control and Prevention analysis found that severely injured patients treated at level 1 trauma centres have a 25% lower risk of death than patients treated at a lower level or non-trauma centre. These figures suggest that the tendency to shift patients secondarily is justified when a level 1 trauma centre is within reach.

Another study found that for improved patient outcomes city hospitals or regional burn centres within a 60-mile radius can be designated as tiered burn disaster-receiving hospitals. These hospitals can be divided into a four-tier system based on clinical resources (Yurt *et al.*, 2008).

However, it is important to remember that transfer is basically undesirable and the good work done in the resuscitation room is undone during the journey (Andrews *et al.*, 1990; Gentleman *et al.*, 1993). Transfer gives rise to certain problems:

- Limited access to the patient;
- Difficulty in making clinical assessment;
- Limited drugs and equipment;
- Equipment failure.

In a mass disaster situation journeys can get delayed and escorts in the ambulances are often inexperienced. These situations can arise in an intra-hospital transfer also (Venkataraman, 1999). Transfer is of three basic types:

1. Primary transfer – Transfer of patients from scene of incident to the primary receiving hospital. Under ideal circumstances, this transfer is made by a fully equipped land ambulance, helicopter or fixed wing aircraft.
2. Secondary transfer – The movement of patients from the primary receiving hospital to a secondary admitting hospital. This is required for specialist care that is unavailable at the primary hospital. In disaster situations this may also be required once space constraints set in.
3. Tertiary transfer is done to allow a patient to be closer to friends and family and sometimes for insurance reasons.

All decisions to transfer require the sending and the receiving hospitals to be in agreement. In a mass disaster situation there are ramifications of transfer. Loss of an ambulance, staff member and a paramedic puts undue pressure on the hospital and the ambulance service.

Transfer due to overflow raises some ethical issues. Transferring a more stable patient to allow a less stable patient the use of an intensive care bed may not be in the best interest of the patient being shifted out but it is the expedient thing to do.

The escorting staff needs to be trained and they should have worked as a team. These prerequisites are not always satisfied in the developing world and the junior-most staff members often accompany the patients during inter-hospital transfer.

The personnel who accompany the patient are also at risk at times. During riots and civil disturbances, these professionals run the risk of being arrested, hurt or even killed. We have experienced the misunderstanding of ambulance insignias in Kashmir by paramilitary personnel as well as the crowds on the streets. This has often caused delays in transporting critically ill patients (Dhar *et al.*, 2011). A study that we conducted on ambulance drivers during mass disaster situations showed significant psychiatric morbidity (unpublished data).

Ambulances in the developing world tend to be used mainly as transport vehicles and are ill-equipped to manage patients during transport. Distances and roads worsen the condition of the patients during transport. Information is almost never passed to the receiving hospital and the hospital response on patient arrival is consequently slow.

Misconceptions

The mass casualty response is often associated with some misconceptions in the general population as well as in the healthcare professionals. These myths often stretch the hospital mass casualty response system further while creating false expectations and fears in the public.

The media sometimes can be blamed for inaccurate, incomplete and sensational coverage that may contribute to public misunderstanding (Drache *et al.*, 2003).

Some of the following problems were mentioned by de Ville de Goyet (2007) after evaluating the lessons learned in the mass disasters occurring in Asia including earthquakes and tsunamis.

1. Dependence on foreign mobile hospitals may be overstated as they rarely arrive on time.
2. Risk of epidemics is overstated.
3. Foreign aid often arrives in the form of inappropriate resources, which are costly and not necessarily useful to the services provided by the local hospitals.
4. Expatriate volunteers are not always helpful as language and cultural barriers are difficult to circumvent in MCIs.

Once a disaster unfolds, an outbreak of disaster mythology is likely to ensue (Alexander, 2007).

Material and resource management

The material management issues pertain to 'stuff, staff and space'. Current hospital reliance on 'just in time' and stockless material management systems to reduce storage and inventory costs leave institutions with vulnerably low reserves of key consumables and durable medical equipment (Moon, 2004).

Amongst the critical components required during mass disasters are ventilators, oxygen, ICUs, vascular access devices, intensive care beds, healthcare providers, transpost and vasopressors.

The answer perhaps lies in storing the more critical items under the supervision of a management system with control groups at the facility, local, regional and national levels to exercise authority. There should be a plan to access, coordinate and increase labour resources along with equipment, pharmaceuticals and supplies.

The US national disaster medical system is capable of providing 7000–8000 volunteers. It also can link together 2000 hospitals and 100,000 beds (Devereaux *et al.*, 2008b).

These figures are not clearly mentioned in disaster preparedness guidelines in India. It is important to prepare on a state and regional level with material management plans for mass disasters.

Optimal allocation of scarce resources in an MCI depends on the ability of public health authorities, government officials, institute leaders, healthcare professionals and the public to embrace the paradigm shift from individual- to population-based care (Joynt *et al.*, 2001).

There is a need to develop a solid healthcare wall against disasters – all these phases need to be focused on (Fig. 30.3).

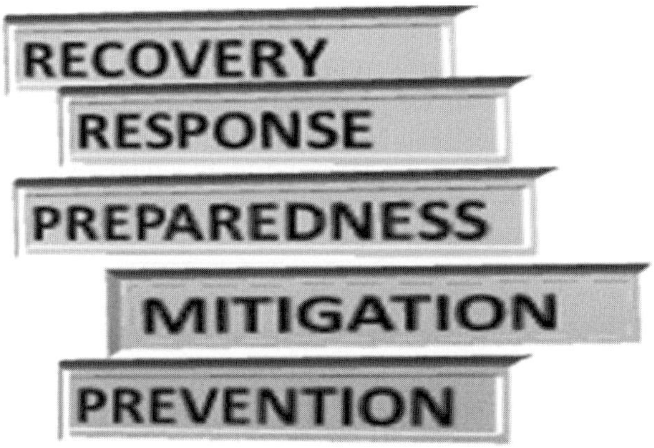

Fig. 30.3. Most of the focus during mass disasters is on hospital response, prevention and mitigation, and preparedness is often relegated to the background. The recovery phase is difficult to focus on from the hospital point of view as a persistent overload of healthcare facilities in the developing world allows very little time for introspection. To develop a solid healthcare wall against disasters all these phases need to be focused on.

Special needs groups

Paediatric and geriatric patients are at special risk in mass disasters. Apart from them, pregnant women as well as the psychologically affected need special attention.

Children are the most vulnerable but there are substantial deficiencies in the preparedness plans in the emergency services for the care of children in an MCI in the USA (Shirm *et al.*, 2007).

Magkos *et al.* (2004) reported that the elderly were at increased nutritional risk during a mass disaster. Pregnant women and their newborns are intimately linked special populations that require continued care despite the community circumstances (Pfeiffer *et al.*, 2008).

Lau *et al.* (2010) reported 22.3% post-traumatic stress disorder, 22.6% depression and 10.6% suicidal ideation in adolescents affected by the Sichuan earthquake. Belfer (2006) stressed the importance of effective mental health programmes for people affected by disaster. Psychologists can play active and important roles within interdisciplinary teams to build self-reliant and self-sustaining systems of care capacities within local communities and to coordinate these local integrated systems with external, humanitarian relief efforts when needed (Margolin *et al.*, 2010).

The health worker is often forgotten in the mass disaster situation. Psychiatric issues pertaining to the health worker include vicarious traumatization and compassion fatigue (Palm *et al.*, 2004). The healthcare worker should also be brought under the ambit of the psychiatric services.

Unexpected issues

Every mass disaster brings new challenges and unexpected issues that have not been reported before.

Health facilities are not immune to structural damage caused by the mass disaster. The 2004 Indian Ocean tsunami damaged 61% of health facilities and killed 7% of the health workers (Gomez *et al.*, 2011). In the aftermath of the Kashmir earthquake of 2005 the management of patients within the hospital building was extremely challenging in the presence of a number of significant aftershocks. In the absence of quakeproof buildings, the healthcare professionals ran the risk of life and limb to keep healthcare delivery going.

Healthcare is also affected by absenteeism during the mass disaster. This is mainly due to concern for themselves and often for their families. Sometimes the mass disaster itself creates a physical obstacle that prevents access of the healthcare worker to the healthcare facilities.

In the subcontinental context politicians need to visit the hospitals to avoid negative publicity. The security issues often cause significant difficulties in patient care and significant manpower is sometimes diverted towards these visits. During the 2005 earthquake we sequestered a small ward for the visit of the dignitaries avoiding major hassles in running the main hospital. An interesting fact that we noticed in the aftermath of these visits was that the patients in the main hospital building complained of being 'left out'. (Dhar *et al.*, 2008, 2009).

In the subcontinent, the attendants of the patient serve very important functions of nursing care during normal times. Mass disasters often separate or wipe out family members. This creates an unusual situation where the critically injured patients are admitted to hospitals without any attendants affecting their day-to-day care significantly. Volunteers can be assigned this function as the hospital staff is already stretched to the limit.

The greater the lead-up time to the reception of the casualties, the higher is the surge capacity (Fig. 30.4). It is not possible to streamline referral from the incident site and the nearest hospitals are affected the most in terms of patient load. Often this can unexpectedly lead to problems. Careful planning can help avert this sort of problem (Dhar *et al.,* 2009).

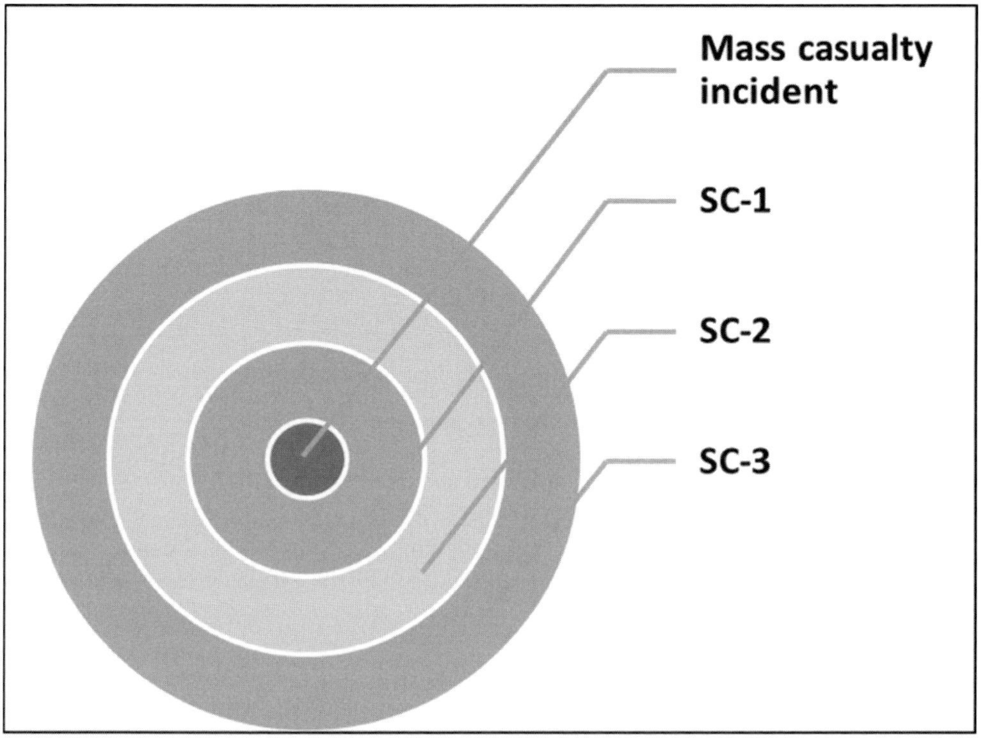

Fig. 30.4. The greater the lead-up time to the reception of the casualties, the higher is the surge capacity. It is not possible to streamline referral from the incident site and the nearest hospitals are affected the most in terms of patient load.

Disaster medicine education

As the science of disaster management is developing, it is important to start preparing students for possible mass disaster management in the future. It is important to incorporate disaster medicine chapters into the curriculum.

Disaster medicine education is an enormous challenge, but indispensable for disaster preparedness (Pfenninger *et al.*, 2010).

In a study of anaesthesia residency programmes it was found that only 37% of residency programmes had any kind of training for mass disaster management. This is against the backdrop of the fact that it is the anaesthesiologists who provide the critical link in care (Candiotti *et al.*, 2005).

India also does not have a defined mass disaster education curriculum for its medical students.

Media

The mass disaster in modern times is inextricably interwoven with media imagery and consequent public judgement.

Journalists and public health officials differ in their perspectives on news relevance in a mass disaster (Anzur, 2000; Shoaf and Rottman, 2000). According to Lowrey *et al.* (2007), journalists are unprepared to cover terrorism and many types of mass disasters in part because of lack of sufficient expertise in science and medicine.

The media indulges in agenda setting with deliberate coverage of topics or events with the goal of influencing public opinion and policy (Barnes *et al.*, 2008). The difference was emphasized by the fact that the reporter is drawn to the danger and drama while health professionals emphasize prevention, reassurance and recovery.

Hospitals in the developing world are not inherently prepared to handle the hungry media and their insatiable desire for information. In such situations it is important for the administration to appoint a public information officer who can keep the media up to date with the facts and figures during a mass disaster.

In such situations, the medical practitioners should be available with core messages, consistent messages and they should be ready to admit that they do not know everything. It is worthwhile to avoid technical language and show sensitivity towards hot buttons (Tinker *et al.*, 2001). Public health practitioners should seek media relationships before, during and after a crisis (Ball-Rokeach and Loges, 2000). However, it must be reiterated that reliable and responsible news coverage should be seen as an integral part of preparedness. Maningas *et al.* (1997) reported that local media can be used effectively to request coordination of volunteer convergence.

Rehabilitation

Rehabilitation is required to minimize complications and restore the physical, emotional, social and intellectual function of the patients affected by disasters. The needs of the patients may range from physical, psychological, functional and social to financial. Many of these will require multidisciplinary management. The rehabilitation team will constitute medical and nursing staff, psychologists, occupational therapists, physiotherapists, speech and language therapists and social workers.

All this produces additional workload for the hospitals especially in dynamic mass disasters.

An important issue in patient management is that while the injured are shifted to the hospitals, their families might be displaced or evacuated. This creates additional problems while rehabilitating the patients. Preparedness plans for mass disasters involving forced mass evacuation and resettlement should place a high priority on keeping families together, even entire neighbourhoods (Jacob *et al.*, 2008).

Interdisaster period

The best time to prepare hospitals for mass disasters is during the interdisaster periods. The average trauma surgeon will not have to deal with a true MCI during his or her career. Healthcare systems are strained on a daily basis and disaster planning is relegated below more urgent needs (Welzel *et al.*, 2010). In this context it is important that focused disaster drills be held by all hospitals to get to know their own capabilities and lacunae. Coordination with the first responders and the regional hospitals has to be developed for these contingencies.

While tiding over a disaster a good community response is confused with a fully functional statewide or regional trauma system and consequently there is a failure to plan for the future.

Conclusion

No one can predict the time, location and complexity of the next MCI. Mass disasters occur sporadically and it is important to learn from the experiences and the mistakes of the others. Those who cannot learn from history are doomed to repeat it (Santayana, 1906).

A modular incident control system needs to be developed alongside a good hospital emergency incident command system. The model of the developed countries can serve as a good starting point, but there are unique issues that exist in the developed world. These exceptional circumstances require open-minded flexibility, a tailored approach and close cooperation between surgeons, anaesthetists and other healthcare professionals to share experiences, opinions and ideas.

It is important to remember that good intentions do not always guarantee a good outcome.

Acknowledgements

The authors are grateful to Zain ul Abidin Adhami (Ilinois, USA) for useful inputs during the compilation of this chapter.

References

Alexander, D.E. (2007) Misconception as a barrier to teaching about disasters. *Prehospital Disaster Medicine* 22(2), 95–103.

Alexander, R.H. and Proctor, H.J. (eds) (1993) *ATLS Student Manual*, 5th edition. American College of Surgeons, Chicago, Illinois.

Amundson, D. (2008) Can there be a consensus on critical care in disasters? *Chest* 133(5), 1065–1066.

Andrews, P.J., Piper, I.R., Dearden, N.M. and Miller, J.D. (1990) Secondary insults during intrahospital transport of head-injured patients. *Lancet* 335(8685), 327–330.

Anzur, T. (2000) How to talk to the media: televised coverage of public health issues in a disaster. *Prehospital Disaster Medicine* 15(4), 196–198.

Ashkenazi, I., Kessel, B., Khashan, T., Haspel, J., Oren, M., Olsha, O. and Alfici, R. (2006) Precision of in-hospital triage in mass-casualty incidents after terror attacks. *Prehospital Disaster Medicine* 21(1), 20–23.

Aylwin, C.J., König, T.C., Brennan, N.W., Shirley, P.J., Davies, G., Walsh, M.S. and Brohi, K. (2005) Reduction in critical mortality in urban mass casualty incidents: analysis of triage, surge, and resource use after the London bombings on July 7, 2005. *Lancet* 368(9554), 2219–2225.

Baker, M.S. (2007) Creating order from chaos: part II: tactical planning for mass casualty and disaster response at definitive care facilities. *Military Medicine* 172(3), 237–243.

Ball-Rokeach, S.J. and Loges, W.E. (2000) Ally or adversary? Using media systems for public health. *Prehospital Disaster Medicine* 15(4), 188–195.

Barnes, M.D., Hanson, C.L., Novilla, L.M., Meacham, A.T., McIntyre, E. and Erickson, B.C. (2008) Analysis of media agenda setting during and after Hurricane Katrina: implications for emergency preparedness, disaster response, and disaster policy. *American Journal of Public Health* 98(4), 604–610.

Beary, J.F. 3rd, Bisgard, J.C. and Armstrong, P.C. (1982) The civilian-military contingency hospital system. *New England Journal of Medicine* 306(12), 738–740.

Belfer, M.L. (2006) Caring for children and adolescents in the aftermath of natural disasters. *International Review of Psychiatry* 18(6), 523–528.

Candiotti, K.A., Kamat, A., Barach, P., Nhuch, F., Lubarsky, D. and Birnbach, D.J. (2005) Emergency preparedness for biological and chemical incidents: a survey of anesthesiology residency programs in the United States. *Anesthesia and Analgesia* 101(4), 1135–1140.

Chamberlain, C. (ed.) (2006) Western Australian department of health disaster preparedness and management: health protection group. *Disaster Medical Assistance Teams: A Literature Review.* Perth, Australia.

Chan, Y.F., Alagappan, K., Gandhi, A., Donovan, C., Tewari, M. and Zaets, S.B. (2006) Disaster management following the Chi-Chi earthquake in Taiwan. *Prehospital Disaster Medicine* 21(3), 196–202.

de Ville de Goyet, C. (2007) Health lessons learned from the recent earthquakes and tsunami in Asia. *Prehospital Disaster Medicine* 22(1), 15–21.

Devereaux, A.V., Christian, M.D., Dichter, J.R., Geiling, J.A. and Rubinson, L.; Task Force for Mass Critical Care (2008a) Summary of suggestions from the Task Force for Mass Critical Care summit, January 26–27, 2007. *Chest* 133(5 Suppl), 1S–7S.

Devereaux, A.V., Dichter, J.R., Christian, M.D., Dubler, N.N., Sandrock, C.E., Hick, J.L., Powell, T., Geiling, J.A., Amundson, D.E., Baudendistel, T.E., Braner, D.A., Klein, M.A., Berkowitz, K.A., Curtis, J.R. and Rubinson, L. (2008b) Definitive care for the critically ill during a disaster: a framework for allocation of scarce resources in mass critical care: from a Task Force for Mass Critical Care summit meeting, January 26–27, 2007, Chicago, IL. *Chest* 133(5 Suppl), 51S–66S.

Dhar, S.A., Halwai, M.A., Mir, M.R., Wani, Z.A., Butt, M.F., Bhat, M.I. and Hamid, A. (2007) The Kashmir earthquake experience. *The European Journal of Trauma and Emergency Surgery* 33(1), 74–80.

Dhar, S.A., Hamid, A., Khan, S.M. and Butt, M.F. (2008) Unforeseen difficulties faced by a hospital in dealing with mass disaster victims. *Tropical Doctor* 38(4), 260.

Dhar, S.A., Mir, M.R., Halwai, M.A., Butt, M.F., Ali, M.F. and Kawoosa, A.A. (2009) Differentiating mass disasters. The barzullah classification. *Ortopedia Traumatological Rehabilitacja*,11(1), 55–60.

Dhar, S.A., Dar, T.A., Wani, Z.A. and Ali, M.F. (2011) Ambulance insignias in a turmoil zone. *Prehospital Disaster Medicine* 26(2), 139.

Drache, D., Feldman, S. and Clifton, D. (2003) Media coverage of the 2003 Toronto SARS outbreak. Roberts Centre for Canadian studies, York University, Toronto, Canada.

Eiseman, B. (2001) Combat casualty management for tomorrows battlefield. Urban terrorism. *Journal of Trauma* 51, 821–823.

Emerman, C.L., Shaele, B. and Kubincanek, J. (1991) A comparison of EMT judgment and prehospital triage instruments. *Journal of Trauma* 31, 1369–1375.

Furbee, P.M., Coben, J.H., Smyth, S.K., Manley, W.G., Summers, D.E., Sanddal, N.D., Sanddal, T.L., Helmkamp, J.C., Kimble, R.L., Althouse, R.C. and Kocsis, A.T. (2006) Realities of rural emergency medical services disaster preparedness. *Prehospital Disaster Medicine* 21, 64–70.

Galson, S.K. (2009) USPHS commissioned corps. A global emergency preparedness and response asset. *Public Health Report* 124(5), 622–623.

Gentleman, D., Dearden, M., Midgley, S. and Maclean, D. (1993) Guidelines for resuscitation and transfer of patients with serious head injury. *British Medical Journal* 307(6903), 547–552.
Gomez, D., Haas, B., Ahmed, N., Tien, H. and Nathens, A. (2011) Disaster preparedness of Canadian trauma centres: the perspective of medical directors of trauma. *Canadian Journal of Surgery* 54(1), 9–16.
Greaves, I., Porter, K. and Garner, J. (eds) (2009) *Trauma Care Manual*, 2nd edition. Hodder Arnold, London, p. 8.
Jacob, B., Mawson, A.R., Payton, M. and Guignard, J.C. (2008) Disaster mythology and fact: Hurricane Katrina and social attachment. *Public Health Reports* 123(5), 555–566.
Jenkins, J.L., McCarthy, M.L., Sauer, L.M., Green, G.B., Stuart, S., Thomas, T.L. and Hsu, E.B. (2008) Mass-casualty triage: time for an evidence-based approach. *Prehospital Disaster Medicine* 23(1), 3–8.
Joynt, G.M., Gomersall, C.D., Tan, P., Lee, A., Cheng, C.A. and Wong, E.L. (2001) Prospective evaluation of patients refused admission to an intensive care unit: triage, futility and outcome. *Intensive Care Medicine* 27(9), 1459–1465.
Ko, P.C., Ma, M.H., Shih, F.Y. and Lin, F.Y. (2000) Urban prehospital emergency medical transportation in Taipei following the Taiwan earthquake. *Prehospital Disaster Medicine* 15(3), 545.
Langworthy, M.J., Sabra, J. and Gould, M. (2004) Terrorism and blast phenomena. Lessons learned from the attack on USS Cole (DDG 67). *Clinical Orthopaedics and Related Research* 422, 82–87.
Lau, J.T., Yu, X., Zhang, J., Mak, W.W., Choi, K.C., Lui, W.W., Zhang, J. and Chan, E.Y. (2010) Psychological distress among adolescents in Chengdu, Sichuan at 1 month after the 2008 Sichuan earthquake. *Journal Urban Health* 87(3), 504–523.
Lowrey, W., Evans, W., Gower, K.K., Robinson, J.A., Ginter, P.M., McCormick, L.C. and Abdolrasulnia, M. (2007) Effective media communication of disasters: pressing problems and recommendations. *BMC Public Health* 7, 97.
Magkos, F., Arvaniti, F., Piperkou, I., Katsigaraki, S., Stamatelopoulos, K., Sitara, M. and Zampelas, A. (2004) Identifying nutritionally vulnerable groups in case of emergencies: experience from the Athens 1999 earthquake. *International Journal of Food Sciences and Nutrition* 55(7), 527–536.
Mahoney, E.J., Harrington, D.T., Biffl, W.L., Metzger, J., Oka, T. and Cioffi, W.G. (2005) Lessons learned from a nightclub fire: institutional disaster preparedness. *Journal of Trauma* 58(3), 487–491.
Maningas, P.A., Robison, M. and Mallonee, S. (1997) The EMS response to the Oklahoma City bombing. *Prehospital Disaster Medicine* 12(2), 80–5.
Margolin, G., Ramos, M.C. and Guran, E.L. (2010) Earthquakes and children: the role of psychologists with families and communities. *Professional Psychology Research and Practice* 41(1), 1–9.
Moon, S. (2004) Taking cost off supply shelf. Healthcare turning to supply chain management techniques honed by retail, manufacturing to limit inventory, slash expenses. *Modern Healthcare* 34(47), 26–28.
Ntuli, A. and Day, C. (2003–2004) Health systems trust 2005. Ten years on – Have we got what we ordered? *South African Health Review* 3–7.
O'Neill, P.A. (2005) The ABCs of disaster response. *Scandinavian Journal of Surgery* 94, 259–266.
Palm, K.M., Polusny, M.A. and Follette, V.M. (2004) Vicarious traumatization: potential hazards and interventions for disaster and trauma workers. *Prehospital Disaster Medicine* 19, 73–78.
Pfeiffer, J., Avery, M.D., Benbenek, M., Prepas, R., Summers, L., Wachdorf, C.M. and O'Boyle, C. (2008) Maternal and newborn care during disasters: thinking outside the hospital paradigm. *The Nursing Clinics of North America* 43(3), 449–467.
Pfenninger, E.G., Domres, B.D., Stahl, W., Bauer, A., Houser, C.M. and Himmelseher, S. (2010) Medical student disaster medicine education: the development of an educational resource. *International Journal Emergency Medicine* 3(1), 9–20.

Rubinson, L., Hick, J.L., Hanfling, D.G., Devereaux, A.V., Dichter, J.R., Christian, M.D., Talmor, D., Medina, J., Curtis, J.R. and Geiling, J.A. (2008) Task Force for Mass Critical Care. Definitive care for the critically ill during a disaster: a framework for optimizing critical care surge capacity: from a Task Force for Mass Critical Care summit meeting, January 26–27, 2007, Chicago, IL. *Chest* 133(5 Suppl), 18S–31S.

Safar, P. (1986) Resuscitation potentials in mass disasters. *Pre-hospital Disaster Medicine* 2, 34–47.

Santayana, G. (1906) *The Life of Reason*. Charles Scribner and Sons, New York.

Shirm, S., Liggin, R., Dick, R. and Graham, J. (2007) Prehospital preparedness for pediatric mass-casualty events. *Pediatrics* 120(4), e756–e761.

Shoaf, K.I. and Rottman, S.J. (2000) The role of public health in disaster preparedness, mitigation, response, and recovery. *Prehospital Disaster Medicine* 15(4), 144–146.

Simon, R. and Teperman, S. (2001) The World Trade Center attack. Lessons for disaster management. *Critical Care* 5(6), 318–320.

Sprung, C.L., Zimmerman, J.L., Christian, M.D., Joynt, G.M., Hick, J.L., Taylor, B., Richards, G.A., Sandrock, C., Cohen, R. and Adini, B.; European Society of Intensive Care Medicine Task Force for Intensive Care Unit Triage during an Influenza Epidemic or Mass Disaster (2010) Recommendations for intensive care unit and hospital preparations for an influenza epidemic or mass disaster: summary report of the European Society of Intensive Care Medicine's Task Force for intensive care unit triage during an influenza epidemic or mass disaster. *Intensive Care Medicine* 36(3), 428–443.

Supe, A. and Satoskar, R. (2008) Health service responses to disasters in Mumbai. Sharing experiences. *Indian Journal of Medical Science* 62(6), 242–251.

Tadmor, B., McManus, J. and Koenig, K.L. (2006) The art and science of surge: experience from Israel and the U.S. military. *Academic Emergency Medicine* 13(11), 1130–1134.

Tinker, T.L., Zook, E. and Chapel, T.J. (2001) Key challenges and concepts in health risk communication: perspectives of agency practitioners. *Journal of Public Health Management and Practice* 7(1), 67–75.

Traub, M., Bradt, D.A. and Joseph, A.P. (2007) The Surge Capacity for People in Emergencies (SCOPE) study in Australasian hospitals. *Medical Journal of Australia* 186(8), 394–398.

Venkataraman, S.T. (1999) Intrahospital transfer of critically ill children – should we pay attention? *Critical Care Medicine* 27, 694–695.

Welzel, T.B., Koenig, K.L., Bey, T. and Visser, E. (2010) Effect of hospital staff surge capacity on preparedness for a conventional mass casualty event. *The Western Journal of Emergency Medicine* 11(2), 189–196.

World Health Organization (WHO) (2008–2009) Hospitals safe from disasters. Reduce risk, protect health facilities, save lives. World disaster reduction campaign. WHO, Geneva.

Yurt, R.W., Lazar, E.J., Leahy, N.E., Cagliuso, N.V. Sr, Rabbitts, A.C., Akkapeddi, V., Cooper, A., Dajer, A., Delaney, J., Mineo, F.P., Silber, S.H., Soloff, L., Magbitang, K. and Mozingo, D.W. (2008) Burn disaster response planning: an urban region's approach. *Journal of Burn Care Research* 29(1), 158–165.

Section 10

Post-disaster Relief, Rehabilitation and Recovery

Chapter 31

The Immediate Post-disaster Reconstruction Phase: Alternate Care Site Settings and Vulnerable Populations

James C. Hagen and Scott P. Hagen

Introduction

All nations of the world have experienced disasters of one type of another throughout recorded history. They are tragic tales of populations being caught unprepared or unaware of impending catastrophe. In that respect, little has changed throughout the ages. With all of our records of historic patterns, weather predictions, more advanced knowledge of the geology of the earth and seismic instruments, natural catastrophes still occur with little or no warning. In fact, it is somewhat disturbing that these events are becoming more frequent and more severe when they do occur.

Natural and man-made disasters affect increasing numbers of people around the world (Kahn, 2005). The recent trend has been for more frequent and more severe global disasters (Freeman *et al.*, 2003; Block, 2008). Concomitantly, the cost of these national disasters has risen enormously (Independent Evaluation Group, 2010). The majority of deaths have occurred in nations who were the poorest (Kahn, 2005; Bandyk, 2010). In his study examining data from 73 nations, Kahn (2005) concluded that natural disasters hit wealthy and poor nations alike, although richer nations suffer less death. Logic follows that the wealthier nations have the means to prepare, mitigate and evacuate if necessary, while the poor live in extremely vulnerable locations and conditions, and have no ability to mitigate against future events. The presence of stronger institutions in the area of the disaster can lead to lower death counts. Not surprisingly, larger countries with higher risk environments have suffered more deaths from their disasters.

Historically, a great deal of money has been spent on mitigation and preparedness activities, while until recently little attention in the USA was spent in the area of post-disaster recovery. That might be, in part, because the USA is a relatively young nation, and has had the advantages of wealth and privilege. It was not until a disaster the size of Katrina hit America that issues concerning lack of coordination, the relationship of disaster and discrimination, and lack of understanding of reconstruction and recovery became abundantly clear. In the USA, the majority of disasters have resulted in the deaths of less than 100 people, many with death tolls less than ten. Our greatest death tolls have come from hurricanes and the San Francisco earthquake of 1900, although the actual numbers of dead are difficult to determine with accuracy in earlier disasters. Hurricane Katrina, although a true disaster from many perspectives including recovery efforts, has been the most costly, costing an estimated US$84 billion thus far.

It is most interesting that efforts to mitigate damage and loss of life in disaster may in fact have provided a false sense of security to residents who feel safe in building behind levees and dams, or on flood plains and major fault lines (Mileti, 1999).

One of the most complete global studies on natural disaster mitigation ever performed was led by the Chinese Academy of Sciences, and carried out by an international panel of experts (InterAcademy Panel on International Issues, 2009). One of the three main disasters addressed was earthquakes, and the document provides a complete description of the causes of earthquakes and their effects. Annex 4 specifically addressed the Wenchuan earthquake and details an intense scientific study of mitigation and actions that need to be taken for a geological disaster. Mitigation is one aspect of disaster reconstruction, and the document provides important information as recovery and reconstruction plans are created.

It is necessary that we extend our measurement of disaster effects beyond easily quantifiable aspects: number of dead and injured, people displaced, homes and businesses destroyed, cost, loss of income and other discrete measures. Increased attention must be paid to aspects of disaster that are far more difficult to understand and measure. This is what Ismet Fanany (2010) called a reconstruction of the 'invisible landscape'. He said that the 'wreckage of the physical aspects of people's lives lay all around where their homes and villages once stood, but the wreckage of the psyche of the Achenese lay inside each person, where it was not easily accessible and where it could not be perceived by the eye alone'. Concerning the Achenese following the Indian Ocean tsunami, he suggests that internal reconstruction lags behind the physical, and that rebuilding the internal environment of the survivors may be beyond the ability of the aid workers. Perhaps more likely than creating a new reality is the integration and reconciliation of what came before and the new reality – a new normal, rather than a return to what existed prior to the disaster. We need to have a better understanding of those invisible factors to foster creation of the new normal.

Another important aspect to consider when rebuilding a 'community' is the psychological vulnerability of some of its residents. Whether these individuals suffer from depression or one of many anxiety or psychosis-related disorders, a disaster within their community has a high probability of exascerbating their symptoms and placing them in a state where they struggle with any form of recovery (Kessler *et al.*, 2008). Within this category of vulnerable populations are individuals with diagnosed psychological conditions that may affect their cognitive functioning, their ability to cope with a disaster or process the recovery process. In addition, it should be noted that there may also be other individuals within a community who have an undiagnosed pre-existing psychological condition that may be brought to attention as a result of disaster. Then, there are also others who may develop symptoms of a psychological disorder, such as post-traumatic stress disorder, as a result of the disaster. Recovery teams and relief efforts need to be aware of the impact of psychological factors in the rebuilding process and must address them as vital components to the community's recovery needs (Benight, 2004). In order to accomplish this, recovery teams should collaborate their efforts with psychologists, social workers and other mental health professionals. Without addressing psychological factors as a part of the community rebuilding process, members within these vulnerable populations may feel disconnected or permanently estranged from their surroundings and inhibited, or even prevented, from regaining a sense of community.

What is Reconstruction?

Each nation or discipline within countries uses the term reconstruction differently. In order to build upon a foundation or understanding and identify lessons learned from activities following disaster, it is first important to have a common understanding of what disaster reconstruction means.

Reconstruction is not just about rebuilding of structures and physical aspects of a culture, but rather rebuilding a multilayered society in all of its complexities. This includes a consideration of historical, cultural, religious, socio-political and interpersonal relationships, as well as international interactions that take place (World Bank, 2008a,b).

There were eight core principles identified for recommendations (Federal Emergency Management Agency, 2010):

1. Individual and family empowerment;
2. Leadership and local primacy;
3. Partnership for recovery;
4. Partnerships and inclusiveness;
5. Communications;
6. Unity of effort;
7. Timeliness and flexibility;
8. Resilience and sustainability.

All sectors need to participate in the recovery process with clarity of purpose and goal. It is understood that far beyond the parameters of rebuilding physical structures and infrastructure, there is a need to reconstruct the social, natural and economic frameworks as well. These parameters are:

- Leadership with clarity of roles and responsibilities on a local, state/province and federal level;
- Coordination of recovery assistance, whether that be on a national and/or international level;
- Promotion of local economic recovery;
- Successful transition from international aid and assistance to reconstruction and recovery;
- Role of public–private partnerships;
- Role of community organizations, faith-based involvement and societal factors in healing;
- Importance of mitigation, resilience and sustainability in recovery activities;
- Difficulty of transitioning from recovery to recovered.

The disaster cycle is a continuum of overlapping activities, including aspects of preparedness, planning, response, recovery and mitigation. There is no absolute time frame associated with the shift from response to recovery. In fact, Mileti (1999) has noted that populations and governments are in so much of a hurry to get back to what was considered normal that they lose the opportunity for community improvement and increasing resiliency. There is focus only on responding and not on long-term planning.

An early document focusing on activities following disaster was published by Hass *et al.* (1977). They identified four post-disaster phases:

- *Phase 1* – Emergency recovery, occurring hours or days after the event, when coping with loss of lives, property, and dealing with injuries.
- *Phase 2* – Restoration, a time when urban services such as transportation are being returned, and when evacuees begin to return.
- *Phase 3* – Replacement and restoration, when things begin to return to pre-disaster levels and a semblance of 'normalcy' returns.
- *Phase 4* – Commemorative, betterment and development, when people begin to look forward again and development occurs.

The World Bank has been involved in disaster recovery and reconstruction for over 25 years. Approximately 10% of its commitments have been for natural disaster assistance. The World Bank (2008a) also provides a similar framework but divided into:

- *Phase 1* – Disaster response;
- *Phase 2* – Disaster relief (Hass phases 1–3);
- *Phase 3* – Damage and loss assessment (Hass phase 1);
- *Phase 4* – Recovery and reconstruction (Hass phases 2–4);
- *Phase 5* – Risk reduction (Hass phases 2–4);
- *Phase 6* – Development (Hass phase 4).

Clarke *et al.* (2010) define three overlapping stages of reconstruction. First, it can be the immediate relief to ensure saving lives; second, it can mean the later and longer term restoration and recovery to what has been termed 'normalcy'; third is the even longer concept of not only rebuilding, but renewing. It is encouraging that current thought is that this last stage should not necessarily be to return to pre-disaster levels, but should be in improvement. If the pre-disaster situation was sufficient and a healthy community existed prior to the event, returning to that level might be sufficient. However, if as we saw in Haiti, the situation was socioeconomic failure, abject poverty, unrest and poor construction, it is not sufficient.

Consistent in all models is that phases, steps or stages are not distinct time periods. There is always overlap and a great variation in time frames. For the purposes of this chapter, we will use the terminology of the four-phase model of Hass *et al.* (1977). Rather than examining longer-term disaster recovery, this work concerns what must be done immediately following disaster to save lives, to provide shelter and care to the vulnerable, and to prepare survivors to rebuild community.

Lessons from Indigenous Cultures

There is much work to be done in the reconstruction phase of disasters, not just within sectors, but between nations and cultures. What is most often neglected and forgotten is that there are cultures within all of our borders that have been struck by, and survived, natural disasters innumerable times in the past. So-called modern management must merge the new with the old to take advantage of lessons embedded with the collective wisdom of the population, especially concerning resilience and sustainability.

As management science has grown to understand that disaster management is a new and specialized field of study, the importance of including all organizations and subcultures has been realized. There is a growing sense of urgency as to the vital need to provide for those subpopulations that might be vulnerable during disaster. One of the most neglected subpopulations thought to be vulnerable is that of indigenous (autochthonous) peoples. Within these groups, it is common to find marginalization, poverty, lack of services and heightened medical/psychological issues. However, there has been a growing realization and intense scrutiny of the special insight that these populations have into how communities can best prepare for recovery and reconstruction following natural disasters. We have learned through many painful experiences that all disasters are local and we must initially, as individuals and communities, be able to handle the disaster on our own. There is a great deal to learn from those who have a history of survival in adverse conditions (Zoujing, 2009). However, Grenier (1998) has warned that because of cultural homogenization and increased modernization, indigenous knowledge was threatened with extinction.

Western scientists have begun to recognize the importance of understanding and valuing indigenous native knowledge systems (Baumwoll, 2008). It is not surprising that it was originally thought that others needed to impose modern western methodologies on how they handled disasters. Barnhardt and Kawagley (2005) maintain that through external relationships, the 16 distinct indigenous cultures of Alaska have had their knowledge systems marginalized and their cultural integrity eroded. However, these knowledge systems have not disappeared. There have been several initiatives in recent years by the USA to examine and integrate indigenous knowledge. The American Association for the Advancement of Science (Lambert, 2003) invited 20 Native American scientists to their 2003 Annual Conference. Presentations focused on how to prepare Native Americans for the future while treasuring the wisdom of the past. Hagen (2008) examined the structure of the emergency management system in the Alaska indigenous peoples and found that special attention needed to be paid to the unique situation of the Native elderly in the family structure during times of disaster. There was great value in respect for indigenous knowledge and cultural belief systems. In 2000, Stephens developed a visual representation to assist in understanding the overlap between traditional native knowledge and western science. In that common ground are found four general areas: organizing principles, habits of mind, skills and procedures, and knowledge. Study of these areas and their application to existing indigenous populations and indigenous knowledge systems can be invaluable in better preparing ourselves for emergencies and disasters that have been faced by native cultures in the past, or providing lessons from which we can mitigate and recover from disasters we have not yet faced. Although often dismissed, this embedded knowledge can teach us much about how to manage and survive extreme events when we must first help ourselves in the hope that other assistance will arrive.

It is disappointing that Julie Dekens (2007) noted that perhaps because of the perception that recent academic work has provided effective disaster response mechanisms, local knowledge has remained as marginalized as the people from whom the knowledge might be gained. Her work provides a framework for understanding local knowledge and lessons learned. However, we must continue our study of how local knowledge can be integrated into all of the policies, procedures and plans associated with the discipline of disaster management.

Cultural and emotional competence

When working with indigenous cultures, two very distinct concepts can be realized as necessity when working with individuals from these groups. The first concept is cultural competence; the ability to recognize certain actions and reactions as culturally based norms and determine how to most effectively interact with individuals from that community (Phillips *et al.*, 2010). For instance, recognizing how an indigenous population has traditionally responded to natural disaster scenarios in the past will improve the ability of an individual worker to work alongside members of that population and create an effective response plan. Phillips *et al.* (2010) also maintain that cultural competence amongst disaster relief workers will not only improve the effectiveness of the relief plan but also improve the community's response to that plan.

The second concept, as stated by West and Albrecht (2007), is one known as emotional competence; a belief that grounds itself in the fact that communities facing a disaster will have very emotional reactions to the destruction and chaos that follows. Individuals may become injured, homes may be destroyed, and cultural or ethnic traditions will likely be disrupted or damaged. Thus, West and Albrecht (2007) claim that it is important for relief workers to be able to identify these emotional responses and be able to address any outward signs of anger or sadness. It is important to also note that any emotional outbursts are not intentionally directed at relief workers, but rather, are displaced reactions as a result of the disaster (West and Albrecht, 2007). The more readily professionals can identify emotional competence, the more effective they will become at working with a population that has been ravaged by disaster.

Alternate Care Sites

There are several types of alternate delivery settings that are commonly utilized immediately following disaster. These include the shelter, the alternate care facility and the alternate hospital facility. Shelters are defined in disaster plans as locations pre-designated as providing safe and secure housing for those individuals who are capable of taking care of themselves. They are not meant for anyone with medical needs or who would be defined as vulnerable or special needs residents. At the other end of the spectrum would be the alternate hospital facility. Hospitals in the USA are required by accrediting bodies to have a secondary location that can be utilized as a hospital should their primary site be forced to evacuate, or if the site is at risk or inoperable. The focus of our work is the designation of a site as an alternate care facility. This location is for temporary housing of individuals who have urgent medical needs, who have special needs, or for those in need of specific in-patient services. One point of discussion is whether home care constitutes a form of alternate care setting. It might be appropriate if that home care consists of palliative care, quarantine (in the case of infectious disease) or mild illness. Home care is not an alternate care facility if there was need of chronic medical care or distribution of medical countermeasures such as vaccines.

Functions

The Agency for Healthcare Research and Quality (AHRQ, 2009; Document, #09-0062) defines the following as potential functions served by an alternate care facility (ACF):

- Bed capacity and surge relief by offering non-acute (ward) in-patient services to allow for decompression of existing hospitals or to augment in-patient ward care capacity.
- Primary medical care and behavioural/mental health services for persons and residents with pre-existing chronic diseases who, as a result of the event, are unable to access their routine sources of healthcare, including supportive care for family members and pets.
- Primary medical care and behavioural/mental health services for displaced or sheltered special needs persons with chronic diseases, limited mobility or other impairments making them unqualified for general population shelters, including supportive care for family members and pets.
- Pre-hospital evaluation and triage services to determine the need for hospital care.
- Evaluation and support to isolation and quarantine operations.
- Provide a site for mass immunization and prophylaxis and point of dispensing services for mass medication distribution.
- Bed capacity and surge relief by offering acute, intensive care-level services to allow for decompression or existing hospitals or to augment in-patient intensive care unit capacity.
- Community outreach to, and assessment of, affected populations.
- This includes assisting with needs such as:

  – Conditions that require observation, assessment, or maintenance;
  – Chronic conditions that require assistance with the activities of daily living and do not require hospitalization;
  – Medications and vital sign monitoring that cannot be provided at home;
  – Conditions that require the level of care provided by the ACF.

An ACF is not, in most cases, a substitute for an acute care hospital or emergency department. However, the American College of Emergency Physicians (2011) has provided a minimum list of special medical needs individuals:

- Individuals with severe respiratory problems (oxygen or ventilator dependent) that require a power source and/or ambu bag;
- Individuals dependent on airway suctioning (tracheotomy dependent);
- Individuals on intravenous therapy;
- Individuals requiring tube feedings;
- Individuals requiring assistance with insulin dosing;

- Individuals requiring wound care or help with injections on a daily basis;
- Individuals with physical or mental conditions that require daily medical supervision.

Vulnerable populations

The populations that have been shown to comprise the residents of the alternate care facilities are a mixture of those with pre-existing conditions that can be predicted, those with injuries or conditions existing as a result of the disaster, and a large group of those with unmanaged mental health conditions or functional issues previously unrecognized, undiagnosed, or where care was unavailable.

There are several needs other than medical that would be defined as special needs or at-risk populations. These would include individuals who have a condition that would interfere with them having access or acquiring medical care. These would include individuals who have issues in one or more of the following six functional areas:

1. Communication (e.g. non-English speaking);
2. Independence (e.g. frail elderly or children, physically impaired);
3. Physically impaired (deaf, blind, mobility impaired, chemical or drug-dependent);
4. Supervision (e.g. cognitive disorders or other mental health issues);
5. Geographic or cultural isolation;
6. Transportation.

Staffing

As with all considerations of large-scale or multi-site disasters, medical surge capacity or MCIs, staffing is of over-riding concern. While there has been a great deal of literature describing the alternate care sites, few have discussed staffing needs or where staff is to be acquired. Although not the purpose of this chapter, two sources that describe these issues and provide templates are: Disaster Alternate Care Facilities: Selection and Operation (Agency for Healthcare Research and Quality, 2009) and the National Center for Medical Readiness programs (National Center for Medical Readiness, 2009).

Psychological Considerations

Immediate post-disaster environment

While there is a good deal of literature and information linked to the development of psychological trauma as a result of a disaster, there is very little credence given to those with pre-existing conditions that are exacerbated during a disaster scenario (Lopez-Ibor, 2006). Some of these individuals may be seeking treatment and developing new coping tools, while others may have an underlying condition that is undiagnosed. In either instance, these individuals are already struggling to some degree concerning their functioning within society; an aspect which will be greatly affected by the onset of a disaster. Suddenly, the individual's support network may be affected or unavailable, and that person's comfort zones may be temporarily or permanently violated. When this occurs, an individual may become highly distressed or panicked making it very difficult for relief services to properly address his or her needs (Lopez-Ibor, 2006). Thus, psychological considerations must be taken into consideration and assessed before individuals within this population can truly participate in and benefit from the reconstructive process.

To properly address these concerns, one must first focus on psychological trauma that is intensified by the effects of the disaster (Lopez-Ibor, 2006). For instance, it is not uncommon for a person who suffers from an anxiety disorder such as obsessive compulsive disorder (OCD) to develop a highly specific daily routine that must be accomplished in a specific order and within clear time parameters in order for that individual to feel a sense of normalcy. In the instance of a natural disaster, such as an earthquake that resulted in severe damage to a community's physical structure, a person struggling with this disorder may find it impossible to continue with his or her routine. Since these routines are often used as coping mechanisms for those suffering from an anxiety disorder, relief efforts must be willing to help these individuals with temporary alternative coping methods to reduce anxiety levels and improve their current cognitive functioning.

Reconstruction and alternative care

The second area of focus should relate to the involvement of members in this vulnerable population with alternative care sites. Workers providing relief and reconstruction services need to be made aware that certain anxiety-related disorders may hinder the functioning and well-being of certain individuals being treated in the alternative care sites (West and Albrecht, 2007). For instance, individuals suffering from agoraphobia who do not normally leave their residences may find it highly difficult to spend large amounts of time surrounded by hundreds of other people in an alternate care site. Similarly, individuals who have an intense fear of microbes may be highly resistant to maintaining themselves in a public facility.

Overall, in the instances of both immediate response and alternative care, the goal should not be to work on long-term care with these individuals but rather to achieve enough stability that they are able to cognitively function well enough to address the immediate concerns of the disaster.

Another important factor to consider when focusing on reconstructive efforts is the idea that a community can meet its basic, natural needs while working to improve livelihood within its infrastructure through concerted efforts as a group (Benight, 2004). This theory is referred to as collective efficacy, which has been studied as a highly relevant factor in the community rebuilding process.

Once the initial danger of a disaster has been overcome, it becomes essential not only for the community to begin a process of physically rebuilding itself, but also to repair its sense of functioning through collective efficacy (Benight, 2004). Because this concept consists of a collective competence amongst members of the community, psychological concerns should, ideally, be considered and managed before a strong sense of collective efficacy can be attained. If these factors can be addressed, individuals within cognitively vulnerable populations will have a greater chance of successfully contributing to the rebuilding of a community's well-being.

Post-disaster Reconstruction Lessons Learned from Specific Disasters

Hurricane Katrina

A quote from Mario J. Rizzo, Professor of Economics at New York University at the front of a recently published book by Emily Chamlee-Wright (2010) states that 'she shows that the micro social networks are often more important for recovery than large government programs'. In this insightful work on post-disaster recovery by Chamlee-Wright (2010), the non-governmental issues involved in disaster recovery from Hurricane Katrina were critically examined. She maintains that coordination necessary following disaster comes from commercial and civil society.

As so often happens with the wide area of destruction that occurs with hurricanes, the residents of New Orleans often returned not only to destroyed homes, but to the loss of entire neighbourhoods and social structures that defined their lives. All of those social and economic structures that surround us and support us were also gone. Gone were jobs and employment, basic services and grocery stores, hospitals and schools, churches – everything that roots a person in their everyday existence.

Some very basic questions had to be asked and answered before the coordination of recovery could begin. For example:

- Would or could the residents return? This was one of the poorest cities in the country and had little to entice residents back. The crime rate was high and safety issues were a constant concern.
- Where would the funding be found to rebuild?
- Should the city even be rebuilt? It was still high risk and effectiveness of the levee system was still in question.
- How soon could basic services be restored?
- When would jobs be available to support those returning, especially the poor and vulnerable?
- Why would businesses return to the area, since many had already been struggling to survive?

These were just some of the questions that needed to be addressed as courses of action were considered. Chamlee-Wright and others (Antunes, 2005; Sparks, 2009) used this event to critically examine factors that promote, and those that inhibit, long-term recovery efforts. It became clear from this example, and from other major disasters in Gujarat, India, Pakistan, Haiti and China, that effective government solutions do not always emerge. Her work is a major contribution to the growing body of scientific inquiry and knowledge being gained as the number of major disasters increases. What do people do when the government is not the solution expected or hoped for (Antunes, 2005)? This was one of the greatest shocks for the American people after Hurricane Katrina! Risk awareness, risk acceptance and personal responsibility in time of crisis were abrogated to government. Although many systems failed, and there is enough blame to provide some for all, ultimately residents must take some personal responsibility for assuring resilience and the ability to rise to the challenges following disaster. Even if money and external resources become available, how are the internal social networks and structures brought back to life? In large-scale disasters, why are some areas able to demonstrate resilience and rapid recovery, while others never do? These are some of the questions being examined from the experience with Katrina and other large magnitude disasters.

One of the most powerful observations made in this work (Chamlee-Wright, 2010) is that private civil society contains within it tremendous capacity to foster resilience. It is maintained that civil society must rapidly occupy the civil society vacuum created by disaster. It is this anchor around which recovery occurs.

Katrina caused the residents of southern Louisiana, especially New Orleans to leave their homes and evacuate throughout a wide area of our nation. Major cities welcomed refugees, as did small cities and communities, churches and other places of refuge. People did not know if their neighbours and other community residents would return. If this expectation did not exist, it is unlikely that they would return as well (Kunreuther *et al.*, 2006).

In an effort to aid in redevelopment and recovery, it was decided that government would designate specific areas for recovery efforts. In this manner, what has been called the jack-o-lantern effect could be avoided. This American colloquialism means that it would be best not to have single, isolated homes or businesses rebuilt surrounded by ruined homes and no support system. Surprisingly, and despite the logic, some areas did start to recover, even in areas that it had been decided were not best to target. Chamlee-Wright (2010) provides specific examples of how private citizens even in the most damaged areas utilized socially embedded resources to promote change. The author identified three specific strategies to utilize this social capital: mutual assistance, cooperation through commercial networks and development of key community resources.

Through personal interviews and research, it was determined that small works of mutual support are vital to a recovery movement. It is all about how those who survived the storm can help one another in areas such as child support, exchange of ideas and expertise, shelter and even tools. This is an example of a social fabric being rewoven, one thread at a time. It also serves as an external signal to others that return is a viable option, that hope remains, and that support, both physical and psychological, is there. All those needs of clean water, power, limited food and resources, debris removal that could not be handled individually could and were addressed by mutual assistance. Numbers grew, community groups and faith-based groups emerged to help the elderly and others in most need. In some cases, it is a school that serves as the trigger for allowing the adults to get to the business of recovering. Just as in the larger cities such as Chicago, one's identity flows from being from a 'neighbourhood'. There is a parallel concept when living in very small communities or rural villages. These areas often survive disasters best because of the concept of 'being in this together'. Americans have become increasingly disconnected from one another and have lost many of the bonds that lead to social connectedness and civic society (Putnam, 2000).

The second strategy focused on the importance of business in recovery and reconstruction. There is no question that many businesses, most notably Wal-Mart and Home Depot, were credited with being the most influential players in responding to Katrina (Horowitz, 2008, 2009). Places of business that related to providing building supplies also provided much-needed professional advice to most of the folks who did not have insurance and could not afford help, but were forced to do the construction and repairs themselves. It is necessary that plans for post-disaster recovery place commercial enterprise at the core, and involve them not only in the response, but recovery and reconstruction planning. Depending on the situation and location, these businesses may have very close ties to the community, so that employees are friends and neighbours as well. It is most interesting that after Katrina commercial spaces were often offered for social gatherings or places to meet, blurring the traditional lines between business and social networking.

The third strategy noted by Chamlee-Wright (2010) was that in more rare cases, it was community organizations, such as churches, that would be the focal point for rebuilding. Many church congregations returned to their communities, and with the help of their religious leaders provided leadership and a foundation for recovery (Sparks, 2009). A myriad of community organizations returned, another notable example being the Musician's Village Project, an effort to use the rich musical heritage of New Orleans to encourage residents to return (National Building Museum, 2010).

Banda Aceh

At approximately 8:00 local time, a massive earthquake of magnitude 9.0 on the Richter scale occurred in the Indian Ocean 30 km below sea level. The quake lasted an incredible 10 min and ruptured the earth for 1200 km at the plate juncture. At closest landfall in Banda Aceh, an estimated 170,000 people died, and the earth's geography was changed. Clarke *et al.* have written a detailed text on the perspectives and experiences of Aceh survivors as viewed not only from a physical infrastructure viewpoint, but political, religious and socioeconomic and cultural aspects as well (Clarke *et al.*, 2010)

In response to the tsunami and incredible death toll and destruction, there was an unprecedented outpouring of international aid (US$13 billion) as well as material and volunteers. Unfortunately, as often happens, aid was organized and delivered more on the basis of what the donor countries and institutions wanted to give rather than any clear needs assessment or appropriate distribution. As with all disasters, international media coverage played a major role in capturing global interest and sympathy.

Some models of reconstruction call for the return to normalcy as a goal. However, this is not always appropriate, especially if normalcy was poverty, and non-functional government and society such as we saw in Haiti. Another reason for changing that goal can be seen in Banda Aceh. There was no way to return to the formal normalcy, since so many people died. A new normal needed to be defined. If the political will, international aid and planning skills can be brought together, this is an opportunity to improve the condition of the people and their environment. The body of knowledge is increasing in this area, although much work yet needs to be done to define appropriate steps to be taken.

Another classic aspect of the time frame of reconstruction is that aid and interest remains very high early in the process, but wanes over time as new emergencies and events take place in the media and minds of the world. As is typical in disaster response from international organizations, the emphasis is often on helping to rebuild, to create something tangible to help those in need. Much less often is there a consideration of what the buildings will house and how they will become and remain functional. This has been a situation often seen in US organizations trying to assist the American Indians, indigenous peoples who can often be very poor and in great need. Well-meaning organizations will build nice homes on reservations to house those who have never had them. However, they neglect to consider that the homes aren't near any source of water or electricity. There is no education of those on the reservation as to how to make use of, and maintain a residence. Examples in Banda Aceh were libraries built with no consideration of books, schools with no teachers or supplies with which to teach, and houses with no infrastructure to allow residents to live there.

Conclusion

Our world continues to be a risky place in which to live and work. Disasters will and do occur, apparently with ever-increasing frequency. Although natural disasters have been the focus of work thus far, strategies that enhance our resilience, sustainability and ability to reconstruct after disaster would also apply to man-made disasters. Regardless of the model used, reconstruction is often separated into phases to allow planning of activities, events and expectations, while fully understanding that it is a flowing and an evolving process. It begins with crisis orientation by the saving of lives, stabilizing locations involved and lastly protecting property. Over time, physical structures, businesses and government begin recovery and reconstruction. It is only in the later phases (and time frames) of disaster management that thoughts and actions normally turn to relationships, social constructs and to re-creating community. Recognition of these needs should occur much earlier in the recovery process. There are many commonalities and lessons that have been learned from recent major natural disasters, including Wenchuan and other massive earthquakes, Hurricane Katrina and Banda Aceh. There are several cross-cutting issues affecting post-disaster reconstruction:

1. There is an increasing number of natural disasters, and they are becoming more violent and unpredictable. There has also been an increased interest in and attention to the recovery and reconstruction phase of disaster management. Sadly, this has been due to the increased need for reconstruction in several locations. Louisiana, Indonesia, Haiti and Japan are the most obvious visual representations of the recovery phase.
2. Although all four aspects of disaster management (preparedness, response, recovery and mitigation) have all been recognized as needing research and study, there has most recently been recognition of the importance of the immediate post-disaster phase of reconstruction. Emergency managers in the USA and those training them have done a wonderful job in addressing emergency management by compartmentalizing the phases. This allows them to be defined, to be studied, and for plans to be made to address each one. In most cases, however, the physical manifestations of disaster have received all of the attention, funding and study. The immediate post-disaster phase of reconstruction has been addressed by meeting the physical needs of those involved, but too little attention has been made to recognize the importance to this time frame concerning invisible factors.
3. In poignant observations made by Suaedy in *Silence can be Deafening and Emptiness can be Blinding* (Clarke *et al.*, 2010), the 'destruction of the soul' has received much less attention than the physical destruction and loss of life so evident in the surroundings. Physical destruction is so much easier to see, to define, to quantitate and correct than issues of the psyche. It is not surprising that it is often ignored, neglected or denied. It is difficult, if not impossible to quantitate loss of what people define as community, the people and social connections that make one 'belong'. Buildings and places can be imbued with meaning. Sights, sounds and smells invoke belonging. How do you quantify helplessness, hopelessness, loss and uncertainty? The blank looks after treasured possessions and important people have been ripped away by a tornado or flood

waters, or crushed by earthquakes or landslides let you know how much the soul has been affected.

4. Indigenous populations need to be included and involved in planning, response and reconstruction efforts. Indigenous knowledge databases currently exist, and global recognition of the value of this information is rapidly increasing. In areas of great diversity, attention must be paid to providing information in appropriate languages, and orally when educational level is low or there is no written form of communication. Cultural values and traditions must be respected and valued. The indigenous peoples have much to gain from our modern knowledge of disaster warning systems, response procedures and reconstruction. Likewise, we must ensure that priceless indigenous knowledge is not ignored or lost. Their oneness with nature and survival over millennia alongside the disasters that have occurred has led to a wealth of indigenous knowledge. On a global basis, we are now only beginning to realize how much has been lost and how much there is to be gained.
5. Alternate care facilities play a vital immediate post-disaster role in providing for vulnerable populations. This role has traditionally been viewed as one of medical care for physical needs. However, disaster not only causes physical effects, but can cause or exacerbate mental health issues and needs, both recognized and unrecognized.
6. It is concluded that through a better understanding and recognition of the role of invisible factors in reconstruction, and concomitant improvement in our treatment of mental health needs in these vulnerable populations, rebuilding of the community can be enhanced and time needed for recovery minimized.

As our knowledge of the relationship between disaster and destruction of community grows, so must the care of our residents in alternate care facilities also improve. This knowledge must be incorporated not only into the design and operation of alternate care facilities, but into care planning and staffing requirements. We must improve the recovery/reconstruction likelihood of not only physical artefacts, but of physical and mental well-being as well. The resiliency of the human condition can be incredible. It is up to those responsible for governing and caring for these populations to optimize the conditions in which this can happen. A study of commonalities between recovery and reconstruction following earthquakes will provide those lessons from which we can incorporate what works best, and avoid actions that delay our goal. Inclusiveness in our plans, especially valuing and incorporating indigenous populations, is vital to this process.

References

Agency for Healthcare Research and Quality (2009) Disaster alternate care facilities: selection and operation. AHRQ Publication No. 09-0062, Denver Health, Denver, Colorado. Available at: http://www.hsdl.org/?view&doc=119176&coll=limited (Accessed 13 February 2013).

American College of Emergency Physicians – Disaster Medical Section (2011) Special medical needs sheltering. Available at: https://www.acep.org/content.aspx?id=38594 (Accessed 13 February 2013).

Antunes, G. (2005) Homeowners left on their own in battered New Orleans. MediaNews, 4 December. Available at: http://www.mail-archive.com/medianews@twiar.org/msg06815.html (Accessed 13 February 2013).

Bandyk, M. (2010) Why natural disasters are more expensive – but less deadly. *US News and World Report*, 24 March. Available at: http://money.usnews.com/money/business-economy/articles/2010/03/24/why-natural-disasters-are-more-expensivebut-less-deadly.html (Accessed 13 February 2013).

Barnhardt, R. and Kawagley, A.O. (2005) Indigenous knowledge systems and Alaska native ways of knowing. *Anthropology and Education Quarterly* 36(1), 8–23.

Baumwoll, J. (2008) The value of indigenous knowledge for disaster risk reduction: A unique assessment tool for reducing community vulnerability to natural disasters. Submitted to Webster University, Vienna, in partial fulfillment of the requirements for the Degree of Master of Arts in International Relations, St Louis, Missouri.

Benight, C.C. (2004) Collective efficacy following a series of natural disasters. *Anxiety, Stress, and Coping* 17(4), 401–420.

Block, B. (2008) Natural disasters becoming more frequent. Worldwatch Institute, 14 July. Available at: http://www.worldwatch.org/node/5825 (Accessed 13 February 2013).

Chamlee-Wright, E. (2010) *The Cultural and Political Economy of Recovery*. Routledge, London and New York.

Clarke, M.C., Fanany, I. and Kenny, S. (eds) (2010) *Post-disaster Reconstruction: Lessons from Aceh*. Earthscan, London.

Dekens, J. (2007) *Local Knowledge for Disaster Preparedness: a Literature Review*. International Center for Integrated Mountain Development (ICIMOD), Kathmandu, Nepal.

Fanany, I. (2010) Afterward: reconstructing the invisible landscape. In: Clarke, M.C., Fanany, I. and Kenny, S. (eds) *Post-disaster Reconstruction: Lessons from Aceh*. Earthscan, London, pp. 235–249.

Federal Emergency Management Agency (2010) National disaster recovery framework (draft). 1-58. FEMA, Washington, DC.

Freeman, P.K., Keen, M. and Mani, M. (2003) Being prepared: Natural disasters are becoming more frequent, more destructive, and deadlier, and poor countries are being hit the hardest. *Finance and Development* 40(9). Available at: http://www.imf.org/external/pubs/ft/fandd/2003/09/pdf/freeman.pdf (Accessed 9 March 2013).

Grenier, L. (1998) *Working with Indigenous Knowledge: a Guide for Researchers*. International Development Research Centre, Ottawa, Canada.

Hagen, J.C. (2008) Emergency management structure for use in the Alaska native (AN) elderly population. *International Journal of Emergency Management* 5(3/4), 279–283.

Hass, J.E., Kates, R.W. and Bowden, M.J. (eds) (1977) *Reconstruction Following Disaster*. MIT Press, Cambridge, Massachusetts.

Horowitz, S. (2008) Making hurricane response more effective: Lessons from the private sector and the coast guard during Katrina. Mercatus Policy Series, Policy Comment No. 17. George Mason University, Arlington, Virginia.

Horowitz, S. (2009) Wal-Mart to the rescue: private enterprise's response to Hurricane Katrina. *The Independent Review* 13(4). Available at: http://www.independent.org/pdf/tir/tir_13_04_3_horwitz.pdf (Accessed 14 February 2013).

Independent Evaluation Group (2010) Facts and figures on natural disasters. World Bank. 10 March. Available at: http://www.worldbank.org/ieg/naturaldisasters/docs/natural_disasters_fact_sheet.pdf (Accessed 14 February 2013).

InterAcademy Panel on International Issues (2009) *Natural Disaster Mitigation: a Scientific and Practical Approach*. Science Press, Beijing. Available at: http://www.interacademies.net/File.aspx?id=10292 (Accessed 14 February 2013).

Kahn, M.E. (2005) The death toll from natural disasters: the role of income, geography, and institutions. *The Review of Economics and Statistics* 87(2), 271–284.

Kessler, R.C., Galea, S., Gruber, M.J., Sampson, N.A., Ursano, R.J. and Wessely, S. (2008) Trends in mental illness and suicidality after Hurricane Katrina. *Molecular Psychiatry* 13(4), 374–384.

Kunreuther, H., Kettl, D., Daniels, R. and Gosselin, P.G. (2006) On their own in battered New Orleans. In: Daniels, R.J., Kettl, D.F. and Kunreuther, H. (eds) *On Risk and Disaster: Lessons from Hurricane Katrina.* University of Pennsylvania Press, Philadelphia, Pennsylvania.

Lambert, L. (2003) From 'savages' to scientists: mainstream science moves toward recognizing traditional knowledge. *Tribal College Journal of American Indian Higher Education* 15, 10–13.

Lopez-Ibor, J.J. (2006) Disasters and mental health: new challenges for the psychiatric profession. *The World Journal of Biological Psychiatry* 7(3), 171–182.

Mileti, D.S. (1999) *Disasters by Design: a Reassessment of Natural Hazards in the United States.* Joseph Henry Press, Washington, DC.

National Building Museum (2010) Civic innovator: New Orleans habitat museums' village. 11 May. Available at: http://www.nbm.org/about-us/national-building-museum-online/musicians-village-jim-pate-interview.html (Accessed 9 March 2013).

National Center for Medical Readiness (2009) NCMR programs. Available at: http://www.medicalreadiness.org/mems (Accessed 14 February 2013).

Phillips, B.D., Thomas, D.S.K., Fothergill, A. and Blinn-Pike, L. (eds) (2010) *Social Vulnerability to Diasters*. CRC Press, New York.

Putnam, R.D. (2000) *Bowling Alone.* Touchstone Books, Simon and Schuster, New York.

Sparks, R.J. (2009) 'An anchor to the people': Hurricane Katrina, religious life, and recovery in New Orleans. *The Journal of Southern Religion.* After the Storm: A Special Issue on Hurricane Katrina. Available at: http://jsr.fsu.edu/Katrina/FrontKatrina.htm (Accessed 10 March 2013).

Stephens, S. (2000) *Handbook for Culturally Responsive Science Curriculum.* Alaska Native Knowledge Network, Fairbanks, Alaska.

West, N.T. and Albrecht, K. (2007) Building emotional competence: a strategy for disaster preparation and recovery. *Exchange* 175, 20–27.

World Bank (2008a) Short-term plan of action re: the Sichuan Wenchuan Earthquake of 12 May 2008. 27 May. The World Bank Global Facility for Disaster Reduction and Recovery. Good Practice Notes V1.1. World Bank, Washington, DC.

World Bank (2008b) Disaster risk reduction (DRR). July. The World Bank Global Facility for Disaster Reduction and Recovery. World Bank Good Practice Notes. World Bank, Washington, DC.

Zoujing, S. (2009) People above the clouds: confidence recovery and culture preservation in a post-catastrophic ethnic village, Taoping, China. MA Thesis, University of Washington, Seattle, Washington.

Chapter 32

Management of Dead following Disasters and Mass Casualty Incidents: Critical Operational Issues Revolve around Human Resources and Logistics

Preeti Arora, Rajesh Arora, Raman Chawla, Rupa Gunaseelan and J.R. Bhardwaj

Managing the Dead and the Missing

For certain is death for the born
And certain is birth for the dead;
Therefore, over the inevitable
Thou should not grieve.

Chapter 2, verse 27 of the Srimad Bhagavad-Gita

In the aftermath of a disaster, the missing ones are neither alive nor dead and this uncertainty can be a cause for grave and continued suffering for the grieved families.

Morbidity or mortality resulting from any natural or man-made event cascading towards a crisis, an emergency, a disaster or a mass casualty incident (MCI) acts as a primary governing factor in assessment of the gravity of situation. Death initiates a cascade of human suffering, which is further worsened by lack of information and unorganized practices adopted by authorities. This has been realized as a long-term consequence involving social, psychological, emotional, cultural, economic and legal repercussions.

As per the Government of India Disaster Management Act, 2005, these situations are defined with respect to the perspective loci of the managing body or simply by the coping capacity of stakeholders/service providers. A situation that arises due to natural disasters in a city like Mumbai or a region like Bhuj (struck by an earthquake) differs from that caused by a tsunami or a supercyclone in a remote area. The Fukushima incident of 2011 in Japan presented altogether different types of challenges as compared with a terrorist attack within city boundaries (e.g. 26 November Mumbai attack), which in turn differs widely from low-intensity conflicts in the border areas of Jammu and Kashmir (India),

Bangladesh, Nagaland, etc., or Naxal (a generic term used to refer to various militant Communist groups operating in different parts of India under different organizational envelopes) internal conflicts. The gravity and dynamics completely change if a 'contamination' factor is involved, e.g. sarin gas attack and the Fukushima incident in Japan and the Bhopal gas tragedy are some of the important examples of such situations (Ajmani, 1998). It is imperative to develop strategies supported by essential advance technologies for mitigation against the impact of failure of effective management of the dead. Air crashes or terrorist bombing are events in another set of categories requiring comprehensive tasks to achieve the set goals of providing effective care to relatives in the shortest possible time.

The present forensic science involving identification of disaster victims was started back in 1897 by a dentist. The International Humanitarian Law (IHL), International Human Rights Law, Guiding Principles on Internal Displacement, Operational Guidelines on Human Rights and Natural Disasters, INTERPOL's Disaster Victim Identification Guide and the Standard of the International Civil Aviation Organization are some of the international directives that provide a basis for international cooperation in identification of the missing and management of the dead during disasters. All such humanitarian factors have consensus on the following issues: (i) respect for the dead person; (ii) the right to family life; (iii) the right to know the fate of their relatives; (iv) freedom of religion and belief/culture; (v) indigenous people's rights; and (vi) obligations to prosecute serious violations. Global societal bindings and linkages are joined amongst all nations through initiatives undertaken by the International Red Cross and Red Crescent societies as well as other related organizations. The major governing principles include: (i) promoting and supporting dignified recovery; (ii) appropriate management of forensic analysis of human remains; and (iii) considering the needs of affected families and communities during all phases. Rule 112-117 adopted as the customary law of IHL accounts for management of the missing and dead (http://www.icrc.org/ihl.nsf). The International Red Cross and Red Crescent societies have released a field manual for first responders on managing the dead in post-disaster situations (Knight, 1996). The various international practices promote the use of the phrase 'human remains' instead of 'dead bodies', which is associated with panic; however, due to the ease of understanding of the latter term, it is still used worldwide.

Factors governing severity of incidences

Mass casualty incidents (MCIs) often lead to collapse of forensic services, thereby limiting the adoption of systematic procedures. Thus, it is essential to develop a basic awareness of easy-to-use procedures in non-specialists to ensure proper and defined management of the dead without unnecessary complexity. However, this is not as simple as it seems to be. It depends upon the severity of the incident itself and related governing factors and variables. The severity of the incident can be ascertained by evaluation of critical factors including: (i) number of deaths; (ii) remoteness of area, which limits resource availability/logistics; (iii) climatic conditions/temperature, which defines the decay rate; (iv) time constraints; (v) non-availability of large number of mortuaries and other related infrastructure; (vi) religious issues that might create a state of panic; (vii) myths with respect to dead bodies; and (viii) whether deaths of foreigners in another nation raise problems due to relative differences in rules and regulations between countries that might create unnecessary confusion and associated delays (Knight, 1996; Bhardwaj *et al.*, 2007).

Systematic procedure(s) should be in place

It is necessary to have systematic procedures in place for effective management of the dead. On humanitarian grounds, the family of the deceased needs to know the facts related to the death and in the case of a person missing and presumed dead the information provided should be linked to the circumstances involved, otherwise the situation can worsen further. The reappearance of a person thought dead after a specific period is a psychological trauma and, conversely, if already dead and the body was not found, a long-term psychological trauma related to acceptance as well as related legal financial procedures can create secondary problems. It is a moral obligation as a civilized human race to give due respect to the deceased and their relatives. The legal issues linked with: (i) correct identification; (ii) post-mortem examination; (iii) investigation into the circumstances of death; and (iv) evidence gathering/preservation are important aspects of the management of the dead. In the case of chemical, biological, radiological and nuclear (CBRN) emergencies, protective equipment is required to be in place to prevent cross-contamination; there are multiple religious concerns related to various ceremonies, and various issues related to medical treatment administered/medical equipment uses and, eventually, process sustenance. A basic procedure applicable to identifying the missing or dead prior to delivering news to concerned relatives is given in Fig. 32.1. It has been accepted worldwide that mock exercises should be conducted keeping in mind the complexities related to management of the dead (Binz, 2007).

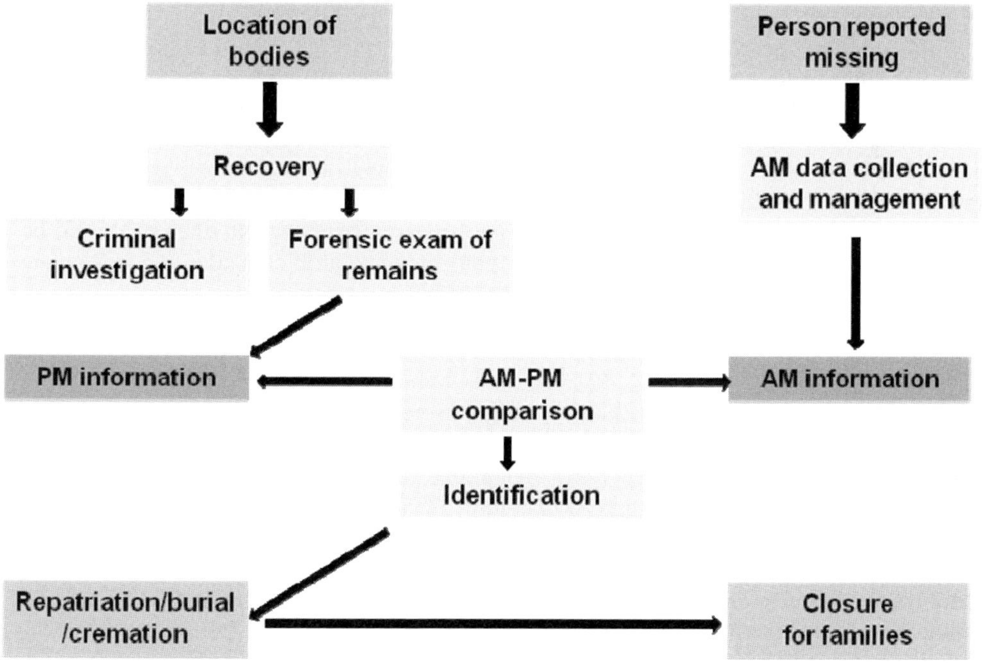

Fig. 32.1. Management of identified dead: basic procedures.

Managing the dead during MCIs

During disasters/MCIs such as tsunamis or supercyclones in India, the September 11 attacks, Hurricane Katrina in the USA or the Fukushima incident in Japan, the events have led to an enhanced burden of casualty management on the complete operational system with defined operational logistics/resources. During such incidents, from the viewpoint of managing the dead, the basic components of the operational system include: body recovery, identification, preservation, repatriation (across cities, states or nations) and burial/cremation, etc. (Arora *et al.*, 2010). The ensuing section provides an insight into each procedure and the criticality linked to the subject matter.

Body recovery

Body recovery procedures should not restrict the process of recovery of survivors. Therefore, they may last a few days, weeks or even be prolonged depending upon the area, the nature and gravity of the disaster, etc. The volunteers, if involved, should follow acceptable procedures. A unique reference number should be allotted to every deceased person, with their related associated and non-associated properties that might help in identification in later stages. Associated properties refer to items or articles found within the clothes of the deceased; however, non-associated properties are those that are collected in the vicinity of the deceased which might belong to the deceased. These articles can help in identification and cross-matching based on input from relatives. The number should be given on waterproof labels to avoid likelihood of misinterpretation in the future. Body bags are essential for carrying the bodies to avoid trauma during transition, and the location of the body and the date it was found should be noted to assist with identification. As an essential standard operating procedure (SOP), personal belongings and notes separated from the body should be put together, or body parts and the location they have been found in with respect to the body should be given an identification number. Every body part should be treated as individual, and having a certain body part in the vicinity of the dead doesn't necessarily mean that it belongs to that body unless and until it has been identified by various means. No attempt should be made to match the body parts in the field as it may enhance problems later and will create confusion (Arora *et al.*, 2010).

Control of body

During a non-MCI, the police (in India) generally take control over the bodies. The body should be placed in a body bag as soon as possible with a unique identification number. Provisional identification can be done by taking photographs from different angles; recording all details, i.e. gender, age, skin colour, various distinguishing features, clothes, etc.; and collecting and numbering of materials around the victim. It is essential to remember that the photo range number of the camera should be mentioned on the first identification form to link it to the complete identification process. The site should be outlined and cordoned off to preserve evidence. It is important to collect forensic evidence and send it to laboratories with its respective unique identification number. On the other hand, during an MCI, the police will take control and bodies should be covered immediately with suitable coverings. In the case of natural disasters such as tsunamis, finding the cause of death is not of concern and relative criminal investigation is not necessary. Provisional identification/documentation should be done based on available resources and minimal numbering is an essentiality, along with noting the date and location where the body was found. As per the regulatory framework in India, the district collector possesses numerous powers to take the ultimate decisions over the issues of whether to practise mass temporary burials to avoid panic or whether to store bodies in temporary mortuary facilities or carry out mass cremations after suitable identification procedures. Rescue service providers are at risk due to working with contaminated bodies and this can lead to spread of contamination amongst them (Arora *et al.*, 2010; Bhardwaj *et al.*, 2010). Necessary decontamination might be needed to allow continuous proximity with dead bodies.

Identification of body

There are various ways of identifying the dead in MCIs such as sex, height, identification by next of kin, face (if not mutilated), medals (worn by military personnel or pilots), identification discs worn by pilots, personal belongings, e.g. necklaces, metal chains, rings and dentition (Gresham, 1979). During a non-MCI, visual identification procedures are generally considered as vital, however, this is erroneous. Experts caution that such visual identification procedures are sometimes correct but otherwise might not even come close to the actuality. Extreme caution should be practised based on the condition of the body and impact of disasters. Post-mortem examination is a well-accepted procedure; however, it is a lengthy forensic procedure and time constraints restrict its utility. Identification requires comparative analysis of post-mortem data with ante-mortem data collected on the basis of information available from relatives. If doubt remains, the adoption of DNA fingerprinting is an ultimate resort (Gresham, 1979). During MCIs, the adoption of temporary mass burial is a well-accepted procedure that provides time to identify each and every body during long-term operations. However, burial is against the beliefs of particular religious communities, therefore if adopted without stringent procedures in place to manage mass hysteria, it might cause significant panic. Mass cremation without identification leads to numbers of people still missing being considered dead, adding further problems to the related issues. The generally accepted procedures adopted during MCIs include visual identification, post-mortem–ante-mortem comparative analysis and DNA-based identification.

Teeth are the most durable organs in the human body, and persist long after the decay of other skeletal structures, often withstanding destruction by other means such as fire, etc. Odontology has been widely accepted as one of the balanced procedures for effective identification if relatives are able to supply sufficient reliable ante-mortem data. Odontology has been in existence since AD 66, however it has only commonly been practised since 1897 (Kinra, 2006).

Dental identification has also been accepted as one of the primary points in the INTERPOL disaster victim identification protocol. Caution needs to be exercised while identifying a body as 'any non-identified deceased buried/cremated adds a gap in the missing/morbidity matrix' and 'any mis-identified deceased buried/cremated leads to another cross mis-identification and supposedly if the person is alive, the situation will be further complex to resolve'. Thus, mistaken identification adds more panic than non-identification. A well-accepted procedure for identification of a body is given in Fig. 32.2. The relative figures provided by these procedures are given in Fig. 32.3.

Visual recognition
(fresh cadavers)

+

Circumstantial evidences
(including garments, etc.)

+

Strong AMD-PMD match

+

Scientific–fingerprints:
odontology, unique medical conditions, X-rays,
genetics, including DNA

Fig. 32.2. Identification procedure.

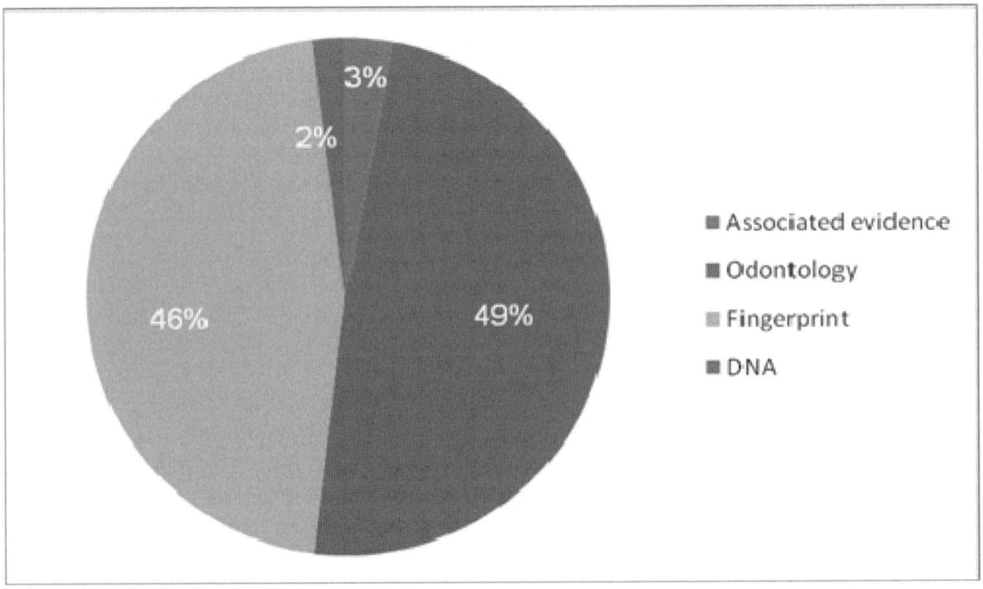

Fig. 32.3. Indicative percentage contribution of commonly used procedures in the identification process.

Preservation of body

In the event of an MCI, various resources can be pooled; alternatively, temporary mortuaries can be created to preserve the bodies for later identification. This could be in the medical facility or other areas could be created by the response forces for effective management of the disaster. Such practice was undertaken for management of mass casualties during the London bombing. Temporary burial is also an important alternative. Dry ice (in areas with good natural ventilation) or ice (in plastic bags) are essential requirements to store the bodies (PAHO, 2004; Morgan *et al.*, 2006; Government of India, 2007, 2010; Leung, 2008). In resource-poor situations, commercial ice is usually used for short-term storage of dead bodies.

Repatriation (across cities, states or nations – burial/cremation)

Repatriation is the process of returning a deceased person back to his or her place of origin or citizenship. Repatriation across cities, states or nations involves strictly laid down procedures, which should be followed to the letter. In case of the Armed Forces of almost all nations, a systematic procedure is practised in a disciplined and honourable manner. Similarly, everybody is an important element of society and adoption of systematic procedures at district, state or national level for both Indian/foreign nationals is a moral obligation (Parikh, 1985). Prior to repatriation, the body needs to be properly reformed to reduce the associated trauma related to post-mortem examination and impact of the event itself. Burial/cremation will be conducted by the relatives according to their religious beliefs. Such religious ceremonies need to be documented for all the diverse religions of the country in question so that necessary precautions can be taken by various stakeholders/service providers. The comparative profiling of such activities is enumerated below: (i) army settings – specified protocol for escorting and proper ceremony; (ii) civilian settings – city/state connections (relatives come and claim the body, followed by taking the body in a mortuary van to the place of burial or cremation); and (iii) MCIs – only a few claims might be entertained, especially if contamination is involved.

Infrastructural facilities required to be developed

The medical facility should have additional supportive structures in place to facilitate smooth certification of death; adoption of formal visual identification procedures; information exchange provisions to search for the deceased; manpower to facilitate identification of images taken by concerned relatives; X-ray/CT scanners; post-mortem/anti-mortem comparison; sealed bags with unique identification numbers for transportation, if necessary. In addition, storage facilities should be in place and bodies should be secured in breathable bags at 2–4°C. In the case of burial, as per religious norms, make-up should be applied and restoration of the facial features is required to make the body ready for the coffin. The unique identification number should be checked with respect to documentation at every stage to avoid mismatch and associated delays (Bhardwaj *et al.*, 2010).

Safety aspects

Dead bodies do not pose a direct risk as microorganisms and causative factors for various diseases are unable to survive beyond 48 h, except for human immunodeficiency virus (HIV), which is found even 6 days post-mortem. Thus, safety precautions must be practised while handling blood, body fluids and faeces leaked after death as they may contain causative factors for HIV, tuberculosis (TB) and diarrhoeal diseases. Use of gloves and boots is imperative while practising common sanitation and hygiene practices. Body handlers should not be allowed to be in confined spaces for long periods as, with the passage of time, toxic gases might develop. Disinfection of all clothes prior to switching over to a new job assignment is a necessity. Face masks, though not required, can reduce chances of infection and anxiety. Psychosocial care of the work force, especially if mass burial is undertaken, should be available as the work can fill them with grief and 'survivor guilt syndrome', which should not be ignored. Prolonged hours of working with the dead can cause psychosocial trauma. The disinfection of bodies and local burial without barriers might cause pollution of nearby drinking water supplies. Use of body bags can reduce psychological trauma. As body recovery teams work in the debris of buildings, necessary basic first aid and trauma care equipment should be made available to manage field casualties.

Critical issues in operations

There are numerous rate-limiting factors in the management of dead bodies. Post-mortem examination requires efforts by a team of specialists to be performed completely and adequately. In some cases, where the causative factor is known to be a disaster, it is essential to ascertain the cause of individual's death to fulfil the criteria of medico-legal issues. A body control officer/escort should identify the body to the pathologist concerned to avoid any confusion. In India and other contiguous South Asian countries, generally such activity is conducted by a member of the police force. In the case of an MCI, sometimes a full forensic post-mortem examination is not feasible, in which case a partial reporting system is practised as per the directions of the Chief Medical Officer, working under the aegis of the Office of the District Collector. However, identification and forensic evidence are required for settling legal matters and other linked issues. For example, any person missing for > 7 years can be considered as dead, but for those who are not confirmed to be dead, legal issues become more complex with respect to transfer of property and other related items, and the beneficiaries can face a number of problems because of this. Thus, identification of the dead is one of the most important aspects to reduce psychological, social and economic trauma (Polson, 1985).

DNA-based identification has been highlighted as one of the most efficient methods of providing proof of identity. However, it requires a sufficient number of samples with a strong chain of evidence and one of the challenges during disastrous situations is contamination/co-mingling, which may cause problems and increase time taken to carry out these tests. The other limiting factor is that there are very few recognized certified laboratories in most developing countries and for such matters, speed is essential. Thus, it is important to develop disaster victim identification cells and a chain of network of such laboratories for sample collection, processing and cross-matching analysis (Gresham, 1979).

As mentioned above, odontology can provide some specific solutions. It requires ante-mortem dental records for cross-comparison and one should always take a second opinion to remove false positives; it is quicker than the DNA method. However, perfect teeth make identification more difficult (Kinra, 2006). The definite establishment of identity based on odontology requires application of logic as it is not usually the case that a person dies after providing a recent dental report to their relatives. Thus, the justification of ascertaining the need for this modality is a matter of experience and varies on a case-to-case basis. However, in cases where ante-mortem data are not available, odontology can provide information on age, ancestral background, sex and the socio-economic status of the deceased by adoption of a process known as post-mortem profiling. It narrows the search towards a focused group. It includes adoption of various newer techniques associated with odontology. Facial reconstruction and facial superimposition of skeletal and teeth fractures restrained by angulations and magnification-related issues can help in identification of an individual. Teeth act as an excellent source of DNA material that can be cross-matched with samples including stored blood, hairbrushes, clothing, cervical smears, etc. Advancements in the extraction of mitochondrial DNA also guide in the identification process. Odontology provides reliable input in age assessment with an approximate accuracy of 1.6 years, while utilizing newer techniques including aspartic acid racemization and translucent dentine. Bite mark identification needs to be immediate, if coupled with DNA identification, it eliminates subjectivity, and cross-matching with suspects guides a criminal investigation in cases such as rape attempts, child abuse, etc. The above-mentioned critical issues taken together classify forensic odontology in disaster victim identification into three basic categories: (i) examination and evaluation of teeth and oral tissue injuries; (ii) examination of marks to enable subsequent elimination or identification of suspect as a perpetrator; and (iii) detailed examination of dental remains including fragments, complete teeth and dental restorations from the deceased for post-mortem–ante-mortem data comparison. The methodology is widely accepted and has been practised for centuries, thus is an important tool in disaster victim identification (Kinra, 2006).

The identification is initiated with visual identification, odontology, pre-existing disorders, post-mortem and ante-mortem comparisons and DNA-based processes – a combination of such methodologies both in parallel and sequentially can avoid confusion and prevent delays.

Social issues also limit the rate of operations during post-disaster scenarios. Management of the dead is generally linked to religious beliefs, e.g. the dead should be buried within 24 h or should be cremated in daytime only, or should not be buried, or should be buried only on ancestral land (remote areas) and many other microvariants as per various cultural values. A degree of knowledge of such aspects needs to be made available to teams to avoid unrest in the targeted community (Bhardwaj *et al.*, 2007).

Human resources and logistics for management of the dead and missing

Human resources and logistics are another challenge in the management of the dead and missing. Trained human resources are often in short supply and supportive equipment for recovery and transportation to storage sites requires a large number of vehicles. It is essential to have facilities for storage, and associated human resources for its proper maintenance. The private sector is required to be integrated to develop infrastructure for managing MCIs. There is an urgent need to have an adequate number of teams of pathologists to carry out post-mortems and supportive trained teams to collect ante-mortem data. In addition, a group of analysts for comparative analysis utilizing advanced decision-making tools can speed up the process. The probable use of the IT sector for error checking is of paramount importance to hasten the identification process. Mobile sample collectors and disaster victim identification cells (including DNA fingerprinting) with trained manpower need to be developed. Identification of trained escorts or police teams for handing over of bodies to relatives, with contingency provisions to provide material support to relatives, e.g. transportation and guidance in documentation, etc. is also needed (Knight, 1996).

Management of contaminated dead bodies

Management of contaminated dead bodies poses various challenges. These include fear of getting contaminated or being infected by diseases held by the dead body. The fear of chemical and radiological contamination can be mitigated by using appropriate protective clothing while managing such contaminated bodies, and decontaminating them prior to disposal. However, in the case of airborne infection, in addition to protective clothing, these dead bodies should be incinerated at a significantly higher temperature so that the infective agent is destroyed. Another aspect with contaminated bodies is an administrative issue linked to return back to the concerned relatives. During an MCI, it is expected that resources will not be adequate to provide necessary assistance in decontamination and then monitor the burial or cremation of the dead by the relatives. Thus, during such events, the district collector can exercise his or her emergency powers to carry out temporary burials; however, mass cremation is not recommended as it precludes the possibility of identification in the long term. During events involving lesser numbers of casualties, proper identification and decontamination procedures should be followed prior to burial or cremation under strict monitoring conditions. However, in the case of bioterrorism activity with airborne infection, such practices should not be permitted, standard disposal procedures should be practised after taking adequate evidence of identification. The above-mentioned procedures are additional to the various basic operations that are routinely practised for non-contaminated dead bodies at the hospital level (Ripmeester, 2005).

Lessons from the Great East Japan Earthquake

Japan was hit by a powerful earthquake and tsunami in March 2011, causing loss of many lives and severely devastating the coastal regions (Arora, 2011). Following the disaster, the management of the dead during the 2011 Japan megadisasters was a big issue as the number of people that died was huge. During interviews with some of the Japanese experts taken in Japan by one of the authors of this chapter during May and June 2013, it was revealed that the administration decided to bury the dead bodies there on the disaster site as there was no other option in view of the unprecedented level of the disaster; after a period of 3 months, when the debris was cleared, a formal funeral was held for the dead. This was a practical solution that they utilized to manage the dead under trying circumstances. It becomes essential to cremate the bodies in time, otherwise there is a risk of spread of infections. Infectious disease surveillance assumes importance under such conditions. In the aftermath of the 2011 Japan megadisasters, gastroenteritis cases were found only sporadically and not epidemically. However, in developing nations this can be a major problem.

In Iwate, Miyagi and Fukushima prefectures, which were the worst affected along the Pacific coast of the north-eastern part of Honshu, the main island of Japan, body remains of a large number of victims (more than 15,000) were recovered and nearly 90% of the victims were positively identified. DNA profiling was established in some cases and more extensive identification attempted using a computer-assisted dental comparison system and kinship analysis of DNA profiles (Kubo, 2012).

One problem faced in taking direct overseas help in identification of bodies of victims was the language barrier. Another problem faced was reaching the spot due to damage of connectivity links. The temporary body inspection facility had to be suspended at sunset due to lack of electricity and water supply. Preparing for such problems in a disaster setting is difficult, but other provisions can be made.

The Indian National Disaster Response Force (NDRF) was sent by the Government of India to Japan. They operated in Onagawa in the aftermath of the 2011 disaster to help in rescue and relief operations. Upon extrication of dead bodies by the NDRF, they showed respect to the dead according to the Indian tradition and offered prayers, thereby creating an environment of empathy and real concern for fellow citizens of the world. This act of showing immense respect to the deceased in India was appreciated during the Japan 2011 Tōhoku earthquake and tsunami.

Lessons from the June 2013 Uttarakhand Floods Disaster (Himalayan Tsunami, India)

While this book was in final revision (June 2013), the states of Uttarakhand and Himachal Pradesh in the North of India were severely hit by heavy rainfall, unprecedented floods and landslides resulting in the loss of a large number of lives. An area of nearly 40,000 km^2 has been affected. As of 25 June 2013, more than 15,000 people have died and a large number of people are missing. Extensive damage to roads and connecting bridges has left nearly 80,000 pilgrims and tourists trapped and stranded in remote inaccessible areas. The Indian Army, Indian Air Force and Indian Navy, along with Indo-Tibetan Border Police, Border Security Force, Border Roads Organization, National Disaster Response Force, Public Works Department and local administrations, NGOs and other agencies are relentlessly participating in the response missions. Unfortunately, a number of people, estimated to be in the thousands, have perished.

Officials of the Uttarakhand State Government along with forensic experts, sub-divisional magistrates and police officials have started an operation to identify dead bodies and, in cases where this is not possible, preserve their DNA, as officials admit that several of the bodies have decomposed beyond identification. Particularly in Gaurikund and Kedarnath region, several bodies had decomposed and stood no chance of being identified. A large number of people perished in the region as a result of cold, sickness, lack of water and food, after surviving the deluge. Inaccessibility to several areas has impeded rescue missions, which are still in progress at the time of writing. It is therefore anticipated that a large number of dead bodies will be found in the coming days and months. The state government is making all-out efforts to preserve whatever personal belongings they are able to find, along with preservation of DNA for establishing their identities.

A large-scale disaster of this kind, which has been branded as the 'Himalayan tsunami', poses problems in a country where a lot of religious significance is attached to disposal of the dead bodies. The government agencies and priests of the region plan a mass cremation of the hundreds of victims 1 week after the tragedy. It is imperative to preserve the DNA of the dead for future identification.

Human resources need to be sensitively trained for such eventualities, doing the needful in times of disasters, yet at the same time respecting the dead and the feelings of the families and the communities. If we adopt the age-old Indian concept of Vasudhaiva Kutumbakam – the world is a family – we would definitely learn to respect humans and all living beings not only in life, but also in death.

Conclusions

To conclude, it is essential to dispel myths associated with the management of the dead. The most common belief is that dead bodies cause epidemics; however, this is not true for either humans or animals. The surviving population on the other hand, is more likely to spread diseases further. Any processes involved in management of the dead need to comply with humanitarian principles and cultural values. The process should be adopted in accordance with the locally prevalent local customs, traditions, practices and regulations. It is necessary to maintain a sympathetic attitude towards the bereaved families under all circumstances. A body should only be released: (i) when identification is certain; (ii) by the responsible authority; and (iii) with a letter or a death certificate. Ambulances should not be used to transport the dead as they are more useful for transportation of sick and injured people. Separation of vehicles for both purposes reduces social and psychological trauma and allows the community to restore its resilience towards disasters.

Acknowledgements

The authors are grateful to several of their colleagues for help in multifarious ways. The views expressed are those of the authors and not necessarily those of their respective organizations. Preeti Arora is grateful to Japan Institute for Labour Policy and Training (JILPT) for award of a Visiting Researcher position and for sponsoring her visit to the Tōhoku region, which was badly affected during the 2011 Japan megadisasters.

References

Ajmani, M.L. (1998) *Embalming – Principles and Legal Aspects*. Jaypee Publishers, Delhi, pp. 81–91.

Arora, P. (2011) The 2011 Tōhoku earthquake and tsunami of Japan: Lessons learnt and implications for effective disaster management. Dissertation submitted to the Center for Disaster Management Studies, Guru Gobind Singh University, Kashmere Gate, Delhi, p. 156.

Arora, R., Basu, M., Chawla, R., Goel, R., Kaushik, A., Kaushik, V., Ravishanker, L., Syed Raza, K., Rakesh, K.S., Silambarasan, M., Tripathi, R.P. and Vijayaraghavan, R. (2010) CBRN casualties management in hospitals. In: Sharma, R.K., Chawla, R. and Tripathi, R.P. (eds) *A Publication of Division of Chemical, Biological, Radiological and Nuclear Defence (CBRN)*. Institute of Nuclear Medicine and Allied Science (INMAS), DRDO, Delhi, p. 177.

Bhardwaj, J.R., Chawla, R. and Sharma, R.K. (2007) Chemical disaster management: current status and perspectives. *Journal of Scientific Industrial Research* 66, 110–119.

Bhardwaj, R.J., Sharma, R.K., Khanna, B.K., Kumar, S. and Chawla, R. (eds) (2010) *Chemical (Industrial) Mock Exercises: Good Practices and Lessons Learnt.* National Disaster Management Authority, Government of India, New Delhi.

Binz, M.T. (2007) Managing the dead in catastrophes: guiding principles and practical recommendations for first responders. *International Review of the Red Cross* 89, 421–442.

Government of India (2007) National disaster management guidelines – medical preparedness and mass casualty management. National Disaster Management Authority, Government of India, New Delhi.

Government of India (2010) National disaster management guidelines – psychosocial support and mental health services. National Disaster Management Authority, Government of India, New Delhi.

Gresham, G.A. (1979) *Postmortem Procedures.* World Medical Publications Ltd, London, pp. 16–28.

Kinra, P. (2006) The use of mitochondrial DNA and short tandem repeat typing in the identification of air crash victims. *Indian Journal of Aerospace Medicine* 50, 54–65.

Knight, B. (1996) *Forensic Pathology*, 2nd edn. Arnold Publishers, London, p. 10.

Kubo, S.I. (2012) Great East Japan Earthquake. Postmortem examinations and personal identifications of victims. *Rechtsmedizin* 22, 12–16.

Leung, C.K.K. (2008) Forensic odontology. *Dental Bulletin* 13, 16–20.

Morgan, O., Binz, M.T. and Alphen, D.V. (2006) *Management of Dead Bodies after Disasters: a Field Manual for First Responders.* PAHO, Washington, DC.

Pan American Health Organization (PAHO) (2004) *Management of Dead Bodies in Disaster Situations*. PAHO, Washington, DC.

Parikh, C.K. (1985) *Medico Legal Postmortems in India*. Medical Publications, Bombay, India, pp. 157–160.

Polson, C.J. (1985) *The Eessentials of Forensic Medicine*, 4th edition. Pergamon Press, Oxford, UK, pp. 677–694.

Ripmeester, N. (2005) Handle with care. *Graduate Recruiter* 22.

Chapter 33

Disaster Management: The Socioeconomic Dimension

Kai-Lit Phua

Introduction

The World Health Organization's (WHO) definition of disaster is 'any occurrence that causes damage, ecological disruption, loss of human life, or deterioration of health and health services on a scale sufficient to warrant an extraordinary response from outside the affected community or area' (WHO, 1999). Disasters can be broadly categorized as natural disasters, technological disasters and human-induced disasters. These are not mutually exclusive since the occurrence of one type of disaster can result in a secondary disaster of another type, e.g. a natural disaster such as a major flood spreading toxic waste widely from an industrial waste dump site into surrounding areas (technological disaster).

Hogan and Burstein said that disaster medicine is related to emergency medicine and public health and deals with the:

> health and medical and emotional issues of disaster casualties. To provide care efficiently, however, the health care provider must be familiar with several elements of disaster management, including planning, mitigation, assessment, response, and recovery (Hogan and Burstein, 2007, p. 2).

Because of this, awareness and understanding of the socioeconomic factors associated with disasters is helpful. Disasters not only affect the health and well-being of individuals and their family members, but can also disrupt the community and larger society they live in for extended periods of time (Phua, 2006, 2008). Health professionals working in the area of disaster medicine should be aware of both short-term and long-term health effects and that these can be magnified or mitigated because of underlying social factors (broadly defined). These social factors include: the pre-disaster political situation, including the effectiveness of the civil service bureaucracy; the economic resources available to the individuals and families living in the community and larger society; pre-existing social tensions, social cleavages and the resulting degree of social solidarity; and cultural norms affecting cooperative behaviour.

Before a disaster strikes

The WHO Regional Office for South-east Asia's document 'Benchmarking emergency preparedness: emergency and humanitarian action' came out with an elaborate list of benchmarks pertaining to emergency and disaster preparedness (WHO, 2007, p. 8). These include:

- Legal framework, active coordinating mechanism and existing organizational structure;
- Regular updates of disaster preparedness and emergency planning;
- Emergency financial, physical and human resources;
- Rules of engagement for external humanitarian organizations;
- Community planning, with risk identification;
- Community-based preparedness, with training, regular simulations and mock drills;
- Local capacity for emergency provision of essential goods and services;
- Good disaster awareness on the part of the public through education and effective use of mass communications;
- Capacity to identify risks and assess vulnerability at all levels;
- Adequate human resources;
- Health facilities built or modified to withstand disasters;
- Early warning and surveillance system in place.

Limpakarnjanarat and Ofrin (2009) note that the United Nations' International Strategy for Disaster Reduction mentions preparedness, prevention, recovery, relief/response and mitigation as part of a cycle. They elaborated on this by mentioning that the cycle and its phases should be considered in terms of managing risks such that there is reduction of vulnerability of individuals and communities, enhanced preparedness, increased relief/response capacity (including local capacity and coordination during or immediately after the event) and increased resilience in post-disaster recovery of communities.

How can social factors affect these phases and, more specifically, the 12 WHO benchmarks? If a country's political leadership does not prioritize disaster management and emergency preparedness, then an active coordinating mechanism and effective organizational structure to handle disasters is unlikely to function effectively or even exist. This would, in turn, affect disaster preparedness and emergency planning. Cuba has one of the developing world's most effective disaster mitigation programmes because of the commitment of top Cuban political leaders to the challenge. This is indicated by the fact that only 28 lives were lost in the 13 hurricanes and tropical storms that struck Cuba from 2001 to 2007 (Mesa, 2008). Steps taken in the programme include the training of health professionals in disaster medicine (with special periodic updating of knowledge and skills of the Henry Reeve Team of Medical Specialists in Disasters and Epidemics), and the provision of disaster planning leadership for specific kinds of disasters (Mesa, 2008).

Financial, physical and human resources need to be allocated and distributed (including geographically) in order to prepare for disasters. In countries where corruption is a significant problem, this would have a negative impact on proper resource allocation and distribution. Corruption would result in significant 'leakages' of financial resources allocated to disaster preparedness programmes. Public sector health personnel in countries where corruption is a major problem may be absent from their posts when disaster strikes because they are engaging in unauthorized private practice, stocks of medical supplies essential for emergency relief may be low or missing because they have been pilfered for sale on the black market, and so on.

In countries where citizens have low levels of trust in the public authorities, citizen participation in community planning would be unenthusiastic at best and non-existent at worst. This would likely be the case in countries with repressive, authoritarian governments where there is great psychological distance between ruling elites and the ordinary citizenry, and the governments are perceived as being unconcerned about the welfare of ordinary people.

Countries that are very poor – such as some of the sub-Saharan countries in Africa and certain countries in Central America and the Caribbean – would not have much local capacity for the emergency provision of essential goods and services. A major disaster would quickly overwhelm the capacity of the community or even the national government to cope with the problem. The Haiti earthquake of 2010 is a good example. In countries where the literacy rate is low and many people are poor, promoting disaster awareness through educational channels and through effective use of mass communications would be a major challenge. Printed material would reach only the functionally literate. The illiterate will need to be reached using radio, television and newer media such as compact discs. This would be affected by the level of individual or community ownership of suitable electrical and electronic equipment (and other factors such as proper supply of electricity and affordable batteries).

The challenge of ensuring adequate human resources to deal with disasters is a major one in developing countries. The most obvious in the area of disaster medicine would be enough health personnel (such as paramedics, doctors and nurses trained in emergency medicine, mental health workers and public health experts) as well as adequate health facilities to handle mass casualties and to prevent subsequent disease outbreaks. In many developing countries – especially the poorer ones – inadequate numbers of health personnel (especially in areas of lower priority such as mental health) are compounded by lopsided geographical distribution and by emigration of health personnel to richer nations. Some are also affected by the problem of significant numbers of health personnel sickened by and dying of HIV/AIDS (Tawfik and Kinoti, 2006).

Ideally, health facilities should be built or modified to withstand disasters. However, due to corruption and lax enforcement, health facilities may be built in a substandard manner with significant violation of building codes. Thus, when a disaster such as an earthquake strikes, the health facilities may be destroyed or rendered non-functional. Personnel working within a health facility that does not meet the standard set by the building code may themselves be at high risk of being seriously injured or even killed during an earthquake.

The lack of an effective early warning system can result in unnecessary suffering and death. One good example is the 2004 Boxing Day tsunami in the Indian Ocean that killed people in areas far away from the epicentre (such as Sri Lanka and parts of East Africa). This was in spite of the fact that authorities knew that tsunami waves had already reached and struck Western and Northern Sumatra and that it would take some time for the killer waves to reach more distant shores.

When a disaster strikes

Hogan and Burstein (2007) mention what to look out for and what can go wrong when a disaster strikes. They mention the 'geographical effect', whereby the health facilities closest to the scene of the disaster will be the most affected by arrival of casualties. The closest facilities may be overwhelmed while facilities that are located further away may be underutilized. This phenomenon manifested itself during the Great Hanshin earthquake that struck Kobe and surrounding areas in Japan in 1995 (Gunn, 1995). Thus, an effective system of communication needs to be in place in order to spread casualties over more health facilities, with the less serious cases transported to more distant locations. Hogan and Burstein (2007, p. 5) note that such 'actions have met with limited success, probably because they go against human nature. How many, after losing their home and means of transport, are going to be willing to be placed on a bus and taken to an unfamiliar hospital on the other side of town?'

A second effect mentioned by Hogan and Burstein (2007) is the 'dual-wave phenomenon', where the first wave of casualties who tend to be ambulatory cases (i.e. the walking wounded) is followed between 30 and 60 min later by a second wave of casualties who are more seriously hurt. The second wave consists of people who are unable to seek help at hospitals by themselves because they need to be extricated or transported by others. Thus, proper organization is necessary in order to ensure that the less seriously hurt first wave cases do not overload the accident and emergency department of hospitals at the expense of the more seriously hurt second wave cases.

A third major effect is the 'Babel effect' – meaning a serious failure of communication (Hogan and Burstein, 2007). Ordinary telephone lines and mobile telephones may become overloaded and jammed. Furthermore, landline facilities and mobile phone towers may be destroyed. The limited number of radio frequencies available to first responders may also become overwhelmed. Social factors may also come into play here, e.g. a culture of bureaucratic neglect or complacency such that equipment that has not been maintained fails to work (such as because of dead batteries), personnel who have not been properly trained to use radio equipment are unable to operate the equipment, absence of shared frequencies between various government agencies such that they are unable to communicate effectively with each other and coordinate disaster relief operations. Even worse, to add further to the confusion, different agencies may use the same code to indicate different phenomena, e.g. 'Code Black' means one thing in a particular agency and a different thing in another agency.

After the occurrence of a disaster

The fourth effect mentioned by Hogan and Burstein (2007) is the 'federation effect', whereby well-meaning individuals (both laypersons as well as voluntary medical personnel) and organizations pour into the disaster area to help but they actually hamper the disaster relief efforts of trained first responders and trained relief workers. Indeed, even the arrival of voluntary medical personnel 'may be both a blessing and a curse. Most health care providers, particularly physicians, are accustomed to a substantial degree of control of their practice environment, and most are unfamiliar with prehospital protocols or capabilities. Such medical practice attitudes do not translate well into the chaotic environment of a disaster site' (Hogan and Burstein, 2007, p. 6). Thus, the authors recommend that (contrary to the normal human impulse to help) 'medical personnel should report to their local hospital in accordance with their hospital disaster plan. They should not report to the disaster site unless they are part of a special disaster response team that has been organized by and that trains regularly with the municipal search and rescue agency' (Hogan and Burstein, 2007, p. 6).

Donated supplies pouring in from outside may also give rise to significant problems, i.e. sorting, storage, distribution and other logistical challenges. Concerned outsiders need to know that donation of money is usually the most helpful and that donations of other material may actually hamper disaster relief operations. Donated disaster relief funds need to be properly managed and with proper accountability for how they are spent. Otherwise, there would be accusations or suspicions of improper spending or improper distribution of relief funds amongst victims of disaster, e.g. as in the case of funds raised from members of the public by a leading political party, supposedly to help the victims of the Nipah virus disaster that struck Malaysian pig-farming communities in the late 1990s (Phua, 2010).

The economic cost of a disaster may be significant, with diversion of scarce resources from other sectors of the economy as a matter of necessity. Rehabilitation costs may also be high in the case of massive infrastructural or environmental damage. As for the public health impact, Noji (2007) mentions disruptions to water supply, excreta disposal, vector control programmes, immunization programmes, basic medical services, and so on. These may increase the risk of disease epidemics in the aftermath of the disaster, e.g. the cholera outbreak in Haiti after the recent earthquake. Crowding in refugee camps may also increase the risk of diseases and conditions such as respiratory infections, measles and even physical and sexual assault.

Social factors mentioned by Noji include the fact that the authorities need to put into place quickly a good system of water supply and excreta disposal. The disaster relief and public health authorities need to know that malnutrition, diarrhoeal diseases, measles, acute respiratory infections and malaria are the greatest threats to the health of disaster victims and should respond accordingly and quickly. There is evidence that giving responsibility to female heads of households to control distribution of relief supplies (especially food) will 'ensure more equitable apportionment of relief items' (Noji, 2007, p. 42).

The so-called Sphere standards for disaster relief with their key indicators for water supply and sanitation, nutrition, food aid, shelter and site management, and health services (Sphere Project, 2004) are useful and comprehensive, but social factors will affect whether they are met adequately.

Summary and Conclusion

Social factors can result in non-fulfilment of the 12 benchmarks as presented in the WHO Regional Office for South-east Asia's document 'Benchmarking emergency preparedness: emergency and humanitarian action' (WHO, 2007). Social factors can also affect the success of disaster management and emergency relief operations even if most of the benchmarks are already in place at satisfactory levels, e.g. if well-meaning people from outside the disaster area and from overseas attempt to assist by pouring into the area in large numbers but they are not properly managed by local authorities. This is also the case with unsolicited donations of physical goods that may give rise to severe logistical challenges for disaster management and emergency relief personnel already in the field. Hogan and Burstein argue that layperson responders need to be properly educated and deployed so that they help rather than hinder professional pre-hospital responders. Similarly, they mention that 'it is a well-known fact that most supplies sent to disaster sites (up to 80% in some cases) intended for the use of responders are eventually lost, unused, and unrecoverable' (Hogan and Burstein, 2007, p. 6).

Earlier, it has been mentioned that social factors that can mitigate or magnify the effects of disasters on individuals, families, communities and the larger society include the pre-disaster political situation; the economic resources available to the individuals and families living in the community and larger society; pre-existing social tensions, social cleavages and resulting degree of social solidarity; and cultural norms affecting cooperative behaviour. These social factors can also make recovery from the disaster, and rebuilding of communities, more problematic. Modified versions of the Haddon Matrix can be used to analyse the impact of these factors before, during and after the occurrence of a disaster (Table 33.1).

In the face of a disaster, some governments have responded inappropriately. Examples include the city of Chicago's initial denial of rising deaths from a heat wave in 1995 as a disaster (Tierney, 2006), the Government of China attempting to cover up the severe acute respiratory syndrome (SARS) disease outbreak (BBC News, 2004) and the reluctance of the Myanmar/Burma government to ask for foreign assistance in the aftermath of the deadly Cyclone Nargis in 2008 (BBC News, 2009).

Psychiatrists have mentioned that disasters have stronger negative effects on the mental health of high-risk individuals (and social groups) such as those directly exposed to life threat, first responders, the bereaved, the injured, single parents, children, the elderly, women, those with pre-existing psychiatric illnesses and those who lack supportive relationships (Ursano *et al.*, 2007). Sociologists have also pointed out repeatedly that disasters have differential impact on different social groups (Rodriguez and Barnshaw, 2006) and that disasters may even exacerbate further the pre-existing social tensions and social cleavages within a community (Tierney, 2006). This seems to be the case with the Hurricane Katrina disaster that struck the city of New Orleans, with accusations of racially motivated efforts (including shootings) to prevent black refugees from fleeing into neighbourhoods inhabited by whites (Thompson and McCarthy, 2010). In the aftermath of disasters, the distribution of relief supplies and other resources (including financial resources) may be discriminatory, with certain ethnic and religious groups or people from the lower classes getting less than their fair share (Rodriguez and Barnshaw, 2006; Tierney, 2006).

Wilkinson's model of the link between a high degree of income inequality and poor quality of social relations may be useful in analysing how certain groups of people may be callously neglected or ruthlessly exploited in the aftermath of disasters. The model posits that greater income inequality leads to increased social distance and a lesser sense of common identity. There is more dominance and subordination, with increased status competition and more emphasis on self-interest and material success. This in turn leads to carelessness of others' welfare coupled with aggressive exploitation of society for individual gain (Wilkinson, 2005). If Wilkinson is correct, then this would mean that in societies with a high degree of income inequality, the aftermath of disasters would be especially unpleasant for people from the lower classes. Phua (2008) has described how disaster victims may be victimized further even long after the disaster is over.

Table 33.1. Using the modified Haddon Matrix to analyse the impact of social factors on disasters.

	Political situation, e.g. corrupt and unresponsive government and civil service	**Economic situation, e.g. poor country with bad infrastructure**	**Social situation, e.g. serious social conflict (ethnic/religious; class; regional); highly unequal income/wealth distribution**	**Cultural situation, e.g. lack of civic-mindedness (due to suspicion of the government)**
Before the disaster	Lack of disaster preparedness (therefore public agencies are ill-equipped to deal with disasters)	Inadequate health facilities; widespread violation of building codes; bad roads, few airports, poor communication system	Resources that can be used for disaster are very unevenly distributed between social groups and geographical regions	Citizen participation in any disaster preparedness activities is poor
During the disaster and right after the disaster	First responders unable to deal effectively with the situation in the field	Emergency medical facilities are overwhelmed quickly; destruction of buildings – including health facilities; rescue and evacuation seriously hampered by bad roads and communication	Maldistribution of resources makes it a challenge to ensure that the social groups and regions most in need actually get access to more resources	Ordinary citizens fail to respond correctly to emergency situation; untrained layperson responders are less able to render assistance effectively
Aftermath of the disaster	Rebuilding is seriously hampered, e.g. money available for rebuilding is stolen, misallocated or misspent	Economic situation deteriorates further; danger of epidemic disease outbreaks due to food, water, sanitation and shelter problems, and public health programme disruptions; poverty of the people is worsened; mass outmigration may occur	Social tensions may be exacerbated	Distrust of the government may increase further

In conclusion, it is necessary for health professionals working in the area of disaster medicine to pay attention to social factors because these can magnify or mitigate the effects of disasters. Good governance in terms of disaster preparedness (as in Cuba), a favourable economic situation (as in rich countries struck by flood disasters such as Australia), a society with a high degree of social solidarity (such as Japan) and trust in the government (such as New Zealand with earthquakes affecting the city of Christchurch in 2010 and 2011) will help to mitigate the effects and also enable the society to have greater resilience and recover more quickly from the disaster.

References

BBC News (2004) China's SARS whistleblower freed. Available at: http://news.bbc.co.uk/2/hi/asia-pacific/3911155.stm (Accessed 1 March 2011).

BBC News (2009) UN warning over Burma cyclone aid. Available at: http://news.bbc.co.uk/2/hi/asia-pacific/8030211.stm (Accessed 1 March 2011).

Gunn, S.W.A. (1995) Health effects of earthquakes. *Disaster Prevention and Management* 4(5), 6–10.

Hogan, D.E. and Burstein, J.L. (2007) Basic perspectives on disaster. In: Hogan, D.E. and Burstein, J.L. (eds) *Disaster Medicine*, 2nd edn. Lippincott Williams & Wilkins, Philadelphia, Pennsylvania, , pp. 1–11.

Limpakarnjanarat, K. and Ofrin, R.H. (2009) Planning for and responding to public health needs in emergencies and disasters. In: Detels, R., Beaglehole, R., Lansang, M.A. and Gulliford, M. (eds) *Oxford Textbook of Public Health.* Oxford University Press, Oxford, UK, pp. 1697–1706.

Mesa, G. (2008) The Cuban health sector and disaster mitigation. *MEDICC Review* 10(3), 5–8.

Noji, E.K. (2007) Public health disasters. In: Hogan, D.E. and Burstein, J.L. (eds) *Disaster Medicine*, 2nd edition. Lippincott Williams & Wilkins, Philadelphia, Pennsylvania, pp. 40–43.

Phua, K.L. (2006) A model for lessening the negative impact of natural disasters and infectious disease outbreaks. *Journal of Emergency Management* 4(5), 69–74.

Phua, K.L. (2008) Post-disaster victimization: how survivors of disasters can continue to suffer after the event is over. *New Solutions* 18(2), 221–231.

Phua, K.L. (2010) The Nipah virus outbreak in Malaysia and its aftermath. *Journal of Emergency Management* 8(1), 77–80.

Rodriguez, H. and Barnshaw, J. (2006) The social construction of disasters: from heat waves to worst-case scenarios. *Contemporary Sociology* 35(3), 218–223.

Sphere Project (2004) Humanitarian charter and minimum standards in disaster response. Sphere Project, Geneva. Available at: http://www.sphereproject.org/content/view/27/84/lang,english/ (Accessed 2 March 2011).

Tawfik, L. and Kinoti, S.N. (2006) The impact of HIV/AIDS on the health workforce in developing countries. WHO, Geneva. Available at: http://www.who.int/hrh/documents/Impact_of_HIV.pdf (Accessed 1 March 2011).

Thompson, A.C. and McCarthy, B. (2010) New clues emerge in post-Katrina vigilante shooting at Algiers Point. Available at: http://www.commondreams.org/headline/2010/04/12-5 (Accessed 1 March 2011).

Tierney, K. (2006) Foreshadowing Katrina: recent sociological contributions to vulnerability science. *Contemporary Sociology* 35(3), 207–212.

Ursano, R.J., Fullerton, C.S., Weisaeth, L. and Raphael, B. (2007) Individual and community responses to disasters. In: Ursano, R.J., Fullerton, C.S., Weisaeth, L. and Raphael, B. (eds) *Textbook of Disaster Psychiatry*. Cambridge University Press, New York, pp. 3–26.

Wilkinson, R.G. (2005) *The Impact of Inequality: How to Make Sick Societies Healthier.* Routledge, London.

World Health Organization (WHO) (1999) Community emergency preparedness: a manual for managers and policy-makers. WHO, Geneva.

WHO, Regional Office for South-east Asia (2007) Benchmarking emergency preparedness: emergency and humanitarian action. WHO, New Delhi. Available at: http://www.searo.who.int/entity/emergencies/documents/9789290223122/en/ (Accessed 1 March 2011).

Chapter 34

Fostering Disaster-resilient Communities through Educating Children and Women for Disaster Preparedness, Response and Recovery in Developing Countries

Yasamin O. Izadkhah and Mahmood Hosseini

Introduction

Based on the United Nations International Strategy for Disaster Reduction (UNISDR) definition, there is no such thing as a 'natural' disaster, only natural hazards. Disaster risk reduction (DRR) aims to reduce the damage caused by natural hazards including earthquakes and floods through prevention. DRR comprises disaster management, disaster mitigation and disaster preparedness, but DRR is also part of sustainable development. In order for development activities to be sustainable they must also reduce disaster risk. On the other hand, unsound development policies will increase disaster risk – and disaster losses. Thus, 'DRR involves every part of society, every part of government, and every part of the professional and private sector' (UNISDR, 2011).

In recent years, 'Community-Based Disaster Preparedness' (CBDP) and training has been declared to be one the most effective ways to ensure successful disaster awareness-raising in various communities. This can also be true in the case of large populated cities, composed of various small communities, where rescue activities can be hindered owing to several factors, including an inappropriate public reaction, which can create adverse situations such as disruption of urban transportation system performance.

In this chapter, first, the vulnerability of children and women are presented. Then the issues related to disaster management in developing countries are addressed. In the next section, the roles of children and women in disaster management-related activities are explained in detail. Then, the education and training issues for children and women are discussed with an emphasis on developing countries. Finally, recommendations are suggested for further studies in this regard.

Vulnerability of Children and Women in Disasters

A community starts from children, as the smallest unit of a family, expanding to various wider levels including women, etc. Although children and women are among the most vulnerable groups in society, there are some main differences between them due to their nature. On this basis, the issues with regard to the high vulnerability of these two groups are discussed separately in the next sections (see Fig. 34.1).

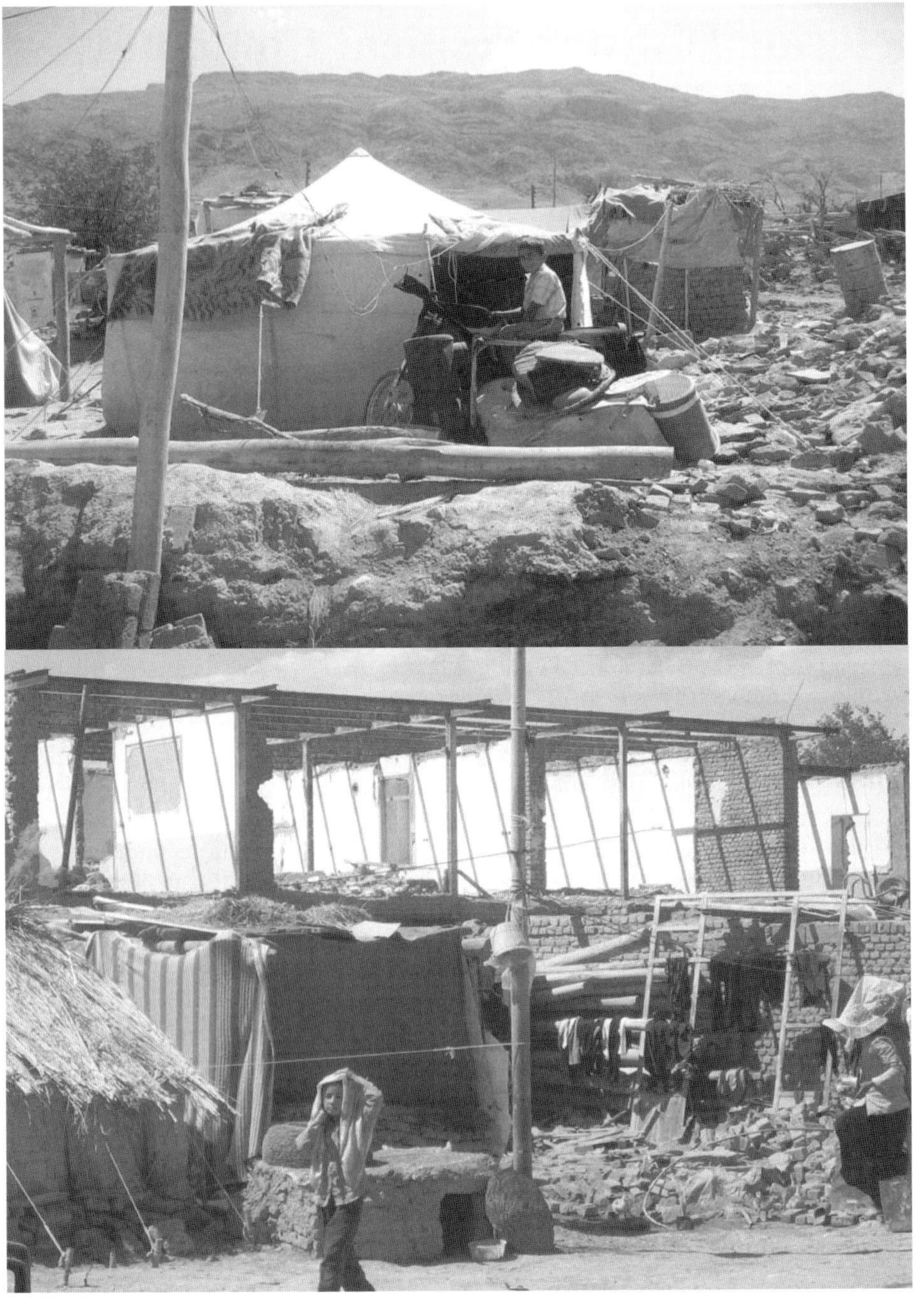

Fig. 34.1. Children and women are classified among the most vulnerable groups in disasters. (Photos: Izadkhah.)

Children

Children are recognized as one of the most vulnerable groups in society. In the years to come, children's vulnerability due to disasters is expected to increase. The impact of global warming is expected to result in up to 175 million children every year being affected by disasters brought about by climate change (IFRC World Disaster Report, 2010). In the 1988 earthquake in Armenia, children suffered more than adults because they were in school at the time of the quake. According to the Armenian National Mental Health Research Center (Miller *et al.*, 1993) almost two-thirds of the total deaths were children and adolescents. School and kindergarten buildings were inadequately designed and could not withstand such a devastating force (Allan, 1989; Noji, 1989; Pomonis, 1990; Hadjian, 1993). In the Bam earthquake, 2003, approximately 10,000 students out of 32,433 died. A total of 1000 teachers out of 3400 died and 131 schools out of 168 were destroyed (Ghafory-Ashtiany *et al.*, 2006). Therefore, there is a need to secure their lives in future disasters. In this regard, educating children, as the future of any community at risk, is an effective strategy to communicate safety messages to the entire community and help in reducing the rate of casualties in upcoming disasters.

Women

Women are among one of the most vulnerable groups in society. Evidence has shown that the number of women who have lost their lives in natural disasters is far more than men and therefore women are considered as one of the main victims of a disaster. For example, the 1992 floods in Bangladesh showed that due to existing traditions, cultural limitations and social prohibitions, women faced difficulties in ensuring their survival and therefore the number of casualties was high among this group (UNDP HD Report, 1995). In the December 2004 South Asian tsunami in Sri Lanka, Indonesia and India (Oxfam, 2005) as well as in the recent South Asian floods in August 2007 in Bangladesh, India and Nepal, it can be seen that many women have lost their lives due to lack of awareness and preparedness or because they faced difficulties in securing their livelihoods after the disaster (Oxfam, 2007).

It has also been recognized that women face a variety of specific hardships during and after natural disasters. Research undertaken in this regard has proved the high degree of women's interest and motivation in learning about disasters. Educating women can not only increase their capability for facing disasters, but also can benefit their families, particularly children, in many ways.

Developing Countries and Disaster Management

There are some problems that are particularly related to developing countries with regard to disaster mitigation. One is the great difference between the level of education in the capital and other cities, especially small towns. This is while, in most cases, the victims of disasters in these countries are the people living in small towns and villages.

In the following subsections, other important factors affecting disaster mitigation in developing countries are mentioned with emphasis on women's issues.

Poverty

Poverty can be defined as shortages of properties for living, including lack of means for protection against the adverse consequences of environmental change. Some 800 million people go hungry every day, and over 1 billion live on less than US$1 a day (Millennium Project, 2006). Without social, economic and scientific progress, one-third of the world's expected population of some 9 billion in the second half of the 21st century could be living in extreme poverty. Women make up two-thirds of the world's poorest people and are nearly twice as likely as men to be illiterate (UNFPA, 1999). They receive less education and less food, and have fewer legal rights. In every part of the developing world, rural and urban, women are primarily responsible for finding water and fuelwood and for the preparation of food. In rural areas, women are often responsible for the care of livestock and for tending the crops. Yet, only rarely do they have an ownership stake in the resources with which they labour.

Gender Inequality

Gender inequality in social, economic and political spheres results in vast differences between men and women in emergency communication; household decisions about use of relief assets; voluntary relief and recovery work; access to evacuation shelter and relief goods; and employment in disaster planning, relief and recovery programmes, among other areas of concern in disaster mitigation. Equal access to education, credit and land, and the enforcement of legal rights would not only benefit women as individuals, but also contribute to the environmental and economic well-being of their families and communities. When women have control over economic resources – whether land, income or credit – they are more likely than men to spend their earnings on food, clothes and other basic needs. This inequality can be classified from different aspects (Fallahi, 1998).

Inequality in education

There are still restrictions in teaching females due to traditions, expenses, early marriage and pregnancy, lack of educational materials and enough education. This can have an indirect effect on all members of the family particularly children.

Inequality in sanitation and healthcare

In spite of improvements in healthcare, the rate of death is still higher among children and women. The latter is due to the lack of sufficient attention to women's health. A mother's weak sanitation can downgrade the level of health in the whole family including in the young members of the family.

Inequality in conflict's consequences

In social conflicts such as wars and disturbances, women are usually more susceptible than men. This is basically because of their nature. In wars, due to the high rate of casualties in men, women will become single mothers and need to take care of the other members of the family. However, this threat can be considered as a source of opportunity for these groups of women which can make them more resilient to facing natural disasters in the future.

Inequality in contribution to economic projects

Although many women contribute actively to economic life in national and international decision making and important activities, they have not been asked to get involved. In some communities, religious and ethical limitations have adverse effects on the activities of women. However, women's self-employment in non-official capacities and management of small units has shown lots of achievements. Women can increase the incomes and product outputs and guarantee sustainable development. In the case of the death of the father of the family, the mother can help in maintaining the economic integrity and sustainability of the family provided that she has the required capabilities in advance.

Inequality in mass media

In spite of the remarkable expansion of the mass media in recent years, they still fail to show a real portrait of women and their value in today's world. This will indirectly limit the scope of women's presence in social activities including those related to disaster mitigation.

Rate of Illiteracy

In most countries, because of the high illiteracy levels of women, they suffer from a lack of awareness with regard to their rights. This is a big obstacle for them to benefit from their contribution in social activities, particularly in the case of disasters. In addition, although women play an important role in maintaining the environment and challenging natural disasters, due to their lack of contributions because of their insufficient knowledge about management and natural resources as well as safety against disasters, they are the first victims in disastrous events.

Population Growth

Research has shown that changes in population growth, age structure and spatial distribution interact closely with the environment and with development. Before the end of this decade, the majority of the world's population will live in urban areas. Urbanization can improve people's access to education, health and other services. However, it can also increase the vulnerability of communities subjected to natural hazards, such as earthquakes.

Cultural Limitations

Because of the local cultural problems and religious beliefs of the people living in developing countries, there is some kind of inherent resistance to every change of manner or diversion from the traditional lifestyles. This decreases the level of acceptance of newly taught materials in general, and even nullifies them in some cases. This obstacle should be overcome in any possible way. For example, it can be suggested to select specific groups of people from each area for a pre-education process. It is believed that school teachers can be the best candidates for these selected groups of people in this regard.

Lack of High-quality Management

Another important challenge in developing countries is poor management in general as well as the frequent replacements at various levels of management in all governmental bodies including disaster-related organizations. This can result in the waste of experience and knowledge gained by managers who have been replaced by a new managerial body. Among the existing deficiencies in this regard, three are more important as follows.

Weakness in emergency management

In many developing countries, managers do not have the related educational background appropriate to their posts; for example, most of the ministers and their deputies are engineers. Therefore, they have not received any specific training for emergency management. Furthermore, there are also some difficulties that can hinder the training process for emergency managers such as insufficient time to train emergency managers mostly due to their daily commitments, lack of appropriate and adequate background knowledge, expertise and experience in emergency management issues, etc. (Hosseini and Izadkhah, 2010). In addition, there are very few females in managerial positions. This is while the number of female casualties in a disaster is generally greater than the number of males.

Lack of assessment

One of the most important factors for improving management quality is assessment. Regular assessment of the effectiveness of all awareness programmes is a necessity. This can be achieved through systematic planning by the involved organizations and related ministries for each of the various disaster awareness programmes that are implemented. When appropriately accomplished, the results of the assessments lead to improved implementation of new and updated initiatives (Hosseini and Izadkhah, 2007).

Lack of documentation

Unfortunately, in many developing countries, there is not much attention paid to the documentation in programmes and projects, including those documents related to disaster mitigation plans and activities. This can therefore result in losing useful experience and know-how gained during the previous management period. In addition, when technical drawings and other related documents are not kept by the authorities, any future evaluation of buildings and facilities for their upgrading or rehabilitation requires new measurements and testing to obtain the corresponding technical specifications. This usually imposes additional costs and requires more time for risk mitigation activities.

Lack of Enough Technological Tools

Another problem in developing countries is the lack of availability of the internet and other information dissemination tools. In a paper by the authors of this chapter, the use of internet communication in increasing earthquake disaster awareness and preparedness has been discussed as a proposed solution for more efficient use of technological tools for disaster mitigation (Izadkhah and Hosseini, 2004). It is evident that the necessity for the contribution of developed countries to developing ones to increase availability is very effective in increasing the capabilities of developing countries to face disasters. In fact, this can be much more effective than the aid given to these countries after a disaster such as a devastating earthquake. It is worth mentioning that lack of technological tools is also crucial in rural areas, where most casualties are recorded. Also, weakness of transportation and communication systems can hinder the emergency response activities after a disaster.

Roles of Children in Disaster Management Issues

In the next sections, the roles that children can play in disaster-related activities as well as in promoting a safety culture are discussed briefly:

Promoting a disaster safety culture

In many developing countries, a large percentage of the population is of school age. Children can communicate the messages they have learned about public safety to their parents, their relatives, their neighbours and to family friends. Through this 'trickle-down' process of dissemination, the wider society may be touched by an effective school safety curriculum. Therefore, if awareness-raising educational programmes for children are effective, then the message is communicated to a broad spectrum of citizens in many communities, making them prepared. However, due to the physical limitations of young children, they are not expected to participate in disaster response and relief activities related to disasters. Nevertheless, children as the next generation of a society can be very useful in learning about disaster-related issues and transferring this knowledge to their families and the wider community.

Other disaster-related activities

Depending on the age of the children, they have different capabilities to cope with disasters and responsibilities in disaster-related issues and activities. Based on this, three categories can be considered:

- Preschoolers;
- School children (7–12 years);
- Young adults (13–18 years).

At preschool level, two things will need to be taught: one is the definition of an earthquake and the other is how to shelter in the event of a disaster. As mentioned earlier, at this age children are not expected to provide any help to their families. They can, however, transfer the messages they learn to the other members of their family. This knowledge can stay with them for years and will automatically upgrade the development of safety in the community.

At school age, children can gradually take care of some roles in disaster risk reduction. Allocating these roles to children may not only speed up the progress of the activities, but also reduce their fear and anxiety in the event of a disaster. Their responsibility can include what they will be asked to do by their parents and/or teachers in order to help the family or other groups of people in disasters. For example, in spite of the high vulnerability of children in this age group, cases have been observed in which they have been useful after a disaster in helping their families. An example can be seen in Fig. 34.2.

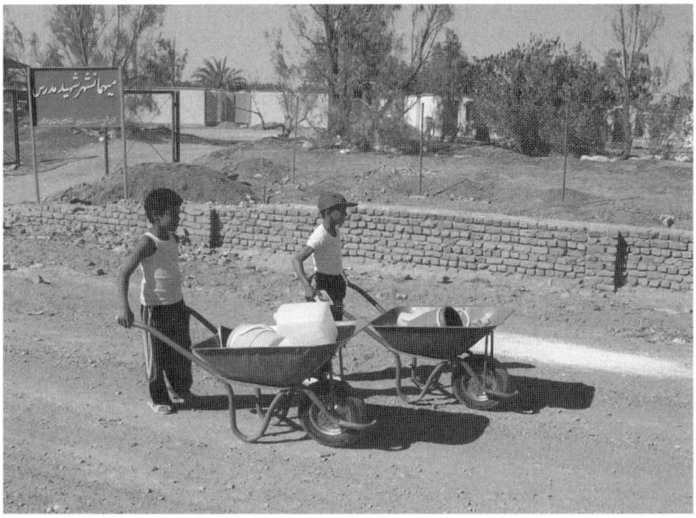

Fig. 34.2. Children help their families after Bam earthquake. (Photo: Izadkhah.)

With regard to young adults, they can play more significant roles in coping with disasters. They can help with planning, decision making and particularly the execution of response activities. They can also help their younger brothers and sisters as well as their grandparents during and immediately after the disaster. It is worth mentioning that with all the help that children can provide in disasters, their assistance will still be less than that from other groups of society.

Roles of Women in Disaster Management Activities

In spite of existing evidence of women's vulnerability to natural disasters, they have shown their capabilities in various activities such as involvement in different stages of the disaster management cycle, resettlement, as well as cooperation in design, decision making and planning for disasters. It is evident that the key role of women in creating a safety culture in a family is crucial, since without convincing the women in a family, other members are not usually capable of following any specific issues related to the whole family.

In addition, research has shown that women are interested in participating in relief activities such as emergency aid alongside men and, most of the time, women can even carry this through independently. For example, in the Iran Manjil-Roudbar earthquake in 1990, most of the families where the wife of the house had survived the disaster were managed perfectly and children's matters were handled properly, temporary houses were built and the overall routine of life went on systematically (Shadi Talab, 1994). Also, after 30 September 1993, in Lature in the south-west of India, a network consisting of 3500 women from the self-drive groups worked on the basic and urgent needs of the affected community such as securing livelihoods, providing water, food and sanitation, healthcare and education (UNISDR India, 2007). In Turkey, after the Izmit earthquake, 'Women and Children Centres' were established in the north-west of the country, which were used as centres for offering services to society and for various other activities (UNISDR Turkey, 2007). Following the Darb-e-Astaneh earthquake in March 2006, women played an important role in the reconstruction process. With regard to emotional support to their families, women are very effective and they also cooperate in various issues such as gathering food, water and fuel. Their effective role in maintaining livelihoods has been recorded as very typical (Hosseini and Izadkhah, 2006). For example, after the Java earthquake in May 2006, women were very active. They worked alongside men in temporary shelters, participated actively in the team work, distributed materials and offered emotional assistance (UNISDR Indonesia, 2007).

There is no need to emphasize that women have a significant role in promoting a disaster safety culture as a mother in the family, as a trainer in the community and as an expert in the disaster management field. In the next section, the roles of women in various phases of disaster mitigation will be addressed separately.

Preparedness phase

Women have demonstrated that they can play a crucial role in the development of a disaster safety culture in society, and can use their capabilities at various stages to assist with managing a disaster. One of women's main activities in earthquake risk reduction is to learn about disasters and their consequences. They should attend related classes and courses regularly and assist in extending the disaster safety culture in home, at work and within the whole community. Sharing and exchanging information and experiences within the family, neighbours and relatives is one of the best ways to expand the seismic safety culture in a society. This neighbourhood network is a method that is very popular in rural areas in Iran between various women societies, and needs to be strengthened in urban areas. Women should use mass media, information technology and educational materials in order to gain the necessary knowledge of disasters and also to try to disseminate this knowledge to the members of various groups in their society.

Some women in the community who have been educated in issues related to disasters are therefore directly engaged in disaster management activities. The cooperation of expert women in education, research and developing comprehensive programmes and activities on disaster risk reduction for various levels of society especially women and children is of great importance. Other women should be given the strength to participate in design, decision making and planning in disaster risk reduction issues. In addition, they should cooperate in research related to economic, cultural, social, environmental and emotional fields in order to identify the vulnerable areas of society and to use the outputs in conducting and implementing appropriate programmes in disaster risk reduction. In many countries, female members of parliament and those with senior positions in the government can act as decision makers and planners in disaster risk reduction issues.

Emergency response

Women, along with men, play a crucial role in emergencies. Women are the first to provide nursing care to the most affected family members whether the disaster is a flash flood or an earthquake, hours before any official relief work begins. Along with the task of providing immediate care, women also take the necessary steps to find food, water and fuel to prepare for the emergency needs of their families. It is evident that the greatest responsibility for immediate rehabilitation also lies with the community members, once temporary relief ends. Again, women can contribute in a variety of ways, alongside their regular routines of preparing food, collecting water, etc. In some developing countries, which have a high number of female nurses, their key and effective roles are automatically highlighted, particularly to assist in the immediate aftermath of disasters.

Recovery and reconstruction

The first days after a disaster are a difficult period for vulnerable groups. They face many problems such as shortages of food, inappropriate nutrition, lack of enough sanitation facilities, insect bites and also mental problems. Women can learn about the health issues and attend first aid classes and courses in order to assist in maintaining health in the environment, the work place and society, as well as personal and family health. Food shortages increase the vulnerability of children and the elderly after a disaster. In this regard, the role of women is very important in producing food and emergency needs in order to prevent malnutrition. This is particularly important in countries with a high percentage of young children and a high rate of population growth. Women can therefore help in preparing and distributing food among children and the elderly, and help injured and affected people in the days after the disaster.

Evidence has proved that women are capable of managing and handling the aforementioned issues, especially providing psychological support to their families and friends after the disasters. For example, in developing countries, since most of the women are housewives, there is more opportunity for training women in order to equip them with awareness of what to do before and in the aftermath of disasters.

As in many disasters in the past, women play a crucial role in all phases of the disaster management cycle, especially in the reconstruction phase (Yonder *et al.*, 2005). In many earthquakes, there has been evidence that women were effective in reconstruction issues, even the physical work. An example can be shown after the Silakhore earthquake in Lorestan (Fig. 34.3).

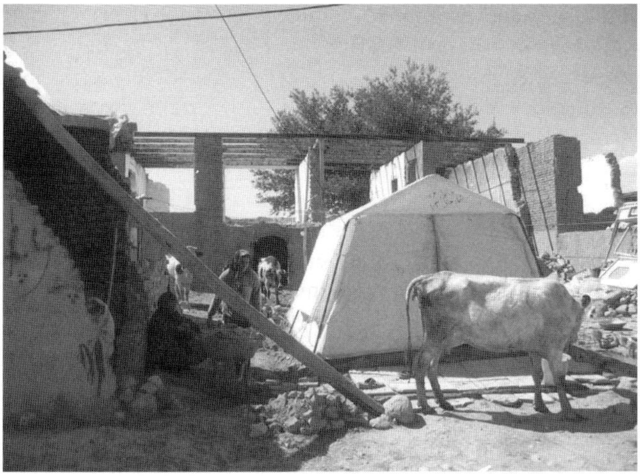

Fig. 34.3. Women help in reconstruction after the Silakhore earthquake. (Photo: Izadkhah.)

Disaster Education and Training

In the next section, a brief background on education and training in disasters is provided. Then education of children and training of women is emphasized and related issues are explained separately.

Background

Over the past decade, there has been a rapid growth in formal and informal attempts to promote learning about disaster threats in order to increase public knowledge and change behavioural patterns to protect lives. Therefore, education and training are recognized as being among the most practical means of enhancing community preparedness and disaster mitigation. Education is the fundamental 'bedrock' of disaster risk reduction.

Disaster education has been implemented effectively in some areas for many years. For example, in the USA, the American Red Cross has a long history of educating the public about natural and technological hazards and about ways to reduce the effects of these hazards on people and their properties. Although printed documents are rarely available, there is evidence of developed public awareness materials from the 1950s onwards. In the 1980s, the responsibility for developing and disseminating disaster safety information was spread. For example, the Federal Emergency Management Agency (FEMA) Earthquake Program wrote and disseminated earthquake-related materials for the people in the 1980s (Lopes, 2001). There is a section on issues in 'earthquake education' in the technical report prepared by the Multi-disciplinary Center for Earthquake Engineering Research (MCEER), formerly the National Center for Earthquake Engineering Research (NCEER), covering articles and case studies relating to earthquake education in general and particularly in the school curriculum (Izadkhah,

2004). At present, the need for greater community disaster preparedness is receiving increasing attention from governments, United Nations (UN) agencies and non-governmental organizations (NGOs), and the emphasis on earthquake education and training is growing.

In Iran, disaster educational activities have been undertaken by various organizations such as the Red Crescent Society of Iran, the National Committee for Disaster Risk Reduction in Ministry of Affairs, the Natural Disaster Center Management, the Tehran Disaster Prevention and Management Centre, Kerman Centre for Disaster, etc., and NGOs such as the Earthquake Hazard Reduction Society of Iran, Mojepishro, etc. The International Institute of Earthquake Engineering and Seismology (IIEES) has attached great importance to public education. The main objectives of the IIEES education department are to expand the safety culture, prevention and earthquake preparedness in all levels of society using all applied research and educational methods (www.iiees.ac.ir).

CBDP and training has also been one the most effective ways for successful disaster awareness-raising in various communities. CBDP is a process in which training for capacity building is one of the major components. Different modules for CBDP are being run by different players like government organizations (GOs), NGOs, multilateral/bilateral organizations and institutes in collaboration with one another as well with other allied agencies. Training forms a vital component of all activities and it requires not only imparting knowledge, but also development of skills and a change in attitudes of the participants. However, such an investment in the development of human resources can only be sustained to the extent that the value of risk reduction is institutionalized. A community should be ready to accept the management of hazards as a way of life and prevent them from becoming disasters (Walia, 2008).

Regarding the important roles of children and women in disaster mitigation discussed in previous sections, education is a key factor in increasing their capabilities to play their roles more effectively. In the following section, this is discussed in more detail.

Educating Children for Disasters

There are a number of significant reasons why children are selected as the target group for learning about disasters (Badalyan, 2003; Tinh, 2003; Izadkhah, 2004):

- Children are one of the most vulnerable groups of society;
- Children are the future of every society;
- Children are more receptive to learning than adults;
- Children have a capacity to influence their parents and can help in disseminating disaster knowledge to their immediate family and then through them to the wider community.

It is believed that schools can be used for disseminating knowledge as well as acting as an interface between those who are willing to reduce the impacts of hazards. Schools are considered as one of the 'prime vehicles for communication'. Schools are also considered as important institutions in forming the culture of a society (Shaw and Kobayashi, 2001). Furthermore, schools can be regarded as one of the ideal places for conducting earthquake awareness activities and an appropriate atmosphere and environment for the learning and transfer process, and these educational centres can be used to disseminate knowledge as well as acting as a forum for those who are willing to participate in reducing the impacts of hazards.

Nursery schools can be an ideal place for children to learn about disasters. They can then pass on to schools basic background knowledge about disasters and their consequences. Besides, safety measures in other sectors are taught to children at preschool level. Issues such as ‘how to cross a street’, ‘how to avoid eating contaminated food’, ‘how to brush teeth’ and ‘how to use dangerous utensils such as knives’ are taught by teachers using their discretion as to what is appropriate for the children. However, in recent years, the scope of teaching earthquake issues has gained a higher priority and is more controlled than the above instructions concerning everyday threats.

At the next level, schools can play a major role in the development of good citizens (Lidstone, 1999). Schools, particularly children, can contribute in developing a culture of prevention and safety. They play a vital role in the community and are considered as a very important institution in forming the culture of a society. During the International Decade for Natural Disaster Reduction (IDNDR), the strategy of supporting school disaster education was developed. The aim was to instruct students with the preparedness guidelines in disaster mitigation. The strategy also aimed to raise public awareness and education about disasters and risk reduction. The challenge was to shift to the culture of prevention through the school system. In accordance, many countries, such as Iran, Nepal, Vietnam, etc. developed strategies for supporting disaster education in schools. The purpose was to include the information that may be used for students as the next generation in order to make them the leaders in raising the awareness of their communities in the future.

Training of Women for Disasters

Women are portrayed as the victims of disaster, and their central role in response to disaster is often overlooked. A woman’s pre-disaster family responsibilities are magnified and expanded by the onset of a disaster or emergency, with significantly less support and resources. Women play a central role within the family, securing relief from emergency authorities, meeting the immediate survival needs of family members and managing temporary relocation. On this basis, training of women is very important in any disaster risk reduction programme, including those in developing countries. In urban areas, this objective can be achieved through establishing community groups of women in schools, mosques, offices, etc. and also training them as representatives to teach larger groups of the society. In rural areas, Participatory Rural Appraisal (PRA) can be used as a tool to carry out the village disaster management plans at the local level.

Education and Training Programmes and Activities

Various factors need to be considered for designing training programmes for children and women. It is necessary, though, to mention that some key topics are common, in principle, to all groups. Issues such as:

- Training materials;
- Training tools and media;

- Training time and the environment;
- Training and teaching methods.

The above-mentioned issues are discussed separately in the following sections.

Training materials

For different phases of a disaster, various materials are needed:

- Before the disaster through preparedness – *Preparedness and safety provisions*;
- During the disaster through proper sheltering – *Correct sheltering*;
- After the disaster by self-help search, rescue and relief activities – *Self-aid provisions.*

Training materials should address all three mentioned issues in detail. The provisions corresponding to each of the above phases are outlined as follows (Hosseini and Izadkhah, 2006).

Preparedness provisions

Some of the preparedness provisions before the disaster are as follows:

- Identify the dangerous spots in a building (such as lifts, the location of wells, and engine rooms in case of earthquakes);
- Learn various sheltering methods;
- Prepare an emergency bag containing water and food especially for children, first aid materials, tents appropriate for the size of the families, toys for children, flashlights and portable radio, whistles, etc. as well as important documents and some money;
- Prepare a special earthquake kit containing identification cards for the family members, and their medical information, blood groups, etc.;
- Identify the responsibility of each family member during and in the aftermath of an earthquake;
- Allocate responsibilities based on the capabilities of the children and women (responsibilities such as turning off of the main pipes, the electricity and gas supplies, rescuing those trapped and offering first aid to the injured;
- Learn the mechanical operation of electrical equipment, e.g. the lifts and the electrical locks at exits, etc.;
- Mark an appropriate route for safe evacuation;
- Identify the places where people should gather after leaving the building.

Correct sheltering

For each disastrous event, there are some specific safety measures that can be followed. For example, some of the main activities during the earthquake include methods for proper sheltering such as:

- Stay in places that are considered as safe, for example under the door frames, beside the main columns and under wooden tables;
- Stay away from dangerous places;
- Cover the head and neck and sit correctly;
- Avoid exiting the building;
- Avoid using the stairs and lifts.

Provisions after the disaster

Some of the activities after the disaster include:

- Make provision to help those who are trapped in buildings or in other critical situations;
- Gather in a safe place;
- Make sure all the family members are gathered in the pre-identified safe places;
- Provide first aid assistance to those in need;
- Help with psychological trauma after the event;
- Help neighbours after making sure that your residence or location is safe enough.

Training tools and media

Different training tools and media should be presented in a way that can be used by children and women. These training materials should be designed by reliable sources and knowledgeable experts, particularly for children and women in rural areas who require more simplified material. Additionally, various forms of media can be employed to be used by children according to their age and sex. Training tools should match the needs of the target group as well. For children, these tools can include textbooks with appropriate materials, films showing aspects from basic knowledge of earthquakes to self-aid measures, regular and wide-ranging 'safety drills' and exhibitions and competitions, displayed paintings and posters in educational environments, booklets, pamphlets, songs, games and peer dialogues used for teaching children on disasters. The internet can also be used by groups of children to learn about disaster preparedness (Izadkhah and Hosseini, 2004).

There are also various tools for teaching women. In rural areas, women can be taught about disasters through various methods such as participatory rural appraisals (PRAs). In the urban community, women can gather in selected groups, e.g. women who live in a residential complex or who are members of a sports group, etc. In addition, women can participate in disaster classes regularly to learn about disaster preparedness through using the internet with the assistance of a disaster expert or a representative member of their complex who has been trained for disaster preparedness, or they can attend sessions taking place in parent–teacher associations (PTAs). Other means of media mentioned above for children can be also employed by women according to their age. For example, women can perform safety drills on some special occasions with their children and the whole family. By performing the drills, a simulated earthquake can be also practised.

Training time and the environment

Children can be taught during school hours about disasters and can learn safety measures through the various tools and media mentioned above through regular teaching by knowledgeable teachers and instructors. Scheduled timetables can be inserted into their school curriculum to continue this process on a regular basis. Other appropriate times for such training include leisure times when school children are taken sightseeing or on scientific field trips/adventurous journeys.

As for women, those who are mothers of school children can attend the regular classes held by the PTA. Also women in residential complexes can participate in disaster preparedness classes in their weekly/monthly gatherings. A series of meetings can also be organized with their children's teachers on a regular basis in which they can talk about their experiences with disasters. In some countries, religious gathering places such as mosques or churches can also be considered as good potential places for teaching women, particularly after the regular religious ceremonies.

Training and teaching methods

There are a variety of approaches and activities for teaching disaster issues to children. One of these is through active participation, which allows the children to make sense of their environment. Ideas applied through play stimulate children to think things through, effectively 'rehearsing' for future application. Play is of course fun, and contains its own incentives for learning. A wide variety of play is seen in preschools, such as discussions and organized conversations, story-telling, theatrical activities, songs and poems, music and movement, play in a closed area, for example with puzzles, play in an open area, play with materials that exist in the environment (e.g. sand, water), puppet plays, group activities, scientific outings and other community field trips. Other groups of older children can be taught through lessons related to disasters, which can be integrated into their school textbooks. Classification of trainees is also very important. Sometimes trainees come from different social/cultural backgrounds and it is not easy to provide useful materials for them.

As for women, there can also be a variety of teaching methods. Women can be gathered in focus groups based on the jobs or skills they are familiar with and can be taught by a representative about disasters such as earthquakes. Women are more experienced but have tighter schedules. Therefore, the PTA can be an ideal place to arrange meetings for them in order to teach about disasters. This is a legal association and women as mothers have enthusiasm to learn about any issues that can be related to protecting their family. Also all the members are selected from the neighbourhood and therefore they are familiar with each other and the place. The safe places for sheltering can be identified, marked and explained to the representatives of the association, so they would know where to gather after a disaster as well how as to guide others on what to do during an event.

Conclusions and Recommendations

With rapid urbanization, developing countries are witnessing an observable change in their socioeconomic structure, which will continue for years and even decades. Education can be regarded as one of the best media for preparing a community for disasters. Unfortunately, in most developing countries educating all levels of society for disaster preparedness is not always easy due to the lack of expertise and materials and social and cultural limitations. Therefore, one of the best ways of publicizing awareness programmes is the education and training of children and women in order to foster disaster-resilient communities. In this respect, extended research has been undertaken in many countries on the key role of children and women in disaster risk reduction, and the response and recovery phases. However, in some developing countries, this work has not been expanded widely so far. There are still issues that should be dealt with to enable successful educational and training programmes for children and women in disasters and to promote their capabilities to demonstrate their key roles in various phases of disaster management.

With regard to this chapter, issues need further research, such as: investigation of the causes of children and women's vulnerability in disasters with regard to the specific characterization of each country (especially developing countries such as Iran); to highlight the role of children and women in planning for earthquake risk reduction activities; to study the role of children and women in disaster management during and after disasters; to examine the successful implementation of disaster reduction strategies through children and women; to explore the key role of women in securing livelihood and resilience after earthquakes; to study the role of women in providing psychological assistance to their families, neighbours and those in need after disasters; to investigate the performance and role of expert women as the decision makers in the disaster risk reduction field; to train women in earthquake risk reduction and support them in attending the related activities and initiatives as well as to investigate the appropriate time, methods and applicable tools for educating them; to identify those people who are responsible for volunteering to teaching disaster strategies to groups of children and women, as well as the type of education and the contents of the educational materials; and to identify specific groups of women who are more active and interested in teaching about disasters to others.

And finally, specific attention should be paid to the cultural aspects that exist in a particular country with regard to the roles of children and women in earthquake risk reduction activities. It is hoped that these activities alongside education and training for children and women can be developed and further expanded in highly disaster-prone countries in the near future.

Acknowledgements

The authors would like to express their gratitude to Mrs Julia Burn, a former colleague of the first author at Cranfield University for editing the whole manuscript.

References

Allan, R. (1989) The Armenian earthquake – the UK response. *Disaster Management* 1(4), 10–17.

Badalyan, S. (2003) The ABCs of survival: disaster training for kids in Armenia. *Living with Risk.* 2003 World Disaster Campaign, UNISDR, Washington, DC.

Fallahi, V. (1998) The role of women in family mental relaxation and sanitation after the earthquakes. First Gathering on the Key Role of Women in Earthquake Hazard Mitigation, IIEES Report, 76-98-12 (in Persian), Tehran, Iran.

Ghafory-Ashtiany, M., Parsizadeh, F., Izadkhah, Y.O. and Petal, M. (2006) School disaster risk reduction, think globally, act locally. IIEES and Risk Red, Published Online.

Hadjian, A.H. (1993) The Spitak, Armenia earthquake of 7 December 1988 – why so much destruction? *Soil Dynamics and Earthquake Engineering* 12, 1–24.

Hosseini, M. and Izadkhah, Y.O. (2006) Training people for disasters in residential complexes – from risk to opportunity. ECEES Conference, September, Geneva.

Hosseini, M. and Izadkhah, Y.O. (2007) On the role of quality management in earthquake disaster risk reduction. Fourth International Conference on Excellence Management and Quality Management Systems, 17–18 June 2007, Tehran, Iran.

Hosseini, M. and Izadkhah, Y.O. (2010) Training emergency managers for earthquake response: challenges and opportunities. *Disaster Prevention and Management Journal* 19(2), 185–195.

IFRC World Disaster Report (2010) Disasters in Asia, the case of legal preparedness. Available at: http://www.ifrc.org/Global/Publications/disasters/idrl/IFRC_IDRL_Report_EN.pdf (Accessed 16 July 2013).

Izadkhah, Y.O. (2004) Bridging the generations: a critical assessment of disaster education in the development of a seismic safety culture in Iran. PhD Dissertation, Cranfield University, Cranfield, UK.

Izadkhah, Y.O. and Hosseini, M. (2004) Using internet communication in increasing earthquake disaster awareness and preparedness. Thirteenth World Conference on Earthquake Engineering, Vancouver, Canada.

Lidstone, J. (1999) Disaster education in the school curriculum. In: Ingleton, J. (ed.) *Natural Disaster Management.*Tudor Rose, Leicester, UK, pp. 235–245.

Lopes, R. (2001) Editorial: Partnerships for disaster education. *Natural Hazards Review* 2(3), 102–104.

Millennium Project (2006) Fast facts: the faces of poverty. Available at: http://www.unmillenniumproject.org/resources/fastfacts_e.htm (Accessed August 2011).

Miller, T.W., Kraus, R.F., Tatevosyan, A.S. and Kamenchenko, P. (1993) Post-traumatic stress disorder in children and adolescents of the Armenian earthquake. *Child Psychiatry and Human Development* 24, 115–123.

Noji, E.K. (1989) The 1988 earthquake in Soviet Armenia: implications for earthquake preparedness. *Disasters Journal* 13(3), 255–262.

Oxfam (2005) The tsunami's impact on women. Available at: http://www.oxfam.org/en/policy/bn050326-tsunami-women (Accessed December 2012).

Oxfam (2007) Hull flood victim sees the extent of disaster for herself. Available at: http://reliefweb.int/report/bangladesh/oxfam-launches-appeal-massive-south-asian-floods (Accessed 9 March 2013).

Pomonis, A. (1990) The Spitak (Armenia, USSR) earthquake: residential building typology and seismic behavior. *Disasters Journal* 14(2), 89–114.

Shadi Talab, J. (1994) Sociology of disasters, case study of Manjil-Roudbar earthquake. Housing Foundation Report, Tehran, Iran.

Shaw, R. and Kobayashi, M. (2001) Role of schools in creating earthquake-safer environment. *Proceedings of the Conference on Disaster Management and Educational Facilities,* Paper presented at the OECD Workshop,Thessaloniki, Greece.

Tinh, D.Q. (2003) Flood kindergarten: community need community solution. In: Living with Risk, 2003 World Disaster Campaign. UNISDR, Washington, DC.

United Nations Development Programme (UNDP) HD Report (1995) Gender and human development. Available at: http://hdr.undp.org/en/reports/global/hdr1995/ (accessed 14 February 2013).

United Nations Population Fund (UNFPA) (1999) Population and sustainable development. Available at: http://www.unfpa.org/6billion/populationissues/development.htm (Accessed 14 February 2012).

United Nations International Strategy for Disaster Reduction (UNISDR) (2007) Grassroots Women Handle Quake Impact Unaided; Gender Perspective: Indonesia; Enabling Women to Play a Lead Role in Disaster-affected Marginal Communities: India; From Makeshift Women's Centers to Sustainable Women's Cooperation: Turkey; Working Together for Disaster Risk Reduction, Good Practices and Lessons Learned. UNISDR, Washington, DC.

United Nations International Strategy for Disaster Reduction (UNISDR) (2011) What is disaster risk reduction? Available at: http://www.unisdr.org/who-we-are/what-is-drr (Accessed July 2011).

Walia, A. (2008) Community based disaster preparedness: Need for a standardized training module. *The Australian Journal of Emergency Management* 23(2), 68–73.

Yonder, A., Ackar S. and Gopalan, P. (2005) Women's participation in disaster relief and recovery, Pamphlet No. 22, Seeds Publication, New Delhi.

Index